Catania's Primary Care of the Anterior Segment

This book has become an iconic textbook in eye care over many years with multiple editions having originally published in 1986. Considered one of the classic, definitive books for comprehensive anterior segment diagnosis, treatment, and management, this new third edition includes pre- and postoperative management of cataract and refractive surgery and glaucoma, which are major parts of primary optometry today, along with updates on proprietary therapeutic drugs, and technology additions such as amniotic membranes, injectables, and minor in-office procedures. It contains high-quality photos, six appendices, 336 clinical photos/diagrams/illustrations, and 74 tables throughout the textbook.

Key Features

- Provides immediate and succinct information necessary for diagnosing, treating, and managing all anterior segment, primary glaucoma, pre- and postoperative management of cataract and refractive surgery, and non-surgical ocular conditions
- Includes 215 color photos to allow the clinician to use the clinical knowledge and assist with diagnosis and treatment options in the clinical setting
- Features a unique presentation format as all the clinical information is organized in the SOAP (Subjective, Objective, Assessment, Plan) format for quick referencing and practical use by primary eye care practitioners

Catania's Primary Care of the Anterior Segment

Third Edition

Brian S. Armitage, OD, MS, FAAO
President, Baymeadows Vision Center
Group Manager, Clinical Sciences, Johnson & Johnson Vision Care

Louis J. (*Lou*) Catania, OD, FAAO, DSc
University of North Florida, Osher Lifelong Learning Institute
Salus University, College of Health Sciences

Contributing Author

Elizabeth Draper (*Beth*) Muckley, OD, FAAO
Director of Optometric Services and Glaucoma Consultant
Northeast Ohio Eye Surgeons
Clinical Associate Professor – Practice, The Ohio State University

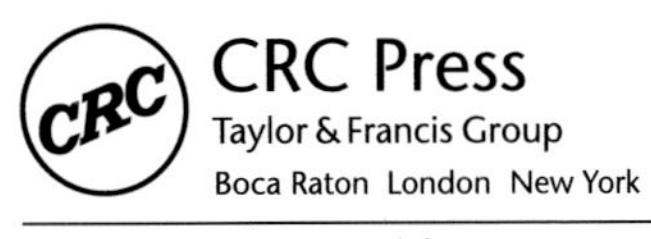

CRC Press is an imprint of the
Taylor & Francis Group, an **informa** business

Third edition published 2023 by CRC Press
6000 Broken Sound Parkway NW, Suite 300, Boca Raton, FL 33487-2742

and by CRC Press
4 Park Square, Milton Park, Abingdon, Oxon, OX14 4RN

CRC Press is an imprint of Taylor & Francis Group, LLC

First edition published by Appleton & Lange, 1988
Second edition published by Appleton & Lange, 1995

ISBN: 978-1-032-18658-0 (hbk)
ISBN: 978-1-032-18656-6 (pbk)
ISBN: 978-1-003-25559-8 (ebk)

DOI: 10.1201/9781003255598

Typeset in Warnock Pro
by Deanta Global Publishing Services, Chennai, India

To my wife, Anne
Thank you for your love, support, and a great life together

Brian Armitage

To my wife, Stephanie
(to whom I dedicated the first edition)
Thank you for your love and your patience
and I promise you, this is my last

Lou Catania

To my always supportive husband Tim, son Max, and parents John and Theresa Draper

Beth Muckley

CONTENTS

PREFACE

Allow me to take you on a quick journey through the history of the book, *Primary Care of the Anterior Segment*.

This book has its roots back in the 1970s and 1980s when the concept of primary eye care was beginning to interest well-trained optometrists. The feeling was that along with vision care, providing medical diagnosis and treatment of common eye diseases for their patients was compatible with their level of professional education and in the best interests of their patients and the public health. All it needed was: (1) commitment from grassroots practitioners; (2) support from state legislatures; and (3) resources to convert professional classroom education into practical clinical skills.

During those early years, I was fortunate to have the opportunity to develop an eye care service in a multidisciplinary healthcare facility (the Joseph C. Wilson Health Center in Rochester, NY), an innovative and experimental primary healthcare delivery model. The medical director (Harold Gardner, MD) and the staff of young, progressive physicians, nurse practitioners, and pharmacists believed that optometry should have a place alongside other primary healthcare professionals. Over the following decades, this atmosphere allowed me to create a model of primary care optometry that has evolved into the practice of optometry we know today. Through those decades and beyond, dedicated optometrists overcame strong political opposition using education as their foundational argument and the primary care optometry model from the Rochester Wilson Health Center as the prototype. What remained was the need for a practical tool to help clinical optometry implement the primary care model in their practices.

By the early 1980s, as the primary care optometry model grew, I was receiving constant requests from an increasing number of optometrists to write a "how-to book" on the treatment and management of common primary eye care presentations. This was being viewed by many as the third leg of the elevated healthcare platform upon which primary care optometry was now standing. As more and more optometric practitioners were embracing the primary care model (leg #1); increasing enabling legislation was allowing practitioners to become certified in an expanding scope of practice (leg #2); the clinical practitioners needed a practical "how-to book" to help them, guide them and, indeed, reassure them on their "in the chair" treatment and management of eye problems (leg #3). This third leg served as my motivation to organize and document the primary eye care that optometry can deliver. It took 3 years to put together (lots of late nights and weekends) and in 1988 the first edition of *Primary Care of the Anterior Segment* was published by Appleton & Lange (referred to by practitioners as "The Red Book" for its red cover).

The book was an instant success and within one year, it had sold over 10,000 copies. Its continued popularity over the following 2 to 3 years causing the publisher to start encouraging (*aka*, pressuring) me to do a second edition. Because of a very busy schedule of practice and lecturing during those years, I remained hesitant (if not procrastinating) about a second edition. However, my increasing interest and involvement in corneal immunology and optometry's role in refractive surgery, as well as advancements in ocular therapeutics motivated me to work on a second edition. In 1995, Appleton & Lange/Simon & Schuster published *Primary Care of the Anterior Segment*, Second Edition (referred to by practitioners as "The Blue Book" for its blue cover) which was a substantially expanded version of the first edition. It contained a new, comprehensive chapter (2) on "Clinical Considerations on Anterior Segment Pathology and Immunology" as well as extensive updating of all the clinical and therapeutic information throughout the remaining 6 chapters. Again, the book was a major success domestically and internationally and it was honored with the Baron's award for "Best Medical Books of 1995."

After about 10 years, the book began to lose its momentum, admittedly as did I in writing another edition. Eventually, reprintings were discontinued, and by 2010, the book was out of print. During that time, Simon & Schuster sold Appleton & Lange and all its inventory and copyrights to McGraw-Hill Publishers. In reviewing their acquired inventory, McGraw-Hill identified about 150 remaining copies of *Primary Care of the Anterior Segment*, Second Edition. Because the book was out of print and 15 years old, rather than attempt to remarket it, McGraw-Hill contacted me and explained that their process was to destroy the remaining copies unless I chose to purchase the books and the copyright. When they quoted the price at $1.00 per book and no additional charge for the copyright, I didn't hesitate to write the check. I donated about half the books to libraries, gave some to friends as gifts, and held on to about 10 copies (still in a box in storage). Over the following 5 to 10 years, I continued to get frequent inquiries and requests for a third edition, all of which I gratefully declined.

In 2019, during a regular lunch date with a colleague, Brian Armitage, a fortuitous discussion ensued. Brian is a brilliant optometrist who had left a 16-year career as director of clinical research at Johnson & Johnson in 2004 to venture into private practice. His bold move proved to be a major success as he grew a large and busy contact lens and primary eye care practice. During our lunch, Brian mentioned that he uses *Primary Care of the Anterior Segment*, Second Edition regularly, but feels it needs updating. I agreed, but admitted my reluctance in tackling it because, at that point, my professional activities had shifted more towards immunology and pre- and post-op management in the multidisciplinary practice that I had been associated with for 20 years. As such, I was too far removed from day-to-day primary care and staying current with new drugs and treatment modalities. But spontaneously, I asked him if he would be interested in working together on a third edition where he can update the clinical chapters and pharmaceutical information and I would update the immunology chapter as well as write a chapter on optometric pre- and post-op management of cataract and refractive surgery patients. We shook hands and the deal was done.

The other additional information we felt was necessary to truly update the book to reflect optometry's clinical "in the chair" needs going forward in the years ahead was a chapter on the practical aspects of glaucoma care, specifically primary open angle glaucoma (POAG). Neither I nor Brian felt sufficiently knowledgeable and experienced enough in day-to-day glaucoma care, so we decided to recruit an expert OD. The person we identified to write the chapter, Dr. Elizabeth (Beth) Muckley, practices in a large multidisciplinary eye care clinic in Ohio where she is the lead practitioner for all primary glaucoma care. Beth is also a scholar in glaucoma and a charter member of the prestigious International Optometric Glaucoma Society. Her contribution to the third edition of *Primary Care of the Anterior Segment* makes it the most comprehensive "how-to book" in primary eye care.

One might interpret this Preface as being a current history of the profession of optometry, and perhaps it is in certain ways. Since optometry's origins in the early 1900s, through its professional education and doctoral degrees in the 1960s, optometry was viewed as an optical science dedicated to the correction of human vision. In the 1970s, through expanding education, the profession began to envision its role in patient care as a vision and biomedical health science. The concept of optometry as a primary healthcare profession evolved naturally from patients' eye care needs and, "the eye as the window to the body" (to paraphrase a saying). Since then, primary care optometry has enhanced public health through the provision of vision and medical eye care to millions of patients worldwide. The three editions of this book have proudly contributed to that goal.

And so, with that history, we are proud to bring you *Catania's Primary Care of the Anterior Segment*, Third Edition published by Taylor & Francis/CRC Press. If you have used the first and/or second editions, you know about the systematic, clinically oriented format for practical "in the chair" use. It incorporates all the information in the SOAP (Subjective, Objective, Assessment [diagnosis], Plan [treatment options] and Follow-Up) format throughout the book. The chapters are anatomically sequenced (including basic anatomy) with each anatomical category organized into *Irritations and Injuries*, *Noninflammatory Conditions*, and *Inflammatory Conditions*. Additional chapters include general considerations in anterior segment care (Chapter 1); immunology and pathology (Chapter 2); post-op cataract and refractive surgery management (Chapter 7); primary open angle glaucoma (Chapter 8); and systemic considerations in anterior segment care (Chapter 9). There are extensive color photos, descriptive diagrams, and tables throughout each chapter and the back section includes 6 voluminous appendices, and a comprehensive subject index. We hope you will find all the information to be valuable to you and to have this book serve as your "go-to resource" and the third leg of primary care optometry's healthcare platform.

Louis J. Catania, OD, FAAO, DSc

ACKNOWLEDGMENTS

The third edition of *Catania's Primary Care of the Anterior Segment* took its authors, Brian Armitage and Lou Catania, and contributing author, Beth Muckley, over a year to complete. Each of us dedicated a significant amount of our personal and professional time to formulate, research, and write the book. It indeed was our genuine commitment to provide a comprehensive and practical, clinical resource for all of our domestic (U.S.) and international colleagues who are providing primary eye care to millions of patients worldwide. It was also an honor and thoroughly enjoyable experience to be able to share our collective expertise (over 130 years of cumulative clinical experience) with our dedicated worldwide colleagues.

As the saying goes, "it took a village" to complete the publishing process of this voluminous body of clinical information. Its ultimate editing, organization, and production ("making it a book") of its extensive textual content, to the vast amount of graphics (photos, figures, tables, etc.) and, finally, to a handsome cover design was the work of highly professional Taylor & Francis/CRC Press editors including Miranda Bromage, Publisher; Shivangi Pramanik, Commissioning Editor; Himani Dwivedi, Editorial Assistant; Lillian Woodall, Project Manager; and Christian Muñoz, cover designer. Working with this first-class group was a professional and personal pleasure for all of us as "demanding" authors.

Lou Catania wants to first offer his special thanks and appreciation to his coauthors, Brian Armitage and Beth Muckley, for being such brilliant optometric physicians. They were a joy to work with during the challenges of coordinating all pieces (texts, graphics, etc.) among the chapters, appendices, and index. It was a real endeavor to get all the updated, edited and new information in chapters, appendices, and previous editions coordinated and integrated in a logical, non-repetitive, and readable format. It actually turned out to be a lot of fun working with such great seasoned and intelligent professionals and especially, good friends. Beyond those very special folks, I also will never forget the support and assistance I got during my first and second edition efforts. That included all the great health professionals of the medical group from the original Joseph C. Wilson Health Center in Rochester, NY; all my outstanding residents over those early years; Randy Beatty, OD, MD, for doing the original oculosystemic chapter; Rodney Gutner, OD, one of the finest ophthalmic photographers for sharing so many of his excellent clinical photos (all in this third edition); and Kimberly Martens and Linda Harris for the outstanding artwork they created for the second edition which is present in this third edition as well. To all of them, I will always be grateful.

Brian Armitage would like to thank his coauthors Lou Catania and Elizabeth (Beth) Muckley. Lou is an icon in the optometric community especially as an advocate for optometric management and treatment of anterior segment ocular pathology and the pre- and post-op management of cataract and refractive surgery. He has played a major role in educating optometrists regarding these topics around the world. We have also become good friends over the years, and I was shocked when he asked for my help with the third edition. Lou and I wanted an OD to author the glaucoma chapter since it was not our forte. Beth was recommended by my good friend and fellow Buckeye, Tom Quinn. Not only is Beth a glaucoma expert working in the trenches every day, but she was also a joy to collaborate with during the writing of the third edition. She has done a fantastic job with her chapter and as a practitioner who is not a glaucoma expert, she wrote a comprehensive chapter that optometrists can use in their day-to-day practice. I have been fortunate to have a long and varied optometric career including contact lens industry researcher (J&J) and primary care practitioner. There are many ODs I would like to thank for teaching me many things about primary eye care. I would be remiss not to mention The Ohio State University College of Optometry faculty; specifically, Kevin Alexander, Arol Augsburger, Joe Barr, Jack King, Jerry Paugh, Mike Polasky, Tom Quinn, and John Schoessler. They provided the educational foundation I was able to use to continue my ongoing optometric education throughout my career. Lastly my wife, Ann, and son, Alex, gave me their love and support not only during the writing of this book but throughout my entire optometric career. I would not have been able to accomplish any of my professional achievements without them right by my side. My only regret is now that the book is completed, I will not be able to get out of my normal household chores!

Elizabeth Muckley would like to especially thank Drs. Catania and Armitage for the opportunity to be a contributing author and for recognizing the importance of glaucoma in primary eye care. It was an extreme honor to have worked with these two legends and pioneers of the optometric profession. I am forever grateful for their guidance, expertise, love for all things Italian, and most of all, their friendship. The second edition was my go-to textbook in 1996 when I was a third-year optometry student. If someone would have told me back then that 25 years later, I would be writing a glaucoma chapter for a new edition, I would have thought they were crazy. It is funny where life leads one. I may not have said yes to this project if my dad had not passed away from ALS shortly before I was asked. It was a tough journey for my family caring for him, but writing this chapter gave me peace during a time of grief as well as a new purpose.

Thank you to Tom Quinn, OD for recommending me to Dr. Armitage as the expert glaucoma clinician to write this chapter and to Mike Earley, OD, MS, PhD, for proofreading the anatomy and visual pathway content. A thank you to Richard Lehrer, MD and Brian Mathie, OD, who developed my early interest in glaucoma through their instruction and teaching. Last, because of the true OD/MD collaboration at NE Ohio Eye Surgeons under the guidance of Lawrence Lohman, MD along with my talented OD and MD practice partners, I have had the opportunity for 22 years to manage medical and post-surgical glaucoma. It is a true privilege to care for patients in our community and prevent vision loss over their lifetime. I am blessed to be an optometrist.

AUTHORS

Brian S. Armitage, OD, MS, FAAO, has recently retired after a 40-year optometric career. He is a 1981 graduate of The Ohio State University College of Optometry. Dr. Armitage completed an MS degree and a 2-year Cornea and Contact Lens Residency from the same institution in 1983. He spent the first half of his career working as a clinical contact lens researcher for Johnson & Johnson Vision Care (aka Vistakon). Dr. Armitage was responsible for protocol development, clinical study design, and clinical data interpretation. He directed and managed domestic and international clinical studies. His clinical team worked directly with chemists, microbiologists, statisticians, engineers, and other professionals which resulted in new product developments such as Acuvue Advance and Acuvue Oasys. He co-authored numerous clinical study reports including FDA 510K and PMA submissions. He spent the second half of his career as a primary care clinician with an emphasis on specialty contact lens prescribing. Dr. Armitage was the first eye care practitioner in Jacksonville to prescribe scleral contact lenses for distorted corneas. He was active in the local optometric society eventually serving as president. Dr. Armitage was an active member of the Jacksonville Chamber of Commerce and served as the president of one of their local chapters. He has served as a member of Johnson & Johnson Vision Care President's Advisory Board and as an Assistant Clinical Professor for The Ohio State University College of Optometry. Dr. Armitage enjoys biking and traveling anywhere around the world with his wife, Anne, at his side.

Louis J. (Lou) Catania, OD, FAAO, DSc (Hon.), is an internationally acclaimed educator, and a recognized expert in eye care, healthcare, artificial intelligence (AI) and immunology. He has authored over 160 journal articles and 12 textbooks including 3 editions of *Primary Care of the Anterior Segment*, which received Baron's Five Star (highest) rating for medical textbooks. He is currently a lecturer with the University of North Florida, Department of Continuing Education, Osher Lifelong Learning Institute; and a visiting Professor at Salus University, College of Health Sciences. During his 52-year clinical and academic career he has taught and lectured extensively worldwide. Dr. Catania's professional accomplishments in eye care, healthcare, and immunology have produced countless honors and awards including two Honorary Doctor of Science degrees; Distinguished Faculty Scholar at three academic institutions; induction into the National Optometry Hall of Fame; and domestic and international keynote and commencement addresses. The third edition of *Catania's Primary Care of the Anterior Segment* is the culmination of a singularly prolific and distinguished professional career. In his personal time, Dr. Catania is an active volunteer with the National Park Service, a sea turtle patrol monitor in his beach community, and involved in multiple humanitarian and human welfare agencies.

Elizabeth (Beth) Draper Muckley, OD, FAAO, is the Director of Optometric Services at NE Ohio Eye Surgeons where she has practiced for over 20 years concentrating in anterior segment disease and the management of medical and post-surgical glaucoma. A recognized leader in the profession of optometry, Dr. Muckley lectures nationally and has contributed articles to journals and mainstream ocular publications. She is an Associate Clinical Professor of Optometry at The Ohio State College of Optometry, Education Chair of the East West Eye Conference, and an 18-year member of the Optometric Glaucoma Society. She is a past President of the Ohio Optometric Association where she was instrumental in the passage of three significant Ohio Laws including scope of practice expansion. Dr. Muckley has received many career awards for her service to the profession and patient care. Notably, she was recognized nationally in 2008 as the American Optometric Association's Young Optometrist of the Year and was named in 2021 as the Ohio Optometrist of the Year by the Ohio Optometric Association. Dr. Muckley enjoys spending time on Lake Erie and traveling overseas with her family. She gardens and maintains a small fruit orchard in her free time. She also is proud of her Italian heritage and preserves those cultural traditions through food and family.

INTRODUCTION

The first and second editions of *Primary Care of the Anterior Segment* were designed as a systemic text with a clinically oriented SOAP (**S**ubjective, **O**bjective, **A**ssessment, **P**lan) format for practical ease of use by the busy clinical practitioner. Retaining this fundamental and popular approach, this new third edition incorporates many new and exciting features that I am pleased to present.

- An entirely new chapter, Chapter 7, has been added, devoted to cataract and refractive surgery pre- and postoperative management. An essential role in primary eye care is the management of cataract and refractive surgery patients. It starts with preoperative evaluation and counseling and extends through the postoperative period with careful assessment of the clinical results of the procedure and any untoward complication. The chapter reviews all types of refractive surgery options and procedures (e.g., PRK, LASIK, Epi-Lasik, LASEK, CK, Intacs, etc) and cataract surgery including specialty IOL options (e.g., monofocal, multifocal, astigmatic, and refractive lens exchange [RLE]).
- An entirely new chapter, Chapter 8, has been added, dedicated to the primary care diagnosis, treatment, and management of glaucoma. This chapter discusses current concepts in glaucoma such as the pathophysiology, clinical assessment, standards of care, and diagnostic testing, as well as the pharmacologic treatment and surgical management options. Glaucoma conditions are detailed in SOAP format to aid the clinician in developing critical thinking skills for differential diagnosis. Clinical pearls in understanding the nuances of key glaucoma testing, treatment algorithms, and patient education are included.
- New and updated primary care pharmaceutical therapies for anterior segment conditions have been added, including drugs (brand and generic), prescribing information, and dosage and duration recommendations. Many new topical medications have been included including a specialty drug section. Oral medications (antibiotics, anti-inflammatory, antivirals, analgesics, and glaucoma) are discussed in greater detail than the previous edition. There is a summary of injectable ophthalmic drugs used for anterior segment care as well.
- The relevant clinical anatomy and practical SOAP format has been retained for all conditions presented (including the new chapters on glaucoma and cataract and refractive surgery).
- Chapter 2, "Clinical Considerations on Anterior Segment Pathology and Immunology," is the backbone of a practical, clinical approach to primary care of the anterior segment.
- Over 200 full-color photographs and many black and white photographs and illustrations of clinical conditions for immediate viewing while reading about any condition.
- The text is organized throughout into Irritations/Injuries, Noninflammatory Conditions, and Inflammatory Conditions. This allows for an easy, quick, and more clinically relevant referencing and understanding.

Every clinician knows we don't have all the answers. Many case presentations just don't fit and defy definitive diagnosis and "cookbook" treatment. The clinician needs a practical way to handle those difficult presentations safely and effectively. A basic and systematic understanding of clinical pathology and immunology is the clinician's way of thinking through the complicated case to arrive at a definite diagnosis or, at the very least, to approach a sensitive situation knowledgeably and with minimal risk of a serious diagnostic or therapeutic error. Chapter 2 provides this information which is used as a foundation for the rest of the book.

Our attempt has been to take the elements from the second edition and modernize them for today's optometric practitioner. We are proud to provide a practical, comprehensive, and up-to-date resource for those of us who must frequently diagnose and manage anterior segment conditions in our day-today primary eye care practices.

Brian S. Armitage, OD, MS, FAAO

Chapter 1
GENERAL CLINICAL CONSIDERATIONS IN ANTERIOR SEGMENT CARE

Chapter Outline

DOI: 10.1201/9781003255598-1

I. Patient Care Considerations

A. Subjective

1. Comprehensive history (Table 1.1)
2. Risk-factor analysis (Table 1.2)
3. Do not skip questions
4. Listen to, and learn from, each response

TABLE 1.1 Questions to Include in Patient History

General Considerations
- Observe and consider patient's general behavior
- Personalize your questioning
- Do not lead patient with loaded questions
- Let the patient talk and expand (within reason)
- Cross-question when indicated or necessary
- Listen

Specific Questions
- Name
- Age
- Occupation
- Habitation
- Cohabitation
- Main statement of complaint (reason for visit?)
- Onset of symptoms (when did it begin?)
- Frequency (recurring, hourly, daily, weekly?)
- Intensity (constant, intermittent, quality, quantity?)
- Duration (how long does it last?)
- Types of symptoms
  - Visual
  - Diplopia
  - Trauma (describe?)
  - Pain or irritation (where?)
- Ocular history
  - Prescription eyeglasses (how long and for what?)
  - Any previous injury, surgery, or diseases?
  - Any family history of eye disease?
- General health
  - Chronic disease
  - Present condition
  - Family history
  - Allergies, asthma
- Medication history
  - Taking any (ocular or other)
  - Allergies or idiosyncratic reactions
    - Topical
    - Systemic
- Nutritional habits
- Stress factors
  - Physical or environmental
  - Mental or psychological
  - Social or economic

TABLE 1.2 Risk Factors to Consider in Diagnosis

- History
- Age
- Sex
- Race
- Incidence or prevalence (frequency of disease: epidemiology)
- Demography (geographic distribution of disease)
- Common etiologies
- Genetic (hereditary) factors
- Predisposing conditions (e.g., systemic diseases, environmental hazards)
- Social, psychosocial, economic factors
- Neurogenic overlay (conversion syndromes)
- Psychogenic overlay (organic)

B. Objective

1. Do not skip appropriate tests (Table 1.3)
2. Entering visual acuities (VAs), a medicolegal essential
3. Systematic approach most efficient
   a. Anatomical categories
      i. Eyelids
      ii. Lacrimal system
      iii. Orbit
      iv. Conjunctiva
      v. Sclera and episclera
      vi. Cornea
      vii. Anterior chamber and aqueous
      viii. Iris and ciliary body
      ix. Crystalline lens
      x. Optic nerve
   b. Pathophysiological etiologies
      i. Allergy/hypersensitivity
      ii. Congenital/developmental abnormalities (versus acquired)
      iii. Degeneration
      iv. Dystrophy
      v. Environmental
      vi. Immunologic (toxic)
      vii. Infectious (bacterial, viral, fungal, parasitic, protozoan)
      viii. Inflammation
      ix. Injury (abrasions, burns, contusion, foreign bodies, laceration)
      x. Metabolic
      xi. Metaplasia (hypoplasia, hyperplasia, hypertrophy)
      xii. Neoplasia (primary, metastatic)
4. Look, listen, and feel (palpate tissue structures)
5. Document findings thoroughly and accurately
   a. Photodocument if possible
   b. Use color coding when indicated (Table 1.4)
   c. Use appropriate abbreviations (Table 1.5)

C. Assessment

1. Differential diagnosis—most important clinical task
2. Rule out (R/O) other involvements (e.g., internal, extraocular muscles, systemic)
3. Consider laboratory workups (e.g., cultures, sensitivities, smears, and systemic testing if indicated) versus clinical observation alone
   a. Newborns
   b. Chronic or unresponsive conditions
   c. Hyperacute conditions
   d. Suspected corneal ulceration
   e. Postoperative involvement

D. Plan

1. Treatment plan should be response to diagnosis (assessment)
2. Variable considerations in a treatment plan
   a. No treatment
   b. Observation (recheck) and monitoring
   c. Placebos if indicated and appropriate
   d. Consultation (another opinion)
   e. Referral (assistance with care)
      i. For technical or professional assistance
      ii. For special forms of care
   f. Procedural care

TABLE 1.3 Objective Tests in Anterior Segment Examination*

Observation (during patient interview)
Head position
Body posture
Scars (from injury or surgery)
Facial symmetry
Ocular and facial motilities
General complexion and skin quality
Quality and quantity of hair, eyebrows, eyelashes
Position of eyelids and lacrimal puncta

Visual Acuities
Distance (with and without correction)
Near (with and without correction)
Pinhole vision
Amsler grid

Orbits and Surrounding Structures
Exophthalmometry
Palpation of bony margins
X-rays or ultrasound, if indicated
Upward gaze test for blowout fracture of orbital floor
Forced ductions test if indicated
Percussion of sinuses (bilateral comparisons)
Transillumination of sinuses
EOM evaluation for intraorbital causes of diplopia
Direct pressure (on globes) for unequal retrobulbar resistance

Eyelids
Palpate for edema, masses, tenderness
Express ("milk") Zeiss, Moll, meibomian glands
Evert (single and double) upper eyelid
Evaluate blink function:
  Rate
  Magnitude (e.g., complete versus lagophthalmos)
  Forced blink
  Bell's phenomenon
  Glabella tap test (in blepharospasm)
Fatigue lids with multiple forced blinks (rule out myasthenia)
Consider tensilon test if indicated
Measure lid apertures and motility (bilateral comparisons)
Examine eyelid margin quality
Evaluate eyelashes (quality, quantity, positioning)

Lacrimal System
Palpate lacrimal gland (superior temporal aspect)
Examine lacrimal puncta (size, position, patency)
Regurgitation of lacrimal sac (nasalward)
Observe for epiphora or hyperlacrimation Schirmer tear testing
Breakup time (BUT) with NaFl
Jones testing (#1 and 2)
Saccharin taste test
Diagnostic dilation and irrigation procedures

Conjunctiva
Examine palpebral and bulbar portions under magnification
Check vascular patterns and surface characteristics
Move vessels and tissue with cotton-tip applicator
Vasoconstrict for differential diagnosis
Palpate preauricular lymph nodes

Cornea and Sciera
Gross observation (e.g., dimensions, curvature)
Transillumination (e.g., for defects, opacities)
Slit-lamp examination (with and without staining:
  NaFI and rose bengal/lissamine green)
Corneal sensitivity with cotton wisp (bilateral comparison)
Evaluate limbal juncture (e.g., vasculature, transition)
Examine scleral anatomy (surface, thickness, color, lesions)

Anterior Chamber
Measure intraocular pressure (tonometry)
Examine aqueous humor for cells, flare, hypopyon, hyphema, foreign body
Estimate depth of chamber
Angle gonioscopy when indicated
Note iris coloration and/or heterochromias (unilateral or bilateral)
Evaluate iris surface and pupil border
Examine pupillary responses carefully

Other Tests
Blood pressure measurement
Pulse (radial)
Carotid bruit ascultation
Ophthalmodynamometry (ODM)
Blood glucose test
Cultures and sensitivities
Laboratory tests (if indicated)

*This list is comprehensive but not all-inclusive. Tests from such a list (and beyond) should be selected based on the examiner's judgment and diagnostic needs.

TABLE 1.4 Color Code for Ocular Diagramming

Red	Hyperemia Hemorrhage Blood vessels
Yellow	Exudate Casseous material Sebum
Orange	Infiltrate
Blue	Edema
Green	Fluorescein /lissamine staining
Black	Opacities
Brown	Pigmentation

   g. Pharmaceutical agents
   h. Prescription writing (Figure 1.1; Table 1.6)
3. Patient education, advice, counsel, and advocacy are essential with all forms of treatment

E. Management and Follow-Up

1. Decisions (when, where, how, and so forth) should be based on each individual case presentation
   a. Diagnosis
   b. Intensity of presentation
   c. Acute versus chronic onset
   d. Risk factors
   e. Prognosis (e.g., time frame, expected outcome)
   f. Psychological and emotional factors and needs
   g. Practical considerations
      i. Geographic (e.g., travel, weather factors)
      ii. Financial hardship
   h. Practitioner comfort and confidence in diagnosis
   i. Perceived patient compliance
2. Accessibility and availability of practitioner
   a. Office accessibility
   b. After-hours and weekend on-call availability
   c. Cross-coverage, answering services, and so forth

TABLE 1.5 **Common Ophthalmic Abbreviations**

Abbreviation	Meaning
AC	Anterior chamber
c̄Rx	With spectacles
s̄Rx	Without spectacles
C/D	Cup-disc ratio
CF	Count fingers vision
D	Diopter (lens power)
dd	Disc diameter (for fundus measuring)
EOM	Extraocular muscles
E	Esophoria (at 20 ft or 6 m)
E'	Esophoria (at 14 in or 33 cm)
ET	Esotropia (distance) or Extraterrestrial
E(T)	Intermittent esotropia (distance)
E(T')	Intermittent esotropia (near)
HM	Hand motion vision
IOP	Intraocular pressure
KP	Keratitis precipitate
L	Left (e.g., LET = left esotropia)
LL	Lower eyelid
LP	Light perception
NLP	No light perception
NPC	Near point of convergence
OD	Right eye
OS	Left eye
OU	Both eyes
PD	Interpupillary distance
PERRLA	Pupils equal, round, reactive to light and accommodation
PH	Pinhole
R	Right (e.g., RET = right esotropia)
R/O	Rule out
RTC	Return check
SVP	Spontaneous venous pulsation
Ta	Applanation tonometry
UL	Upper eyelid
VA	Visual acuity
VF	Visual field
WNL	With normal limits (or "We never looked")
X	Exophoria (distance)
X'	Exophoria (near)
XT	Exotropia (distance)
X(T)	Exotropia (near)
XT'	Intermittent exotropia (distance)
X(T)'	Intermittent exotropia (near)
△	Prism diopter
(+)	Convex lens (for hyperopia)
(-)	Concave lens (for myopia)

(*Continued*)

Elements of Prescription Writing:

A. Doctor information: Name, address, telephone number (minimum); license number, DEA number, practice description, office hours (optional).

B. Patient information: Name, address, date (minimum); age, date of birth, male or female (optional).

C. Rx: Superscription (symbol only).

D. Inscription: Drug prescribed (brand or generic name); include description, concentration, vehicle.

E. Disp.: Amount, size to be dispensed.

F. Sig.: Precise directions to patient (how much, which eye, how often).

G. Label: Request for pharmacist to label container with instructions; the prescription form should include this (required in some states).

H. Refill: Indicate number of times patient allowed to refill (be conservative, do not allow a large number of refills).

I. Generic permission: Law in many states requires appropriate signature placement.

J. Signature: sign on appropriate line (substitution versus no substitution) semi-legibly!

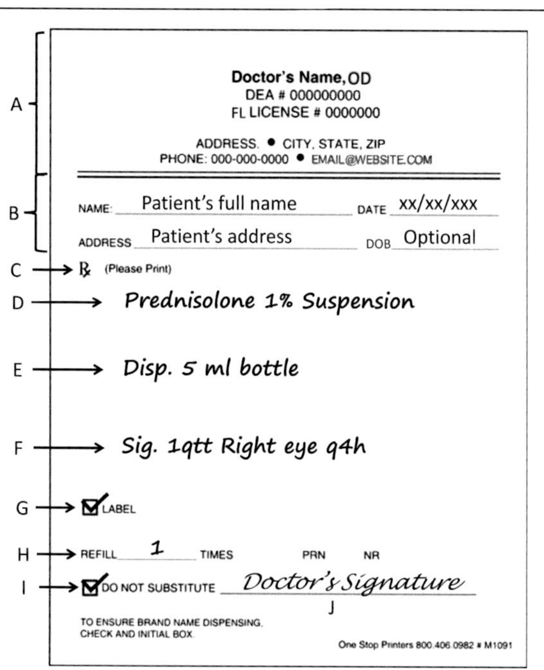

A

Doctor's Name, OD
DEA # 000000000
FL LICENSE # 0000000

ADDRESS • CITY, STATE, ZIP
PHONE: 000-000-0000 • EMAIL@WEBSITE.COM

B

NAME: Patient's full name DATE xx/xx/xxx
ADDRESS Patient's address DOB Optional

C → ℞ (Please Print)

D → Prednisolone 1% Suspension

E → Disp. 5 ml bottle

F → Sig. 1qtt Right eye q4h

G → ☑ LABEL

H → REFILL 1 TIMES PRN NR

I → ☑ DO NOT SUBSTITUTE Doctor's Signature

J

TO ENSURE BRAND NAME DISPENSING, CHECK AND INITIAL BOX.

One Stop Printers 800.406.0982 # M1091

Tips for prescription writing from a pharmacist's perspective:

- Write out as much as you can (instructions, etc.) in words or sentences;
- Print legibly all word elements of the prescription;
- Do not abbreviate drug names (brands or generics);
- Know your area pharmacists well. They are an invaluable resource.

FIGURE 1.1 Sample prescription form.

TABLE 1.6 Prescription (and Pharmaceutical) Abbreviations

Abbreviation	Meaning
a.c.	Before meals
ad lib	At pleasure
ASAP	As soon as possible
bid	Twice a day
Collyr., Coil.	Eyewash
Cum,c̄	With
Disp.	Dispense
gtt	One drop
gtts	Drops
h	An hour
hs	At bedtime
Le, L Eye	Left eye
No., #	Number
OD	Right eye
OS	Left eye
OU	Both eyes
P.C.	After meals
PO	By mouth
PRN	When necessary
q	Each, every (e.g., q4h)
qid	Four times a day
Q.S.	As much as needed
RE, R Eye	Right eye
Rx	Treatment, prescribe
Sig.	Label
Sine,s̄	Without
Sol.	Solution
STAT	Immediately
tid	Three times a day
Ung	Ointment
i	One
ii	Two
iii	Three

3. Patient care versus practitioner education or research
   a. Patients should pay for their doctor's care
   b. Patients should not have to pay for their doctor's ongoing educational or research interests

F. Other Considerations

1. Tools Needed

a. Instruments and equipment (Table 1.7)
b. Consumable supplies (Table 1.8)
c. Pharmaceutical agents (Table 1.9)

2. Accurate and Thorough Record Keeping

a. Neat and organized
b. Record all positives
c. Most important medicolegal consideration

3. Appointment Scheduling

a. For problem-oriented care
   i. Brief office visit (BOV)
   ii. Office visit (OV)
   iii. Extended office visit (EOV)
b. ASAP (as soon as possible)
c. STAT (urgent or emergent)

TABLE 1.7 Equipment and Instrumentation for Anterior Segment Care

Item	Use
Essentials	
Snellen chart	Visual acuity (distance)
Near point card	Visual acuity (near)
Pinhole	Visual acuity
Direct ophthalmoscope	Fundus examination
Tonometer	IOP measurement
Slit-lamp biomicroscope	For diagnosis
Transilluminator	Varied
Penlight	Varied
Plus 20 diopter lens	Magnification
Head Loope	Gross examination
Millimeter rule	Measurement
Jeweler's forceps	Varied
Punctal dilator	In puncta
Lacrimal cannulus (needle)	For lacrimal irrigation
3-cc syringe	For lacrimal irrigation
Hypodermic needles 18-gauge (2 inches) 22-gauge (2 inches) 25-gauge (5/8 inches)	Varied (e.g., cyst drainage, foreign-body removal)
Golf club spud	Foreign-body removal
Sphygmomanometer	Blood pressure
Stethoscope	Pressure and auscultation
Nonessential Essentials	
Binocular indirect ophthalmoscope and 20 D condensing lens	Fundus examination
Burton (UV) lamp	Examination with NaFI
Retinoscope	Refraction
Trial lenses	Refraction
External camera	Photodocumentation
Goniolens (3-mirror)	Angle or fundus gonioscopy
Visual-field instrument	Peripheral fields
Amsler grid	Central fields
Microscope	Cytology
Color plates	Color vision
Ophthalmodynamometer (ODM)	Cerebrovascular diagnoses
Exophthalmometer	Proptosis
Stainless steel tray	For instrument storage
Eyelid evertor (Desmarre)	Eyelid eversion
Eyelid retractors (adult and pediatric size)	Eyelid retraction (for procedure)
Toothed forceps	Grasping procedures
Iris scissor	Varied
Cautery	Varied
Cilia forceps	Epilation
Schirmer tear strips	Tear testing
Foreign-body loop (Bailey)	Foreign-body removal
Metal shield (Fox)	Eye protector
Plus 78 D lens	Nerve head and macula evaluation
Alger B rush	Rust ring removal

4. Economic Factors and Third-Party Considerations

a. Extensive business and practice management aspects must be understood and mastered regarding the financial aspects, economics, and proper management of a primary eye care practice
b. The nature of such a discussion is beyond the scope of this book for three basic reasons:
   i. This book is primarily a clinical text
   ii. The author of this text is neither a business nor practice management authority

TABLE 1.8 **Consumable Supplies**

Item	Use
Sodium fluorescein (NaFI) strips	Stains missing epithelial cells
Rose bengal strips	Stains dead/devitalized cells and mucus
Lissamine green strips	Stains dead/devitalized cells and mucus
Goniofluid or gel	Gonioscopy
2 × 2 gauze pads	Varied
Diagnostic agents (see Table 1.9)	Varied
Culture media (broth and/or agar)	For laboratory work
Microscope slides	Cytology
pH paper	For chemical burns
Irrigating solution	Lavage
Disposable soft lenses (plano or low power)	Corneal bandaging
Cotton-tip applicators	
Sterile	Culturing
Nonsterile	Varied procedures
Alcohol sponges	Antiseptic
Eyepads	Patching
Adhesive tape	Patching
Paper (Micropore)	Moderate adhesion
Plastic (Transpore)	Good adhesion
Cloth (Dermicel)	Good but expensive
Adhesive remover	After taping
Zephiran HCI (1: 750)	Antiseptic
Chlorhexidine gluconate (Hibiclens)	Antibacterial cleanser
Cotton balls	For cleansing surface
Therapeutic agents (see Table 1.10)	Varied
Ammonia ampules	For vasovagal responses
AdenoPlus	Adenoviral diagnostic test
Amniotic membranes	Corneal wound healing

(*Continued*)

TABLE 1.9 **Useful In-Office Pharmaceutical Agents**

Name	Primary Purpose
Drugs Used Primarily for Ocular Diagnosis	
Mydriacyl 0.5%, 1%	Pupil dilation
Cyclogyl 0.5%, 1%, 2%	Cycloplegia
Phenylephrine 2.5%	Pupil dilation
Proparacaine 0.5%	Topical anesthesia
Fluress	Topical anesthesia with NaFI
Sodium fluorescein (NaFI)	Diagnostic stain
Rose Bengal	Diagnostic stain
Lissamine Green	Diagnostic stain
Drugs Used for Various Purposes	
Pilocarpine 2%, 4%	To reverse angle closure
Topical beta blocker	Angle closure
Diamox 250 mg caps	Angle closure
Glycerol 50% soln	Angle closure
Homatropine 2%, 5%	Pupil dilation (with uveitis)
Scopolamine 0.25%	Pupil dilation (with uveitis)
Atropine 0.5%	Prolonged pupil dilation
Muro 128 sol 2%, 5%	Reduce diffuse edema
Muro 128 ointment	Reduce epithelial edema
Antibiotic Agents	
Broad spectrum	Prophylaxis or initiating therapy
Combination drug (antibiotic/steriod)	Drops and ointments
Gentamicin	Drops and ointments
Tobramycin	Drops and ointments
Ciprofloxacin	Corneal ulcer
Besifloxacin	Corneal ulcer
Bacitracin/Polymyxin B	Ointment
Antiviral Agents	
Viroptic	Drops
Anti-Inflammatory Agents	Initiating steroid therapy
Prednisolone 1%	For uveitis
Lotemax 0.5%	For chemical burns/ with glaucoma risk
Hydrocortisone 0.5%, 1%	For allergic reactions
Decongestants	
Brimonidine tartrate 0.025% (Lumify)	Vasoconstriction
Lubricants (Ointments and Drops)	
Mucomimetic drops	Daily use (ad lib)
Ointments	Lubrication

iii. The nature of such material is temporal as compared with the content of this text, and hence is best obtained through contemporary journal literature and lectures by experts in the field

5. *A Primary Care Philosophy (The "Seven C's")*

a. Compassion and communication
b. Clinical competency
c. Comfort and confidence
d. Comprehensive care
e. Coordination and continuity
f. Counseling
g. Cost consciousness

II. General Pharmaceutical Considerations

A. Major Ophthalmic Drug Categories

1. *Autonomics (Autonomic Nervous System Drugs)*

a. Antiglaucoma agents → refer to Chapter 8
b. Atropine group (cycloplegics and dilators)
   i. Atropine (0.5% and 1%)
      - Strongest cycloplegic drug
      - Duration up to 1 to 2 weeks
      - Prolonged immobilization of pupil may increase risk of posterior synechiae in anterior uveitis
   ii. Homatropine (2% and 5%)
      - Duration about 12 to 24 hours
      - Good dilator in treatment
      - No longer available in United States
   iii. Scopolamine (0.2% and 0.25%)
      - Duration about 24 to 48 hours
      - May work better than homatropine in darkly pigmented patients
      - No longer available in United States
   iv. Cyclopentolates (0.5%, 1%, and 2%)
      - Short-acting cycloplegic
      - Popular diagnostic agent for cycloplegic refraction
   v. Tropicamide (0.5% and 1%)
      - Excellent short-acting dilator
      - Good for diagnosis and treatment
c. Phenylephrine (2.5% and 10%)
   i. Short-acting dilator with no cycloplegia
   ii. Excellent sympathomimetic drug to combine with tropicamide (parasympatholytic drug) for maximal short-duration dilation
d. Hydroxyamphetamine
   i. Alternative to phenylephrine
   ii. Combined with tropicamide 0.25% (Paremyd)

2. *Anti-Infective (Antimicrobial) Agents*

Background

Antibiotic resistance has become a major issue in healthcare including ocular treatment. Doctors will treat most presumed infections empirically except sight threatening disease. It is important to remember that infections not responding to treatment may be resistant to the medication being prescribed. Cultures may need to be performed to identify the causative pathogen and appropriate treatment.

Gastrointestinal side effects such as nausea, vomiting, diarrhea, abdominal pain, loss of appetite, and bloating are common with all oral antibiotics. Practitioners should always ask patients about their experience with prior antibiotic use.

a. Antibiotics and antibacterials[1–7]
   i. Aminoglycosides
      - Widely used broad-spectrum topical agents
      - Excellent choice for corneal infection
      - Effective against gram-negative organisms and Staphylococcus (gram-positive)
      - Oral intravenous and intramuscular forms highly toxic which minimizes systemic overuse and subsequent bacterial resistance
      - Popular topical ophthalmic forms
        - Gentamicin
        - Neomycin
          - Approximately 5% to 10% risk of hypersensitivity reaction
          - Neomycin used in combination with polymyxin B (gram-negative including Pseudomonas) and bacitracin (gram-positive) in ointment form (e.g., Neosporin) (gramicidin is solution soluble and replaces bacitracin for solution form)
        - Tobramycin 0.3%
      - Toxic to corneal epithelium if used long term (e.g., > 14 days); gentamicin > tobramycin
      - Other topical, oral, injectable forms
        - Amikacin
        - Kanamycin
        - Netilmicin
        - Streptomycin
        - Vancomycin
      - All forms can be fortified in strength especially for central bacterial ulcers
   ii. Bacitracin
      - Effective against gram-positive (e.g., Staphylococcus)
      - Stable only in ointment form
   iii. Cephalosporin agents (broad-spectrum oral)[8,9]
      - Oral forms used to cover gram-positive and gram-negative bugs
      - First generation cephalexin (Keflex) effective against gram-positive but not MRSA or Pseudomonas
      - 10% cross-sensitivity between penicillin and cephalosporins is probably overestimated
      - Cross-reactivity between penicillin and second (e.g., cefuroxime) and third (e.g., cefotaxime) generation cephalosporin is low
   iv. Chloramphenicol
      - Excellent broad-spectrum topical
      - Infrequent use in eye care (in United States) due to increasing fear of fatal aplastic anemia risks
   v. Fluoroquinolones[10–12]
      - Superior to aminoglycosides and first-line treatment in active bacterial corneal infections
      - Highly effective against gram-negative (including *Pseudomonas aeruginosa*) and better gram-positive in fourth generation
      - Non-toxic to ocular surface
      - Second generation [ciprofloxacin, (Ciloxan) ofloxacin (Ocuflox)], third generation [norfloxacin, levofloxacin (Levaquin)], fourth generation [moxifloxacin, (Vigamox, Moxeza) gatifloxacin (Zymaxid), besifloxacin, (Besivance)]
      - Ciprofloxacin most effective against gram-negative including Pseudomonas
      - Besifloxacin (e.g., Besivance) newest approved fluoroquinolone with low MICs (minimum inhibitory concentration) against Pseudomonas, MRSA and MRSE bacteria

  - No oral med so less resistance than other fluroquinolones
- Levofloxacin (Levaquin) oral use has been reduced due to serious adverse reactions including tendinitis, tendon rupture, aorta dissection, peripheral neuropathy, central nervous system effects, and exacerbation of myasthenia gravis

vi. Macrolides[13,14]

- Erythromycin 0.5% (topical ointment and oral forms)
  - Due to overuse significant bacterial resistance
  - No longer used as a primary antibiotic treatment
  - Used when nighttime lubrication is indicated
- Azithromycin

  Oral (Zithromax)
  - Single-dose, oral antibiotic used in 1-gram dosage or Z-pak (6 250-mg tabs), 500 mg × 1 day, 250 mg × 4 days
  - Effective against chlamydia, some gram-negative (e.g., Haemophilus) and some gram-positive (e.g., Staphylococcus and Streptococcus)
  - Reduces noncompliance

  Topical
  - Azithromycin 1% solution (e.g., Azasite)
  - Effective against gram-positive and *Haemophilus influenzae*
  - High viscosity drop with prolonged half-life and therefore reduced dosing (e.g. bid for 2 days, qd for 5 days)
  - Great choice for pediatric conjunctivitis due to reduced dosing

vii. Penicillins (oral forms only in eye care)[15,16]

- Popular broad-spectrum oral agents
- Use penicillinase-resistant forms against Staphylococcus
  - Cloxacillin
  - Dicloxacillin
  - Methicillin
  - Nafcillin
  - Oxacillin
- Aminopenicillins
  - Developed to add gram-negative coverage
  - Amoxicillin—good gram-positive antimicrobial but not effective against MRSA; some gram-negative antimicrobial but not Pseudomonas
  - Ampicillin
- Organisms become resistant by producing beta-lactamase which inactivates antibiotics
  - A beta-lactamase inhibitor (Clavulanic acid) is combined with Amoxicillin (e.g., Augmentin)
- Penicillin and cephalosporin drug of choice if antibiotic needed for pregnant female
- Beware of allergic patients
  - 10% cross-sensitivity between penicillin and cephalosporins is probably overestimated
  - More common with parental use than oral
- Alternative drugs
  - Cephalosporins (e.g., cephalexin; Keflex)

viii. Polymyxin B

- Effective against gram-negative
- Used in combination with Bacitracin; only available as ointment in United States (e.g., Ak-Poly-Bac)

ix. Sulfacetamide (10%, 15%, and 30%)

- Increasing resistant staphylococcal strains to 10% concentration
- No longer used frequently due to availability of broader coverage with other antibiotics

x. Tetracyclines[17–19]

- Tetracycline, doxycycline, minocycline
- Tetracycline (250, 500 mg capsules dosed qid) rarely used due to poor adsorption
- Useful oral and topical broad-spectrum antibacterial action as well as actions against other pathogenic microbial agents (e.g., chlamydia)
- Also acts as anticollagenolytic agent in corneal disease
- Can cause depression and discoloration of developing bone and teeth
- Avoid in children under 12 to 15 years of age
- Avoid in pregnancy (and even in females of childbearing age)
- Also risk of phototoxic (sun) response
- Adverse effects: doxycycline vs minocycline
  - GI upset more common with doxycycline
  - Cutaneous disorders (e.g., blue pigmentation, lupus-like syndrome), idiopathic intracranial hypertension, and liver damage more common with minocycline
- Good alternative drug: Azithromycin
- Semisynthetic form: doxycycline (20, 50, 100 mg tablets/capsules)
  - 100 mg bid for MRSA skin infections
  - Lower dosages (e.g., 50 mg qd to bid) reduces side effects and increases compliance; used for anti-inflammatory effects for ocular rosacea, meibomian gland dysfunction, recurrent corneal erosion
  - ORACEA qd (30 mg immediate release plus 10 mg delayed release doxycycline)

xi. Trimethoprim[20,21]

Topical
- Effective against gram-positive organisms especially MRSA
- Combined with polymyxin B (Polytrim) as broad-spectrum topical anti-infective solution (similar to Neosporin)

Oral
- Combined with sulfamethoxazole (Bactrim, Septra DS)
  - Sulfamethoxazole/trimethoprim (800/160 mg, 400/80 mg)
- Trimethoprim and sulfamethoxazole effective against gram-positive organisms especially MRSA
- Not first choice in eye care but can be used if allergic to other oral antibiotics (e.g., penicillin)
- Beware of allergic patients—potential severe T cell-mediated reactions including

Stevens–Johnson syndrome and toxic epidermal necrolysis
- Sulfa-containing non-antibiotic drugs (e.g., Diamox) are not cross-reactive

xii. Hypochlorous acid 0.01% (e.g., Avenova, OcuSoft Hypochlor Spray)[22]
- Non-antibiotic, naturally occurring agent produced by immune response
- Reduces staphylococcal strains for blepharitis and meibomian gland dysfunction treatment

xiii. Numerous combinations of anti-infective agents with other compatible anti-infectives and anti-inflammatory agents
- Referred to as "combination or combo" drugs
- Very popular in anterior segment care (e.g., tobramycin/dexamethasone)

b. Antifungal agents[23]
i. Highly toxic drugs
ii. Nonocular drugs are occasionally used (e.g., amphotericin B, nystatin, triazoles)
iii. Only specific ocular drug: Natamycin

c. Antiviral (herpes simplex) agents[24–28]
Topical
i. Stoxil and Vira-A no longer available
ii. Trifluridine 1%. (e.g., Viroptic)
- Toxic with prolonged use

iii. Ganciclovir gel 0.15% (e.g., Zirgan)
- Better tolerated and no less effective than topical acyclovir
- Less toxic than trifluridine 1%

iv. Acyclovir ointment
- Ophthalmic use approved in Europe
- 5% ointment approved for cold sore and genital herpes in United States (e.g., Zovirax)

v. Povidone-iodine 5% and 10% (e.g., Betadine)
- Broad spectrum microbicide solution; toxic against bacteria, viruses, fungi, yeasts, molds, protozoans, parasites
- Used for surgical and laboratory antisepsis
- Used off label to treat epidemic keratoconjunctivitis (EKC)

Orals
i. Acyclovir (Zovirax)
ii. Famciclovir (Famvir)—Penciclovir prodrug
iii. Valacyclovir (Valtrex)—Acyclovir prodrug; better oral availability than acyclovir
iv. Side effects
- GI upset
- Use with caution with liver and kidney disease
- Patients older than 65 have increased risk of central nervous system adverse reactions (e.g., agitation, hallucination, confusion, and encephalopathy) with acyclovir and valacyclovir

d. Pesticidals (antiparasitic agents)[29]
i. Ocular ointments
- Physostigmine 0.25% ointment (Eserine) for *Phthiriasis palpebrarum* (lice)—very toxic to ocular surface
- Yellow mercuric oxide for *Phthiriasis palpebrarum* (lice)
- Pyrethrin ointments for *Phthiriasis palpebrarum*

ii. Solutions
- Tea tree oil (e.g., Cliredex, Ocusoft Oust Demodex Cleanser) for demodex (mites)

iii. Hair products
- Lindane 1% (Kwell) shampoo for *Phthiriasis palpebrarum*
- Permethrin 1% hair lotion
- Nix

e. Acanthomoeba drugs
i. 0.02% biguanides → first-line treatment
- Polyhexamethylene (PHMB)
- Chlorhexidine gluconate (CHX)

ii. 0.1% diamidines
- Propamidine isethionate (Brolene)
- Hexamidine

3. *Anti-Inflammatory Agents (Steroids and Nonsteroidal Anti-Inflammatory Drugs [NSAIDs])*

a. Steroids[30–34]
i. Actions
- Broad anti-inflammatory action
- Inhibit inflammatory cytokines, chemokines, adhesion molecules, and other inflammatory mediators
- Inhibit vasodilation, vascular permeability, leukocytes migration, scar formation
- Inhibit synthesis of histamine, stabilize cell membranes, and inhibit degranulation of mast cells
- Reduce symptoms of photophobia, pain, redness, swelling
- Inhibit adverse tissue changes
- Reduce scarring potential
- Steroids do not cure disease

ii. Indications
- Inflammatory reactions
- Toxic, hypersensitive (allergic) reactions
- Associated inflammatory pain

iii. Contraindications
- Active infection
- Herpes simplex epithelial keratitis
- Active ulcerative process
- During cell regeneration or tissue healing
- Use with caution in glaucoma patient or family history of glaucoma

iv. Adverse reactions
- Worsens microbial infections
- Delays wound healing
- Posterior subcapsular cataract formation with chronic use
- Increase IOP; amount depends on specific steroid medication, dosage frequency, route of administration, patient susceptibility
  - IOP increase more likely with topical vs. systemic treatment
  - Increase more likely in certain patients (i.e., steroid responders)
  - IOP spikes usually 3–6 weeks after use but can occur as early as 1 week

v. Drug selection
Topical ophthalmic

- Anti-inflammatory activity ranking (greatest to least)
  - Difluprednate 0.05% emulsion (e.g., Durezol); no shaking required
  - Prednisolone acetate 1% suspension (e.g., Pred Forte)
  - Loteprednol etabonate 0.25% (e.g., EYseuVIS; nanoparticle suspension), 0.38% (Lotemax SM gel; submicron particles), 0.5% (e.g., Lotemax; suspension, gel, and ointment) and 1% (e.g., Inveltys; suspension)
  - Rimexolone 1% suspension (e.g., Vexol)
  - Fluorometholone acetate 0.1% suspension (e.g., Flarex)
  - Prednisolone sodium phosphate 1% (solution)
  - Dexamethasone alcohol 0.1% (suspension, ointment)
  - Fluoromethalone alcohol 0.1% suspension/ointment (e.g., FML)
  - Loteprednol etabonate 0.2% suspension (e.g., Alrex)
  - Prednisolone acetate 0.12% (suspension)
- Shake suspensions before use
- Potential for IOP increase
  - Prednisolone and Difluprednate penetrate cornea most effectively and have highest potential for IOP increase
  - Ester-based (e.g., Loteprednol) steroids are inactivated faster than ketone-based (e.g., Prednisolone acetate) and minimize potential side effects
  - Ester-based steroid reduces risk of significant IOP spikes (>10 mm) compared to ketone-based in short term (<28 days) and long term (greater than 28 days); Prednisolone was worse than dexamethasone
  - Fluoromethalone alcohol 0.1% ketone-based steroid with least impact on IOP due to poor corneal penetration
  - Rimexolone has limited ocular penetration which limits risks of IOP increase
- Dosage will vary depending on degree of inflammation; standard dosing is usually qid for 7–10 days unless condition is severe; if so, dose every 1–2 hours the first 1–2 days; Some patients may also need a longer tapering schedule if condition is chronic.
- Always taper steroids when terminating
- Reduce gradually over 3 to 5 days or longer if condition is chronic; qh to q2h to qid to tid to bid to 1 × and then off

Topical dermatological

- Triamcinolone cream (0.25%, 0.5%, 0.1%)
- Indicated for relief of inflammatory, red, scaling, itching, and dermatological (skin) conditions (e.g., psoriasis)
- Not indicated for in-eye use but can be prescribed for allergic blepharitis

Oral

- Prednisone—2.5 mg, 5 mg, 10 mg, 20 mg, 50 mg
- Methylprednisolone (e.g., Medrol)—2-mg, 4-mg, 8-mg, 16-mg, 32-mg tablet; Medrol Dosepak 21 4-mg tablets
  - Dosepack has built in tapering plan; 6 tabs day 1; 5 tabs day 2; 4 tabs; day 3; 3 tabs day 4; 2 tabs day 5; and 1 tab day 6
- Side effects include: Cushing syndrome, decrease bone density, growth suppression in children, impaired skin collagen synthesis, cataract, central serous chorioretinopathy, hyperglycemia, infection, effect on central nervous system
- Take with food or milk to minimize GI upset
- Contraindicated in peptic ulcers, diabetics, and pregnant females, or may become pregnant
- Prescribe lowest possible dose to manage inflammation and minimize side effects
  - Typical Prednisone dose 40–60mg/day (80mg maximum daily adult dose); for acute conditions that require maximum 3–6 weeks treatment for inflammation control, taper slowly, decrease 10mg/day for every 1–2 days until done
- Careful evaluation of systemic health should be considered when prescribing oral steroids, especially in high doses. Communication and care coordination with other healthcare providers is important in a multidisciplinary approach in mitigating potential risks.

b. Nonsteroidal anti-inflammatory drugs (NSAIDs)[35–49]

i. Actions
- Inhibit production of prostaglandins
  - Most are non-selective COX inhibitors
- Less effective than steroids for anti-inflammation but with fewer side effects

ii. Indications
- Analgesic (peripheral acting)
- Anti-inflammatory (except Acetaminophen)
- Antipyretic

iii. Contraindications
- Active GI or cerebral vascular bleeding
- Kidney and liver impairment or disease
- Cardiovascular disease (CVD)
- Avoid aspirin in children and adolescents with flulike symptoms

iv. Adverse reactions

Topical
- Redness, burning, stinging
- Corneal epithelial breakdown
- Corneal ulceration and melts have occurred; may be associated with NSAIDS impairing epithelial healing
- Concurrent use with topical steroids, significant inflammation present, history of diabetes, prior ocular surgery, and higher doses are risk factors for corneal erosion and melts

Oral
- Minimize by prescribing the least dose for the shortest time
- GI upset with short-term use, may need gastroprotective agents (e.g., proton pump inhibitors) for higher dosage
- GI bleeding/ulcers, cardiovascular disease (CVD), respiratory, liver and kidney disease with chronic use

- Acetaminophen chronic use causes liver damage especially with alcoholism
- Aspirin → GI ulcers, tinnitus; EXCEPTION to other NSAIDs, potent cardiovascular protective agent
- Celecoxib (e.g., Celebrex) → lower incidence of gastrointestinal complications but highest CVD
- Ibuprofen → GI upset, hypersensitivity reactions

v. Drug selection

Topical

- FDA approved for post-cataract surgery inflammation and pain, used off-label pre-op for cataract surgery, cystoid macular edema (CME); pain from corneal abrasions, post-PRK, foreign-body removals, chemical keratitis, itch from allergic conjunctivitis
- Diclofenac sodium 0.1% (e.g., Voltaren, qid)
- Ketorolac tromethamine 0.4% (Acular LS, qid); 0.45% (e.g., Acuvail, bid); 0.5% (e.g., Acular, qid)
  - Only NSAID FDA approved to treat ocular itch associated with allergic conjunctivitis but others (i.e., diclofenac, indomethacin) are used off-label
- Bromfenac sodium 0.09% (e.g., Bromday qd, Xibrom, bid); 0.07% (e.g., Prolensa, qd dosing)
- Nepafenac sodium 0.3% (Ilevro, qd); 0.1% (e.g., Nevanac, tid)

Oral

- Acetaminophen (e.g., OTC Tylenol 325, 500 mg); Not an NSAID but has analgesic and antipyretic action; maximum acetaminophen dosage 4000 mg/day due to potential hepatoxicity
- Aspirin (OTC 325 mg)
- Celecoxib (e.g., Celebrex Rx 100 mg, 200 mg, 400 mg)
  - Selective Cox-2 inhibitor
- Diclofenac (e.g., Voltaren Rx 25, 50, 75 mg)
- Ibuprofen (e.g., OTC Advil 200 mg, Rx 400, 600, 800 mg) maximum dosage 2400 mg/day
- Indomethacin (e.g., Indocin Rx 25, 50 mg)
- Ketorolac (e.g., Toradol Rx 10 mg)
- Naproxen (e.g., OTC Aleve 220 mg, Rx Naprosyn, Anaprox DS 275, 350, 500, 550 mg) maximum 1100 mg/day
- Ibuprofen and acetaminophen combination provide pain management similar to some opioid analgesics and better than each drug individually

c. Cyclosporin[50–54]

i. An immunotherapy drug that decreases activation and function of T lymphocytes

ii. FDA approved for dry eye treatment

- 0.05% (e.g., Restasis), 0.09% (e.g., Cequa), bid dosing
- Some studies show improvement in signs/symptoms while others show similar performance to artificial tears
- Clinical efficacy may depend on specific dry eye patients since pathology origin is multifactorial in origin

iii. FDA approved for vernal keratoconjunctivitis

- 0.1% (e.g., Verkazia) qid

iv. Most common side effect on instillation: ocular burning

d. Lifitegrast 5% (e.g., Xiidra)[55,56]

i. FDA approved to reduce signs (inferior corneal staining) and symptoms of dry eye

ii. LFA-1 antagonist

iii. Lifitegrast prevents the adhesion, activation, migration, and proliferation of lymphocytes and therefore decrease the inflammatory response

iv. Shorter (approximately 2 weeks) efficacy onset than cyclosporine

v. Most common side effects on instillation: ocular burning and dysgeusia (funny taste in back of throat)

e. Protopic (e.g., Tacrolimus 0.03%, 0.1%)

i. FDA-approved ointment for atopic dermatitis

ii. Inhibits T and B cell activation and therefore inhibits inflammatory cytokine release

iii. Used off-label to treat dry eye, vernal keratoconjunctivitis, atopic keratoconjunctivitis, anterior uveitis, scleritis, corneal graft rejection, and graft vs. host disease

iv. May not be well tolerated when applied to conjunctival sac and therefore needs to be applied transdermally to eyelids

v. Since FDA issued a black box warning in 2005 for potential to cause cancer, ocular approval has been hindered

4. *Antihistamine/Mast Cell Stabilizers*[57–61]

a. Antihistamine: H (1) receptor antagonists block histamine receptors and reduce itch but not redness for acute relief

b. Mast cell stabilizer: prevents mast cell degranulation and release of pro inflammatory mediators; used to prevent symptoms from occurring

c. Combination drugs prescribed more often than individual components

d. Combined agents: OTC olopatadine (e.g., Pataday), ketotifen (e.g., Alaway) 0.025%, and alcaftadine (e.g., Lastacaft) 0.25%; Rx azelastine (e.g., Optivar), epinastine (e.g., Elestat), bepotastine besilate 1.5% (e.g., Bepreve), cetirizine ophthalmic solution 0.24% (e.g., Zerviate)

e. Mast cell stabilizer only: RX lodoxamide (e.g., Alomide) and nedocromil (e.g., Alocril)

f. Antihistamine only: Rx emedastine (e.g., Emadine)

g. Contact lens drug delivery system

i. Acuvue Theravision with Ketotifen

5. *Anesthetic and Analgesic Agents*

a. Topical anesthetic agents[62–64]

i. Proparacaine 0.5%, tetracaine 0.5%, benoxinate 0.4% plus sodium fluorescein (e.g., Fluress)

ii. Anesthetic effect starts within 1 minute of application and maximum effect after 5 minutes

iii. Short-term duration approximately 10–20 minutes

iv. Chronic use delays wound healing and toxic

v. Used for in-office procedures only

vi. Not used for pain management

b. Oral nonnarcotic analgesic agents

i. See NSAIDs

c. Narcotic analgesic agents[65–67]
  i. Central nervous system acting
  ii. Occasional need for Schedule III, IV, V drugs in anterior segment care
  iii. Controlled substances (under the Federal Controlled Substance Act of 1970, Title 21 of the Federal Food, Drug, and Cosmetic Act of 1938) classified by risk of abuse or dependence

Schedule I (C-1)
- Drugs or substances with a high potential for abuse or dependence
- No current acceptable medical use
- Unlawful to prescribe or possess
- Opiates heroin, hallucinogens (e.g., LSD), marijuana, MDMA (ecstasy/molly), mescaline

Schedule II (C-II)
- Drugs or substances with a high potential for abuse or dependence
- Acceptable use with severe restrictions
- Cocaine, morphine, methamphetamine, hydromorphone (Dilaudid), oxycodone (OxyContin), meperidine (Demerol), fentanyl, Adderall, Ritalin, pentobarbital, secobarbital

Schedule III (C-III)
- Less potential for abuse or dependence
- Hydrocodone/acetaminophen (Vicodin); codeine in combination with acetaminophen (Tylenol #3 and #4), aspirin, or ibuprofen, ketamine, anabolic steroids, testosterone

Schedule IV (C-IV)
- Low potential for abuse or dependence
- Phenobarbital, chlordiazepoxide (Librium), diazepam (Valium), Tramadol, Xanax, Ambien, Darvon

Schedule V (C-V)
- Lowest potential for abuse or dependence
- Some are available OTC (e.g., antitussives with codeine, antidiarrheals (Lomotil)

  iv. Must be registered with the Drug Enforcement Administration (DEA) to prescribe Schedules II through V
  v. Examples of oral narcotics in primary eyecare
- Acetaminophen and hydrocodone (e.g., Vicodin)
  - 300 → 750 mg acetaminophen and 2.5 → 10 mg hydrocodone
  - 1–2 tablets q4h to q6h
- Ibuprofen and hydrocodone
  - 200 mg ibuprofen and 2.5/5/7.5/10 mg Hydrocodone
- Acetaminophen and codeine (e.g., Tylenol #3, #4)
  - 300 mg acetaminophen and 15/30/60 mg codeine tablets
  - One tablet q4h
  - Daily maximum 4000 mg Tylenol and 360 mg codeine
- Tramadol (e.g., Ultram), 50 mg tablets
  - Synthetic analogue of codeine
  - Inhibits norepinephrine and serotonin reuptake
  - 50–100 mg q4h to q6h, maximum 300–400 mg/day
  - Least side effects

  vi. Long-term dependence potential
  vii. Side effects: nausea, vomiting, constipation, and sedation; avoid alcohol, muscle relaxants, and depressants

6. *Antihistamines and Decongestants (Vasoconstrictors)*[68,69]

Antihistamines (OTC)

a. Topical
  i. First generation—Antazoline and pheniramine
  ii. Used in combination with vasoconstrictor (Tetrahydrozoline)

b. Oral
  i. First generation with anti-cholinergic properties and side effects (e.g., drowsiness and ocular dryness)
    - Diphenhydramine (e.g., Benadryl)
    - Chlorpheniramine (e.g., Chlor-Trimeton)
  ii. Second generation do not cross blood–brain barrier and reduce side effects
    - Loratadine (e.g., Claritin), Fexofenadine (e.g., Allegra), Cetirizine (Zyrtec)

Decongestants (OTC)

a. Topical agents constrict arterioles and venules to decrease ocular redness with minor ocular irritation
b. Adrenergic receptor agonists: alpha 1, alpha 2, and mixed alpha 1 and 2
  i. Alpha 1—constricts arterioles and venules
    - Associated with tachyphylaxis (i.e., diminishing response to successive doses of a drug) and rebound hyperemia
    - Tetrahydrozoline 0.05%, phenylephrine 2.5%
  ii. Alpha 2 only constricts veins
    - Brimonidine tartrate 0.025% (e.g., Lumify)
    - Reduces redness for up to 8 hours
    - No tachyphylaxis even with higher doses used for glaucoma
    - Negligible rebound hyperemia
  iii. Mixed alpha 1 and 2
    - Naphazoline 0.012% to 0.03%

7. *Lubricants and Tear Substitutes*[70–72]

Solution active ingredients: demulcents and emollients are defined by US Food and Drug Administration

a. Demulcents: "An agent, usually a water-soluble polymer, which is applied topically to the eye to protect and lubricate mucous membrane surfaces and relieve dryness and irritation"
  i. Carboxymethylcellulose (CMC)
  ii. Hydroxypropyl methylcellulose (HPMC)
  iii. Polyvinyl alcohol (PVA)
  iv. Propylene glycol (PPG)
  v. Polyethylene glycol (PEG)
  vi. Dextran
  vii. Glycerin
  viii. Povidone
b. Emollients: "An agent, usually a fat or oil, which is applied locally to eyelids to protect or soften tissues and to prevent drying and cracking"; very common in artificial tears for evaporative dry eye
  i. Lanolin
  ii. Mineral oil
  iii. Petrolatum
  iv. Paraffin
  v. Wax
c. Other ingredients
  i. Sodium hyaluronate (glycosaminoglycan)
  ii. Hydroxypropyl-guar (HP-guar)

d. Agents with greater viscosity are used to increase ocular retention time; increasing viscosity: solutions → gels → ointments
   i. High viscosity agents may cause transient visual blur and therefore better for nighttime use
e. Available preserved, preservative-free unit dose, and multidose preservative-free specially designed bottles to prevent microbial contamination

8. *Hypertonic Saline Agents*[73]

a. Use osmotic gradient to draw fluid (edema) from cornea (more from epithelium than stroma)
b. Solution and ointment, 2% or 5% (e.g., Muro 128)
c. Burns and stings with instillation resulting in reflex tearing and reduce retention time
d. Use 5% ointment at night for longer ocular retention

9. *Specialty Drugs*[74–78]

a. Oxymetazoline hydrochloride 0.1%, ophthalmic solution (e.g., Upneeq)
   i. α-adrenergic receptor agonist that stimulates receptors on Mueller's muscle to cause muscle contraction which results in superior lid lift in acquired ptosis
   ii. 1 drop/day
   iii. Adverse reactions that occurred in 1–5% of subjects treated with UPNEEQ were punctate keratitis, conjunctival hyperemia, dry eye, blurred vision, instillation site pain, eye irritation, and headache
   iv. May lower blood pressure
b. Cenegermin-bkbj 0.002% ophthalmic solution (e.g., Oxervate)
   i. Recombinant human nerve growth factor to restore corneal surface in neurotrophic keratitis
   ii. 1 drop 6×/day (2-hour intervals) for 8 weeks
   iii. Adverse reactions include pain on instillation, redness, tearing, foreign-body sensation
c. Varenicline solution (e.g., Tyrvaya)
   i. Rx nasal spray → One spray in each nostril twice daily
   ii. FDA approved for treatment of signs and symptoms of dry eye
      - Nicotinic acetylcholine receptor activates the trigeminal parasympathetic pathway resulting in increased production of basal tear film
   iii. Adverse reactions → sneezing very common, others include cough, throat and nose irritation
d. Pilocarpine 1.25% (e.g., Vuity)
   i. FDA approved as a daily drop for presbyopia treatment (see also Chapter 7, page 292)
   ii. Miosis increases depth of focus
   iii. Two large Phase 3 clinical studies compared Vuity to a placebo eyedrop; percentage of patients with >3 lines improvement in near mesopic visual acuity and <1 line decrease in distance visual acuity at hour 3 compared to placebo was 31% to 8% and 26% to 11%
      - Improved near vision peaks about 1 hour after instillation and returns to placebo levels after 6–8 hours
   iv. Most common side effects were hyperemia and headache (> 5% of the patients)
   v. Exercise caution in night driving and other hazardous occupations in poor illumination

10. *Injectable Ophthalmic Medications*[79–82]

a. Local anesthetics
   i. Most anesthetics are either esters or amides
      - Topical = ester, injectable = amide
      - No allergic cross reactivity between the amide and ester class anesthetics
   ii. Lidocaine (Xylocaine) 0.5%, 1.0%, or 2.0%
      - Onset of action in 30 seconds to 1 minute
      - Duration of around 30 to 60 minutes
   iii. Bupivacaine (Marcaine) 0.25%
      - Onset five minutes
      - Lasts around twice as long as lidocaine
   iv. Lidocaine with epinephrine (0.5 mL of 1% lidocaine with epinephrine 1:100,000)
      - Epinephrine causes vasoconstriction which reduces bleeding and produces longer anesthetic effect
      - Agent used most commonly by eye care providers since lid/face highly vascularized
      - Entire lid can be anesthetized with less than 1 mL
      - Epinephrine contraindications
         - Contaminated wounds, peripheral vasculature disease
         - If epinephrine contraindicated, use single-agent lidocaine 1–2%
   v. Risks
      - Allergic reaction, infection, bleeding from needle trauma, ischemia, (see epinephrine side effects above)
b. Triamcinolone acetonide (e.g., Kenalog)
   i. Used for chalazion not responding to conventional therapy; 0.1 ml to 0.3 ml (Kenalog 40 mg/ml)
      - Works best if recent chalazia (onset less than 4 months)
      - Risks
         - Skin depigmentation in dark-skinned individuals
         - Retinal infarction due to micro embolization by steroid particles
   ii. Used for treatment of inflammation (Triesence, Trivaris, Kenalog)
      - Recalcitrant anterior uveitis that fails on topical therapy (subconjunctival injection)
      - Pars planitis (sub-Tenon's injection)
      - Macula edema (sub-Tenon's or intra-vitreal injection)
      - Risk of increased IOP
c. Intra-muscular epinephrine
   i. Indicated for anaphylaxis and injected into outer thigh, through clothing if necessary
   ii. Can be drawn up from vial of 1 mg/1 mL 1:1000
      - For those >66 lbs administer 0.3–0.5 mg (0.3–0.5 mL)
      - For those 33–66 lbs administer 0.15 mg/kg (0.15 mL)
   iii. Disposable, prefilled autoinjectors (preferred method)
      - Epipen (available as generic)
         - 0.15 mg indicated for children 33–66 lbs
         - 0.3 mg indicated for those >66 lbs
      - Auvi-Q

- When activated, has automated voice instructions guiding you through injection process
- Pocket-sized
- 0.1 mg indicated for infants/toddlers 16–33 lbs
- 0.15 mg indicated for children 33–66 lbs
- 0.3 mg indicated for those >66 lbs

iv. Side effects
- Fast, irregular, or "pounding" heartbeat, sweating, shakiness, headache, paleness, feelings of over excitement, anxiety, weakness, dizziness, and nausea
- Rare—infection at injection site a few days later

d. Botox (onabotulinumtoxinA)

i. Purified neurotoxin complex made from Botulinum toxin type A (*Clostridium botulinum*)
- Interrupts the normal neuromuscular junction transmission, resulting in muscle paralysis

ii. Used for the reduction of glabellar lines and facial wrinkles falls but also for blepharospasm, strabismus, and migraine headache

iii. Complications include ptosis and exposure problems secondary to incomplete lid closure

11. *Miscellaneous Agents*[83–85]

a. Compresses (warm and cold)

i. Warm for heating meibomian gland contents (e.g., microwavable masks absorb heat and moisture for 15-minute treatment, e.g., Bruder mask)

ii. Hot air (hair blowers) effective heat source for variable causes of corneal edema

iii. Cold for conditions requiring vasoconstriction
- Generalized inflammatory reactions
- Intracellular bleeding

b. Irrigating solutions

c. Pressure patching

d. Soft contact lenses

i. Disposable soft lenses of plano or low power

ii. As bandage in corneal epithelial disease (e.g., abrasion, erosion)

iii. As lubricators (e.g., dry eye disease)

iv. As protective shield (e.g., entropion)

v. As reservoir for drug delivery (e.g., allergic conjunctivitis)

e. Sodium fluorescein (NaFl) stains any missing epithelial cells or cells with damaged cell membranes

i. Preferred dye for cornea

f. Rose bengal (RB) and Lissamine green (LG) stains dead and devitalized cells (cells that have lost their protective mucin coating)

i. LG preferred dye for conjunctiva

ii. RB stings upon instillation and LG does not

g. Amniotic membranes (AM)[86,87]

i. AM is obtained from placentas during elective cesarean section

ii. Epidermal and keratocyte growth factor support its wound healing properties

iii. Promotes epithelial healing, anti-inflammatory, anti-scarring, anti-fibrotic, and anti-angiogenic therapeutic action

iv. Two types
- Inlay (graft) → membrane is grafted (sutured) on the damaged cornea and is integrated into the ocular tissue
- Onlay (patch) → membrane is placed on superficial wound for physical protection and proteins secreted to facilitate wound healing; will be eventually removed or self-degrades with time

v. Patch treatments
- Chemical/thermal burns
- Persistent epithelial defects
- Recurrent corneal erosion
- Stevens–Johnson syndrome (SJS)
- Toxic Epidermal Necrolysis (TEN)
- Graft versus Host Disease
- Ocular Pemphigoid
- Corneal ulcers

vi. Patch products
- Self-containing cryopreserved (e.g., Prokera)
  - Multiple thicknesses available → use thicker membranes for more severe disease
  - Must be thoroughly rinsed prior to insertion
  - Anesthetize cornea before insertion
  - Patient will typically report awareness to PMMA ring for 24 hours
  - Insert with patient looking down; once inserted, have patient look up to place ring in the inferior cul-de-sac
  - To minimize ring ejection and discomfort, do a tape tarsorrhaphy at the temporal margin to slightly raise the lower lid
  - PMMA ring will need to be removed after membrane dissolves
- Dehydrated (e.g., AmbioDisk and BioDOptix)

1. Wash your hands before and after using eye medications.
2. Tilt your head back and look up at the ceiling. You may want to lay down on your back if it is easier.
3. Place a finger on your cheek just under your lower eyelid and gently pull down until a "V" pocket is formed between your eyeball and your lower lid.
4. Put 1 to 2 drops into the eye. Do not let the dropper tip touch the eye or eyelashes. This may contaminate the medication.
5. Do not blink your eyes, simply close them very lightly and leave them closed for approximately one minute. Blinking and closing your eyes hard pushes the drop out of the eye and onto your cheek. We want the drop *in* the eye.
6. If you still have difficulty getting the drops into your eyes, tilt your head back and with your eyes closed, place 1 to 2 drops in the corner of your eye. With your head still tilted backward, open your eyes, and look up at the ceiling. This will then allow the medication to get into the eye.

FIGURE 1.2 Instillation of eyedrops: patient instruction sheet.

1. Wash your hands before and after using eye medications.
2. Tilt your head back and look up at the ceiling-you may want to lay down on your back if it is easier.
3. Place a finger on your cheek just under your lower eyelid and gently pull down until a V pocket is formed between your eyeball and your lower lid.
4. Place a small amount (about 1/4 inch) in the V pocket: Do not let the tip of the tube touch the eye or eyelashes-this may contaminate the medication.

FIGURE 1.3 Instillation of eye ointments: patient instruction sheet.

- Lid speculum may be needed to prevent lid from dislodging graft during insertion
- Graft is smoothed out on the eye and a large BCL is inserted to hold membrane in place
- Remove bandage lens after membrane dissolves

h. AdenoPlus[88]
   i. In-office diagnostic test for adenovirus; results provided in 10 minutes
   ii. Lower palpebral conjunctiva is swabbed with an Adenoplus collector
   iii. Antigen-based immunoassay
   iv. Sensitivity (i.e., to correctly identify patients with a disease) varies among studies: specificity (i.e., to correctly identify people without the disease) has been consistently high

i. Spectacle lenses
   i. As for protection in hazardous conditions
   ii. As for protection for monocular patients
   iii. For UV protection

B. Practical Considerations

1. Determine dosage, concentration, and duration of drug use by diagnosis and degree of presentation
2. Vehicles
   a. Use drops (solutions or suspensions) for ocular surface conditions
   b. Use ointments for superficial lid conditions and prolonged effect on ocular surface
   c. Creams and lotions provide increased skin penetration for allergic lid reactions
3. Hydrochloride versus acetate versus sulfate salts may affect penetration rates in varying disease states (clinically insignificant)
4. Buffering of ophthalmic solutions dictates initial comfort but not a major factor in drug use
5. Sterility required in ophthalmic drugs, but realities of use relate more to aseptic, contamination-free drug and container conditions
6. Drug instillation (for topical ophthalmic agents)
   a. Standard methods are fine but are usually a problem for patients, especially the elderly (Figures 1.2 and 1.3)
   b. Reservoir technique useful for lids and mild ocular surface conditions
   c. One drop is better than two (reduces hyperlacrimation dilution)
   d. If you think you (or the patient) missed first drop, drop again (and again if necessary)
      i. You cannot overdose an eye very easily
      ii. Cul-de-sacs hold only 1 drop
   e. Topical anesthetic instilled first increases drug absorption
   f. Separate instillation of drops or ointments (same or different) by at least 1 minute
   g. Block puncta if drug has systemic implications
   h. Ask pharmacist to help instruct patient
7. Run topical antibiotics for a minimum of 5 to 7 days
8. Always consider a nondrug approach if clinically reasonable

C. Complications and Adverse Reactions

1. Hypersensitivity reactions (common and superficial)
   a. Erythema or hyperemia
   b. Itching and irritation
   c. Treatment
      i. Eliminate source
      ii. Cold, decongestants, steroids (if severe)
2. Vasovagal (syncope) response
   a. Pale, clammy, short blackout
   b. Blood pressure decreases rapidly
   c. Treatment
      i. Position head below the level of the heart (between the knees)
      ii. Ammonia (smelling) salts
3. Prolonged-use reactions
   a. Delayed hypersensitivities
   b. Reduced healing rate (steroids and topical anesthetics)
   c. Medicamentosa (any medicine, any time)
   d. Steroid responses (short and long term)
4. Cardiopulmonary reactions
   a. Hyperventilation
   b. Cardiac arrest
   c. Treatment: cardiopulmonary resuscitation (CPR)
5. Anaphylaxis
   a. Very rare with topical drops but possible with oral meds
   b. Treatment: Call for help immediately
6. Iatrogenic considerations (not you!)

III. Basic Guidelines

A. Ten Simple Philosophies for Safe and Efficient Patient Care

1. "F-1-D approach"
   a. Frequency-intensity-duration (of a condition)
   b. Consider each aspect in the history and your instructions to the patient
2. "Diagnose things by the company they keep and the innocent bystanders"
   a. A single clinical finding by itself means very little diagnostically

   b. A single clinical finding in the company of others becomes a differential clue
   c. If those "other" findings are not directly associated (i.e., "innocent bystanders") with the primary affected structure, think deeper involvement or ulceration (especially corneal)
3. "If you hear hoofs and see stripes, think zebras!"
   a. Do not overlook the obvious
   b. Most diagnoses have one or more definitive signs
4. "It ain't rare if it's in your chair!"
5. "Pharmacists are not just 'counters and pourers'!"
   a. They are perhaps the most accessible, educated, and up-to-date resources available regarding drugs, pharmacology, and toxicology
   b. Readily available to health professionals and patients
   c. Grossly underused by all
6. "When you're a hammer, everything starts looking like the head of a nail!"
   a. An important consideration (especially to your patient) when referring or seeking consultation
   b. The nonsurgical primary eye care provider should counsel their patients carefully on all levels of care and their alternatives
7. "Never be the last to see an eye before it goes blind!"
8. "The 'You can't win' theory"
   a. You prescribe correctly, but they never do it! (Expect a high rate of noncompliance)
   b. You prescribe and they do it, but who's to say it helped? (Post hoc, ergo propter hoc: "after this, therefore because of this")
   c. You do not prescribe, and they get better anyway!
9. "If an undocumented clinical variable could occur, it will occur the first time you manage a condition (probably on a Friday afternoon at 5:45)!"
   a. Murphy's Law: primary care corollary #13
      Do not panic or question yourself too quickly
10. "Crawl, walk, and then run!"
   a. Go from the simple to the complex
   b. Go from the early to the advanced
   c. Go from the chronic to the acute
   d. Go from the lids to the conjunctiva to the cornea

B. Good Luck and Enjoy!

References

1. Tabbara KF. Antimicrobial agents in ophthalmology. *Ocular Infect.* 2014;19–35. Published 2014 Nov 10. doi:10.1007/978-3-662-43981-4_2
2. Wong RL, Gangwani RA, Yu LW, Lai JS. New treatments for bacterial keratitis. *J Ophthalmol.* 2012;2012:831502. doi:10.1155/2012/831502
3. Asbell PA, Sanfilippo CM, Sahm DF, DeCory HH. Trends in antibiotic resistance among ocular microorganisms in the United States From 2009 to 2018. *JAMA Ophthalmol.* 2020;138(5):439–450. doi:10.1001/jamaophthalmol.2020.0155
4. Bremond-Gignac D, Chiambaretta F, Milazzo S. A European perspective on topical ophthalmic antibiotics: current and evolving options. *Ophthalmol Eye Dis.* 2011;3:29–43. Published 2011 Oct 24. doi:10.4137/OED.S4866
5. Azari AA, Barney NP. Conjunctivitis: a systematic review of diagnosis and treatment [published correction appears in JAMA. 2014 Jan 1;311(1):95. Dosage error in article text]. *JAMA.* 2013;310(16):1721–1729. doi:10.1001/jama.2013.280318
6. Fraunfelder FW. Corneal toxicity from topical ocular and systemic medications. *Cornea.* 2006;25(10):1133–1138. doi:10.1097/01.ico.0000240084.27663.fd
7. Padberg S. Anti-infective Agents. *Drugs during Pregnancy and Lactation.* 2015;115–176. doi:10.1016/B978-0-12-408078-2.00007-X
8. de Lalla F. Oral cephalosporins in airway infections. *Clin Microbiol Infect.* 2000;6(Suppl 3):70–72. doi:10.1111/j.1469-0691.2000.tb02048.x
9. Chambers ST, Murdoch DR, Pearce MJ. Clinical and economic considerations in the use of third-generation oral cephalosporins. *Pharmacoeconomics.* 1995;7(5):416–427. doi:10.2165/00019053-199507050-00006
10. Silverstein BE, Morris TW, Gearinger LS, Decory HH, Comstock TL. Besifloxacin ophthalmic suspension 0.6% in the treatment of bacterial conjunctivitis patients with *Pseudomonas aeruginosa* infections. *Clin Ophthalmol.* 2012;6:1987–1996. doi:10.2147/OPTH.S35715
11. Janssen Pharmaceuticals Inc. *Levaquin (Levofloxacin) [Prescribing Information].* Titusville; February 2017.
12. van der Linden PD, Sturkenboom MC, Herings RM, Leufkens HM, Rowlands S, Stricker BH. Increased risk of achilles tendon rupture with quinolone antibacterial use, especially in elderly patients taking oral corticosteroids. *Arch Intern Med.* 2003;163(15):1801–1807. doi:10.1001/archinte.163.15.1801
13. Bremond-Gignac D, Messaoud R, Lazreg S, Speeg-Schatz C, Renault D, Chiambaretta F. A 3-day regimen with azithromycin 1.5% eyedrops for the treatment of purulent bacterial conjunctivitis in children: efficacy on clinical signs and impact on the burden of illness. *Clin Ophthalmol.* 2015;9:725–732. Published 2015 Apr 20. doi:10.2147/OPTH.S78747
14. Katusic D, Petricek I, Mandic Z, et al. Azithromycin vs doxycycline in the treatment of inclusion conjunctivitis. *Am J Ophthalmol.* 2003;135(4):447–451. doi:10.1016/s0002-9394(02)02094-9
15. Bhattacharya S. The facts about penicillin allergy: a review. *J Adv Pharm Technol Res.* 2010;1(1):11–17.
16. Lobanovska M, Pilla G. Penicillin's discovery and antibiotic resistance: lessons for the future? *Yale J Biol Med.* 2017;90(1):135–145. Published 2017 Mar 29.
17. Lebrun-Vignes B, Kreft-Jais C, Castot A, Chosidow O; French Network of Regional Centers of Pharmacovigilance. Comparative analysis of adverse drug reactions to tetracyclines: results of a French national survey and review of the literature. *Br J Dermatol.* 2012;166(6):1333–1341. doi:10.1111/j.1365-2133.2012.10845.x
18. Garner SE, Eady A, Bennett C, Newton JN, Thomas K, Popescu CM. Minocycline for acne vulgaris: efficacy and safety. *Cochrane Database Syst Rev.* 2012;2012(8):CD002086. Published 2012 Aug 15. doi:10.1002/14651858.CD002086.pub2
19. De Benedetti G, Vaiano AS. Oral azithromycin and oral doxycycline for the treatment of Meibomian gland dysfunction: a 9-month comparative case series. *Indian J Ophthalmol.* 2019;67(4):464–471. doi:10.4103/ijo.IJO_1244_17
20. Shah TJ, Moshirfar M, Hoopes PC Sr. "Doctor, i have a sulfa allergy": clarifying the myths of cross-reactivity. *Ophthalmol Ther.* 2018;7(2):211–215. doi:10.1007/s40123-018-0136-8
21. Krantz MS, Stone CA Jr, Abreo A, Phillips EJ. Oral challenge with trimethoprim-sulfamethoxazole in patients with "sulfa" antibiotic allergy. *J Allergy Clin Immunol Pract.* 2020;8(2):757–760.e4. doi:10.1016/j.jaip.2019.07.003
22. Stroman DW, Mintun K, Epstein AB, et al. Reduction in bacterial load using hypochlorous acid hygiene solution on ocular skin. *Clin Ophthalmol.* 2017;11:707–714. Published 2017 Apr 13. doi:10.2147/OPTH.S132851
23. FlorCruz NV, Evans JR. Medical interventions for fungal keratitis. *Cochrane Database Syst Rev.* 2015;(4):CD004241. Published 2015 Apr 9. doi:10.1002/14651858.CD004241.pub4
24. Rowe AM, St Leger AJ, Jeon S, Dhaliwal DK, Knickelbein JE, Hendricks RL. Herpes keratitis. *Prog Retin Eye Res.* 2013;32:88–101. doi:10.1016/j.preteyeres.2012.08.002

25. Fan S, Stojanovic D, Malvankar-Mehta MS, Hutnik C. Treatment of herpes zoster ophthalmicus: a systematic review and Canadian cost-comparison. *Can J Ophthalmol.* 2018;53(2):117–123. doi:10.1016/j.jcjo.2017.08.005
26. Schuster AK, Harder BC, Schlichtenbrede FC, Jarczok MN, Tesarz J. Valacyclovir versus acyclovir for the treatment of herpes zoster ophthalmicus in immunocompetent patients. *Cochrane Database Syst Rev.* 2016;11(11):CD011503. Published 2016 Nov 14. doi:10.1002/14651858.CD011503.pub2
27. White M, Chodosh J. Herpes simplex virus keratitis; June 2014, https://www.aao.org/clinical-statement/herpes-simplex-virus-keratitis-treatment-guideline, Reviewed and endorsed by the Ocular Microbiology and Immunology Group.
28. PubChem [Internet]. *PubChem Compound Summary for CID 3324, Famciclovir.* Bethesda: National Library of Medicine (US), National Center for Biotechnology Information; 2004; [cited 2021 June 9]. Available from: https://pubchem.ncbi.nlm.nih.gov/compound/Famciclovir
29. Karabela Y, Yardimci G, Yildirim I, Atalay E, Karabela SN. Treatment of phthiriasis palpebrarum and crab louse: petrolatum jelly and 1% permethrin shampoo. *Case Rep Med.* 2015;2015:287906. doi:10.1155/2015/287906
30. Sheppard JD, Comstock TL, Cavet ME. Impact of the topical ophthalmic corticosteroid loteprednol etabonate on intraocular pressure. *Adv Ther.* 2016;33(4):532–552. doi:10.1007/s12325-016-0315-8
31. Razeghinejad MR, Katz LJ. Steroid-induced iatrogenic glaucoma. *Ophthalmic Res.* 2012;47(2):66–80. doi:10.1159/000328630
32. Pleyer U, Ursell PG, Rama P. Intraocular pressure effects of common topical steroids for post-cataract inflammation: are they all the same? *Ophthalmol Ther* 2013;2(2):55–72. doi:10.1007/s40123-013-0020-5
33. Stout A, Friedly J, Standaert CJ. Systemic absorption and side effects of locally injected glucocorticoids. *PMR.* 2019;11(4):409–419. doi:10.1002/pmrj.12042
34. Nazir, A., Masih, M. & Iqbal, M. Formulation, optimization, qualitative and quantitative analysis of new dosage form of corticosteroid. *Futur J Pharm Sci.* 2021;7:208.
35. Duan P, Liu Y, Li J. The comparative efficacy and safety of topical non-steroidal anti-inflammatory drugs for the treatment of anterior chamber inflammation after cataract surgery: a systematic review and network meta-analysis. *Graefes Arch Clin Exp Ophthalmol.* 2017;255(4):639–649. doi:10.1007/s00417-017-3599-8
36. Zhao X, Xia S, Wang E, Chen Y. Comparison of the efficacy and patients' tolerability of Nepafenac and Ketorolac in the treatment of ocular inflammation following cataract surgery: a meta-analysis of randomized controlled trials. *PLoS One.* 2017;12(3):e0173254. Published 2017 Mar 2. doi:10.1371/journal.pone.0173254
37. Sahu S, Ram J, Bansal R, Pandav SS, Gupta A. Effect of topical ketorolac 0.4%, nepafenac 0.1%, and bromfenac 0.09% on postoperative inflammation using laser flare photometry in patients having phacoemulsification. *J Cataract Refract Surg.* 2015;41(10):2043–2048. doi:10.1016/j.jcrs.2015.10.061
38. Walters T, Raizman M, Ernest P, Gayton J, Lehmann R. In vivo pharmacokinetics and in vitro pharmacodynamics of nepafenac, amfenac, ketorolac, and bromfenac. *J Cataract Refract Surg.* 2007;33(9):1539–1545. doi:10.1016/j.jcrs.2007.05.015
39. Jones BM, Neville MW. Nepafenac: an ophthalmic nonsteroidal antiinflammatory drug for pain after cataract surgery. *Ann Pharmacother.* 2013;47(6):892–896. doi:10.1345/aph.1R757
40. Moore PA, Hersh EV. Combining ibuprofen and acetaminophen for acute pain management after third-molar extractions: translating clinical research to dental practice. *J Am Dent Assoc.* 2013;144(8):898–908. doi:10.14219/jada.archive.2013.0207
41. Ngo VTH, Bajaj T. Ibuprofen. In: *StatPearls.* Treasure Island: StatPearls Publishing; May 31, 2021.
42. Alfaro RA, Davis DD. Diclofenac. In: *StatPearls.* Treasure Island: StatPearls Publishing; June 3, 2021.
43. Meek IL, Van de Laar MA, Vonkeman EH. Non-steroidal anti-inflammatory drugs: an overview of cardiovascular risks. *Pharmaceuticals.* 2010;3(7):2146–2162. Published 2010 Jul 7. doi:10.3390/ph3072146
44. Pelletier JP, Martel-Pelletier J, Rannou F, Cooper C. Efficacy and safety of oral NSAIDs and analgesics in the management of osteoarthritis: evidence from real-life setting trials and surveys. *Semin Arthritis Rheum.* 2016;45(4 Suppl):S22–S27. doi:10.1016/j.semarthrit.2015.11.009
45. Nissen SE, Yeomans ND, Solomon DH, et al. Cardiovascular safety of celecoxib, naproxen, or ibuprofen for arthritis. *N Engl J Med.* 2016;375(26):2519–2529. doi:10.1056/NEJMoa1611593
46. Tai FWD, McAlindon ME. Non-steroidal anti-inflammatory drugs and the gastrointestinal tract. *Clin Med.* 2021;21(2):131–134. doi:10.7861/clinmed.2021-0039
47. Bindu S, Mazumder S, Bandyopadhyay U. Non-steroidal anti-inflammatory drugs (NSAIDs) and organ damage: a current perspective. *Biochem Pharmacol.* 2020;180:114147. doi:10.1016/j.bcp.2020.114147
48. Conaghan PG. A turbulent decade for NSAIDs: update on current concepts of classification, epidemiology, comparative efficacy, and toxicity. *Rheumatol Int.* 2012;32(6):1491–1502. doi:10.1007/s00296-011-2263-6
49. Ackerman S, Smith LM, Gomes PJ. Ocular itch associated with allergic conjunctivitis: latest evidence and clinical management. *Ther Adv Chronic Dis.* 2016;7(1):52–67. doi:10.1177/2040622315612745
50. de Paiva CS, Pflugfelder SC, Ng SM, Akpek EK. Topical cyclosporine A therapy for dry eye syndrome. *Cochrane Database Syst Rev.* 2019;9(9):CD010051. Published 2019 Sep 13. doi:10.1002/14651858.CD010051.pub2
51. Leonardi A, Messmer EM, Labetoulle M, et al. Efficacy and safety of 0.1% ciclosporin A cationic emulsion in dry eye disease: a pooled analysis of two double-masked, randomised, vehicle-controlled phase III clinical studies. *Br J Ophthalmol.* 2019;103(1):125–131. doi:10.1136/bjophthalmol-2017-311801
52. Willen CM, McGwin G, Liu B, Owsley C, Rosenstiel C. Efficacy of cyclosporine 0.05% ophthalmic emulsion in contact lens wearers with dry eyes. *Eye Contact Lens.* 2008;34(1):43–45. doi:10.1097/ICL.0b013e3180676d44
53. Tuan HI, Chi SC, Kang YN. An updated systematic review with meta-analysis of randomized trials on topical cyclosporin A for dry-eye disease. *Drug Des Devel Ther.* 2020;14:265–274. Published 2020 Jan 17. doi:10.2147/DDDT.S207743
54. Deveney T, Asbell PA. Patient and physician perspectives on the use of cyclosporine ophthalmic emulsion 0.05% for the management of chronic dry eye. *Clin Ophthalmol.* 2018;12:569–576. Published 2018 Mar 23. doi:10.2147/OPTH.S115098
55. Haber SL, Benson V, Buckway CJ, Gonzales JM, Romanet D, Scholes B. Lifitegrast: a novel drug for patients with dry eye disease. *Ther Adv Ophthalmol.* 2019;11:2515841419870366. Published 2019 Aug 22. doi:10.1177/2515841419870366
56. Keating GM. Lifitegrast ophthalmic solution 5%: a review in dry eye disease. *Drugs.* 2017;77(2):201–208. doi:10.1007/s40265-016-0681-1
57. Kam KW, Chen LJ, Wat N, Young AL. Topical olopatadine in the treatment of allergic conjunctivitis: a systematic review and meta-analysis. *Ocul Immunol Inflamm.* 2017;25(5):663–677. doi:10.3109/09273948.2016.1158282
58. Abelson MB. A review of olopatadine for the treatment of ocular allergy. *Expert Opin Pharmacother.* 2004;5(9):1979–1994. doi:10.1517/14656566.5.9.1979
59. Abelson MB, McLaughlin JT, Gomes PJ. Antihistamines in ocular allergy: are they all created equal? *Curr Allergy Asthma Rep.* 2011;11(3):205–211. doi:10.1007/s11882-011-0188-5
60. Ben-Eli H, Solomon A. Topical antihistamines, mast cell stabilizers, and dual-action agents in ocular allergy: current trends. *Curr Opin Allergy Clin Immunol.* 2018;18(5):411–416. doi:10.1097/ACI.0000000000000473
61. Dudeja L, Janakiraman A, Dudeja I, Sane K, Babu M. Observer-masked trial comparing efficacy of topical olopatadine (0.1%), bepotastine (1.5%), and alcaftadine (0.25%) in mild to moderate allergic conjunctivitis. *Indian J Ophthalmol.* 2019;67(9):1400–1404. doi:10.4103/ijo.IJO_2112_18

62. Kumar M, Chawla R, Goyal M. Topical anesthesia. *J Anaesthesiol Clin Pharmacol.* 2015;31(4):450–456. doi:10.4103/0970-9185.169049
63. Aksoy A, Başkan AM, Aslan L, Aslankurt M. Topical proparacaine abuse resulting in evisceration. *BMJ Case Rep.* 2013;2013:bcr2013009539. Published 2013 Apr 22. doi:10.1136/bcr-2013-009539
64. Wang L, Shankarappa SA, Tong R, et al. Topical drug formulations for prolonged corneal anesthesia. *Cornea.* 2013;32(7):1040–1045. doi:10.1097/ICO.0b013e31828cbfe6
65. Gaynes BI, Barkin RL. Analgesics in ophthalmic practice: a review of the oral non-narcotic agent tramadol. *Optom Vis Sci.* 1999;76(7):455–461. doi:10.1097/00006324-199907000-00020
66. Lewis KS, Han NH. Tramadol: a new centrally acting analgesic. *Am J Health Syst Pharm.* 1997;54(6):643–652. doi:10.1093/ajhp/54.6.643
67. Gabay M. The federal controlled substances act: schedules and pharmacy registration. *Hosp Pharm.* 2013;48(6):473–474. doi:10.1310/hpj4806-473
68. McLaurin E, Cavet ME, Gomes PJ, Ciolino JB. Brimonidine ophthalmic solution 0.025% for reduction of ocular redness: a randomized clinical trial. *Optom Vis Sci.* 2018;95(3):264–271. doi:10.1097/OPX.0000000000001182
69. Hosten LO, Snyder C. Over-the-counter ocular decongestants in the United States: mechanisms of action and clinical utility for management of ocular redness. *Clin Optom.* 2020;12:95–105. Published 2020 Jul 23. doi:10.2147/OPTO.S259398
70. Code of Federal Regulations Title 21, Food and drugs chapter I: food and drug administration department of health and human services subchapter D: drugs for human use, Part 349, ophthalmic drug products for over-the-counter human use. April 1, 2020.
71. Pucker AD, Ng SM, Nichols JJ. Over the counter (OTC) artificial tear drops for dry eye syndrome. *Cochrane Database Syst Rev.* 2016;2:CD009729. Published 2016 Feb 23. doi:10.1002/14651858.CD009729.pub2
72. Kathuria A, Shamloo K, Jhanji V, Sharma A. Categorization of marketed artificial tear formulations based on their ingredients: a rational approach for their use. *J Clin Med.* 2021;10(6):1289. Published 2021 Mar 21. doi:10.3390/jcm10061289
73. Feizi S. Corneal endothelial cell dysfunction: etiologies and management. *Ther Adv Ophthalmol.* 2018;10:2515841418815802. Published 2018 Dec 7. doi:10.1177/2515841418815802
74. Slonim CB, Foster S, Jaros M, et al. Association of oxymetazoline hydrochloride, 0.1%, solution administration with visual field in acquired ptosis: a pooled analysis of 2 randomized clinical trials. *JAMA Ophthalmol.* 2020;138(11):1168–1175. doi:10.1001/jamaophthalmol.2020.3812
75. Deeks ED, Lamb YN. Cenegermin: a review in neurotrophic keratitis. *Drugs.* 2020;80(5):489–494. doi:10.1007/s40265-020-01289-w
76. Sheha H, Tighe S, Hashem O, Hayashida Y. Update on cenegermin eye drops in the treatment of neurotrophic keratitis. *Clin Ophthalmol.* 2019;13:1973–1980. Published 2019 Oct 7. doi:10.2147/OPTH.S185184
77. Oyster Point Pharma Inc. *Tyrvaya (Varenicline) Solution, Prescribing Information.* Princeton; October 2021.
78. Abbvie Inc. *VUITYTM (Pilocarpine Hydrochloride Ophthalmic Solution) 1.25% [Prescribing Information].* Chicago, IL; October 2021.
79. Ing EB, Philteos J, Sholohov G, Ta Kim D, Nijhawan N, Mark PW, Gilbert J. Local anesthesia and anxiolytic techniques for oculoplastic surgery. *Clin Ophthalmol.* 2019;13:153–160.
80. Ben Simon GJ, Huang L, Nakra T, Schwarcz RM, McCann JD, Goldberg RA. Intralesional triamcinolone acetonide injection for primary and recurrent chalazia: is it really effective? *Ophthalmology.* 2005;112(5):913–917. doi:10.1016/j.ophtha.2004.11.037
81. Sicherer SH, Simons FER, Section on allergy and immunology. Epinephrine for first-aid management of anaphylaxis. *Pediatrics.* 2017;139(3):e20164006. doi:10.1542/peds.2016-4006
82. Wan MJ, AlShaker S, Hunter DG. Use of botulinum toxin in ophthalmology published correction appears in *Handb Exp Pharmacol.* 2021;263:283. *Handb Exp Pharmacol.* 2021;263:147–160. doi:10.1007/164_2019_325
83. Daphna O, Mimouni M, Keshet Y, et al. Therapeutic HL-contact lens versus standard bandage contact lens for corneal edema: a prospective, multicenter, randomized, crossover study. *J Ophthalmol.* 2020;2020:8410920. Published 2020 Sep 21. doi:10.1155/2020/8410920
84. Miller DD, Hasan SA, Simmons NL, Stewart MW. Recurrent corneal erosion: a comprehensive review. *Clin Ophthalmol.* 2019;13:325–335. Published 2019 Feb 11. doi:10.2147/OPTH.S157430
85. McDonnell C, Murphy O, Cochrane A, Martin E, Wolffsohn J, Maldonado-Codina C, Vianya-Estopa M, Gibson E, Dunning D, Oehring D, Nagra M, Huntjens B. Lissamine green: where have we been and where are we now? *Optomet Pract.* 2020;21(2). ISSN 1467-9051.
86. Walkden A. Amniotic membrane transplantation in ophthalmology: an updated perspective. *Clin Ophthalmol.* 2020;14:2057–2072. Published 2020 Jul 22. doi:10.2147/OPTH.S208008
87. Ryff K, Ryff B, Lighthizer N. Insert and remove an amniotic membrane graft. *Rev Optomet.* February, 2015;152:60–71. www.reviewofoptometry.com/article/how-to-insert-and-remove-an-amniotic-membrane-graft.
88. Holtz KK, Townsend KR, Furst JW, et al. An assessment of the adenoplus point-of-care test for diagnosing adenoviral conjunctivitis and its effect on antibiotic stewardship. *Mayo Clin Proc Innov Qual Outcomes.* 2017;1(2):170–175. Published 2017 Jul 25. doi:10.1016/j.mayocpiqo.2017.06.001

Chapter 2
CLINICAL CONSIDERATIONS ON ANTERIOR SEGMENT PATHOLOGY AND IMMUNOLOGY

Chapter Outline

DOI: 10.1201/9781003255598-2

We should try to make things as simple as possible, but not simpler.

—**Albert Einstein**

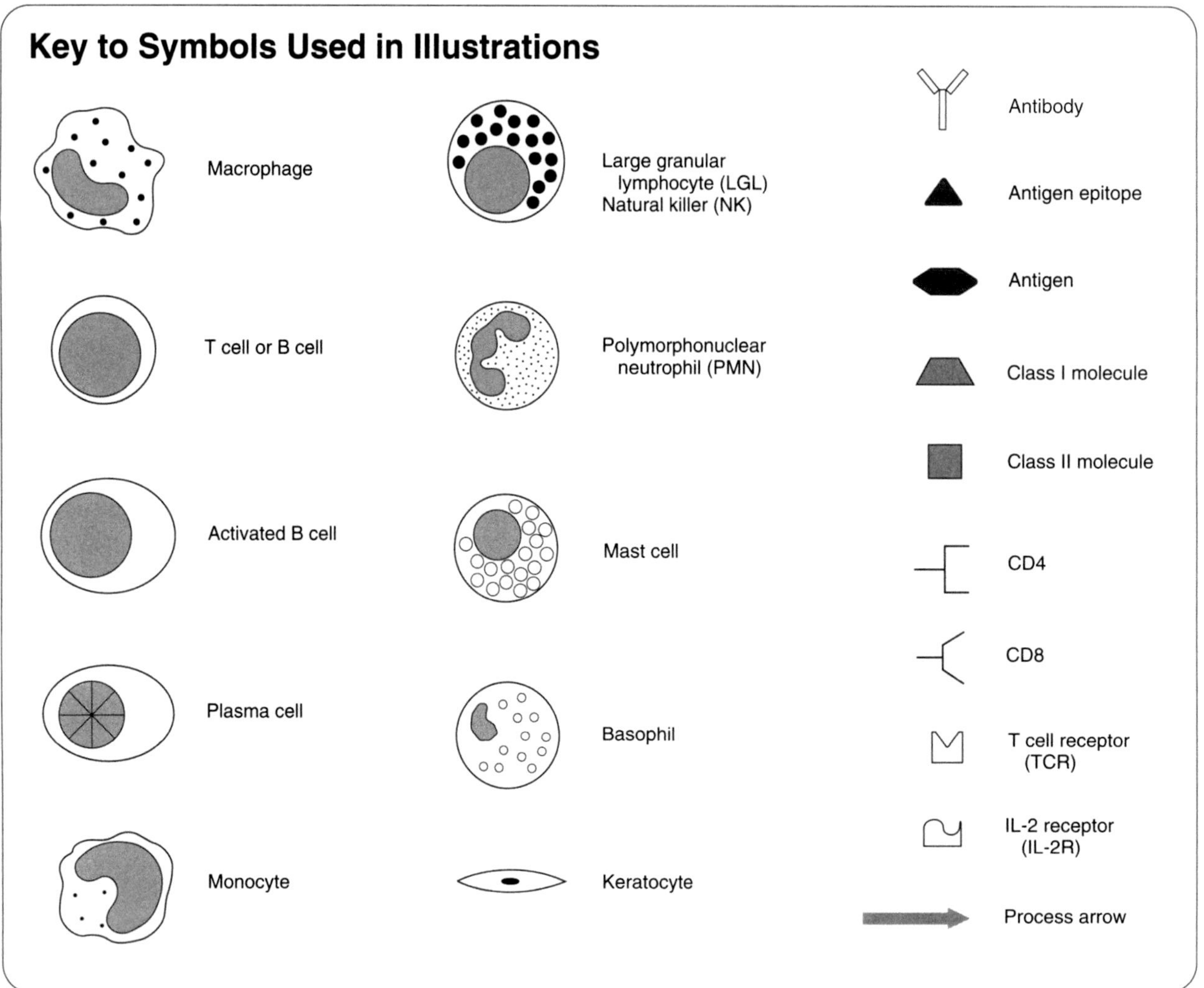

I. Current Concepts, Terminology, and Abbreviations

A. Definitions

1. The *anterior segment* of the eye may be considered the eyelids and adnexa, and the front (anterior) one-third of the globe (eyeball)
   a. Eyelids and adnexa (orbit and lacrimal system)
   b. Conjunctiva
   c. Anterior sclera and episclera
   d. Cornea
   e. Anterior chamber angle structures
   f. Anterior chamber and aqueous humor
   g. Ciliary body
   h. Iris
   i. Crystalline lens
2. *Pathology* is the study of abnormal structures, tissues, or functions that may produce disease
   a. Clinicopathology: abnormal structures
   b. Histopathology: abnormal tissues
   c. Pathophysiology: abnormal function
   d. Immunopathology: abnormal function involving the immune system
3. *Pathological processes* are those specific abnormal activities of or to the body that can cause disease. These include, but may not be limited to (in alphabetical order):
   a. Allergy/hypersensitivity: immunopathophysiological response to environmental antigens
   b. Congenital/developmental abnormalities: multiple pathological etiologies from birth
   c. Degeneration: clinicopathological deterioration of tissue or function
   d. Dystrophy: multiple pathological etiologies from biological deficiencies
   e. Environmental: external elements and conditions that can produce a disease state
   f. Infection: histopathology from invading, multiplying, and toxin-producing microorganisms
   g. Inflammation: the fundamental immunopathophysiological process

h. Injury: clinicopathology inflicted by an external force
   i. Abrasions: superficial cutting or scraping
   ii. Burns
      - Chemical
      - Radiation (e.g., ultraviolet)
      - Thermal (heat)
   iii. Contusion or concussion (blunt)
   iv. Foreign bodies
      - Superficial
      - Embedded
   v. Laceration
      - Penetration: into tissue layer
      - Perforation: through tissue layer
i. Metabolic: pathophysiology of physical and chemical processes of the body
j. Metaplasia: histopathology from changes in cell and tissue type
   i. Hyperplasia: increased number of cells
   ii. Hypertrophy: increased size of cells, tissue, or organ
   iii. Hypoplasia: incomplete development of tissue or organ
k. Neoplasia: histopathology from abnormal, progressive, uncontrolled multiplication of cells (cancer)
   i. Primary
   ii. Metastatic (secondary)
l. Neurological: multiple pathological etiologies involving the nervous system
m. Nutritional: pathophysiological changes associated with food intake, assimilation, and utilization
n. Systemic manifestations: multiple etiologies caused by interrelating pathologies between bodily tissues, organs, or systems

4. *Immunology* is the study of the highly complex biological system that defends the human body ("self") against foreign substances, stress, and/or stimuli ("non-self")
   a. Occasionally, this imperfectly understood system functions in such a way as to produce organ or tissue dysfunction and pathology
   b. Categories of immunology include (but may not be limited to):
      i. Allergy/hypersensitivity: a type of pathological reaction of the immune response
      ii. Clinical immunology
         - Observable positive and negative effects of the immune system
         - Inflammation is the fundamental process in clinical immunology
      iii. Immunochemistry
      iv. Cellular immunology
      v. Immunopathology
      vi. Immunopharmacology
      vii. Tumor immunology
      viii. Transplantation immunology
      ix. Molecular immunology (and molecular biology)
      x. Immunogenetics and immunogenomics

B. Defense Mechanisms of the Anterior Segment

1. *Prevention* of negative stimulation (toxic, mechanical, physiological), more than any defense system, is the foremost means of protecting and defending our bodies and the anterior segment of our eyes
2. Normal anatomy and physiology serve as the primary defense systems
   a. Bony orbit and orbital rims protect against injury
   b. Skin of the eyelids prevents penetration of toxins and infectious agents
   c. Eyebrows and eyelashes protect against particulate invasion
   d. Blinking function serves multiple protective functions:
      i. Protects against rapid attack or invasion of the ocular surface (the "menace reflex")
      ii. Cleans and swabs the ocular surface
      iii. Spreads tears evenly over the ocular surface (Marangoni effect)
      iv. Closes to protect mucocutaneous ocular surface tissue from drying
      v. Lacrimal tear film serves multiple protective functions:
         - Antibacterial
         - Lubrication to ocular surface
         - Nutrition to ocular surface
         - Dilutes and flushes toxins from ocular surface
         - Serves as medium for superficial ocular surface immune activity
      vi. Corneal epithelium with tight cell junctures protects against penetration into the corneal stroma by most bacteria
      vii. Bowman's layer of the corneal stroma resists many stimuli (mechanical, physiological, toxic) from penetrating into and disrupting the stromal matrix
3. Immune system
   a. A regulated defense system protecting the body ("self") against antigens ("immunogens"), or foreign ("non-self") substances or stressors
   b. Natural or innate immunity
      i. Genetic, anatomic, or physiological defenses
      ii. Provides immediate defenses against antigens
      iii. Primitive functioning cells
         - Natural killer (NK) cells
         - Neutrophils
         - Macrophages
      iv. System can be enhanced by acquired immunity
      v. Clinical response time: within minutes
   c. Acquired immunity
      i. The most clinically relevant system functioning through its fundamental process of inflammation
         - Depends on the body's vascular system
         - Uses specialized functions of white blood cells
         - Humoral and cellular systems
            – Humoral relates to the system that works through the fluids (blood and serum) and the chemicals and molecules (mediators, cytokines, and proteins) they carry
            – Cellular relates to the series of vascular and avascular cells active in the immune response: vascular cells-basophils (polymorphonuclear neutrophil: PMNs), eosinophils (PMNs), lymphocytes, monocytes, natural killer cells,

neutrophils (PMNs), and platelets; and avascular cells—lymphocytes, macrophages, mast cells, and natural killer cells

ii. Attempts to develop an effective response to an antigen occur in three ways:
   - The *afferent arc*, where immunocompetent cells recognize the antigen and become sensitized to it
   - *Central processing*, where the cells differentiate and produce the evolution of new sensitized cells and specific antibodies
   - The *efferent arc*, where these new sensitized cells and antibodies attack and neutralize the antigen

iii. Acquired response has two clinical patterns
   - Positive memory (anamnestic), where memory cells from a first antigen encounter rapidly enhance a response on subsequent encounters with the same antigen
     - Reaction will generally increase with subsequent exposure to the antigen
     - Booster injections of vaccines can maintain this increased response level
   - Negative memory (immunologic intolerance) is believed to be produced by low-level antigen dosages that trigger a special type of immunocompetent (T) cells or immune complexes that suppress reactions
     - Vaccination by weak (attenuated) dead or genetically engineered organisms
     - Vaccination by mRNA
     - Desensitization therapy
     - Clinical problems and challenges arise with rapidly mutating (changing) organisms such as the human immune deficiency virus (which attacks T_h cells)

d. Functional components of the acquired immune response:

i. Specific cellular elements, protein molecules, enzymes, and chemical mediators must interact "cooperatively" for the immune system to function properly

ii. The foundation of this cooperative interaction is the unique "specificity" of surface receptor configurations (disulfide-linked heterodimers) on each specialized white blood cell (WBC) involved that allow it to react with only one specific antigen

iii. Among the trillions of specialized WBCs with specific surface receptor configurations, only a very small fraction ("clones") created genetically by somatic mutation or by gene splicing can react with a specific antigen

e. Key clinical components of the immune system (a limited alphabetical list):

i. *Allergen*: a large protein antigen that produces a hypersensitivity (Type I), immediate, humoral, or anaphylactic reaction

ii. *Antibody*: protein molecules synthesized by plasma cells derived from B lymphocytes and having specific configurations for combining with antigen to form antigen–antibody or immune complexes

iii. *Antigen*: any substance (or stressor), usually a protein (never lipid) of a foreign nature ("nonself") to the body ("self") that can combine with an antibody to produce an immune response. The greater the antigen's complexity (greater molecular weight) the more antigenic it becomes

iv. *Antigen-antibody complex*: see "Antibody" (ii, above) and "Immune Complex" (later in the chapter)

v. *Autoantigen*: the body's ("self") own proteins (tissues or cells) or dynamic (physiological or mechanical) factors (stressors), which abnormally produce an antigenic (or autoimmune) effect

vi. *Autoimmunity*: a poorly understood phenomenon of an immune response to self (autoantigen) caused by a bodily substance or stress factor, or a dysregulation of the immune system

vii. *Cells*
   - *Antigen-presenting cells (APCs)*: cell types (sometimes called accessory or dendritic cells) that provide appropriate receptors and mediators to process antigen and communicate with B cell antibodies and T cells for antigen binding and lymphocyte response
   - *B cells (B lymphocytes)*: multifunctioning cells derived from bone marrow that can synthesize antibodies or serve as an APC functioning "dependent" or "independent" of T cells.
     - *T-dependent B cells* serve as APCs to activate T cells that secrete mediators (lymphokines) that together with the antigen, trigger the B cell to develop into an antibody-secreting cell (plasma cell) first to make immunoglobin M (IgM), and later ("positive memory") IgG, IgA, or IgE.
     - *T-independent B cells* are triggered by weak antigens (T-independent antigens, e.g., polysaccharides) without T cell help to provoke IgM antibody production with little memory
   - *Basophils*: small circulating polymorphonuclear (PMN) cells (about 1% of total PMNs) arising in bone marrow from stem cells and releasing mediators (histamine and small quantities of arachidonic acid) in response to prostaglandin D2. Usually associated with the early phase (onset within 4 to 6 hours and peaking at 10 to 24 hours) of the IgE-mediated or immediate (Type I) hypersensitivity response
   - *Dendritic cells*: non-lymphocyte antigen-presenting cells (APCs)
   - *Eosinophils*: large, non-phagocytizing, polymorphonuclear (PMN) cells activated by components of complement and releasing major basic protein (MBP), peroxidase, and proteolytic enzymes that attack microorganisms
   - *Granulocytes*: see "Polymorphonuclear Cell" below

- *Histiocytes*: resident macrophages in the spleen, lymph nodes, lung (Kupffer's cells), skin (Langerhans cells), thymus, peritoneum, nervous system, and other tissues (e.g., conjunctiva and peripheral cornea)
- Immunocompetent cells: specialized white blood cells (WBCs) that participate in the immune response
- *Langerhans cells*: non-lymphocyte antigen-presenting cells (APCs) found in skin, vascular endothelium, and conjunctival, limbal, and corneal epithelium
- *Leukocytes*: white blood cells (WBCs)
- *Lymphocytes*: unique leukocytes associated with immunologic specificity-dependent antigen receptors
- *Macrophages*: nonlymphocytic, principle antigen-presenting cells (APCs) of the mononuclear phagocyte system, residing in connective tissue and around small blood vessels (as "adherent cells") and critical in the humoral and cellular response. Four essential functions include:
  - Antigen presentation for T cell proliferation
  - Principal control by immune response gene
  - Receptors to augment phagocytosis
  - Secretion of a wide range of active molecules for afferent arc of immune response
- *Mast cells*: large, abundant cells found in many tissues of the body (*excluding* the cornea, iris, retina, and optic nerve) with a granulated surface bound with IgE and several intracellular preformed mediators (e.g., histamine, serotonin, heparin, and chemotactic factors for eosinophils, neutrophils, and lymphocytes) whose release is responsible for the IgE, immediate (Type I) anaphylactic response. Mediators' modulation of polymorphonuclear (PMN) cell activity provides inflammatory stimulus within seconds of the early phase of anaphylaxis, also during its late phase (up to 24 hours), and possibly as a "gatekeeper" to the cell-mediated immune (CMI or type IV in old terminology), delayed inflammatory response
- *Monocytes*: circulating, nonlymphocytic, antigen-presenting cells (APCs) of the mononuclear phagocyte system, a portion of which exit the blood to develop into histiocytes (resident macrophages) in the spleen, lymph nodes, lung (Kupffer's cells), skin (Langerhans cells), thymus, peritoneum, nervous system, and other tissues
- *Mononuclear cells*: two subtypes of phagocytic, antigen-presenting cells (APCs) including monocytes and macrophages, and constituting the mononuclear phagocyte system
- *Natural killer (NK) cells*: primitive, nonphagocytic, cytotoxic cells of the natural (innate) immune system, requiring no antibodies or major histocompatibility complex (MHC) products to act against antigens. Secrete cytokines are activated by interleukin 2 (IL-2) and interferon. Capable of killing tumor cells and highly effective against viruses, they can also function as mediator cells in antibody-dependent cellular cytotoxicity (ADCC), activated by specific IgG antibody
- *Neutrophils*: most numerous type of phagocytic polymorphonuclear (PMN) leukocyte in the blood, existing briefly between formation in bone marrow to phagocytic and microbicidal activity. Primary cellular element in acute inflammation (especially early stage)
- *Phagocytes*: any cells that engulf (phagocytosis) and ingest (pinocytosis) foreign matter
- *Plasma cells*: mature B cells responsible for production of large quantities of immunoglobins
- *Platelets*: smallest circulating cells, which aggregate intravascularly and generate preformed inflammatory mediators
- *Polymorphonuclear (PMN) cells*: three subtypes of cells (also called granulocytes) including neutrophils, basophils, and eosinophils
- *Stem cells*: undifferentiated cells with the ability to self-replicate and differentiate into all forms of circulating cells
- *T cells (T lymphocytes)*: principal regulatory lymphocytic cells of the adaptive immune system, derived from thymus and having four subsets:
  - T-helper (T_h) cells activate other effector cells (T and B) in the immune response by binding to the antigen complex on the antigen-presenting cell (APC) and producing mediators and differentiation factors (see cytokines). In cell-mediated immunity (CMI) or delayed-type hypersensitivity (DTH) inflammation where the individual has been sensitized, the T_h cell is labeled the T_{dh} cell
  - T-cytotoxic (T_c) or T-killer cells (triggered by T_h cells) "kill" the antigen by the release of cytotoxins
  - T-suppressor or regulatory (T_s or T_{reg}) cells suppress the activity of T_h and B cells (origin is poorly understood and under intensive research)
  - Memory T cells capable of rapid self-renewal on re-exposure to an antigen years, even decades after primary stimulation

viii. *Cell-mediated immunity (CMI)*: see Section II., "Inflammation"

ix. *Chemotactic factors and mediators*: chemicals or "cytokines" released by lymphocytes (lymphokines) and monocytes or macrophages (monokines) that modulate other inflammatory cells to amplify the effects of phagocytes, or that directly affect the target cells. These chemicals include (listing is partial):

- Arachidonic acid
- B cell-activating factor (BAF)
- B cell differentiation factor (BCDF)
- B cell growth factor or interleukin-4 (IL-4 or BCGF)
- Bradykinin
- Colony-stimulating factor (CSF)
- Colony-stimulating factor of granulocytes and macrophages (CSF-GM)
- Cyclic adenosine monophosphate (cAMP)
- Cytotoxin
- Endothelial leukocytic adhesion molecule (ELAM)
- Eosinophil chemotactic factor (ECF)
- Eosinophil chemotactic factor of anaphylaxis (ECF-A)
- Growth-inhibitory factory (GIF)
- Heparin
- High-molecular-weight neutrophil chemotactic factor (HMW-NCF)
- Histamine
- Histamine-sensitizing factor (HSF)
- Homologous restriction factor (HRF)
- Interferon
- Interleukins 1 to 8 (IL-1 to 8)
- Intrinsic/initiating factor (IF)
- Leukocyte inhibitory factor (LIF)
- Leukocyte-activating factor or interleukin-1 (IL-1 or LAP)
- Leukotriene
- Lymphocyte-derived chemotactic factor (LDCF)
- Lymphotoxin
- Macrophage chemotactic factor (MCF)
- Macrophage-activating (arming) factor (MAF)
- Migration inhibitory factor (MIF)
- Mitogenic factor (MF)
- Neutrophil chemotactic factor (NCF)
- Peroxidase
- Phospholipids
- Platelet-activating factor (PAF)
- Prostaglandin
- Serotonin
- T cell-activating factor (TAF)
- T cell-growth factor or interleukin-2 (IL-2 or TCGF)
- Thromboxane
- Transfer factor (TF)
- Transforming growth factor (TGF)
- Tumor necrosis factor (TNF)

x. *Clotting system*: a plasma component in inflammation that produces fibrin and fibrinopeptides, which interact with the complement, fibrinolytic (plasmin), and kinin systems to promote clotting factor and vasodilation

xi. *Complement system*: a group of plasma and cell membrane proteins that can cause cell or bacterial lysis, envelop viruses, mediate opsonization, and generate peptides that regulate features of inflammation and immune response. These more than 25 proteins ("components") including Cl through C9, properdin, factors B, D, I, H operating through two major plasma pathways (classic complement and alternative complement pathway), help in inflammatory vasodilation, phagocyte exudation, migration, and direction, and ultimately in clearing infectious agents from the body

xii. *Cytokines*: see "Chemotactic factors and mediators" above

xiii. *Epitope*: part of an antigen that combines with a specific antibody or T cell

xiv. *Fibrinolytic (fibrin or plasmin) system*: a plasma component mediator forming system in inflammation that activates complement, helps generate bradykinin, and increases proteolytic activity through complex interactions with the complement, kinin, and clotting systems

xv. *Hapten*: a substance that is not immunogenic but can react with an antibody of appropriate specificity

xvi. *Human leukocytic antigen (HLA)*: see "Major histocompatibility complex (MHC)" later in this list

xvii. *Idiotype*: part of an antibody that binds with a specific antigen. B cells produce genetically cloned antibodies with unique profiles of idiotypic epitopes (idiotopes) that increase on immunogenic stimulation. This stimulation induces anti-idiotype and anti-anti-idiotype antibodies (called antibody-2 and antibody-3), which ultimately suppress continued stimulation by binding with compatible lymphocytes (T_s cells?) producing a regulatory closed-loop suppressor system in the lymphoid system. (Poor understanding of this area has produced extensive research efforts resulting in multiple Nobel Prizes)

xviii. *Immune complex*: antigen–antibody complex that can activate the complement system and deposit in various tissues, producing cutaneous arthus reactions, systemic serum sickness, or autoimmune responses

xix. *Immunogen*: any substance (or stress) that can stimulate an immune response independently or in combination with antibody

xx. *Immunoglobins*: glycoproteins produced from induced immune responses to function as antibodies making up the humoral arm of the immune system. Each molecule is specific for one antigen, but also possesses secondary biological activities such as complement fixation of phagocytosis. Immunoglobins (lg) are subdivided by antigenic determinants in the Fe region of the H (polypeptide) chain into five classes:

- *Immunoglobin G (IgG)*: 75% of total serum immunoglobin, with four subclasses (IgGl-4) that cross the placenta to protect newborns during first month of life, fix complement, and bind with macrophages (IgG1 and 3), "arming" them for cytotoxic function and phagocytosis of opsonized bacteria

- *Immunoglobin A (IgA)*: 15% of total immunoglobin and predominant mucosa, secretory immunoglobin (e.g., tears) for defense against local infection (bacteria, virus, etc.)
- *Immunoglobin M (IgM)*: 10% of total immunoglobin, prominent in early immune responses, expressed on B cell surfaces, and most efficient complement-fixing immunoglobin
- *Immunoglobin D (IgD)*: trace (0.2%) amounts in serum present on B cell surfaces during their development with poorly understood function (possibly B cell differentiation)
- *Immunoglobin E (IgE)*: only 0.004% of total serum immunoglobin, but very high affinity to bind with mast cells in combination with allergens to release preformed mediators involved in allergic disease

xxi. *Kinin system*: mediator-forming system in blood that generates a potent inflammatory factor, bradykinin, activated by four elements—Hageman factor, clotting factor XI, prekallikrein, and high-molecular-weight kininogen. System acts with the complement, clotting, and fibrin system to serve as a potent inflammatory activator

xxii. *Lymphoid system*: extravascular tissues throughout the body, including lymph nodes, spleen, bone marrow, thymus gland, and mucosal-associated lymphoid tissue (MALT), daily producing (in bone marrow) lymphocytes (immunocytes, about 10^{12} cells or 1% of total body weight) found most in the spleen, and circulating and recirculating in blood vessels and lymphatic channels from one lymphoid organ to another (Figure 2.1)

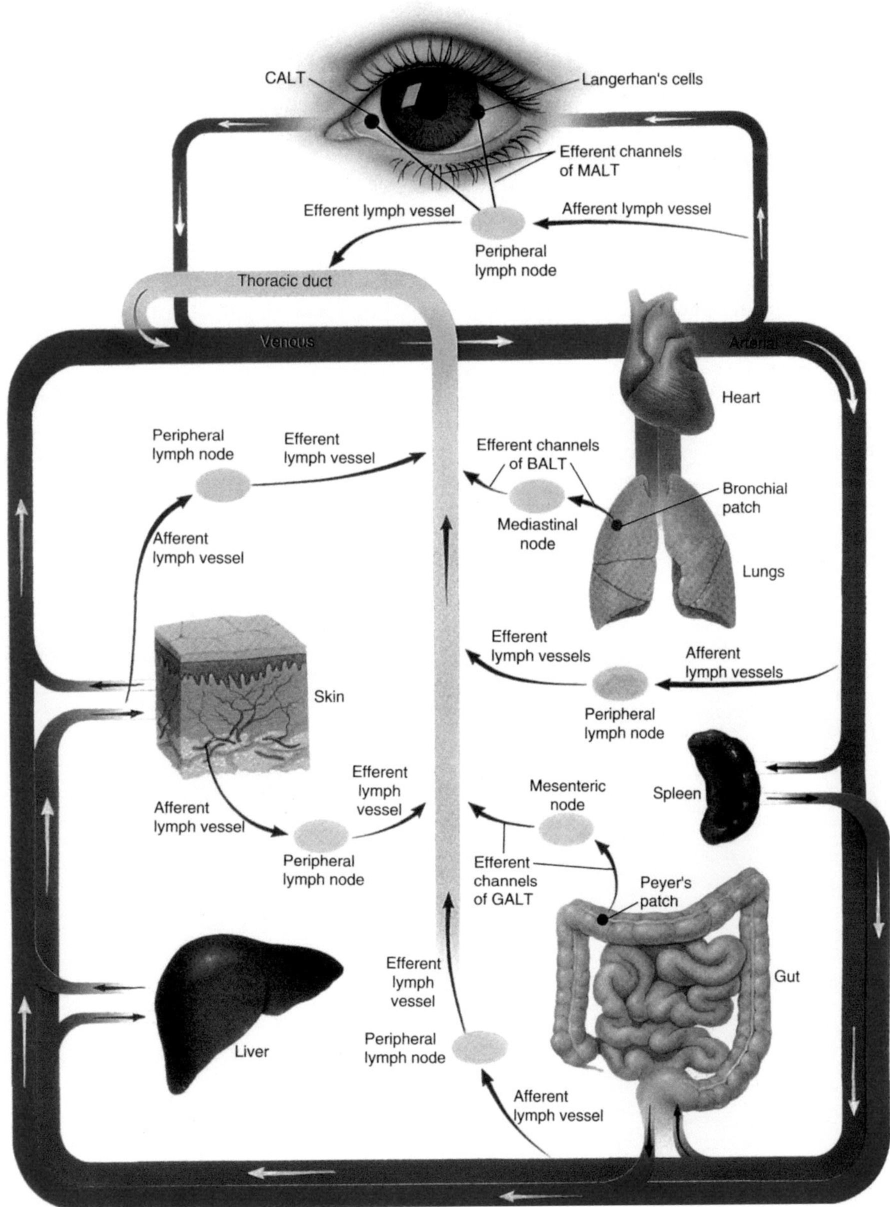

FIGURE 2.1 The lymphoid system includes lymph nodes, spleen, bone marrow, thymus gland, and mucosal-associated tissue (MALT). *Abbreviations*: GALT, gut-associated lymphoid tissue; CALT, conjunctival-associated lymphoid tissue; BALT, bronchial-associated lymphoid tissue.

xxiii. *Major histocompatibility complex (MHC)*: a complex of molecules present on cells of some individuals in a species (genetically predetermined) that serve as antigens (alloantigens) in a system human leukocytic antigen (HLA) system that recognizes "self" (syngeneic) from "non-self" (allogeneic) and, along with the complement system, processes and presents, on antigen-presenting complexes (APCs), antigens to T cells. There are three categories of HLA molecules:
- Class I molecules possess selective binding sites for antigen epitopes and function only in combination with CDS antigenic markers on cytotoxic T_c cells (called HLA restriction)
- Class II molecules, found on B cells, APCs, and activated T cells, possess selective binding sites for antigen epitopes and function in combination with CD4 antigenic markers on activated helper T_h cells
- Class III molecules possess C2, C4, and properdin factor B of the complement system and have no antigen-presenting properties.

xxiv. *Mononuclear phagocyte system*: circulating monocytes and tissue macrophages (previously termed the reticuloendothelial system)

xxv. *Opsonization*: coating of bacteria by antibody (opsonin) and sometimes called complement, which binds with macrophages to facilitate phagocytosis

xxvi. *Reticuloendothelial system*: see "Mononuclear phagocyte system" above

xxvii. *Stressor*: any environmental, emotional, psychological, physiological, or mechanical (physical) factor of a nonsubstance nature that may produce an immunogenic stimulus

C. The "Clinical Immune Matrix"

A key to the symbols used in the illustrations may be found at the beginning of this chapter.

1. Basic steps in the acquired immune response
2. Ten "not-so-easy" steps to understanding the immune system

Afferent Arc Stage

Step #1

Immunogen (antigen) enters the system (Figures 2.1 and 2.2)

a. Through bloodstream (to the spleen)
b. Through skin (to lymphatic channels and lymph nodes)
c. Through mucosal system (to lymphoid system) diffusely distributed as the mucosal-associated lymphoid tissue (MALT)
   i. Gut-associated lymphoid tissue (GALT)
      - Peyer's patches
   ii. Lymphoid follicles
   iii. Bronchial-associated lymphoid tissue (BALT)
   iv. Conjunctival-associated lymphoid tissue (CALT)
d. "Clinical clock" (clinical response time)—"zero point" of entry or contact

Step #2

APC captures immunogen by recognizing it as foreign and processing it in association with its class I HLA molecules and CD4 receptors (Figure 2.3)

a. APCs include
   i. Macrophages in avascular tissue
   ii. Dendritic cells in lymphoid tissue
   iii. Langerhans cells in skin (and CALT)
   iv. Kupffer's cells in liver
   v. Microglial cells in central nervous system
   vi. B cells may also act as antigen-specific APCs

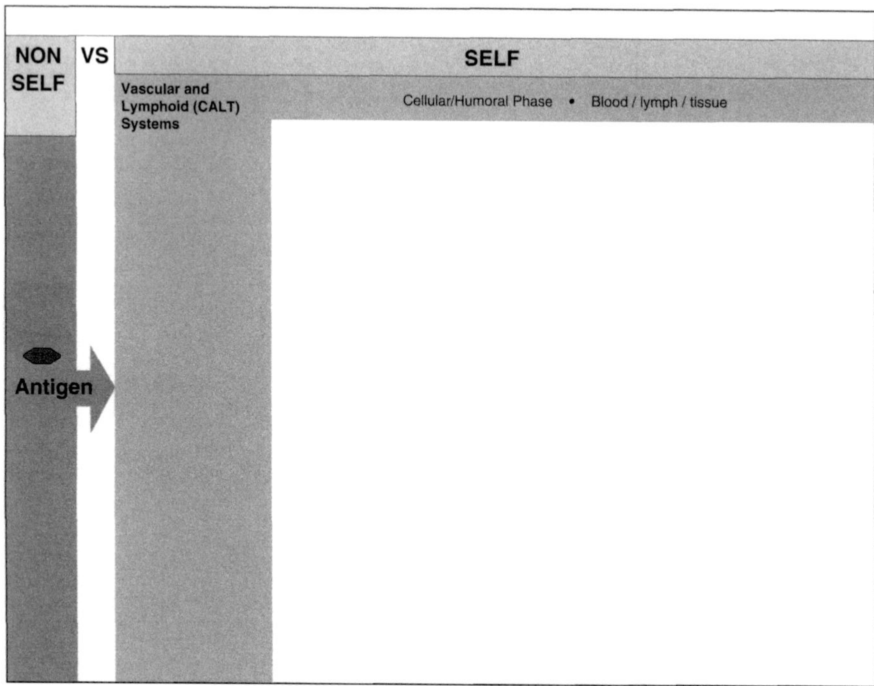

FIGURE 2.2 Immunogen enters the system. Step #1 of clinical immune matrix.

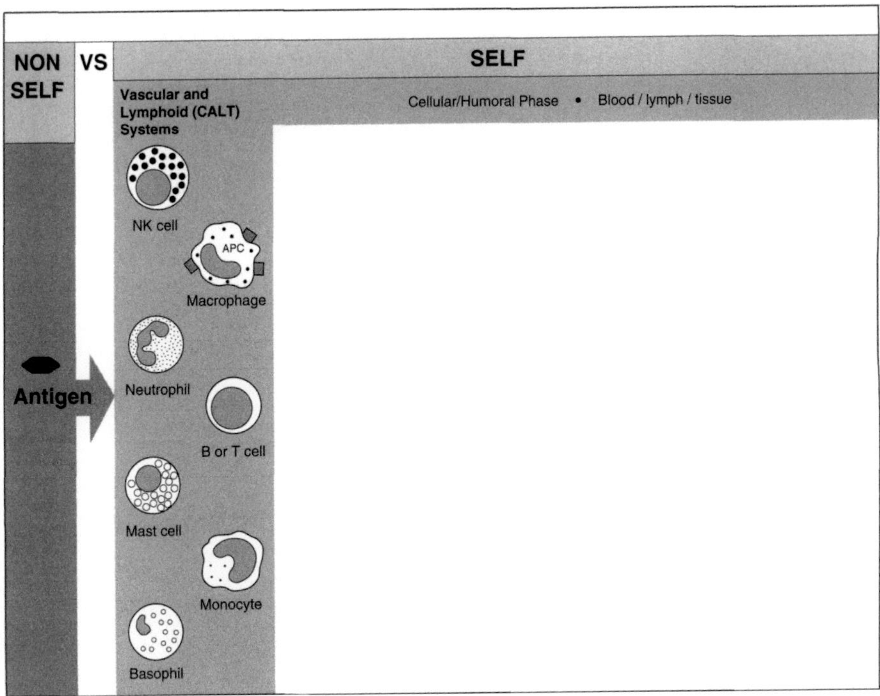

FIGURE 2.3 Antigen-presenting cells (APCs) capture immunogen. Step #2 of clinical immune matrix.

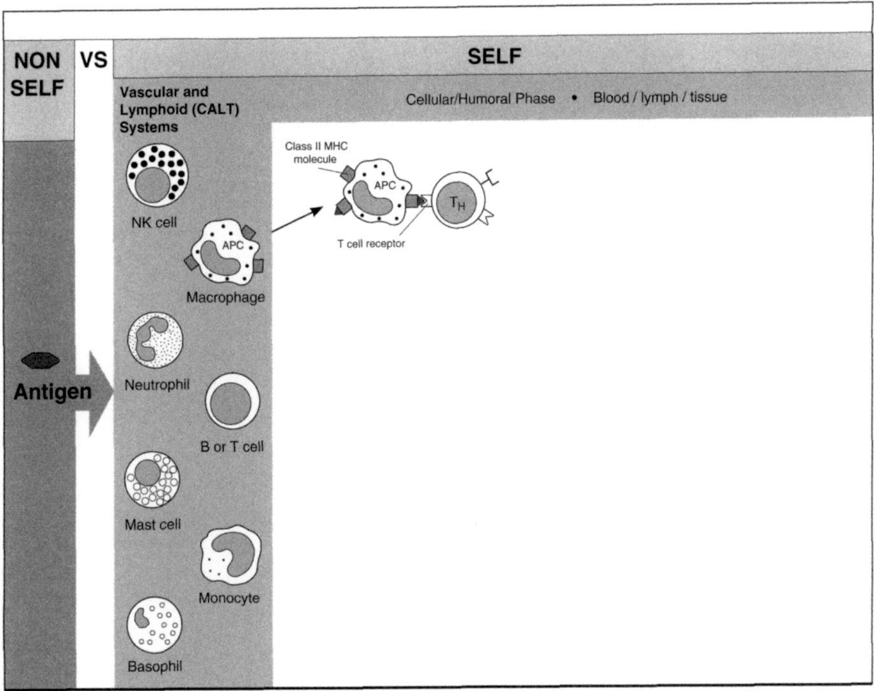

FIGURE 2.4 Immunogenic complex is bound by helper T cells. Step #3 of clinical immune matrix.

b. Clinical clock
   i. Primary response: hours, up to a day or so
   ii. Secondary (anamnestic, memory) response: minutes to a few hours

Step #3

a. Specific epitope of antigen associates with class II HLA molecule to form immunogenic complex, which is recognized and bound by a specific helper T cell (T_h; Figure 2.4)
   i. B cells activated by monocytes and suppressor Ts cells may express immunoglobin and also bind certain antigens (T cell-independent antigens) on these surface immunoglobins, independent of APC and T_h cells
b. T cell-dependent antigens require B and T cell activity
   i. T_h cells recognize antigen and secret interleukin 4 and 5 (IL-4 and IL-5) and other cytokines
   ii. B cells are then activated to produce antigen-specific immunoglobin (Figure 2.5)

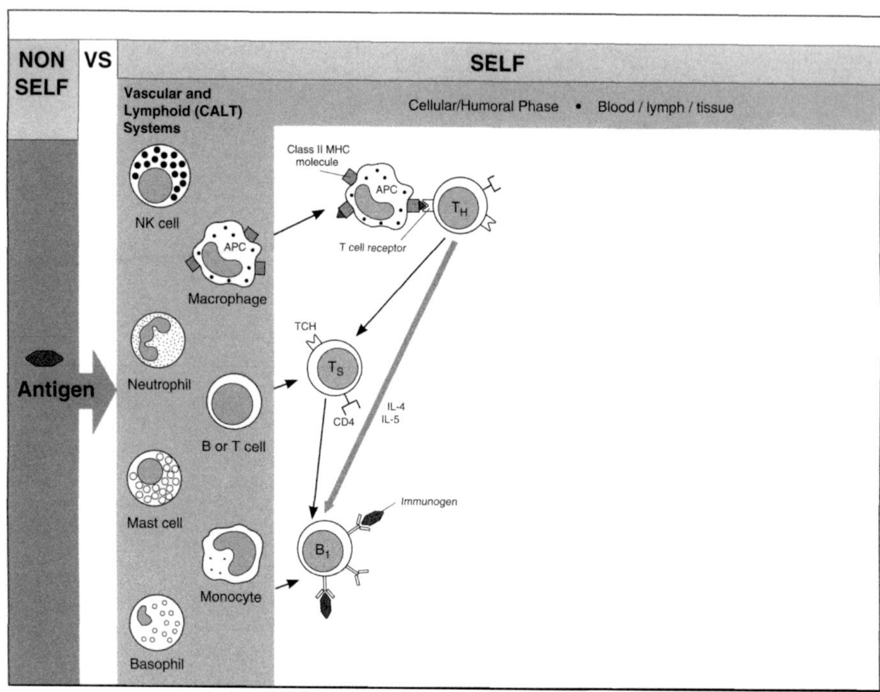

FIGURE 2.5 B and suppressor T cell activity. Step #3 of clinical immune matrix.

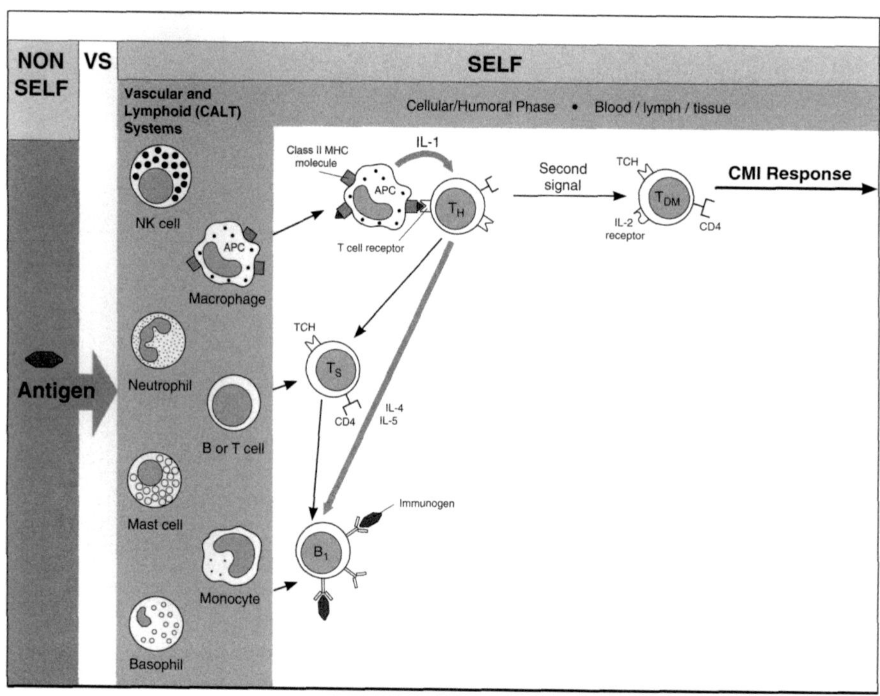

FIGURE 2.6 Interleukin-1 is produced and cell-mediated immune response initiated. Step #4 of clinical immune matrix.

c. Clinical clock
   i. Primary response: minutes, up to a day or so
   ii. Secondary (anamnestic, memory) response: minutes to a few hours
   iii. IgE-mediated response: minutes

Central Processing Stage

Step #4

T_h cells orchestrate immune reactions by two signals:

a. First signal is produced by the HLA-antigen complex (steps #2 and #3 above)
b. Second signal is produced by the production of interleukin 1 (IL-1) secreted by APC and initiating the cell-mediated immune (CMI) inflammatory (delayed hypersensitivity) response (Figure 2.6)
c. Together, the two signals induce receptors on T cells for lymphokine, interleukin-2 (IL-2), and a battery of cell growth and differentiating factors (cytokines, BCGF, and BCDF)

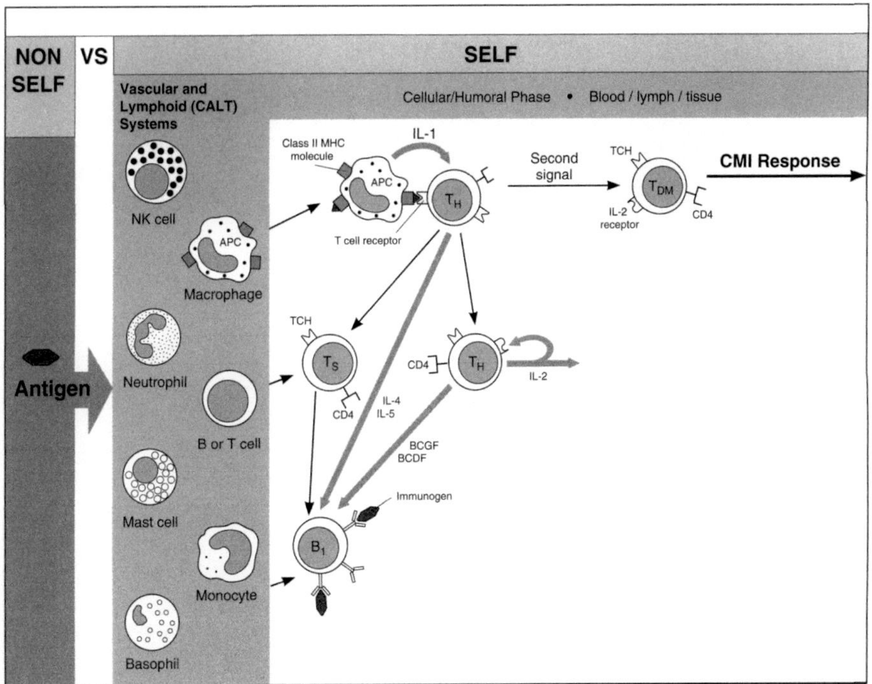

FIGURE 2.7 Interleukin-2 is produced. Step #4 of clinical immune matrix.

i. IL-2 will also become the second signal for cytotoxic T cell activity
ii. BCGF and BCDF will become the principal initiating mediators for B cell and plasma cell development and activity (Figure 2.7)

d. Clinical clock
   i. Primary response: 1 to 2 days
   ii. Secondary (anamnestic, memory) response: minutes to a few hours
   iii. IgE-mediated response: minutes

Efferent Arc Stage

Step #5

T_h cell activation leads to four general immune pathways (or combinations) to eliminate the foreign immunogen

a. T cell-mediated responses
   i. "Feedback inhibition" (see step #9, below)
   ii. Delayed hypersensitivity or cell-mediated immune (CMI) inflammation
b. Antigen–antibody (immune)-mediated responses
   i. Antigen-specific regulatory loop
   ii. Idiotype-specific regulatory circuit
   iii. Immune complement-mediated inflammation
c. IgE-mediated responses
d. Anamnestic ("rapid recall") response
   i. Memory T_h cells
   ii. Memory T_c cells
   iii. Memory B cells

Step #6

Cytotoxic T cells (T_c), triggered by T_h cells, function to kill antigen (on APC complex) by two signals (Figure 2.8)

a. First signal is produced by the recognition and binding of antigen to T_c cell class I HLA molecules and CDS receptors (versus T_h cell class II HLA molecules and CD4 receptors)
b. Second signal is furnished by IL-2 produced by activated T_h cells
c. Activated T_c cell (by the two signals) releases cytotoxins, which phagocytize and pinocytize the target cell (APC-MHC-antigen complex)
d. After antigen neutralization, T_c cells contribute to a subset of memory T and B cells to provide years of "rapid recall" or anamnestic response to antigen re-exposure.
e. Clinical clock
   i. Primary response: about 36 hours
   ii. Secondary (anamnestic, memory) response: minutes to a few hours

Step #7

Antibody-mediated responses are triggered by activated B cells and their differentiation into antibody-producing plasma cells (Figure 2.9)

a. B cells are activated by class II HLA antigen processing molecules and two lymphokines from proximal T_h cells
   i. B cell growth factor (BCGF) stimulates proliferation of B cells
   ii. B cell differentiating factor (BCDF) induces differentiation of activated B cells into antibody-producing plasma cells
b. A fraction of activated B cells do not differentiate (insufficient BCDF?) and form a pool of "memory B cells," which along with antigen-specific memory T_c and T_h cells provide years of "rapid recall response" or anamnestic response to antigen re-exposure

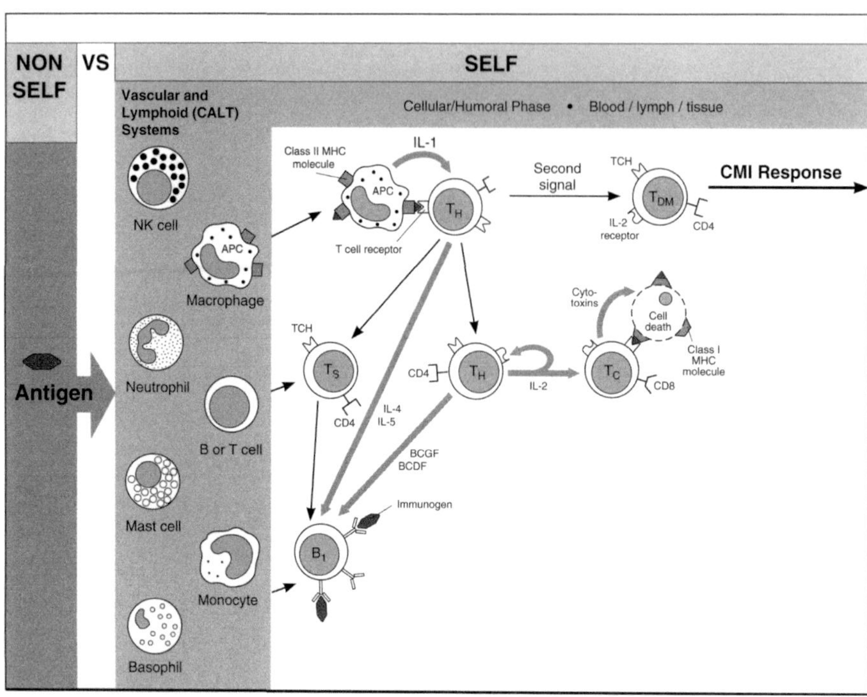

FIGURE 2.8 Cytotoxic T cells kill antigens. Step #6 of clinical immune matrix.

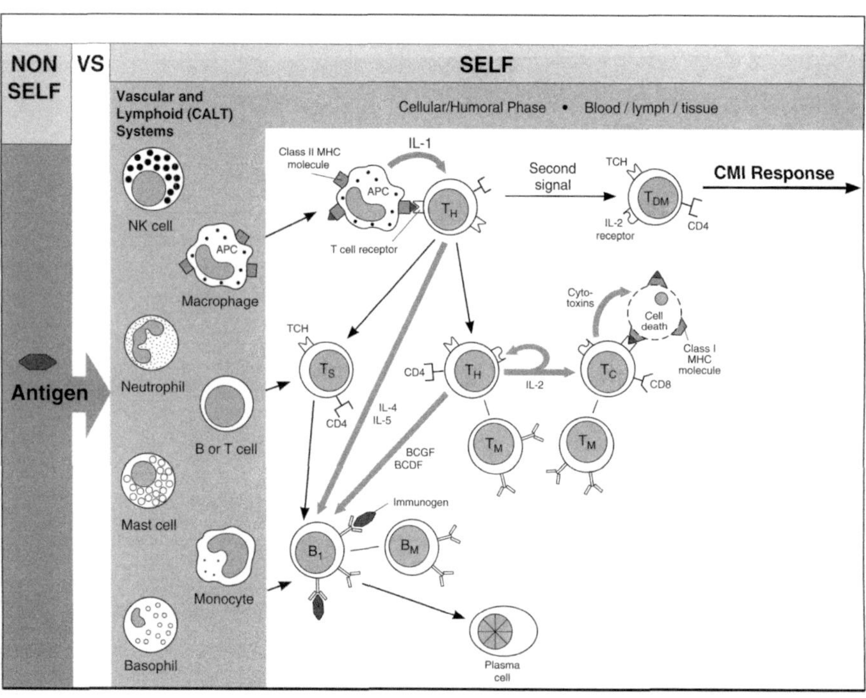

FIGURE 2.9 Plasma cells and memory cells are produced. Step #7 of clinical immune matrix.

c. Formation of antigen–antibody (from antigen-producing plasma cell complexes, or immune complexes) leads to immune complex-mediated inflammation or immune response regulation (Figure 2.10)

d. Clinical clock
   i. IgA- and M-mediated response
      - Primary: about 8 hours
   ii. Secondary: minutes
   iii. IgE-mediated response
      - Immediate phase: about 15 minutes
      - Late phase: about 6 hours

Regulation Stage

Step #8

Elimination of the antigen is the principal means of regulating activity of the immune system

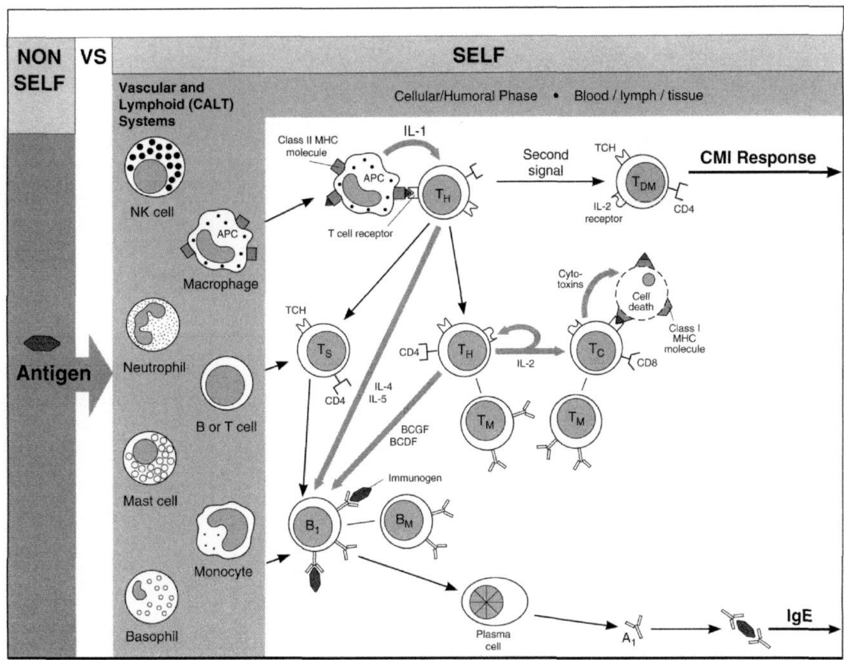

FIGURE 2.10 Immune complexes are formed. Step #7 of clinical immune matrix.

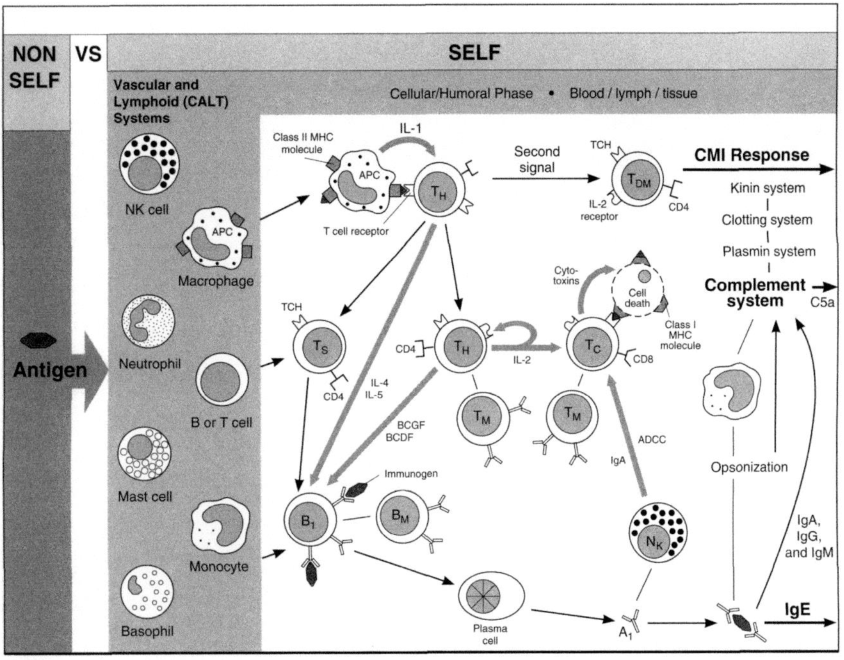

FIGURE 2.11 Complement system is activated. Step #8 of clinical immune matrix.

a. Cytotoxic destruction of the antigen
b. Inactivation of the antigen through antigen–antibody immune complexes
c. Opsonization of bacteria through complement system to promote phagocytosis by macrophages
d. Activation of the complement system by antibodies IgA, IgG, or IgM in immune complexes, and the kinin, clotting, and fibrinolytic (plasmin) systems, produce enzymatic lysing activity, opsonic activity, chemotaxis with PMN phagocytosis, as well as subacute or acute immune complex-mediated inflammation
e. Antibody-dependent cellular cytotoxicity (ADCC) uses NK cells to bind IgA to kill bacteria and tumor cells with cytotoxins
f. Classical and alternative complement pathways activated by immune complexes use the inflammatory factor Csa from the complement cascade to attract neutrophils (PMNs) to phagocytize the immune complex, with resultant toxic by-products capable of blood vessel wall destruction (vasculitis) and hemorrhage (Figure 2.11)
g. Clinical clock averages about 2 to 5 days (time frame determined by circulating antibodies)

Step #9

Control of intensity and duration of response(s) is poorly understood, with three mechanisms believed to be interrelated:

a. Production of antibody results in inhibition of continued production of the same antibody ("feedback inhibition") by removal of antigen and by reduction in circulating antibody level (antigen-specific regulatory loop; Figure 2.12)
b. Suppressor T cells (T_s), also poorly understood, turn off T_h cells and may also affect B cells by secreting chemical factors that suppress B and T_h cell activity and/or by binding epitopes or idiotypes of B and T_h cells through participation in the "idiotypic-specific regulatory circuits." (Now, please try and stay with me on this!)
c. On immunogenic stimulus, idiotopes (antigen-specific B cells) increase by genetic cloning and create an immunogenic stimulus of their own, which induces an anti-idiotype antibody (antibody-2) response with its own set of idiotopes, resulting in anti-anti-idiotype antibody (antibody-3) production. This circuit of anti-antibodies (Figure 2.13) seems to function by stimulating T_h and T_s cells, which close the loop to turn off further immunogenic effects. (Needless to say, a very complicated process with a very delicate balance—all poorly understood by the "immunology gurus" and most of the rest of us)
d. Clinical clock for regulation averages about 1 week

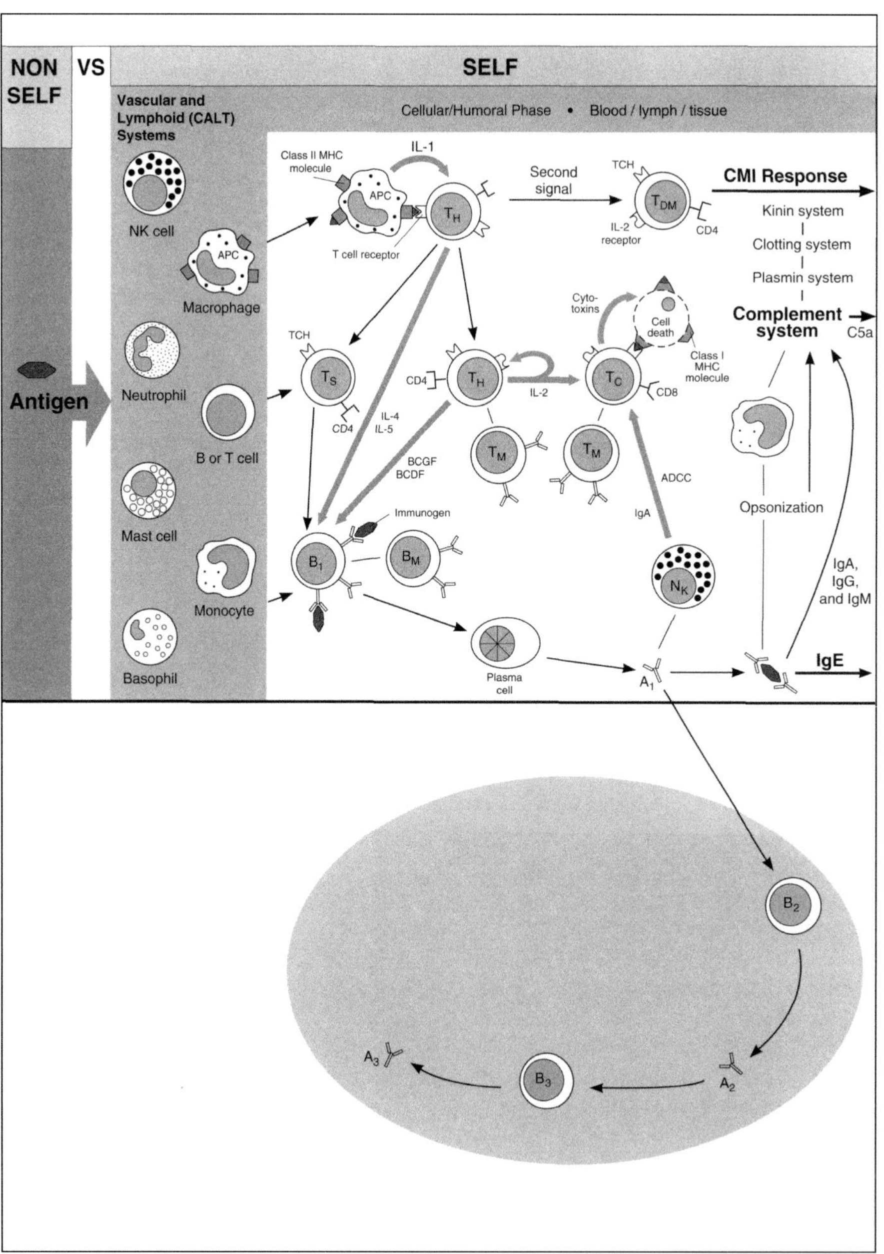

FIGURE 2.12 Antigen-specific regulatory loop removes antigens and reduces circulating antibody levels. Step #9 of clinical immune matrix.

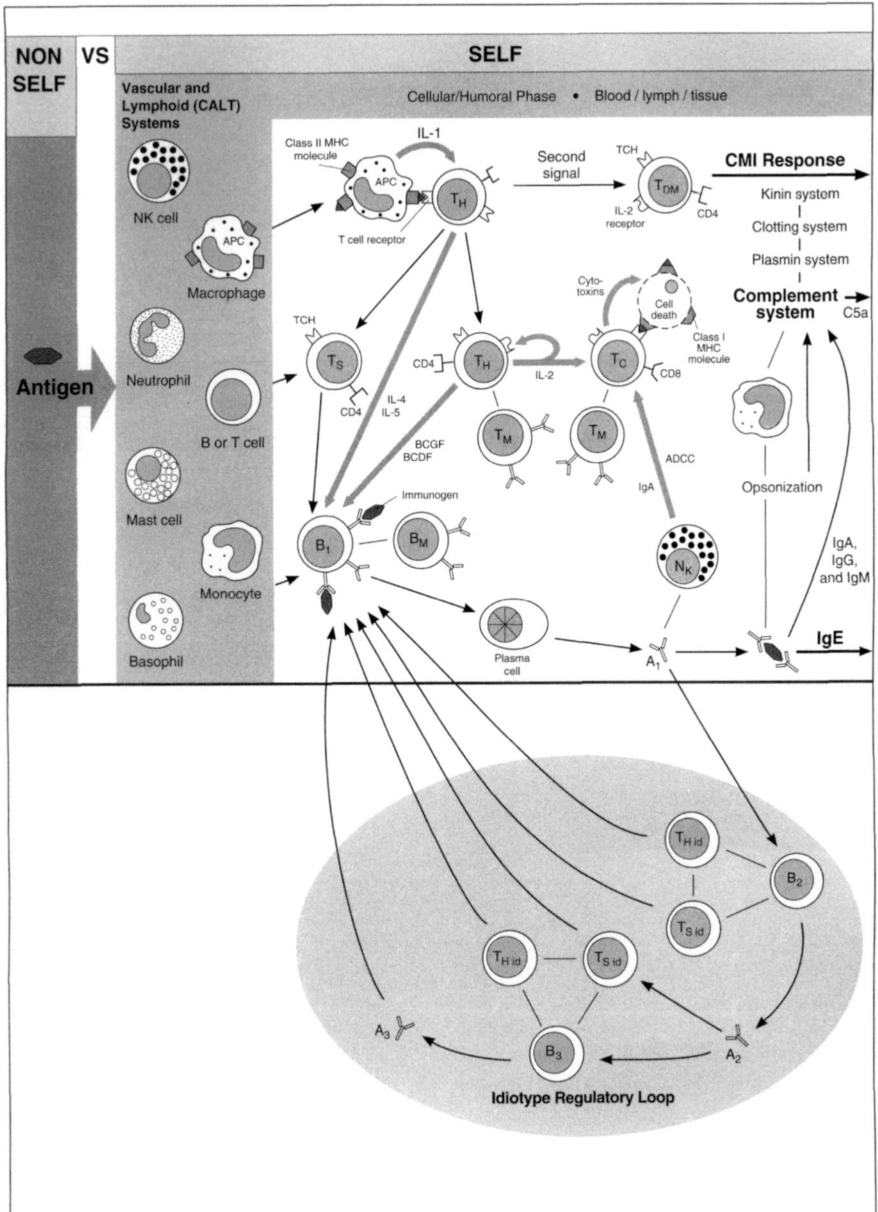

FIGURE 2.13 Idiotypic regulatory loop. Step #9 of clinical immune matrix.

"Dysregulation"

Step #10

The most poorly understood aspects of the entire immune system are those factors (extrinsic and intrinsic) that cause "dysregulation" and improper immune function and response.

a. Some extrinsic factors affecting dysregulation include (but are not limited to):
   i. Genetic defects
   ii. Aging
   iii. Nutrition
   iv. Environment
   v. Stress
      - Emotional
      - Psychological
      - Mechanical
   vi. Physiological
   vii. Hormonal imbalance
   viii. Neoplasia
   ix. Infectious disease (e.g., acquired immune deficiency disease [AIDS])
b. Some intrinsic dysregulating factors include (but are not limited to):
   i. Allergy/hypersensitivity (negative inflammatory responses)
   ii. Immunodeficiency disorders
   iii. Loss of "self-non-self" discrimination
   iv. Dysregulation of homeostasis
   v. Autoimmunity
c. Clinical clock: from minutes to weeks depending on the antigenic stimulus and the cause of dysregulation

II. Inflammation

A. Definitions

Defined as the fundamental, clinical process of the immune system, consisting of reactions that occur in affected blood vessels and adjacent tissues in response to injury or abnormal stimulation.

1. Antigen activation (abnormal stimulus) of T cells and/or antibodies (in affected blood vessels and adjacent tissues) produces the recruitment of inflammatory cells and chemical mediators
2. These inflammatory cells and mediators produce multiple reactions (see below), all of which are initiated by portions of (in some cases, possibly all of) the "Clinical Immune Matrix"
3. Inflammation is an efficient, though non-specific defense mechanism of the body, producing an observable clinical response (the "inflammatory cascade") that "usually" (+/– 95% of the time?) self-limits and resolves through the "regulation phases" of the immune response
4. Clinical response may, however, from time to time (+/– 5% of the time?) not self-limit or resolve and may produce tissue changes, damage, and interfere with tissue or organ function
    a. Negative inflammatory process
        i. Hypersensitivity/allergic response
        ii. Autoimmune response (poorly understood)
        iii. Regulatory dysfunction
    b. Negative responses can be natural (innate) or acquired (induced)
        i. Allergy can be natural or acquired
        ii. Hypersensitivity is usually acquired
    c. In avascular tissues and structures (e.g., cornea and anterior chamber), sometimes called "privileged immune sites" (misnomer), inflammatory changes at any degree or duration potentiate abnormal changes in the tissue/structure and can serve to produce permanent alterations, reshaping, remodeling, and damaging the tissue/structure's integrity or function (e.g., corneal transparency)
        i. In vascular tissue, inflammation can be considered an asset (in removing antigen) with nominal potential risk of secondary negative effects through hypersensitivity, autoimmunity, tissue damage, or regulatory dysfunction
        ii. In avascular tissue, however, inflammation should always be considered a liability
            - In spite of its positive, helpful, and perhaps necessary antigenremoval function, it presents significant potential for adverse tissue changes and damage
            - The corneal stromal matrix and its associated transparency are particularly at risk
    d. Thus, the inflammatory process presents a therapeutic challenge in clinical management due to its positive, beneficial, defensive effects versus its potential for negative, damaging, and destructive results
        i. In vascular tissue, clinical management of inflammation can be passive and conservative on effective removal of the cause
        ii. In avascular tissue, clinical management of inflammation must be watchful, carefully measured, and active to protect tissue and structural integrity and function, sometimes even after removal of the primary cause

B. The Inflammatory Cascade

General term for the set of dynamic clinical events activated by any portion of the immune response for any one of the three classes (or four types) of inflammatory reactions (Figures 2.14 and 2.15).

1. Acute versus Chronic

Clinical inflammation can occur in an acute phase (hours to days) and/or a chronic phase (weeks, months, or years), both of which have clinical and biological differences

a. The inflammatory cascade in acute inflammation is produced by certain cells and mediators leading to distinct yet dynamic clinical events that the clinician must appreciate as an unfolding process (a "clinical cascade") rather than as separate clinical entities
    i. Vasodilation producing "rubor" or redness, and "calor" or increased temperature
    ii. Increased vascular permeability leading to "tumor" or swelling, and "dolor" or pain
        - Transudation of fluids (inflammatory edema)
    iii. Exudation of leukocytes (infiltration)
    iv. Ulceration (tissue destruction)
    v. Loss of function ("functio laesa")

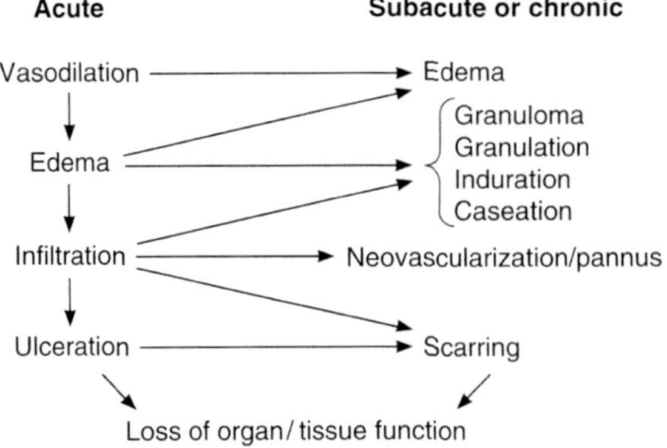

FIGURE 2.14 The inflammatory cascade occurs in both acute and chronic forms

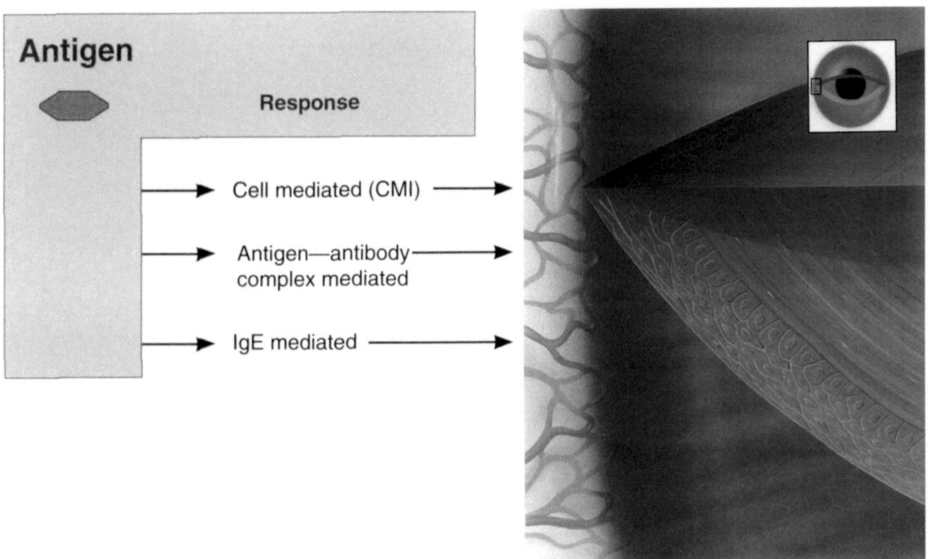

FIGURE 2.15 Clinical immune matrix summarized in schematic representation.

b. Chronic inflammation can occur in 4 ways:
   i. Secondary to acute inflammation
      - Persistent antigenic stimulation
   ii. Persistent inflammatory by-products
   iii. Without acute inflammatory phase
      - Idiopathic disease (e.g., sarcoidosis)
   iv. Autoimmune disease (e.g., multiple sclerosis)
   v. It is believed that chronic inflammation may be the pathophysiological basis of all diseases based on its propensity towards destroying the perivascular lining of blood vessels, thus producing both diffuse and organ specific pathology
c. The chronic inflammatory phase includes additional biological and clinical features with or without initial acute phase events
   i. Fibrinization secondary to accumulated inflammatory cells converting to fibroblasts
   ii. Granulomatous formation (granulomas)
      - Focal accumulation of inflammatory cells monocytes, lymphocytes, neutrophils, plasma cells, and epithelioid (giant) cells (from monocytes and macrophages)
   iii. Chronic inflammation is the end result of the CMI response
   iv. Production and deposition by the fibroblasts of connective tissue elements (sometimes referred to as granulation tissue)
      - Smooth muscle fibers
      - Collagen and elastin
   v. Proteoglycans (ground substance)
   vi. Tissue hardening (induration) secondary to chronic edema, infiltration, fibrinization, connective tissue, and granulomatous formation
   vii. Tissue destruction (from leukocytes, enzymes, and antigen) including caseation necrosis (tissue liquefaction)
   viii. Neovascularization
      - From vasogenic factors
   ix. Newly formed deep, poorly endothelially lined, "leaky" capillaries
   x. Pannus
      - Superficial blood vessel formation with an associated fibrous tissue bed
      - Frequently associated with phlyctenule formations (immune complex clinical reactions) of the cornea and/or conjunctiva, which include focal accumulations of inflammatory cells and tissue ulceration
d. Loss of body (organism), organ and/or tissue function in chronic inflammation is quite common from the above mentioned clinical sequelae ("functio laesa")

2. *Control Mechanisms*

Clinical events of the inflammatory cascade in all classes (or types) are controlled by complex neurogenic and nonneurogenic (cellular and humoral) mechanisms. These will be partially listed and charted below (to help complete the clinical immune matrix), but will not be described in detail.

a. Neurogenic mechanisms control the larger vessels
b. Cellular and humoral mechanisms control the smaller capillaries and arterioles
   i. Cytokines
   ii. Vasoactive and smooth muscle constricting mediators and mediator-producing systems
      - Kinin system
      - Fibrinolytic system
      - Clotting system
      - Complement system
   iii. Chemotactic factors to attract other cells
   iv. Enzymes, hormones, and proteoglycans
   v. Reactive molecules (Figure 2.16)

3. *Vasodilation ("Rubor" and "Calor")*

a. Antigen initiates immune response leading to two general possibilities:
   i. Elimination of the antigen and regulation of the immune reaction
   ii. Activation of at least two systems that initiate vasodilation and the inflammatory cascade

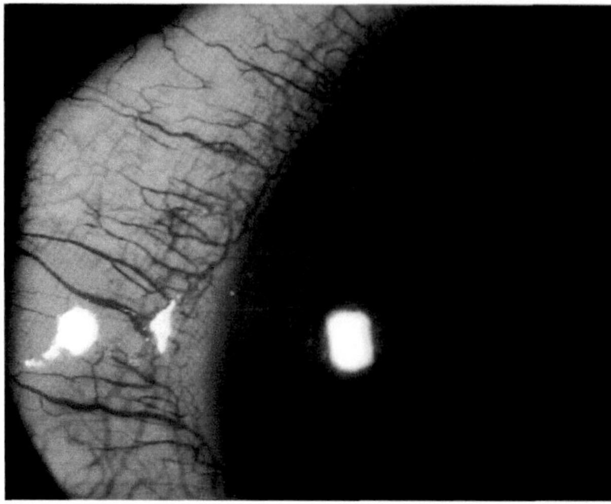

FIGURE 2.16 Vasodilation of limbal vessels secondary to antigen stimulus to cornea.

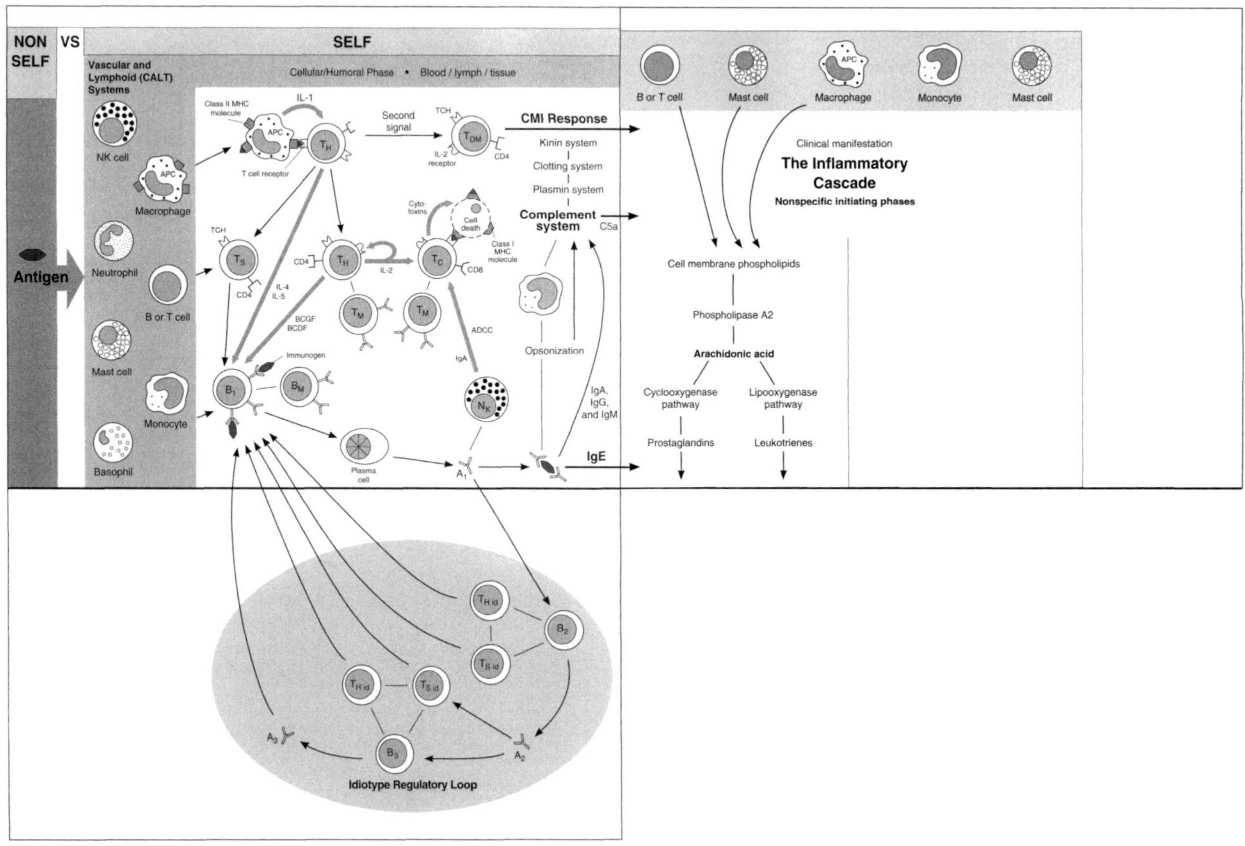

FIGURE 2.17 Arachidonic acid initiating system.

b. Non-specific vasodilatory-initiating systems
   i. Arachidonic acid (derived from cell-wall phospholipids) metabolizes through two enzymatic pathways (Figure 2.17)
      - Cyclo-oxygenase pathway acting on tissue-type mast cell walls produces prostaglandin D_2
        - Prominent in anterior segment inflammation
        - Also augments infiltration
      - 5-Lipo-oxygenase pathway acting on mucosa mast cells produce leukotrienes
        - Potent systemic activators (e.g., bronchoconstriction, hypotension, allergy)
        - Leukotrienes are several hundred times more potent than histamine
   ii. Endothelial leukocytic adhesion molecule (ELAM) activation by cytokines (IL-2, tumor necrosis

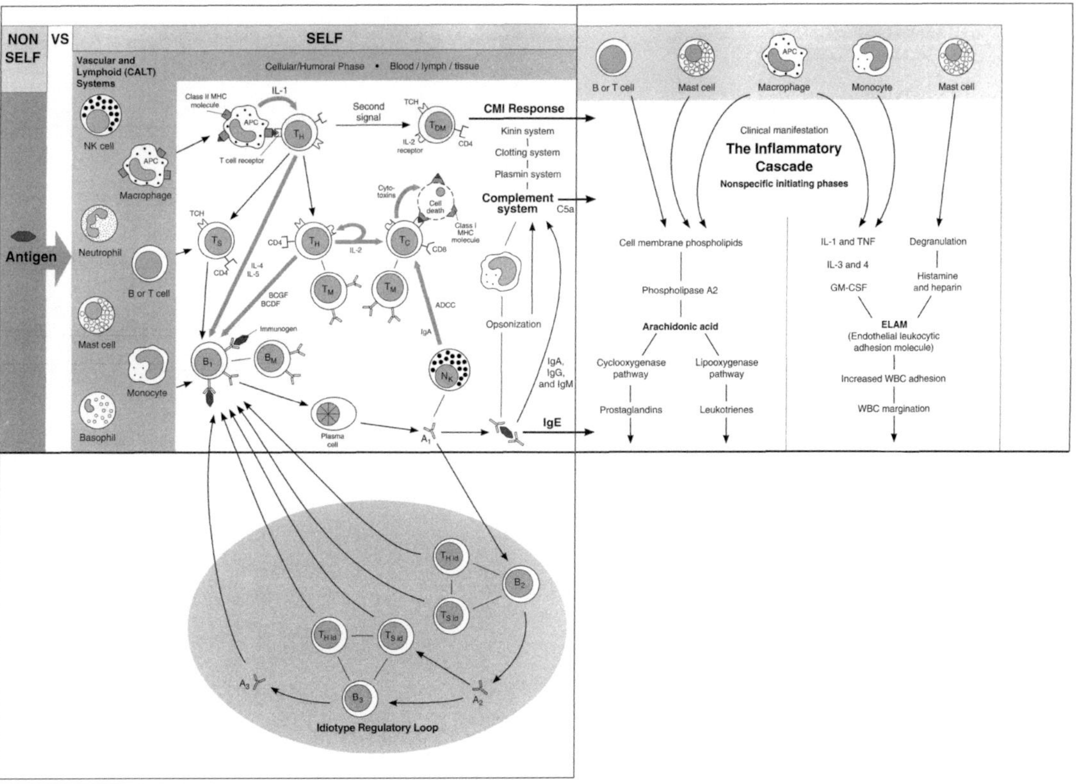

FIGURE 2.18 ELAM. Initiating system is activated by cytokines.

factor alpha, and possibly IL-3, IL-4, and GM-CSF) (Figure 2.18)
- Recruits inflammatory cells to the site of involved tissue
- Aids in WBC adhesion to vessel wall for diapedesis (migration) and extravascular emigration
- Mast cell may also be the "gatekeeper" for this vasodilatory system

c. Blood vessels begin to dilate (mediator induced) increasing volume of blood (with associated increased temperature—"calor") in the vicinity of antigen, to provide more WBCs to eliminate antigen
d. Clinical redness ("rubor") appears
e. Greater in acute inflammation
   i. In deeper vessel dilations and chronic inflammation (Figures 2.19 and 2.20), redness may be imperceptible
f. Clinical clock
   i. Almost instantaneous in injury (prostaglandin-E_2 stimulated)
   ii. IgE mediated: 15 to 30 minutes

4. *Increased Vascular Permeability (Edema or "Tumor" and "Dolor")*

a. Vasodilation causes endothelial pores of vessels to open wider, increasing permeability, with the goal of allowing polymorphonuclear WBCs (PMNs) to emigrate (diapedesis) extravascularly to reach and eliminate antigen
b. The dilation of endothelial pores in the blood vessel wall also allows the escape or leakage of fluids (serum transudation) from the blood vessel into avascular tissue, producing clinical swelling ("tumor") and pain ("dolor")
   i. Termed *inflammatory edema* and defined as the presence of abnormally large amounts of fluid in the intercellular tissue spaces of the body
      - Versus noninflammatory (physiological) edema, a separate clinical entity defined as edema without redness or pain (e.g., white eye edema) occurring from passive congestion or from lowered serum osmolarity
      - Noninflammatory edema is commonly produced from tissue or cellular abnormalities
        - Dystrophies (e.g., Fuchs' endothelial)
        - Degeneration (e.g., endothelial loss secondary to aging)
        - Biochemical disturbances (e.g., contact lens hypoxia)
   ii. Inflammatory edema produces clinical swelling and pain (relative to the amount of nerves in affected area; Figures 2.21 to 2.23)
   iii. Clinical clock
      - Progresses over 1 hour to 1 day
      - Prolonged (for days) if injury induced
c. Ironically, inflammatory edema presents a bit of a dilemma due to its simultaneous value in the inflammatory process along with its numerous adverse clinical effects and risks to the tissue and the system
   i. The value of inflammatory edema is its "loosening" effect on the tightly compacted avascular tissue through which the WBCs must travel to reach and eliminate the antigen. Also in chronic edema, these spaces may provide avenues for new blood vessels (neovascularization) to gain proximity to antigenic sites, allowing for more effective leukocytic activity

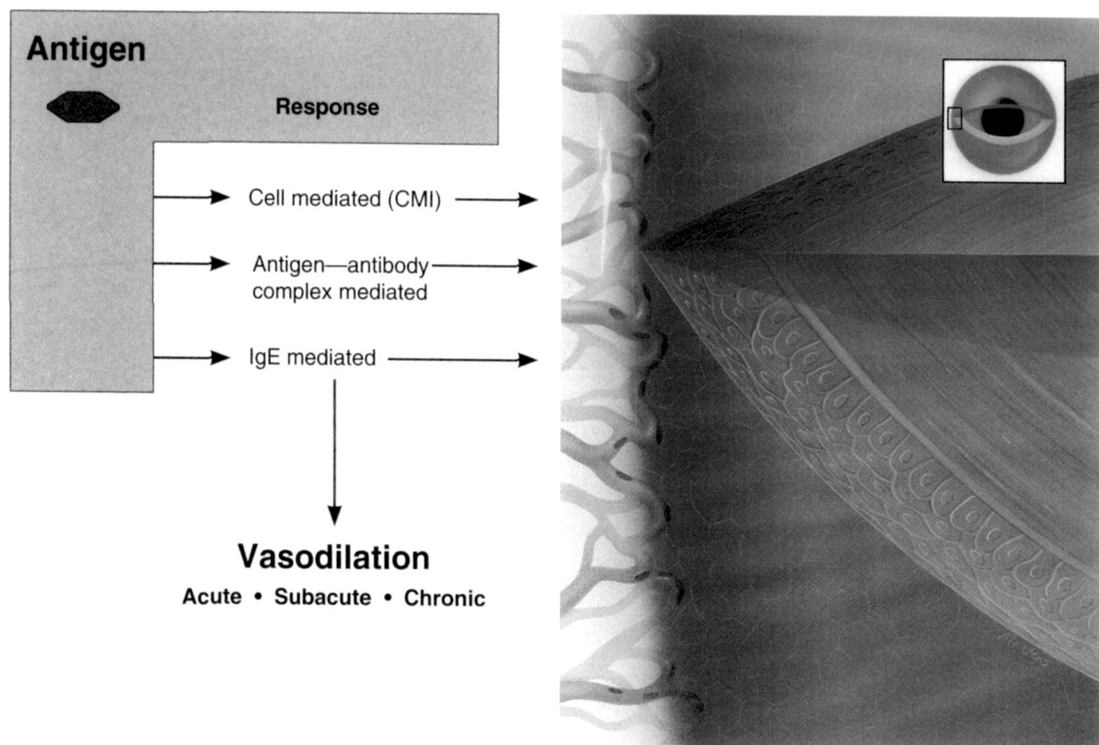

FIGURE 2.19 Vasodilation (limbal vessel) shown in schematic representation.

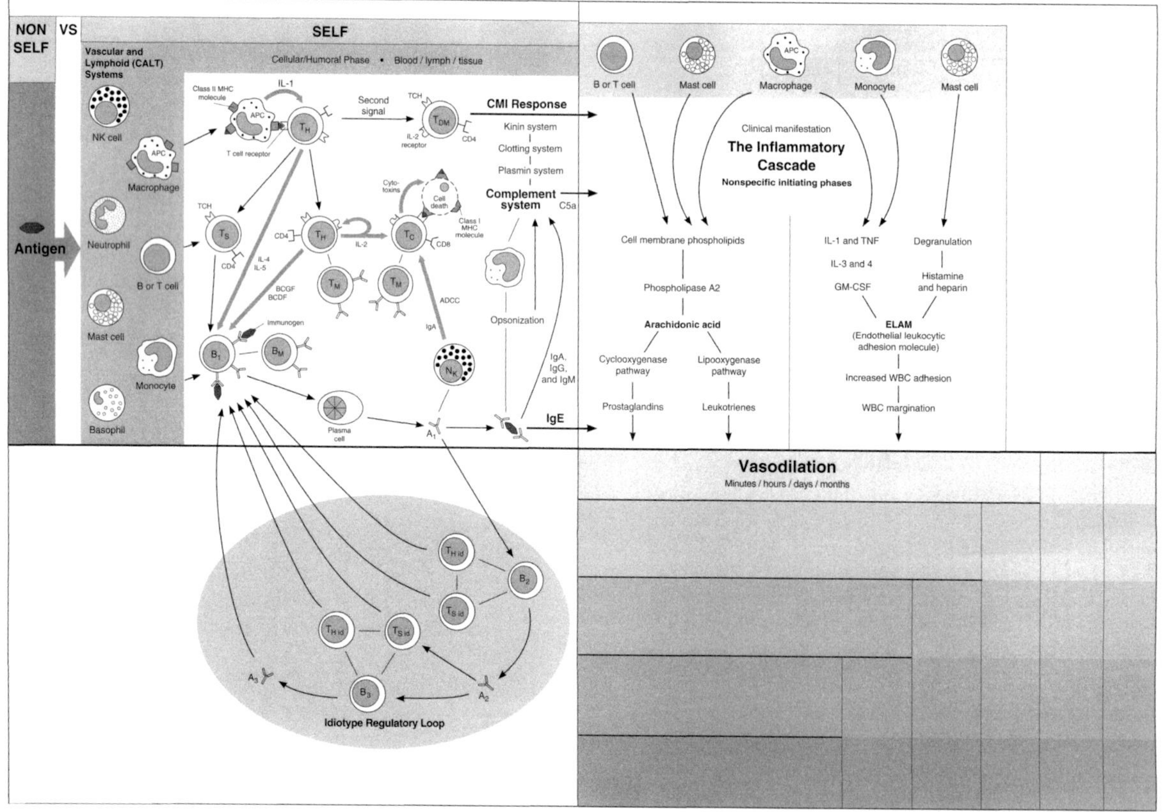

FIGURE 2.20 Inflammatory cascade (vasodilation).

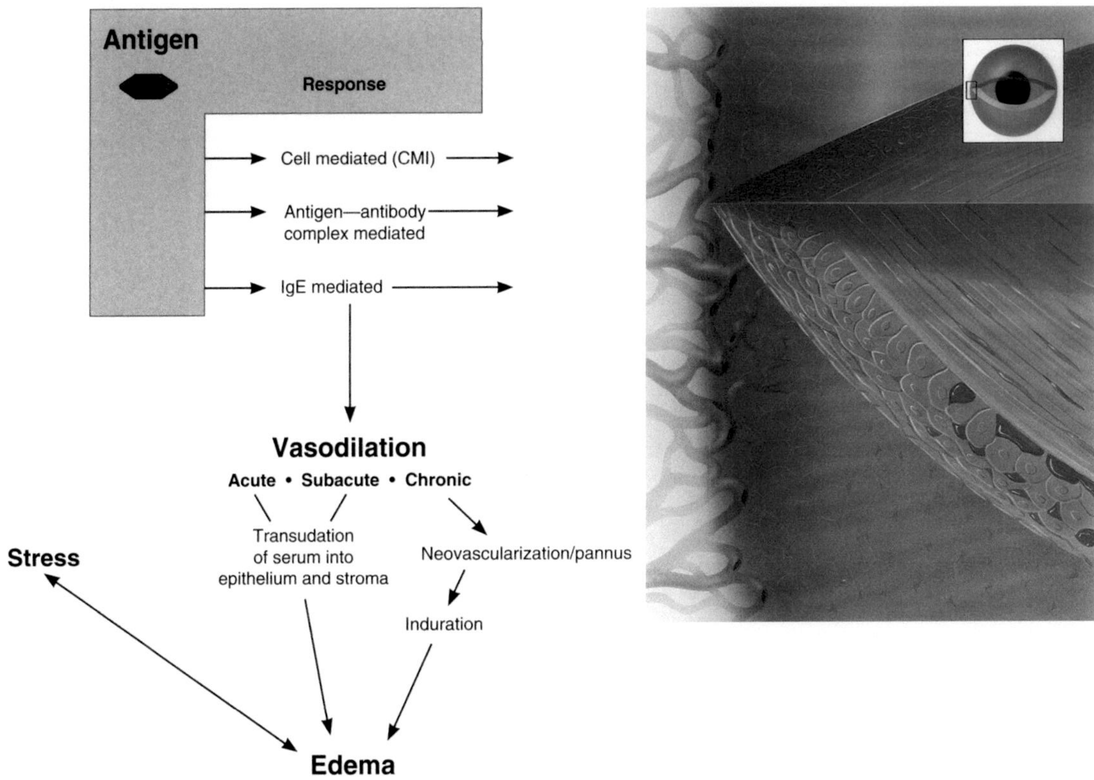

FIGURE 2.21 Inflammatory edema (corneal epithelium) shown in schematic representation.

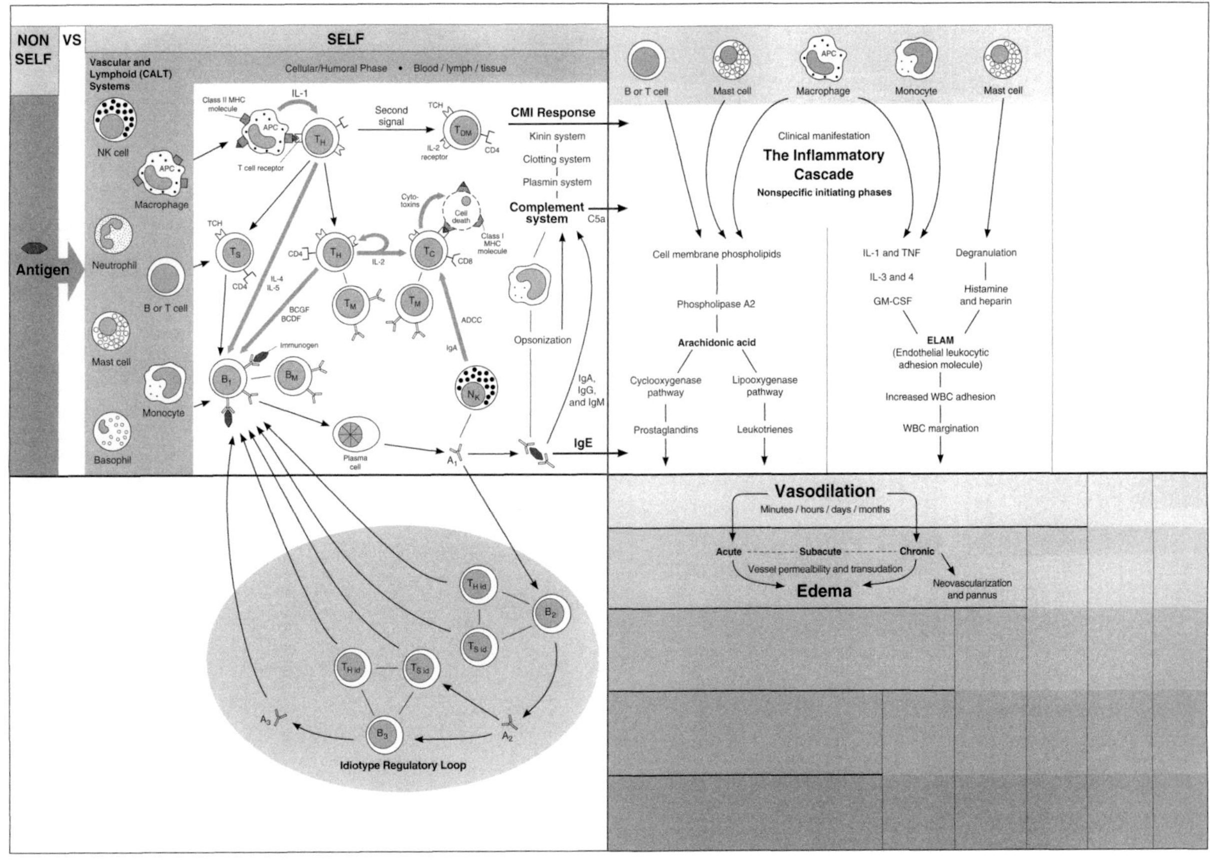

FIGURE 2.22 Inflammatory cascade (edema).

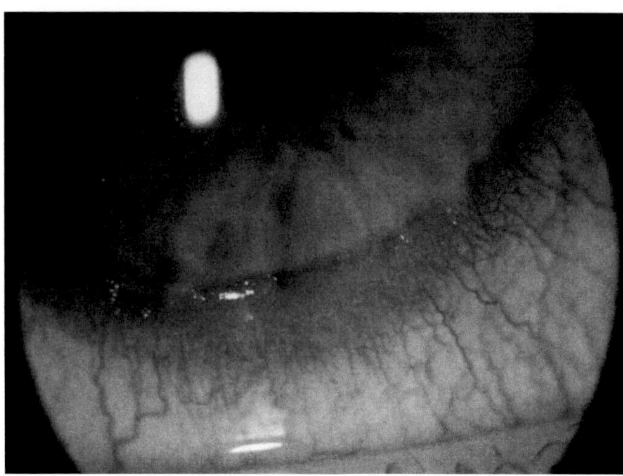

FIGURE 2.23 Inflammatory edema associated with the inflammatory cascade accumulating at the inferior corneal limbus.

ii. Negative effects of inflammatory edema include:
   - Subjective clinical pain in tissues (especially tissue with rich nerve supply)
   - Abnormal stress on, and disruption of avascular tissue integrity (e.g., corneal stromal matrix), with the risk of irreversible damage (especially in chronic inflammatory edemas)
   - Avascular tissue spaces and "pockets" allowing for increased focal accumulations of fibrin (especially in chronic responses), antigen and potential toxins from inflammatory by-products including WBCs, chemicals, and necrotic debris (from destruction of antigen, normal host tissue, and WBCs)
     - Any of the stressors (pain, tissue disruption, mechanical and physiological factors) and cellular or chemical substances described above may serve as autoantigens to elicit an autoimmune response

5. *Infiltration*

The process of extravascular emigration of WBCs is termed exudation or, clinically, *infiltration.*

a. Infiltration is defined as the diffusion or accumulation in a tissue or cells of substances not normal to it or in amounts in excess of the normal
b. Escaping WBCs (PMNs) are referred to as infiltrative or inflammatory WBCs
c. Infiltrative WBCs, in conjunction with other immune/inflammatory cellular and humoral components, demonstrate efficiency of function and purpose by moving directly to the level and site of the antigen they are to attack
   i. Emigration may occur
      - Into the eyelid tissue
      - Through the tears, to conjunctival sites (e.g., follicles) or superficial corneal sites (e.g., superficial punctate keratitis)
      - Into the corneal epithelium and/or stroma
        - Intraepithelial infiltrates
        - Subepithelial infiltrates
        - Stromal infiltrates
        - Intraocularly into aqueous humor and beyond (into posterior segment of the eye)
   ii. This exudation and emigration of WBCs often results in clinically apparent blood vessels as well as producing a clinical presentation of more dramatic, deeper, and diffuse (due to vasodilation of tributary vessels to adjacent tissues and structures) edema and infiltration
   iii. "Innocent bystander" effects to the lids, conjunctiva, deep corneal stroma, and anterior chamber structures
d. The loss, destruction, or disruption of tissue in the ulcerative response usually (always in the corneal example) leads to permanent scarring of tissue (Figure 2.29) accumulations of edema and infiltrative WBCs at the site(s) or in the vicinity of antigen stimulation (Figures 2.24 to 2.26)
e. Clinical clock
   i. PMNs: 6 to 12 hours
   ii. Mononuclear cells: 12 to 48 hours

6. *Ulceration*

a. Defined as a local defect, or excavation, of the surface of an organ or tissue, which is produced by the sloughing of inflammatory necrotic tissue (Figures 2.27 and 2.28)
b. This destructive process generally occurs in the late acute stages (beyond 48 hours) or chronic phase of inflammation, unless the antigen is highly virulent and attacking highly specialized, poorly defended tissue (e.g., pseudomonal infection of the corneal stroma)
c. The process can occur from four primary sources:
   i. The antigen
   ii. WBCs (particularly PMNs) that are attacking the antigen
   iii. Toxic or necrotic by-products produced by the immune response but not effectively eliminated by the body (e.g., cellular debris, enzymes, etc.)
   iv. Chronic inflammation
d. On destruction of deeper tissues in ulceration, vasodilation of deeper (larger diameter) blood vessels also occurs producing a clinical presentation of more dramatic, deeper, and diffuse (due to vasodilation of tributary vessels to adjacent tissues and structures) edema and infiltration

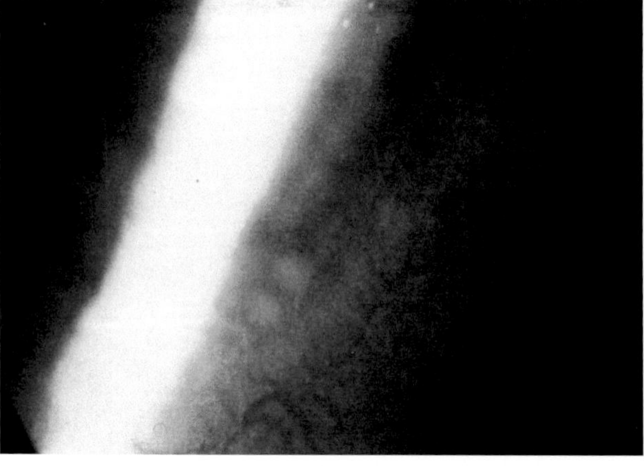

FIGURE 2.24 Intraepithelial infiltrates associated with the inflammatory cascade in the peripheral cornea.

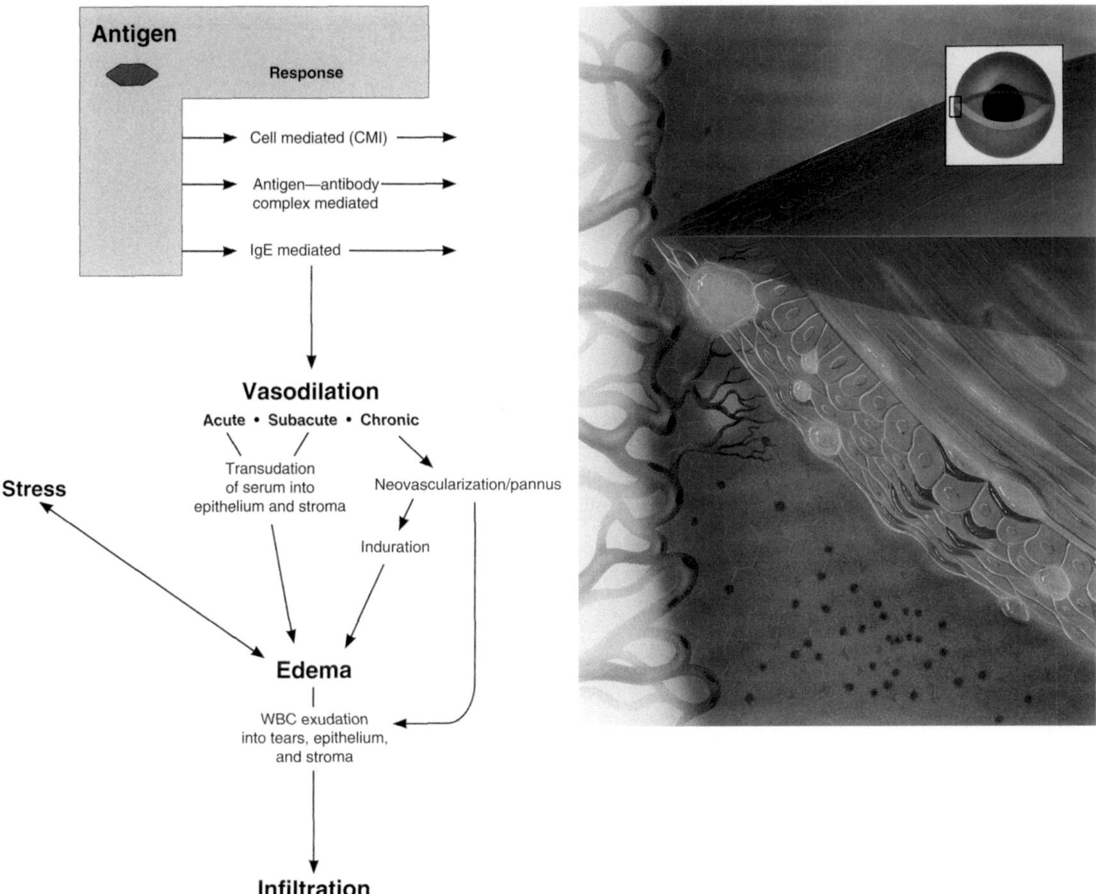

FIGURE 2.25 Infiltration (corneal epithelium) shown in schematic representation.

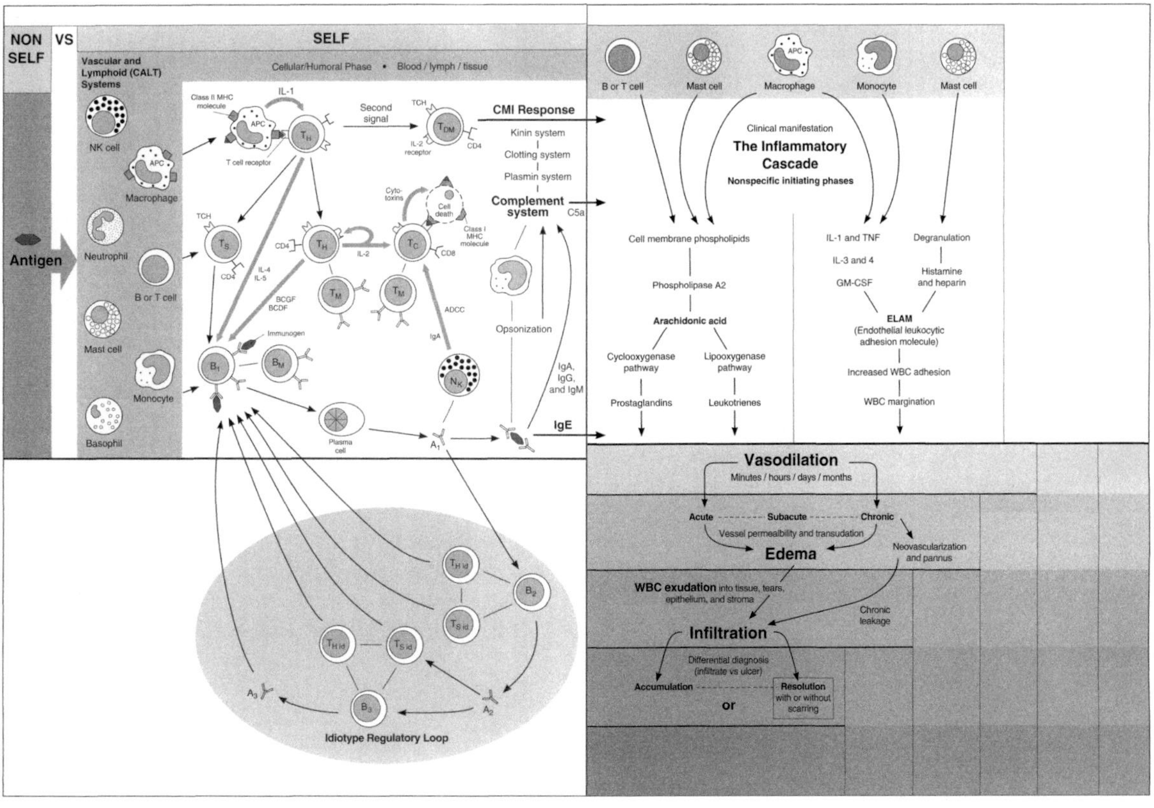

FIGURE 2.26 Inflammatory cascade (infiltration).

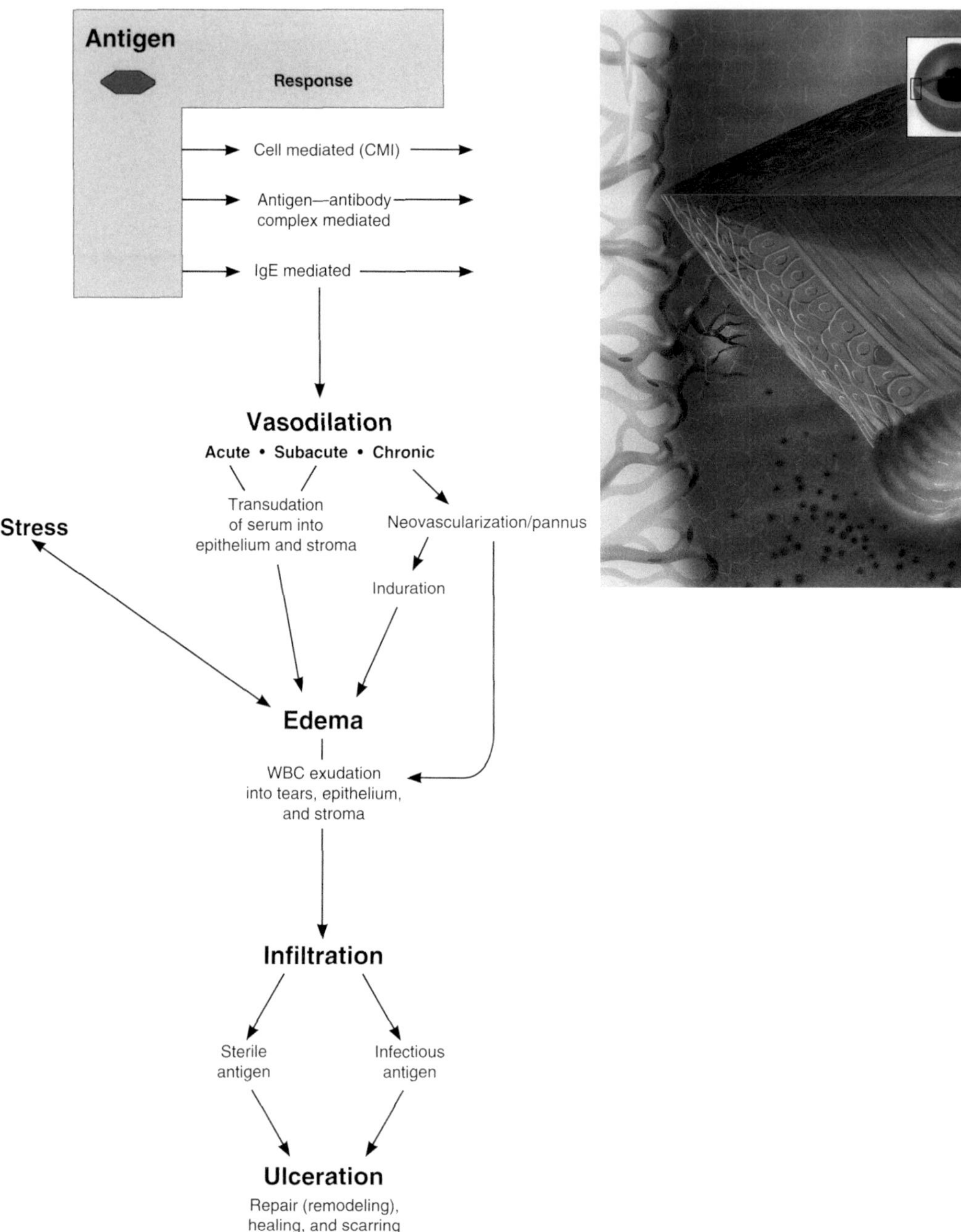

FIGURE 2.27 Ulceration (corneal stroma) shown in schematic representation.

  i. Increased "rubor, calor, dolor, tumor"
  ii. "Innocent bystander" effects to the lids, conjunctiva, deep corneal stroma, and anterior chamber structures
e. The loss, destruction, or disruption of tissue in the ulcerative response usually (always in the corneal example) leads to permanent scarring of tissue (Figure 2.29)

7. *Loss of Function ("Function Laesa")*

a. All of the combined effects of the inflammatory cascade produce an inability of the affected tissue, organ, or organism (body) to continue to function in its normal mechanical and/or physiological manner
b. This loss of function may be temporary or permanent depending on degree and duration of inflammation

8. *Repair, Healing, and Scarring (Cicatrization)*

a. Repair is the replacement of lost or disrupted tissue by connective and fibrous tissue
  i. Macrophages clear and remove damaged tissue and cells
  ii. Fibroblasts begin to wall off the periphery of the inflammatory focus (early scar formation)
    - If the repair process occurs simultaneously with active inflammation, fibrin walls can cause an "abscess"
    - Such a clinical occurrence requires dissection of the wall and drainage of the inflammatory focus
b. Newly forming lymphatic channels (and new blood vessels in chronic inflammation) help clear the site of inflammatory cells and necrotic debris

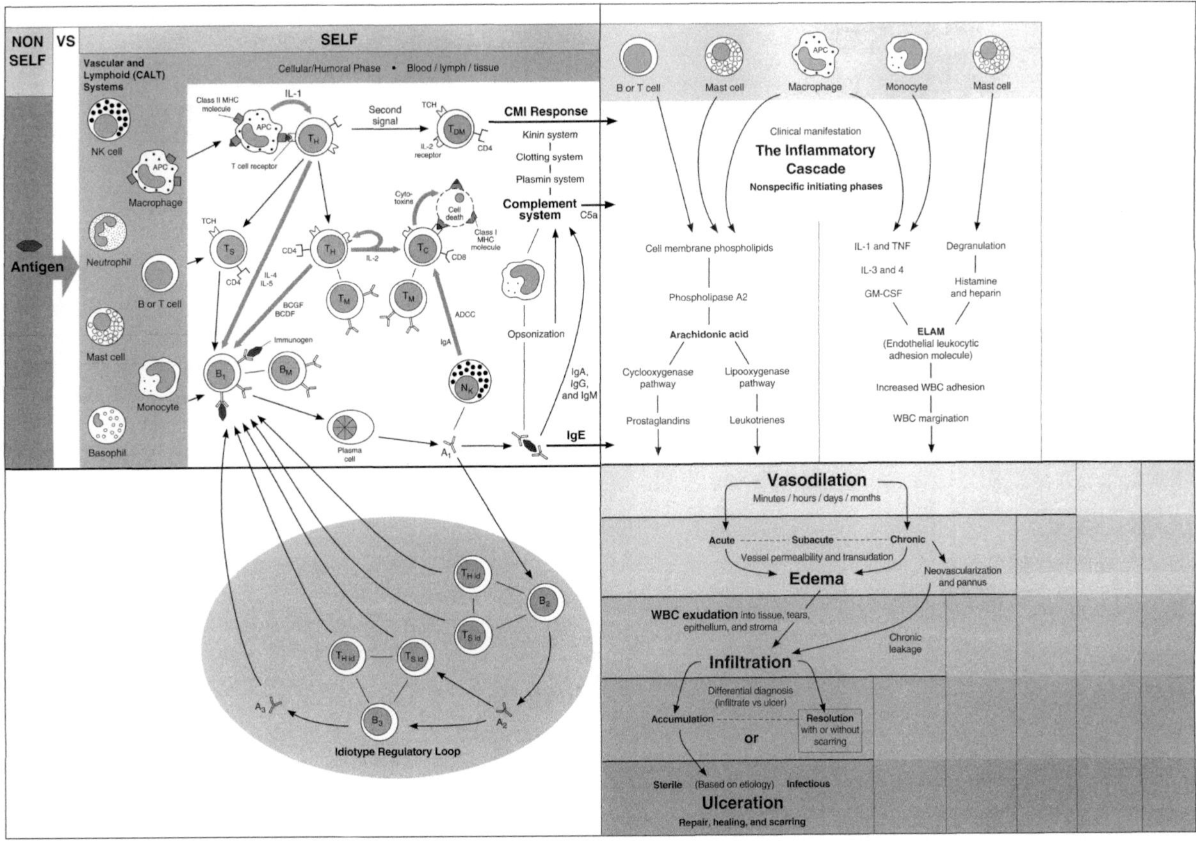

FIGURE 2.28 Inflammatory cascade (ulceration and scarring).

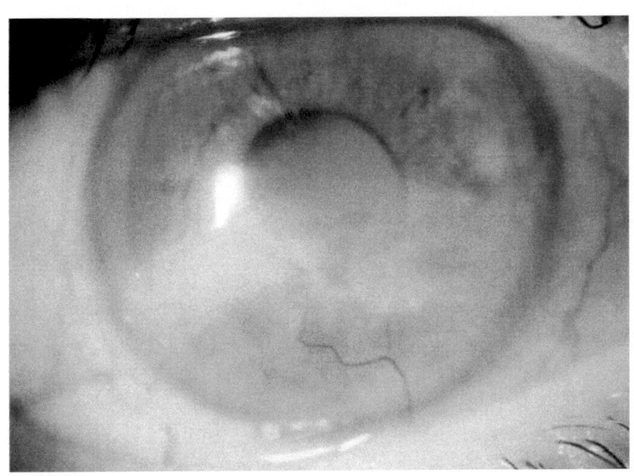

FIGURE 2.29 Stromal ulceration representing the endpoint and destructive portion of the inflammatory cascade leading to corneal neovascularization and scarring.

c. Fibroblasts (myofibroblasts) lay down new elements of structural matrix (connective or granulation tissue) which begin to pull together to produce shrinkage (contraction) and closure of the wound
   i. Collagen fibers
   ii. Elastin
   iii. Proteoglycans (ground substance)
d. Wound healing occurs as a result of the events of the repair process
   i. As fibroblasts multiply and hypertrophy at the edges of each side of a wound, the connective tissue produced begins to migrate into and across the wound gap
   ii. Epithelial cells at the margins (under a cover of dried red blood cells, a scab, in dermal tissue) undergo mitosis and migrate over the wound and replace connective and fibrous tissue
      - This can occur within days
      - Can be delayed by poor circulation to the area, or poor nutrition, and immunosuppression
e. This repair and healing process may leave a visible, raised, or depressed fibrous marking called a scar
   i. Subcutaneous tissue under the scar is completely healed, perhaps stronger than original tissue
   ii. Excessive production of collagen in the dermis during repair may produce a sharply elevated, irregularly shaped, progressively enlarging scar called a keloid (more prominent among Black patients)
f. The overall process of wound healing and scar formation is termed cicatrization; the scar itself is called a cicatrix
g. In mucocutaneous tissue (e.g., corneal stroma) this "remodeling" process (as it is referred to in the cornea) will produce a cosmetically apparent opacification (scar), and functional compromise if in the visual axis

C. Hypersensitivity/Allergic Responses

Hypersensitivity or allergic inflammatory responses have been classically categorized into four "types" following the Coombs-Gell classification

1. ***Type I: Immediate or Anaphylactic Reaction***
   a. Most common ocular reaction
   b. Potential allergens include dust, pollen (seasonal), microbes, and drugs
   c. Allergen attaches to two adjacent IgE molecules on the surface of a mast cell or basophil
   d. T_h and T_s cells modulate reaction, initiating IgE (T_h cells) and regulating its production (T_s cells)
   e. Cell membrane degranulation produces immediate release of preformed vasoactive amines and chemotactic factors for PMNs and lymphocytes
      i. Histamine
      ii. Leukotrienes
      iii. Platelet-activating factor (PAF)
   f. "Early phase" response (within a few minutes to a few hours) is mediated by histamine and leukotrienes (humoral phase), resulting in "immediate" clinical response
      i. Erythema
      ii. Localized edema ("wheal and flare" [hive or welt] formation and pruritis)
      iii. Tearing
      iv. Conjunctival edema (chemosis)
   g. "Late phase" (6 to 12 hours) is mediated by arachidonic acid metabolites (leukotrienes and prostaglandins) and platelet-activating factor (PAF) producing inflammatory cascade (cellular phase) lasting hours to days
      i. Erythema
      ii. Induration (lids)
      iii. Heat and "soreness"
      iv. Burning and itching
   h. Examples of systemic conditions
      i. Hay fever
      ii. Asthma
      iii. Atopic dermatitis
      iv. Allergic urticaria (hives)
      v. Anaphylactic shock

2. ***Type II: Cytotoxic Reaction***
   a. Produced by exogenous (e.g., microbes) or endogenous (e.g., drugs) antigens
   b. IgG, IgM, and complement bind (and opsonize) antigen, which is then phagocytized by macrophages and natural killer cells through the antibody-dependent cellular cytotoxicity (ADCC) reaction
   c. Associated with corneal graft rejection, ocular drug reactions, and Mooren's ulcer
   d. May also have direct relationships to autoimmunity
   e. Example of systemic reactions:
      i. Drug reactions
      ii. Transfusion reactions
      iii. Acute nephritis or endocarditis
      iv. Organ transplant reactions
      v. Autoimmune diseases

3. ***Type III: Immune-Complex Reaction***
   a. Antigens associated are generally diffusible through blood vessels including microbes, ingested food, drugs, and injected toxins (e.g., insect bites, stings)
   b. IgG and IgM activate complement, and when exposed to large amounts of antigen and/or for long durations, can produce large antigen antibody (immune) complexes, which persist in circulation, or smaller immune complexes, which deposit in tissue inducing macrophage and PMN phagocytosis and cellular inflammation (e.g., peripheral corneal diseases)
   c. Small quantities of immune complex are formed normally in the body (secondary to environmental antigens, ingested food, and possibly autoantigens), which are promptly eliminated by the normal functioning mononuclear phagocyte system
   d. Three classic clinical reactions
      i. Rapid onset (12 to 24 hours or less) and short duration (5 to 7 days) "Arthus reaction" caused by excess antibody producing localized tissue inflammation with no vasculitis (e.g., insect sting)
      ii. "Serum sickness" is a more disseminated, systemic, vascular inflammatory response (including fever, lymphadenopathy, and arthralgia) caused by large amount of antigen and beginning over 5 to 7 days and lasting weeks (e.g., penicillin or drug reaction)
      iii. Autoimmune diseases
   e. Generally associated with ocular infiltrative and infectious disease (with Types II and IV)
      i. Marginal infiltrates and ulcers
         - From organism (e.g., Staphylococcus)
         - From sterile exotoxins such as staphylococcal alpha toxin; most common marginal infiltrative keratitis
      ii. Bacterial and fungal corneal ulceration
      iii. Viral infections
         - Herpes simplex virus (HSV)
         - Adenovirus
      iv. Contact lens-related infiltrates
         - Wessely ring phenomenon ("immune ring")
         - White infiltrative ring in corneal stroma
      v. Elicited by any antigen or autoantigen

4. ***Type IV: Cell-Mediated Immunity (CMI) or Delayed-Type Hypersensitivity (DTH) Reaction***
   a. CMI infers protective inflammation whereas DTH infers harm
   b. The principle effector cell is the T (T_{dh}) cell, which functions similarly to the T_h cell in the step-by-step clinical immune matrix described earlier
   c. Antigens are numerous, including foreign substances, topical drugs, and stressors (?), and produce clinical responses over a 24- to 48-hour period
   d. CMI is acquired over time by the buildup of sensitized memory T cells to many antigens
   e. Hallmark clinical manifestation of CMI includes granuloma formation (focal accumulation of inflammatory cells)
   f. A special type of DTH reaction called the cutaneous, basophil type (previously termed Jones-Mote reaction) demonstrates abundant basophils and mast cells activated by antigen-specific T cell factors
      i. This poorly understood type of reaction suggests a "gatekeeper" function of the mast cell in inflammation
      ii. Such a theory blurs the distinctions between the classical Type I and Type IV inflammatory reactions

D. Current Models of Inflammation

Contemporary models choose to eliminate the Type I through IV categories of reactions (due to the strong likelihood of combined and simultaneous reactions) and now use three classes for immunologically induced inflammation

1. *Cell-Mediated Immune (CMI) Response*

a. Predominantly Type IV, delayed-type hypersensitivity (DTH)
b. "Gatekeeper" mast cell and/or basophil participation (cutaneous basophil response) suggests the possibility of combined or simultaneous Type I (IgE-mediated) and Type IV (CMI) responses
   i. Systemic example would include contact dermatitis
   ii. Anterior segment example would include giant papillary conjunctivitis (GPC)
c. Lymphokines (MIF, MAF, IFN, CF, IL-2) activated by T_h cells initiate inflammatory cascade

2. *Antigen-Antibody (Immune) Complex-Mediated Response*

a. Type III, immune-complex response
b. Associations with ocular diseases include particular emphasis on peripheral corneal disease (limbal tissue-based complexes) and recurrent uveitis (vasculitis or aqueous based complexes) termed the Auer reaction
c. Again, concepts of autoimmune responses to tissue and circulating immune complexes suggest the combined and simultaneous activity of antigen–antibody-mediated responses along with classical Type II, cytotoxic reaction CMI, and IgE-mediated responses

3. *IgE-Mediated Response*

a. Type I, immediate or anaphylactic reaction with probable relationships to CMI reactions (and other "type" reactions?) through its direct and indirect mast cell activities
b. "Late phase" causes inflammatory cascade to persist for hours to days resulting in increased potential for clinical confusion (i.e., "immediate" or "early phase") and possible conversion of reaction into secondary responses

III. Clinical Theories on Variable Immunopathological Responses

A. "Most Things Get Better by Themselves"

1. The vast majority (author's guess, greater than 95%) of antigenic stimuli, with or without clinical manifestations, probably get better without awareness of, or practitioner intervention in, the process
2. These events would include each time an antigen comes in contact with or enters the surface, tissue, or cells of the body or the anterior segment
   a. Impossible to determine amount of times
   b. There are believed to be over 100 trillion (100,000,000,000,000 or 1×10^{13}) substances that are antigenic to the body and anterior segment
      i. Nonsubstance (stress) antigenic stimulation can double or triple this number
      ii. Autoimmune theories would justify an argument for an "infinite" number of antigenic stimuli
   c. No way of calculating how many antigenic events occur in each person, each day that do not manifest an observable clinical response
      i. The clinical immune matrix with its regulatory loops usually succeeds in eliminating the antigen
      ii. The cellular/humoral phase is successfully regulated without an inflammatory response or with subclinical activity
   d. Even most clinically manifested events usually get better by themselves
      i. Each time a patient's history includes a subjective or objective finding that they report as self-limiting, one can assume some level of immune response
      ii. Each time we see a clinical variable that we monitor without treatment and observe its disappearance, it probably was immune related
      iii. The three probable reasons why, and causes of most things getting better by themselves, are as follows
         - Antigen self-limits
           – Loses virulence
           – Loses contact with host
         - Antigen is removed
           – By patient (probably most common)
           – By recognition (diagnosis) and action by a clinician (probably less common—sorry!)
         - Successful immune system activity

B. "Sometimes Things Don't Get Better"

1. *Causes*

Although things usually do get better by themselves, approximately less than 5% of the time, something goes wrong.

a. Antigen does not self-limit
b. Antigen is not removed by patient or clinician (no examination or misdiagnosis)
c. Abnormal immune system activity
   i. Allergy and hypersensitivities
   ii. Antigen elimination process dysfunction
      - Suppressor T cell abnormalities
      - Idiotype specific dysregulation
   iii. Suppression of part or whole system
      - Immunodeficiency disorders and diseases (e.g, AIDS)
      - Metabolic, physiologic, and environmental disorders
      - Infection (e.g., HIV, the AIDS virus)
   iv. Regulatory process problems (dysregulation)
      - Hypoactivity of system, causing elimination of problems
      - Hyperactivity of system causing persistence of immune/inflammatory activities
   v. Autoimmune disorders and diseases
   vi. Cancers, which represent a complex of neoplastic antigenicity (autoimmunity), consequences of its immune responses, and corresponding immune system modulation to recognize and control neoplasia

2. *Clinical Theories*

From the above list of causes and reasons why some things don't get better (in anterior segment disease), three relevant clinical theories can be considered for the causes most related to variable clinical responses in anterior segment disease (if not the body at large).

a. The "stress immunogen" theory to address the effects of stress on normal homeostasis (balance of bodily forces) and resultant dysregulation problems in immune system activity

b. The "conversion" theory to address the cause of potential variable clinical outcomes or misdiagnosis
c. The "clinical autoimmune cycle" theory to attempt to address and better understand the concept of autoimmune disorders

3. *The "Stress Immunogen" Theory*

The "stress immunogen" theory proposes that the mechanical and physiological stress factors produced by the inflammatory cascade disrupt normal tissue homeostasis (the equilibrium and stability of bodily forces) resulting in a dysregulation of control mechanisms in the immune system.

a. This theory has long been recognized in other forms of stress, including emotional and psychological
b. Central and peripheral physiological systems provide regulation of homeostasis
   i. Counterregulatory elements to control and self-limit immunopathology can be lost, resulting in a "vicious cycle" of clinical unresponsiveness to therapy
   ii. Imbalances (overactive or underactive) in homeostasis produced by stress can initiate pathophysiological changes in these regulatory systems
c. Overaction (hyperregulation) of the immune system leads to increasing clinical inflammation and potential tissue changes and scarring
   i. Clinically, this produces obvious or persistent subjective and objective signs and symptoms
   ii. Usually causes the patient to seek initial or continuing care
d. Underaction (hyporegulation) of the immune defense system (immunodeficiency) may produce a clinically innocent (e.g., white eye) appearance, but an increased vulnerability to antigen stimulus such as opportunistic microbes, or even otherwise nonpathogenic parasites or synergists
   i. Patient may be without clinical subjective symptoms or objective physical signs
   ii. Such a "preclinical" vulnerable stage without patient (or practitioner) awareness usually results in delayed, late, or acute presentations (frequently for infectious ulcerative care)

4. *The "Conversion" Theory*

The "conversion" theory proposes that all major categories of anterior segment pathological, diagnostic etiologies convert during their clinical course into immunopathologies, thus making each of them a complex form of immunogen to the anterior segment.

a. The three-principle diagnostic etiological categories of anterior segment disease (particularly in primary care) are as follows:
   i. Toxic/immune etiologies
      - These represent the antigenic substances that activate the immune system in the standard, traditionally understood antigenic manner
      - Substances include (but are not limited to):
        - Sterile toxins: proteins, carbohydrates, hydrocarbons, chemicals, and allergens
        - Infectious agents: bacteria, viruses, parasites, fungi, protozoa, and other microbes
   ii. Mechanical etiologies
      - Irritation
      - Injury
      - Environmental factors
        - Pollution
        - Wind
        - Heat
      - Chemicals (really toxins)
   iii. Physiological etiologies
      - Metabolic
        - Congenital
        - Degenerative
      - Nutritional
        - Dystrophic
        - Systemic
      - Biochemical
      - Cellular
        - Metaplasia
        - Neoplasia
b. The conversion theory does not apply to toxic/immune etiologies in that they are, by definition, immunopathologies (Figure 2.30)
c. Mechanical etiologies convert to immunopathology in three possible ways (Figure 2.31)
   i. Prostaglandin E_2 induction
      - Irritation and injury to tissue produce immediate production of prostaglandins which serve as potent vasodilators resulting in rapid clinical hyperemia (redness)
      - Absent of "substance" antigen and the primary steps of the clinical immune matrix, secondary activation of the inflammatory cascade may occur

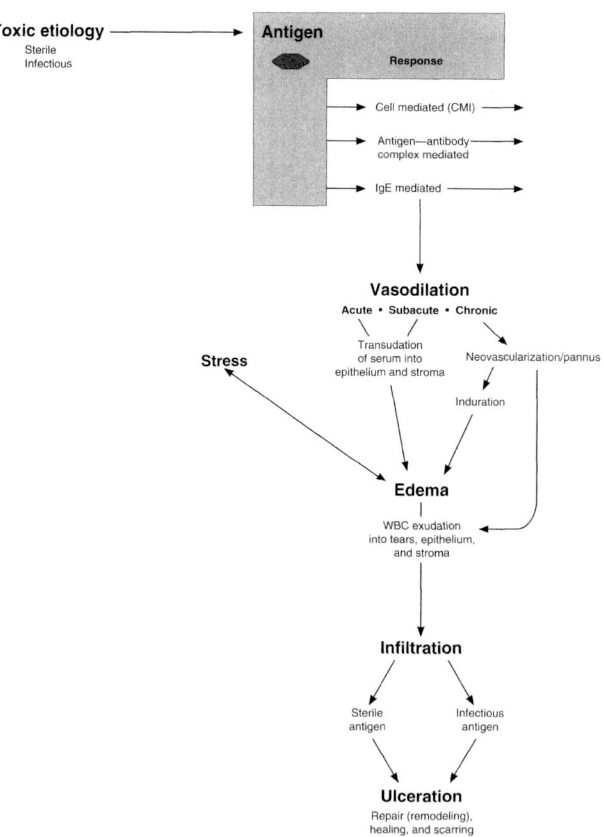

FIGURE 2.30 Toxic etiological stimuli shown in schematic representation.

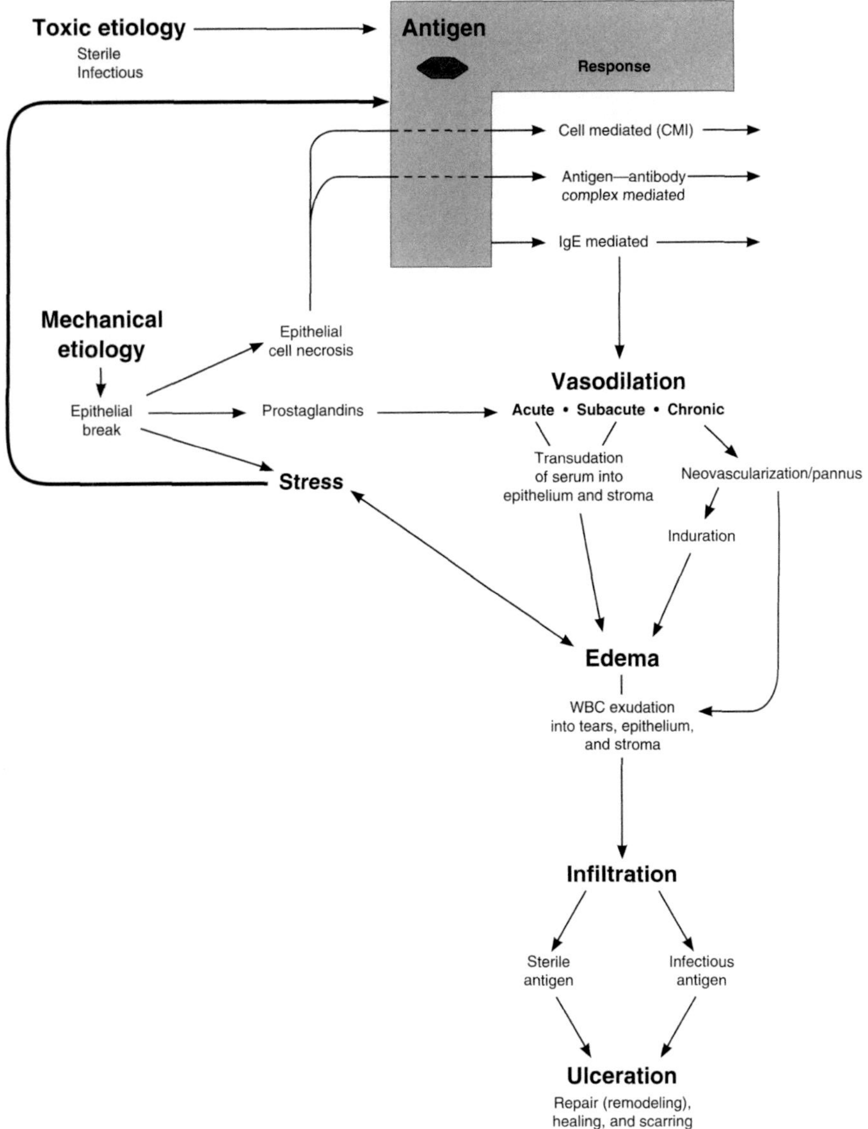

FIGURE 2.31 Mechanical etiological stimuli and conversion effects shown in schematic representation.

- The primary prostaglandin-induced redness is clinically indistinguishable from the vasodilatory (hyperemic) stimulation of the secondarily triggered and continuing immune-driven inflammatory cascade
  - The clinician diagnosing (accurately) and managing a red eye caused by mechanical injury must recognize that on removal of the mechanical cause (removal usually being de facto in injury), persisting hyperemia may be more a product of secondary immune-stimulated inflammation than acute injury-related (prostaglandin-related) vasodilation
  - On certainty of removal of the mechanical cause, management decisions for persisting inflammatory signs and symptoms should be based on immunopathological therapeutic considerations
- Secondary necrotic debris antigen stimulation mechanical irritation or injury to surface tissue and cells produces a destructive process leading to cell death and necrosis
- Necrotic debris is no longer "self" and may be recognized as foreign ("nonself") by the body, which activates an immune response producing a potential immunopathological process
- Persistence of necrotic, toxic debris from the irritation or injury will result in an initiation of the inflammatory cascade, converting the etiology (if not the characteristics) of the clinical red reaction from a mechanical etiology to an immunopathology

ii. Secondary stress immunogen stimulation
  - Mechanical etiologies can be considered as stressors to anterior segment tissue (particularly ocular surface epithelium)
  - These stressors serve as immunogenic activators and may initiate and prolong the inflammatory cascade, producing a persisting clinical red eye, which should be recognized and "rediagnosed" as immunopathological in spite of an

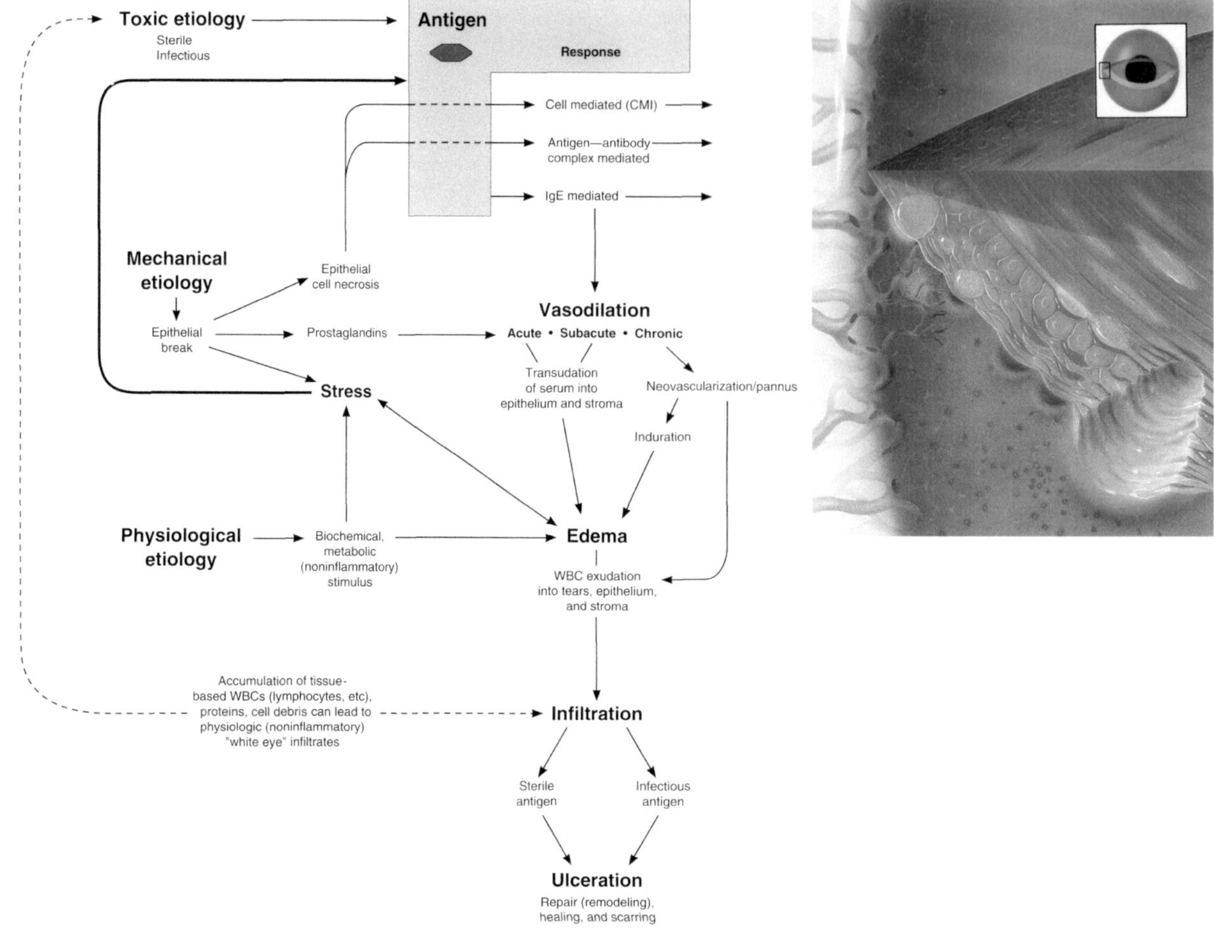

FIGURE 2.32 Physiological etiological stimuli and conversion effects shown in schematic representation.

antecedent, primary mechanical etiology and diagnosis

d. Physiological etiologies convert to immunopathology in four ways (Figure 2.32)
   i. Physiological edema (white eye edema) produces "stress" on normal cell and tissue junctures, thus dysregulating homeostasis and initiating immune-induced inflammatory effects
   ii. Physiological edema provides tissue and cellular "space" for resident tissue lymphocytic WBCs, proteins, cellular debris, and so forth, to begin to accumulate ("nature abhors a vacuum")
      - In the noninflammatory state, these infiltrative elements can accumulate to a visible level in the cornea, referred to as "white eye infiltrates"
      - These accumulations, although "self" in nature, are abnormal in amount and represent abnormal forces being exerted (especially in larger accumulations) on surrounding cells and tissue
         – In such histopathological situations, "self" (e.g., lymphocytic WBCs) may be recognized by the immune system as "non-self" to produce an autoantigen stimulus, leading to an immunopathological response
         – The abnormal forces of this physiologically induced infiltrate in the edematous tissue can also further add to the stress antigenic stimulus
   iii. Whether remaining noninflammatory (as in white eye infiltrates), or on secondary immune/inflammatory stimulation, these accumulations of infiltrative lymphocytes, proteins, cellular debris, and so forth, and their eventual by-products (toxic necrotic debris and enzymes) in noninflammatory, physiological (or inflammatory) edematous tissues could become destructive to the normal surrounding tissue and produce a destructive proteolytic stromal response
      - Termed sterile ulceration
      - An obvious precipitator and component of the inflammatory cascade
      - These physiological (white eye) infiltrates usually progress in a slow, insidious manner
      - Inflammatory (PMN) or red eye infiltrates have more potential to more rapidly progress to ulceration due to the increased virulence of phagocytic PMN WBCs (foreign to avascular tissue) versus nonphagocytic lymphocytic WBCs resident and normal to avascular tissue
   iv. The classical biochemical imbalances associated with physiological edematous environments in tissues (lactate buildup, glycogen deprivation, etc.) may also play a role in the conversion of physiological etiologies into immunopathologies
      - Chemical accumulations could effectively function as both "self" or autoantigens (produced by the body) as well as "non-self" antigenic toxins

- Also, chemical imbalances in the tissue, again relate directly to a dysregulation in homeostasis

e. The clinical sum total of the "conversion" theory can be simply stated:
   i. A diagnosis of mechanical or physiological etiology should improve rapidly with removal of the cause and appropriate supportive therapies
   ii. Prolonged, delayed, or resistant resolution of a properly diagnosed mechanical or physiological etiology, after definitive removal of the cause, may be considered a condition that has converted into a secondary immunopathology that should effectively become the new working diagnosis

f. The clinical conclusion of this theory (along with consideration of the other two theories discussed) presents two interesting clinical diagnostic and management premises for primary care of the anterior segment (and perhaps beyond?)
   i. All clinical conditions can be considered either primary or secondary immunopathologies
   ii. Many clinical conditions, especially those which don't improve with removal of the cause and/or standard therapies, should be considered as probable autoimmune disorders

5. *The "Clinical Autoimmune Cycle" Theory*

The "clinical autoimmune cycle" theory proposes that substances and stress factors produced by the inflammatory cascade itself, provide autoantigenic stimuli creating a self-sustaining clinical cycle of autoimmune responses.

a. Such a cycle can occur in the presence or absence (on removal) of the primary inciting antigenic source
b. Risk of development and the degree of intensity of the resultant clinical response would be directly proportional to the duration of the primary antigenic stimulus
c. The inflammatory cascade, in spite of its protective and reparative functions, also produces a series of potential negative effects including the classical adverse clinical reactions previously described and some histopathophysiological, antigenic/immunogenic (or autoantigenic/autoimmunogenic) effects just beginning to be better understood (Figure 2.33)
   i. Substances produced that can act as autoimmunogens
      - Necrotic debris from antigen destruction by the immune response
      - Debris from the destruction of normal tissue by polymorphonuclear WBCs, macrophages, and even lymphocytes
      - Excess amounts of circulating and focal inflammatory/infiltrative WBCs in the tissue
      - Enzymes and necrotic debris from dying WBCs in the tissue
   ii. Stress and dysregulation of homeostasis
      - Physiological stress factors
        - From edema disruption of intracellular and intercellular forces
        - From imbalances in tissue hemodynamics
      - Mechanical stress factors
        - Breaks in cell junctures from inflammatory edema

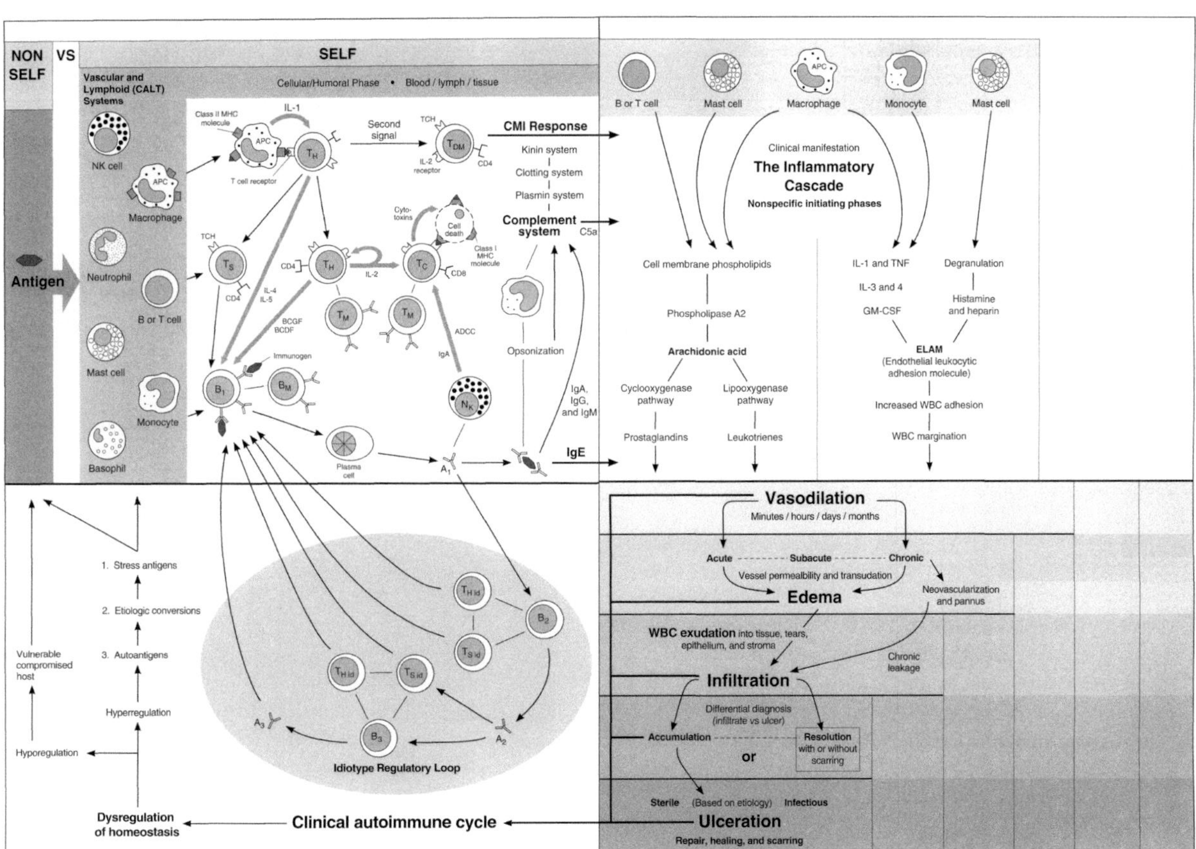

FIGURE 2.33 Autoimmune cycle, clinical immune matrix.

  - Increase vector forces in tissue at sites of focal accumulations of inflammatory/infiltrative WBCs

d. The effects of these immunogenic (autoimmunogenic) stimuli can thus initiate a self-sustaining cycle of clinical immunopathological events
   i. Potentially increasing magnitude (virtually exponential in potential), resulting in a worsening acute inflammatory condition
   ii. Thus, this autoimmune cycle can produce a clinical condition that, even with successful removal of the primary diagnostic etiology, can continue to deteriorate unless recognized and rediagnosed as a secondary immunopathology

IV. Clinicoimmunopathological Diagnosis of Anterior Segment Disease

A. Anatomical Perspective

Classical education teaches disease diagnosis strictly from an anatomical perspective.

1. It works very well, especially for the busy clinical practitioner
2. It is comfortable, efficient, and generally a comprehensive approach
   a. In diagnostic care, comprehensive equals safe
   b. A comprehensive diagnostic workup covers all possibilities so that the specific condition in question (definitive diagnosis) will not be omitted nor mismanaged

B. Immunopathological Basis

Our growing understanding of the immunopathological basis of disease now gives us a system that proves to be equally comfortable and efficient, while more comprehensive (safer) in diagnostic assessment than the classical anatomical approach.

1. Results of a clinicoimmunopathological workup of anterior segment disease (or any category) may not yield a higher degree of accurate definitive diagnoses
2. It will, however, produce a significantly lower percentage of failures to diagnose, or misdiagnoses (two leading causes of professional liability)
3. This value in the system is achieved by allowing the clinician to narrow the assessment of a condition to a general pathological category through recognition of its set of clinically observable findings, as well as the ruling out of other general pathological categories through the lack of their relatively identifiable clinical characteristics
4. The clinician can now establish a general pathological category, a category within which the definitive diagnosis must fall, even though the clinician may not have established the disease's specific etiology or "label"
   a. Toxic/immune category
   b. Mechanical category
   c. Physiological category
5. Treatment and management decisions become safer within the diagnostic, categorical framework established for the pathological (not specific disease) entity in the chain
   a. Safe categorical management steps can be administered until a definitive diagnosis is established (if ever)
   b. These safe management regimes are the established and accepted approaches developed by clinical experts and documented in the literature and textbooks

C. Clinicoimmunopathological Categories

Table 2.1 lists the clinicoimmunopathological categories by traditional clinical diagnostic criteria (subjective and objective findings), so practitioners can become comfortable with their use in a diagnostic workup and clinical care.

D. Anterior Segment Care by Clinicoimmunopathological Categories

Table 2.2 lists the traditional clinical criteria by clinicoimmunopathological categories, so an interested practitioner can begin to "think categories" in his or her day-to-day diagnostic and management decision-making.

E. Summary

In summary, primary care of the anterior segment centers around three comprehensive clinicoimmunopathological diagnostic categories (Table 2.3). The three categories are reflected in the structure of Chapters 3 through 6:

1. *Irritations and injuries*, usually determined through history and symptoms
2. *Noninflammatory conditions* (of varying etiologies), determined clinically by the relative absence of redness (the initial clinical phase of inflammation-vasodilation or "rubor")
   a. This category includes all pathologies except infection, inflammation, and injury
      ii. Congenital/developmental abnormalities
      iii. Degeneration
      iv. Dystrophy
      v. Environmental or external elements
      vi. Metabolic processes
      vii. Metaplasia
      viii. Neoplasia
      ix. Nutritional factors
      x. Physiological factors
      xi. Systemic manifestations
   b. Most are subacute or chronic
   c. Rarely imminently eye- or sight-threatening
   d. Immediate definitive diagnosis is usually not critical
3. *Inflammatory conditions*
   a. Red eyes
   b. Definitive etiological diagnosis
      i. Toxic
         - Sterile
         - Infectious
      ii. Physiological
      iii. Mechanical
      iv. "Autoimmune cycle"
   c. A "label" is not critical
   d. The critical consideration is establishing a differential diagnosis:
      i. What is the etiological category?
      ii. If it is a toxic etiology, is it sterile or infectious?
      iii. Is it an infiltrate or an ulcer?
      iv. Has the cause (antigen) been removed?

TABLE 2.1 Diagnosing Clinicoimmunopathological Categories in Anterior Segment Disorders by Standard Clinical Examination Criteria

Subjective Examination
(History and symptoms)

1. Allergy/hypersensitivity
   History: previous episodes
   Symptoms: itching, burning, soreness
2. Congenital/developmental abnormalities
   History: since birth or childhood
   Symptoms: "FLK" (funny-looking kid)
3. Degeneration
   History: usually secondary to aging
   Symptoms: none or secondary complications
4. Dystrophy
   History: developed during childhood
   Symptoms: none or complications
5. Environmental
   History: exposure
   Symptoms: frequently allergic
6. Infection
   History: risk factors for infection
   Symptoms: usually inflammatory pain
7. Inflammation
   History: immunogenic stimulus
   Symptoms: pain
8. Injury
   History: abrasion, burn, contusion, laceration
   Symptoms: pain, loss of function
9. Metabolic
   History: medical or family history
   Symptoms: varies with involvement
10. Metaplasia
    History: anomalous tissue growth
    Symptoms: varies with involvement
11. Neoplasia
    History: anomalous tissue growth
    Symptoms: varies with involvement
12. Neurological
    History: congenital or acquired
    Symptoms: motor or sensory
13. Nutritional
    History: usually dietary
    Symptoms: secondary irritations (e.g., dry eye)
14. Systemic manifestation
    History: positive medical or family
    Symptoms: related to primary system and secondary manifestation

Objective Examination
(Physical findings by anatomical structure)

1. Eyelids/adnexa
   a. Allergy/hypersensitivity
      i. Erythema ("rubor")
      ii. Edema ("tumor")
   b. Congenital/developmental abnormalities
      i. Coloboma
      ii. Blepharoptosis
   c. Degeneration
      i. Blepharochalasis
      ii. Keratoses
   d. Environmental
      i. Contact allergy
      ii. Injury
   e. Infection
      i. Purulent discharge
      ii. Inflammation
   f. Inflammation
      i. Dramatic swelling (edema) in acute forms
      ii. Hardening (induration) in chronic forms
   g. Injury
      i. Ecchymosis (intracellular hemorrhage)
      ii. Blowout fracture (of orbital floor)
   h. Metaplasia
      i. Hyperplasia (papilloma)
      ii. Cysts (sudoriferous, sebaceous)
      i. Neoplasia
      i. Basal cell carcinoma
      ii. Others
   j. Neurological
      i. Blepharoptosis
      ii. Blepharospasm
2. Lacrimal system
   a. Congenital/developmental abnormalities
      i. Dacryostenosis
      ii. Dacryocystitis
   b. Degeneration
      i. Lid/punctal ectropion
      ii. Punctal atresia
   c. Environmental
      i. Mechanical blockage of puncta
      ii. Mechanical blockage of canaliculi
   d. Infection
      i. Dacryocystitis
      ii. Dacryoadenitis
   e. Inflammation
      i. From infection
      ii. Secondary to blockage
   f. Injury
      i. Laceration
      ii. Punctal obliteration
   g. Neoplasia
      i. Bloody tears
      ii. Metastatic
   h. Systemic manifestations
      i. Dacryoadenitis
      ii. Mikulicz's syndrome
3. Conjunctiva
   a. Allergy/hypersensitivity
      i. Mucoid discharge
      ii. Chemosis (edema)
   b. Congenital/developmental abnormalities
      i. Dermoids
      ii. Pigmentation
   c. Degeneration
      i. Pinguecula
      ii. Calcification
   d. Environmental
      i. Ultraviolet irritation
      ii. Foreign body
   e. Infection
      i. Discharge
      ii. Inflammation (conjunctivitis)
      f. Inflammation
      i. Hyperemia (papillae)
      ii. Follicles (infiltration)
   g. Injury
      i. Laceration
      ii. Subconjunctival hemorrhage
   h. Metaplasia
      i. Squamous epithelial cell (in severe dry eye)
      ii. Hyperplasia (papilloma)
   i. Neoplasia
      i. Carcinoma
      ii. Kaposi sarcoma (in AIDS)

(*Continued*)

TABLE 2.1 (CONTINUED) Diagnosing Clinicoimmunopathological Categories in Anterior Segment Disorders by Standard Clinical Examination Criteria

j. Nutritional
  i. Vitamin A deficiency (dry eye)
  ii. Xerophthalmia
k. Systemic manifestations
  i. Roth spots (in anemias)
  ii. Hypoxia (in occlusive vascular disease)
4. Sclera/episclera
  a. Congenital/developmental abnormalities
    i. Melanosis
    ii. Blue sclera
  b. Degeneration
    i. Scleromalacia
    ii. Scleral thinning (staphyloma)
  c. Inflammation
    i. Episcleritis
    ii. Scleritis
  d. Injury
    i. Penetration
    ii. Perforation
  e. Systemic manifestations
    i. Icteric sclera (jaundice)
    ii. Collagen vascular diseases
5. Cornea
  a. Congenital/developmental abnormalities
    i. Micro/megalocornea
    ii. Rubella
  b. Degeneration
    i. Arcus senilis
    ii. Marginal furrowing
  c. Dystrophy
    i. Epithelial/endothelial
    ii. Stromal
  d. Environmental
    i. Exposure keratitis
    ii. Keratoconjunctivitis sicca
  e. Infection
    i. Gram-positive (especially Staphyloccus)
    ii. Gram-negative (especially Pseudomonas)
  f. Inflammation
    i. Sterile
    ii. Infectious
  g. Injury
    i. Epithelial
    ii. Stromal
  h. Metabolic
    i. Mucopolysaccharidosis
    ii. Amyloidosis
    i. Nutritional
    i. Vitamin deficiencies
    ii. Liver disease
  j. Systemic manifestations
    i. Venereal diseases
    ii. Hyperlipidemias
6. Anterior angle and ciliary body
  a. Congenital/developmental abnormalities
    i. Axenfeld–Rieger (A–R) syndromes
    ii. Narrow angles
  b. Inflammation
    i. Neovascularization
    ii. Cyclitis
  c. Injury
    i. Angle recession
    ii. Hyphema
7. Anterior chamber and aqueous
  a. Infection
    i. Hypopyon
    ii. Herpes simplex virus (HSV)
  b. Inflammation
    i. Acute anterior uveitis (AAU)
    ii. Anterior chamber associated immune deviation (ACAID) response
  c. Injury
    i. Traumatic uveitis
    ii. Hyphema
  d. Systemic manifestations
    i. Recurrent uveitis
    ii. Chronic uveitis
8. Iris
  a. Congenital/developmental abnormalities
    i. Iridocorneal endothelial (ICE) syndromes
    ii. Aniridia
  b. Degeneration
    i. Iris atrophy
    ii. Iridoschisis
  c. Inflammation
    i. Iritis
    ii. Iridocyclitis
  d. Injury
    i. Rupture of iris root (iridodialysis)
    ii. Rupture of the sphincter pupillae muscle
  e. Metaplasia
    i. Brusfeld's spots
    ii. Nevi
  f. Neoplasia
    i. Primary
    ii. Metastatic
  g. Neurological
    i. Adie's tonic pupil
    ii. Pupil abnormalities
  h. Systemic manifestations
    i. Albinism
    ii. Diabetes mellitus (rubeosis iridis)
9. Crystalline lens
  a. Congenital/developmental abnormalities
    i. Congenital/developmental cataract
    ii. Down syndrome
  b. Environmental
    i. Ultraviolet radiation
    ii. Injury
  c. Injury
    i. Traumatic cataract
    ii. Luxation
  d. Metabolic
    i. Homocystinuria
    ii. Turner's syndrome
  e. Nutritional
    i. Hypervitaminosis
    ii. Galactosemia
  f. Systemic manifestations
    i. Endocrine disorders
    ii. Multiple syndromes

TABLE 2.2 Anterior Segment Care by Clinicoimmunopathological Categories

Allergy/Hypersensitivity

1. Subjective (history and symptoms)
   History: previous episodes
   Symptoms: itching, burning, soreness
2. Objective (physical findings by anatomical structure)
   a. Eyelids/adnexa
      i. Erythema ("rubor")
      ii. Edema ("tumor")
   b. Lacrimal system: usually not involved
   c. Conjunctiva
      i. Mucoid discharge
      ii. Chemosis (edema)
   d. Sclera/episdera: usually not involved
   e. Cornea: see text at II., "Inflammation"
   f. Anterior angle and ciliary body: usually not involved
   g. Anterior chamber and aqueous: see text at II., "Inflammation"
   h. Iris: usually not involved
   i. Crystalline lens: usually not involved

Congenital/Developmental Abnormalities

1. Subjective (history and symptoms)
   History: since birth or childhood
   Symptoms: "FLK" (funny-looking kid)
2. Objective (physical findings by anatomical structure, with clinical examples)
   a. Eyelids/adnexa
      i. Coloboma
      ii. Blepharoptosis
   b. Lacrimal system
      i. Dacryostenosis
      ii. Dacryocystitis
   c. Conjunctiva
      i. Dermoids
      ii. Pigmentation
   d. Sclera/episclera
      i. Melanosis
      ii. Blue sclera
   e. Cornea
      i. Micro/megalocornea
      ii. Rubella
   f. Anterior angle and ciliary body
      i. Axenfeld–Rieger (A–R) syndromes
      ii. Narrow angles
   g. Anterior chamber and aqueous: usually not involved
   h. Iris
      i. Iridocorneal endothelial (ICE) syndromes
      ii. Aniridia
   i. Crystalline lens
      i. Congenital/developmental cataract
      ii. Down syndrome

Degeneration

1. Subjective (history and symptoms)
   History: usually secondary to aging
   Symptoms: none or secondary complications
2. Objective (physical findings by anatomical structure, with clinical examples)
   a. Eyelids/adnexa
      i. Blepharochalasis
      ii. Keratoses
   b. Lacrimal system
      i. Lid/punctal ectropion
      ii. Punctal atresia
   c. Conjunctiva
      i. Pinguecula
      ii. Calcification
   d. Sclera/episclera
      i. Scleromalacia
      ii. Scleral thinning (staphyloma)
   e. Cornea
      i. Arcus senilis
      ii. Marginal furrowing
   f. Anterior angle and ciliary body: usually not involved
   g. Anterior chamber and aqueous: usually not involved
   h. Iris
   i. Iris atrophy
      ii. Iridoschisis
      i. Crystalline lens: usually not involved

Dystrophy

1. Subjective (history and symptoms)
   History: developed during childhood
   Symptoms: none or complications
2. Objective (physical findings by anatomical structure, with clinicalexamples)
   a. Eyelids/adnexa: usually not involved
   b. Lacrimal system: usually not involved
   c. Conjunctiva: usually not involved
   d. Sclera/episclera: usually not involved
   e. Cornea
      i. Epithelial/endothelial
      ii. Stromal
   f. Anterior angle and ciliary body: usually not involved
   g. Anterior chamber and aqueous: usually not involved
   h. Iris: usually not involved
   i. Crystalline lens: usually not involved

Environmental

1. Subjective (history and symptoms)
   History: exposure
   Symptoms: frequently allergic
2. Objective (physical findings by anatomical structure, with clinical examples)
   a. Eyelids/adnexa
      i. Contact allergy
      ii. Injury
   b. Lacrimal system
      i. Mechanical blockage of puncta
      ii. Mechanical blockage of canaliculi
   c. Conjunctiva
      i. Ultraviolet irritation
      ii. Foreign body
   d. Sclera/episclera: usually not involved
   e. Cornea
      i. Exposure keratitis
      ii. Keratoconjunctivitis sicca
   f. Anterior angle and ciliary body: usually not involved
   g. Anterior chamber and aqueous: usually not involved
   h. Iris: usually not involved
   i. Crystalline lens
      i. Ultraviolet radiation
      ii. Injury

Infection

1. Subjective (history and symptoms)
   History: risk factors for infection
   Symptoms: usually inflammatory pain
2. Objective (physical findings by anatomical structure, with clinical examples)
   a. Eyelids/adnexa
      i. Discharge
      ii. Inflammation
   b. Lacrimal system
      i. Dacryocystitis
      ii. Dacryoadenitis
   c. Conjunctiva
      i. Discharge
      ii. Inflammation (conjunctivitis)
   d. Sclera/episclera: usually not involved

(*Continued*)

TABLE 2.2 (CONTINUED) Anterior Segment Care by Clinicoimmunopathological Categories

e. Cornea
  i. Gram-positive (especially Staphyloccus)
  ii. Gram negative (especially Pseudomonas)
f. Anterior angle and ciliary body: usually not involved
g. Anterior chamber and aqueous
  i. Hypopyon
  ii. Herpes simplex virus (HSV)
h. Iris: none
i. Crystalline lens: usually not involved

Inflammation

1. Subjective (history and symptoms)
   History: immunogenic stimulus
   Symptoms: pain
2. Objective (physical findings by anatomical structure, with clinical examples)
   a. Eyelids/adnexa
      i. Dramatic swelling (edema) in acute forms
      ii. Hardening (induration) in chronic forms
   b. Lacrimal system
      i. From infection
      ii. Secondary to blockage
   c. Conjunctiva
      i. Hyperemia (papillae)
      ii. Follicles (infiltration)
   d. Sclera/episclera
      i. Episcleritis
      ii. Scleritis
   e. Cornea
      i. Sterile
      ii. Infectious
   f. Anterior angle and ciliary body
      i. Neovascularization
      ii. Cyclitis
   g. Anterior chamber and aqueous
      i. Acute anterior uveitis (AAU)
      ii. Anterior chamber associated immune deviation (ACAID) response
   h. Iris
      i. Iritis
      ii. Iridocyclitis
   i. Crystalline lens: usually not involved

Injury

1. Subjective (history and symptoms)
   History: abrasion, burn, contusion, laceration
   Symptoms: pain, loss of function
2. Objective (physical findings by anatomical structure, with clinical examples)
   a. Eyelids/adnexa
      i. Ecchymosis (intracellular hemorrhage)
      ii. Blowout fracture (of orbital floor)
   b. Lacrimal system
      i. Laceration
      ii. Punctal obliteration
   c. Conjunctiva
      i. Laceration
      ii. Subconjunctival hemorrhage
   d. Sclera/episclera
      i. Penetration
      ii. Perforation
   e. Cornea
      i. Epithelial
      ii. Stromal
   f. Anterior angle and ciliary body
      i. Angle recession
      ii. Hyphema
   g. Anterior chamber and aqueous
      i. Traumatic uveitis
      ii. Hyphema
   h. Iris
      i. Rupture of iris root (iridodialysis)
      ii. Rupture of the sphincter pupillae muscle
   i. Crystalline lens
      i. Traumatic cataract
      ii. Luxation

Metabolic

1. Subjective (history and symptoms)
   History: medical or family history
   Symptoms: varies with involvement
2. Objective (physical findings by anatomical structure, with clinical examples)
   a. Eyelids/adnexa: usually not involved
   b. Lacrimal system: usually not involved
   c. Conjunctiva: usually not involved
   d. Sclera/episclera: usually not involved
   e. Cornea
      i. Mucopolysaccharidosis
      ii. Amyloidosis
   f. Anterior angle and ciliary body: usually not involved
   g. Anterior chamber and aqueous: usually not involved
   h. Iris: usually not involved
   i. Crystalline lens
      i. Homocystinuria
      ii. Turner's syndrome

Metaplasia

1. Subjective (history and symptoms)
   History: anomalous tissue growth
   Symptoms: varies with involvement
2. Objective (physical findings by anatomical structure, with clinical examples)
   a. Eyelids/adnexa
      i. Hyperplasia (papilloma)
      ii. Cysts (sudoriferous, sebaceous)
   b. Lacrimal system: usually not involved
   c. Conjunctiva
      i. Squamous epithelial cell (in severe dry eye)
      ii. Hyperplasia (papilloma)
   d. Sclera/episclera: usually not involved
   e. Cornea: usually not involved
   f. Anterior angle and ciliary body: usually not involved
   g. Anterior chamber and aqueous: usually not involved
   h. Iris
      i. Brushfeld's spots
      ii. Nevi
   i. Crystalline lens: usually not involved

Neoplasia

1. Subjective (history and symptoms)
   History: anomalous tissue growth
   Symptoms: varies with involvement
2. Objective (physical findings by anatomical structure, with clinical examples)
   a. Eyelids/adnexa
      i. Basal cell carcinoma
      ii. Others
   b. Lacrimal system
      i. Bloody tears
      ii. Metastasis
   c. Conjunctiva
      i. Carcinoma
      ii. Kaposi sarcoma (in AIDS)
   d. Sclera/episclera: usually not involved
   e. Cornea: usually not involved
   f. Anterior angle and ciliary body: usually not involved
   g. Anterior chamber and aqueous: usually not involved
   h. Iris
      i. Primary
      ii. Metastasis
   i. Crystalline lens: usually not involved

(Continued)

TABLE 2.2 (CONTINUED) Anterior Segment Care by Clinicoimmunopathological Categories

Neurological

1. Subjective (history and symptoms)
   History: congenital or acquired
   Symptoms: motor or sensory
2. Objective (physical findings by anatomical structure, with clinical examples)
   a. Eyelids/adnexa
      i. Blepharoptosis
      ii. Blepharospasm
   b. Lacrimal system: usually not involved
   c. Conjunctiva: usually not involved
   d. Sclera/episclera: usually not involved
   e. Cornea: usually not involved
   f. Anterior angle and ciliary body: usually not involved
   g. Anterior chamber and aqueous: usually not involved
   h. Iris
      i. Adie's tonic pupil
      ii. Pupil anomalies
   i. Crystalline lens: usually not involved

Nutritional

1. Subjective (history and symptoms)
   History: usually dietary
   Symptoms: secondary irritations (e.g., dry eye)
2. Objective (physical findings by anatomical structure, with clinical examples)
   a. Eyelids/adnexa: usually not involved
   b. Lacrimal system: usually not involved
   c. Conjunctiva
      i. Vitamin A deficiency (dry eye)
      ii. Xerophthalmia
   d. Sclera/episclera: usually not involved
   e. Cornea
      i. Vitamin deficiencies
      ii. Liver disease
   f. Anterior angle and ciliary body: usually not involved
   g. Anterior chamber and aqueous: usually not involved
   h. Iris: usually not involved
   i. Crystalline lens
      i. Hypervitaminosis
      ii. Galactosemia

Systemic Manifestations

1. Subjective (history and symptoms)
   History: positive medical or family
   Symptoms: related to primary system and secondary manifestation
2. Objective (physical findings by anatomical structure, with clinical examples)
   a. Eyelids/adnexa: usually not involved
   b. Lacrimal system
      i. Dacryoadenitis
      ii. Mikulicz's syndrome
   c. Conjunctiva
      i. Roth spots (in anemias)
      ii. Hypoxia (in occlusive vascular disease)
   d. Sclera/episclera
      i. Icteric sclera
      ii. Collagen vascular diseases
   e. Cornea
      i. Venereal diseases
      ii. Hyperlipidemias
   f. Anterior angle and ciliary body: usually not involved
   g. Anterior chamber and aqueous: usually not involved
   h. Iris
      i. Albinism
      ii. Diabetes mellitus (rubeosis iridis)
   i. Crystalline lens
      i. Endocrine disorders
      ii. Multiple syndromes

TABLE 2.3 Differential Diagnosis of Anterior Segment Conditions by Three Pathological Categories

Irritations and injuries
- Abrasions
- Burns
- Contusion or concussion (blunt)
- Foreign bodies
- Lacerations

Noninflammatory conditions: White eyes
- Congenital/developmental abnormalities
- Degeneration
- Dystrophy
- Environmental or external elements
- Metabolic processes
- Metaplasia
- Neoplasia
- Nutritional factors
- Physiological factors
- Systemic manifestations

Inflammatory conditions ("itis"): Red eyes
- Toxic
  - Sterile
  - Infectious
- Physiological
- Mechanical
- "Autoimmune cycle"

Conversion (Stress) [bracket linking Irritations and injuries to Mechanical]

Conversion (Autoantigen or stress) [bracket linking Physiological factors to Physiological]

V. Clinicoimmunopathological Considerations in Managing Anterior Segment Disease

A. General Principles

1. Remove the cause (the antigen or immunogen)
   a. The overriding consideration in all therapy is to identify and understand the nature of the problem, and then to remove the problem
      i. Identification of the problem equals diagnosis, the clinician's primary and most important duty (and the primary objective of this book)
      ii. Understanding the problem includes the knowledge of what is normal, and what is abnormal—the reason for professional and continuing education (and the primary reason for this chapter)
   b. Removal of the cause in a health-related problem is tantamount to its cure
      i. All other treatment and management approaches are to protect and defend the host against damage, to support the host through a pathological process (supportive therapy), and to attempt to relieve discomfort associated with a pathological process (palliative therapy)
      ii. Curative therapy can only be considered removal of the cause, or prevention (preventive therapy)
   c. Conscientious care throughout the management of disease should always include reassessment of cause, and continued concern and consideration of its successful elimination, especially in conditions that are not responding appropriately
   d. No therapeutic measures should ever be introduced, added, or adjusted in a management plan without reassessing the cause (diagnosis) of the disorder and all available attempts at its removal
      i. Without such a philosophy of disease management, measures to defend, support, and/or relieve pain may be counterproductive and harmful
      ii. The most significant example of such counterproductive effects includes management or suppression of the apparent adverse clinical effects of immune system activity and inflammation
         - Though such effects may appear to distress the patient, those same effects are attempting to remove the cause of the disease—sometimes the most potent and/or the only effort being conducted in the body
         - Suppression of such intrinsic bodily defenses and elimination efforts, without successful clinical removal of the cause, could result in significantly more damage than the secondary adverse effects the immune system might have produced
2. Removal of the cause in anterior segment disease includes three primary approaches:
   a. Diagnosis
   b. Nonpharmacological measures
   c. Pharmacological therapies
3. The balance of this book will provide specifics in each of these three areas for anterior segment disorders common to primary eye care practitioners
   a. A brief listing below outlines the general, accepted nonpharmacological and pharmacological measures used in primary care of the anterior segment
   b. These common therapeutic measures are also clinically correlated to the pathological processes described in this chapter, with an emphasis on the inflammatory process due to its significance in anterior segment care

B. General Nonpharmacological Measures

1. Prevention
2. Hygiene (preventive therapy)
   a. Lid wipes (e.g., anti-staphylococcal therapy)
   b. Irrigation of the ocular surface
      i. To flush out immunogens
      ii. To dilute antigenicity
      iii. To neutralize toxins
      iv. To remove necrotic and/or inflammatory debris
3. Lubrication of ocular surface with artificial tear preparations (non-preserved) or other lubricating agents (e.g., ointments, gels, hydrophilic lens materials, lipids, hyaluronidase) that can enhance or substitute for tear film elements or serve as a mucomimetic agent mimicking the functions of the mucin layer of the tears (supportive/palliative therapy)
   a. To protect the ocular and corneal surface from antigenic attack
   b. To soothe the corneal epithelium from mechanical irritation (and resultant prostaglandin production)
4. Warm or cold application to tissue or structure (supportive/palliative therapy)
   a. Heat
      i. Vasodilates and thus is used to enhance circulation and blood-borne elements in and to vascularized tissues and organs where increased blood supply (and WBCs) would be an asset, or of assistance, in eliminating an antigen
      ii. Dehydrates tissue and can be used to remove (noninflammatory) edema when its cause is physiologic and/or its cause cannot be removed (e.g., dystrophy, degeneration, blunt injury)
   b. Cold
      i. Vasoconstricts and thus can be used to reduce circulation, bleeding, volume of blood, and blood-borne elements to vascular tissue, and avascular tissue into which blood and its elements may permeate in certain pathological states (e.g., inflammation)
      ii. Whereas cold does not dehydrate as heat does, its vasoconstrictive effects reduce vessel wall permeability and thus reduce resultant inflammatory edema (versus physiological edema) and its sequelae (edema and infiltration)
      iii. Other therapeutic benefits of cold
         - Reduces inflammatory edema and WBC exudation (infiltration)
         - Cools ocular surface (diminishing favorable environment for infectious microbes)
         - Decreases lactate accumulation in tissue

- Reduces clinical effects of the inflammatory cascade ("rubor, calor, dolor, and tumor")

5. Nutritional therapies (preventive therapy)
   a. Dietary considerations
   b. Vitamin and mineral supplementation
      i. Topical and oral considerations
      ii. Significant research is being conducted in this area with strong indications of unrecognized relationships in numerous pathological and immune responses
6. Environmental (preventive therapy)
   a. Primarily prevention and industrial safety
   b. Environmental protection
      i. Earth and elements
      ii. Air and atmosphere
   c. Ultraviolet radiation has been recognized as a potent environmental immunogen requiring our serious concern for the future of our air and atmosphere
7. Patient counseling and education (preventive therapy)
   a. Genetic counseling (e.g., dystrophies, systemic manifestations) provided or referred to a consultant
   b. Education on prevention may be the most valuable service a clinician can offer patients (before the fact!)
8. Future nonpharmacological therapies
   a. Therapeutic lasers (curative therapy)
   b. Molecular biology and genetic therapies (preventive therapy)
      i. Science can map the genes of the body to determine the causes of pathologies and diseases, and correct the problems before they manifest clinically
      ii. Progress in this field has led one of this book's authors (Lou Catania) to write a book on the advances in molecular biology, immunology, and genetic therapies developed since the second edition of this book. Catania's new book is *The Paradox of the Immune System* (Elsevier, 2023; ISBN 9780323951876)

C. General Pharmacological Anterior Segment Measures (See Also Chapter 1)

1. Anti-infective pharmaceutical agents to remove infectious causes of disease (curative therapy—removal of the cause)
   a. Antibacterials and antibiotics
   b. Antifungals
   c. Antiparasitics
   d. Antivirals
2. Antihistamines and decongestants (supportive/palliative therapy)
   a. Topicals and orals to inhibit inflammatory mediators (antihistamine) and vasoconstrict (decongestants) to reduce the vascular permeability leading to pathological processes
   b. Antihistamines combined with decongestants are synergistic in preventing or inhibiting the release and activation of cells and mediators in the allergic/hypersensitivity responses
   c. Reduces effects of clinical inflammatory cascade ("rubor, calor, dolor, and tumor")
   d. Works synergistically with cold
3. Hypertonic saline (2% and 5%, ointment or drops); supportive/palliative therapy)
   a. Reduces epithelial edema (inflammatory or noninflammatory)
      i. Works by Donnan's equilibrium
      ii. Reduces "stress immunogen" effect and potential for "clinical autoimmune cycle"
      iii. Works synergistically with cold
4. Immunosuppressive pharmaceutical agents (supportive/palliative therapy)
   a. Anti-inflammatory agents—steroidal
      i. Corticosteroids block the cyclooxygenase and lipooxygenase pathways in the inflammatory cascade to inhibit prostaglandins and leukotrienes
      ii. Most potent clinical anti-inflammatory agent in primary eye care
      iii. Should be withheld whenever doubt exists as to pathological diagnosis, persisting antigen (e.g., infection), active infection, and the need for continuation of the defense mechanisms of the immune system (e.g., ulceration)
   a. Nonsteroidal anti-inflammatory agents or drugs (NSAIAs or NSAIDs)
      i. Block only prostaglandin production (cyclooxygenase pathway) in the inflammatory cascade, and thus are less effective than steroids (but clinically quite effective, especially for inflammatory pain
      ii. Aspirin (oral)
      iii. Ibuprofen (topical and oral)
      iv. Naproxen (oral)
      v. Diclofenac (topical and oral)
      vi. Ketorolac (topical and oral)
   b. Antihistamines/Mast cell stabilizers
      i. Inhibits mast cell degranulation to prevent IgE-mediated inflammation
      ii. See antihistamines above
      iii. If mast cell plays additional role(s) as "gatekeeper" to other forms of inflammation, mast cell stabilizers may have additional roles as a future NSAID
   c. Other immunosuppressive therapies and drugs to date do not have a place in primary care of the anterior segment due to their specialized and toxic nature
      i. Cytotoxic drugs
         - Azathioprine
         - Cyclophosphamide
         - Methotrexate
      ii. Therapies for cancers, and systemic immune and autoimmune disorders (e.g., lymphoid irradiation, plasmapheresis, antilymphocyte antibodies)
5. Analgesic agents (supportive/palliative therapy)
   a. Noncontrolled substances
      i. Topical agents
      ii. Anti-inflammatories
         - Steroidal
         - NSAIDs
   a. Controlled substances (narcotic agents)
      i. Federal schedules II through V
      ii. Generally avoidable

D. Summary of Anterior Segment Therapies by Preventive, Curative, and Supportive/ Palliative Classification (Alphabetical)

1. Preventive therapies
   a. Counseling/education
   b. Environmental
   c. Genetic therapies
   d. Hygiene
      i. Irrigation
      ii. Lid scrubs
   e. Nutrition
2. Curative therapies
   a. Anti-infectives
   b. Diagnosis and removal of the cause (basis of all curative therapy)
   c. Therapeutic lasers
3. Supportive/palliative therapies
   a. Analgesic agents
   b. Antihistamines
   c. Anti-inflammatory agents
      i. Corticosteroids
      ii. Nonsteroidals (NSAIDs)
   d. Cold (temperature) therapies
   e. Decongestants
   f. Heat therapies
   g. Hypertonic saline
   h. Lubrication
      i. Antihistamine/mast cell stabilizers

E. General Anterior Segment Therapeutic Measures by Specific Pathological Process

1. Allergy/hypersensitivity
   a. Nonpharmacological measures
      i. Prevention (avoid known allergens)
      ii. Cold compresses
      iii. Patient education
      iv. Genetic therapies (coming!)
   b. Pharmacological measures
      i. Antihistamine/decongestants
      ii. Hypertonics
      iii. Steroids (if necessary)
      iv. Antihistamine/mast cell stabilizers
   c. Other
      i. Allergy testing
      ii. Desensitization therapy
2. Congenital/developmental abnormalities
   a. Nonpharmacological measures
      i. Genetic counseling
      ii. Genetic therapies (coming!)
   b. Pharmacological measures per complications
3. Degeneration
   a. Nonpharmacological measures
      i. Lubrication
      ii. Nutritional considerations
      iii. Genetic therapies (coming!)
   b. Pharmacological measures per complications
4. Dystrophy
   a. Nonpharmacological measures
      i. Per complications
      ii. Nutritional considerations
      iii. Genetic counseling
      iv. Genetic therapies
   b. Pharmacological measures per complications
5. Environmental
   a. Nonpharmacological measures
      i. Prevention
      ii. Hygiene
      iii. Protection and safety
      iv. Patient education
   b. Pharmacological measures per complications
   c. Other
      i. Industrial consultation
      ii. Environmental awareness (e.g., ultraviolet)
6. Infection
   a. Nonpharmacological measures
      i. Prevention
      ii. Hygiene
      iii. Hot for vascularized tissue
      iv. Cold for avascular tissue (e.g., cornea, anterior uveitis)
      v. Environmental awareness (to contamination)
   b. Pharmacological measures per nature of infectious agent
      i. Anti-infective pharmaceutical agent
      ii. Anti-inflammatory upon removal of infectious antigenic agent
7. Inflammation (see F)
8. Injury
   a. Nonpharmacological measures
      i. Prevention
      ii. Hygiene (irrigation)
      iii. Lubrication
      iv. Warm compress (for contusion)
      v. Cold compress (for cornea or bleeding)
      vi. Nutrition and vitamins (for burns)
      vii. Environmental protection (UV)
      viii. Patient education
      ix. Laser "welding"
   b. Pharmacological measures
      i. Anti-infective agents (antibiotic)
      ii. Hypertonics (for any type of edema)
      iii. Anti-inflammatories (in burns)
      iv. Analgesics if indicated
   c. Other
      i. Dress (bandage) wounds
      ii. Soft lens bandage
      iii. Cycloplege and dilate pupil
      iv. Surgical repair if indicated
9. Metabolic
   a. Nonpharmacological measures
      i. Nutritional considerations
      ii. Genetic counseling
      iii. Genetic therapies
   b. Pharmacological measures per complications
10. Metaplasia
   a. Nonpharmacological measures
      i. Nutritional considerations
      ii. Genetic counseling
      iii. Laser obliterations
      iv. Genetic therapies (coming!)
   b. Pharmacological measures per complications
   c. Other
      i. Cosmetic surgical repair if indicated or desired
      ii. Monitor for neoplastic changes
11. Neoplasia
   a. Nonpharmacological measures

i. Genetic counseling
ii. Environmental considerations
iii. Laser obliterations
iv. Genetic therapies (here already for malignant melanoma!)

b. Pharmacological measures per complications
c. Other
i. Biopsy
ii. Surgical excision
iii. Radiation therapies if indicated
iv. Systemic medical evaluation for metastasis
v. Careful, watchful monitoring

12. Neurological
a. Nonpharmacological measures
i. Genetic counseling
ii. Patient education
iii. Genetic therapies
b. Pharmacological measures (by neurological specialist)
c. Other
i. Careful primary care diagnostic evaluation
ii. Referral to appropriate specialist

13. Nutritional
a. Nonpharmacological measures
i. Prevention
ii. Nutritional considerations
iii. Genetic counseling
iv. Patient education
b. Pharmacological measures (generally contraindicated)
c. Other
i. Careful primary care diagnostic evaluation
ii. Referral to appropriate nutritional specialist

14. Systemic manifestations
a. Nonpharmacological measures
i. Prevention
ii. Nutritional considerations
iii. Genetic counseling
iv. Patient education
b. Pharmacological measures per complications
c. Other
i. Careful primary care diagnostic evaluation
ii. Referral to appropriate healthcare specialist

F. General Anterior Segment Therapeutic Measures for the Inflammatory Process

1. Nonpharmacological measures
a. Hygiene (to reduce antigenic volume and potency)
b. Lubrication (to reduce mechanical stimulus to corneal epithelium)
c. Warm compress on vascularized tissue until antigen is removed (then switch to cold)
d. Cold compress on avascular tissue and on removal of antigen from vascular tissue
i. Highly effective, non-invasive vasoconstrictor
ii. Should be included with all pharmacological and/or nonpharmacological anti-inflammatory treatment regimes
e. Nutritional considerations (including vitamins and minerals)
f. Genetic therapies (coming!)

2. Pharmacological measures
a. Decongestants (topical and oral)
b. Hypertonic saline (5%, qid)
c. Steroids
i. Rule out persistent antigen (infection) and ulceration
ii. On appropriate clinical decision to introduce steroid, use no less than 1% prednisolone or its equivalent, qid
iii. Based on the fact that the inflammatory process is considered an asset in vascular tissue and a liability in avascular tissue, clinical management decisions in the use of steroids for anterior segment inflammatory disorders (and their clinical features—"rubor, calor, tumor, dolor") must be judged according to involved structures
iv. Vascularized anterior segment structures: eyelids, lacrimal system, conjunctiva, episclera/sclera, iris, anterior angle, and ciliary body
- Avascularized ("privileged sites") anterior segment structures: cornea, anterior chamber and aqueous, and crystalline lens
v. Use of steroids for vascularized structures should be passive and conservative, with removal of cause being primary
- Prior to certain removal of cause, support of vascular (immune system) response with heat will protect tissue/structure and promote elimination of antigen.
- Although histopathologically beneficial, heat will exaggerate negative clinical inflammatory effects through its vasodilatory stimulation. Too intense an inflammatory stimulation (by antigen or heat) can become an intolerable experience for the patient and may also precipitate or aggravate the clinical autoimmune cycle. An intense or chronic inflammatory process in vascularized tissue (with or without antigen removal) may occasionally require careful anti-inflammatory, immunosuppressive therapy (steroids) with simultaneous, aggressive steps towards removal of the cause (e.g., antibiotic/anti-inflammatory steroid combination drug for acute bacterial blepharitis).
- Limit to chronic or subacute reactions; contraindicated in acute or hyperacute infection
vi. The aggressive use of steroids (anti-inflammatory/immunosuppressive therapy), preferably with removal of the primary cause, is critical and essential in the management of avascular tissues and structures to protect them from the potential irreparable damage and destruction produced in avascular tissue by the inflammatory process
- Use of steroids should be in lieu of contraindications. Continuing and active antigen (especially infection): bacterial, viral, fungal, and parasitic; active ulceration where the immune system is the primary source of antigen elimination (PMNs) and defense against continued tissue destruction (by

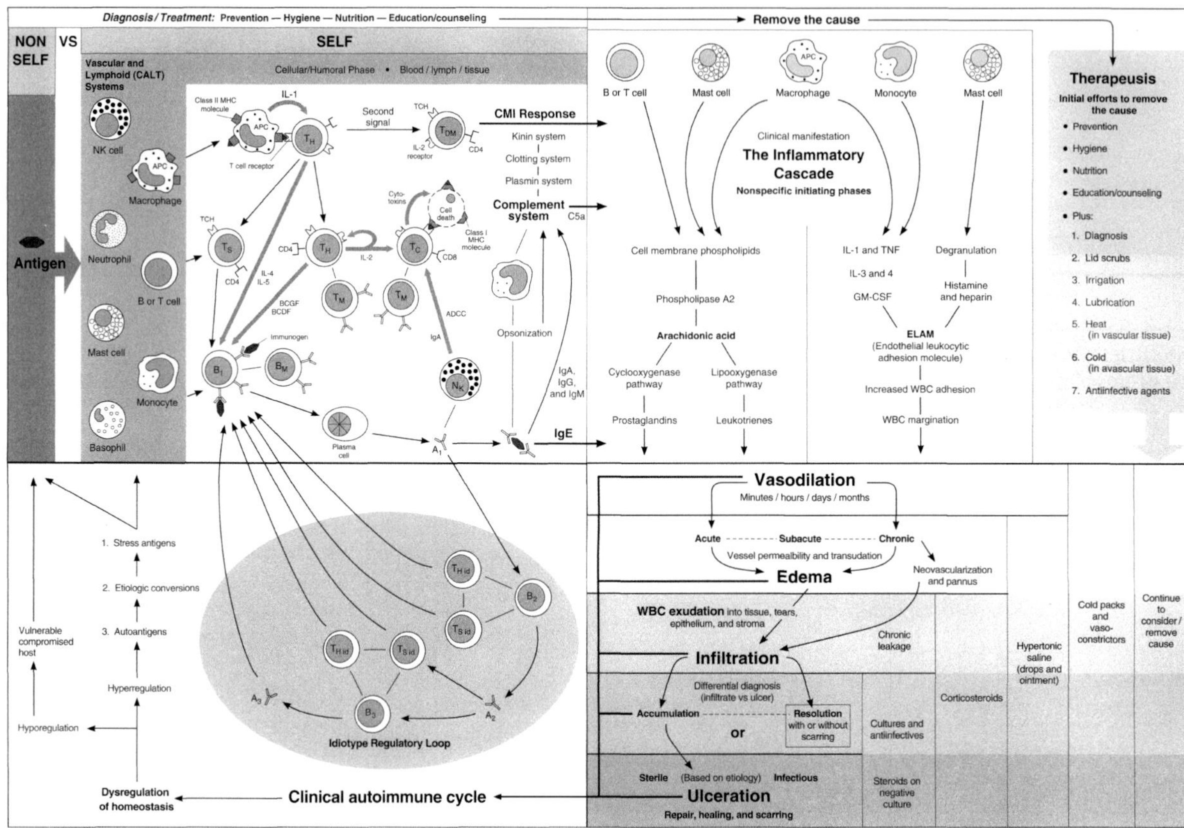

FIGURE 2.34 Therapeutic cycle, clinical immune matrix.

antigen) and potential scarring through the repair and wound healing process. Continuing clinical research is suggesting that steroids may also be indicated in certain inflammatory conditions in avascular tissue, even in the presence of traditional contraindications

- Inflammatory/infiltrative cells (particularly PMNs) appear to be equally or more destructive than the antigen in chronic corneal ulceration and corneal ulcers secondary to staphylococcus. Use of combination drugs (antibiotic/steroid agents) has been shown to provide effective simultaneous action against infectious agents and "autoantigenic," destructive PMNs. Such combination therapies have not been shown equally effective in acute gram-negative, fungal, or parasitic corneal ulceration. Removal of cause continues to be superior form of treatment prior to steroid introduction (in all forms of inflammation and ulceration)

d. Oral nonsteroidal anti-inflammatory drugs (NSAIDs) effective in anterior segment care
   i. Aspirin (2 5-grain tablets, q4h)
   ii. Ibuprofen (400 to 600 mg, qid)
   iii. Naproxen (220 to 440 mg bid, not to exceed 1100 mg daily)
   iv. Serve as anti-inflammatory as well as analgesic

e. Topical NSAIDs
   i. Ketorolac (Acular)
   ii. Diclofenac sodium (Voltaren)
   iii. Bromfenac sodium 0.09% (e.g., Bromday qd, Xibrom); 0.07% (e.g., Prolensa)
   iv. Nepafenac sodium 0.3% (Ilevro, qd); 0.1% (e.g., Nevanac)

3. Therapeutic steps should be additive, based on multiple factors (Figure 2.34)
   a. The dynamics of the clinical inflammatory cascade
      i. Introduction of antigen
      ii. Vasodilation
      iii. Inflammatory edema
      iv. WBC infiltration
      v. Ulceration (tissue destruction)
   b. At what point within the clinical cascade of inflammatory events does the patient present?
   c. What is the degree of inflammation?
   d. Have any or all of the secondary inflammatory complications ("theories") been activated?
      i. "Conversion"
      ii. "Stress immunogenicity"
      iii. The "clinical autoimmune cycle"

VI. Postscript

A. The balance of this book will expand on the traditional and clinicoimmunopathological diagnostic and management approaches presented in this chapter, with specific clinical findings, diagnoses, treatments, and management techniques (SOAP) for the primary care of the most common anterior segment disorders

1. Subjective
2. Objective
3. Assessment
4. Plan

B. Thank you for reading this chapter! I hope you enjoyed it, found it clinically relevant and valuable, and mostly, I hope it helps you and your patients

Bibliography

This chapter was conceptualized, constructed, and written back in 1995 from information and ideas gathered through my (L.J. Catania) clinical experience in anterior segment eye care; personal, collaborative, and cooperative clinical research efforts over the years; and extensive reading and studying of definitive works in the field by preeminent scientists and authors. As mentioned in this chapter, I wrote a book on immunology (*The Paradox of the Immune System*, Elsevier, 2022) updating the advancing applications of immunotherapies, molecular biology, and genetic therapies. But notwithstanding those advances, the basic science of immunology remains unchanged. In fact, all of the new knowledge and developments in autoimmune diseases and cancers are based on this scientific foundation. I offer my sincere appreciation on behalf of all primary healthcare practitioners, to each of those authors and research scientists who were and continue to be responsible for the stable and growing fields of clinical pathology and immunology. Their outstanding contributions towards improving our knowledge and understanding of these critically important areas deserve our deepest gratitude and respect.

The following list includes some of the pioneers in immunology and primary sources I used in writing this chapter (in 1995) with some of the recent literature used to explain advancements.

Allansmith MR. How the cornea defends itself. *Trans Ophth Soc UK.* 1978;98:361–362.

Allansmith MR. Immunology of the external ocular tissues. *J Am Optom Assoc.* 1990;61(6 Suppl):S16–22.

Allarakha S, Suyog Uttekar P. *What Are the Four Types of Allergic Reactions?* MedicineNet; 13 August 2020.

Allergy and the Immune System. *Johns Hopkins Health.* Allergy and the Immune System; 2019.

Catania LJ. *The Paradox of the Immune System.* Academy Press; July 2022.

Chen Liu, Yu Lan, Bing Liu, et al. T cell development: Old tales retold by single-cell RNA sequencing. *Trends Immunol.* Feb 2021;42(2):165–175.

Chrousos GP, Gold PW. The concepts of stress and stress system disorders. *JAMA.* 1992;267:1244–1252.

Claman HN. The biology of the immune system. *JAMA.* 1987;258(20):2834–2840.

Foster CS. Ocular immunology. *Semin Ophthalmol.* 1988;3:211–220.

Friedlaender MH. Immunologic aspects of diseases of the eye. *JAMA.* 1992;268:2869–2873.

Furman D., Campisi J., Verdin E. et al. Chronic inflammation in the etiology of disease across the life span. *Nat Med.* 25 Dec 2019;12:1822–1832.

Hemad R, Tauber J, Foster CS. Immunosuppressive drugs in immune and inflammatory ocular disease. *Surv Ophthalmol.* 1991;35:369–385.

Klein LM, Lavker RM, Matis WL, et al. Degranulation of human mast cells induces an endothelial antigen central to leukocyte adhesion. *Proc Natl Acad Sci USA.* 1989;86:8972–8976.

Kuchroo VK, Ohashi PS, Sartor RB, et al. Dysregulation of immune homeostasis in autoimmune diseases. *Nat. Med.* 2021;18:42–47.

Meyer PAR. The circulation of the human limbus. *Eye.* 1989;3:121–127.

National Institute of Environmental Health Science. *Autoimmune Disease.* NIH; 2019. USA.gov.

Netea MG, Schlitzer A, Placek K, Joosten LAB, Schultze JL. Innate and adaptive immune memory: An evolutionary continuum in the host's response to pathogens. *Cell Host Microbe.* 9 Jan 2019;25(1):13–26.

Orbai AM. *Autoimmune Disease: Why Is My Immune System Attacking Itself?* Johns Hopkins Health; 2019.

Robbins SL. *Basic Pathology.* 4th ed. Philadelphia: Saunders; 1987.

Ryan GB, Majno G. *Inflammation.* Kalamazoo: Upjohn Company; 1987.

Serhan CN, Ward PA, Gilroy DW. (2011) Fundamentals of Inflammation. *Yale J Biol Med.* Mar 2011;84(1):64–65.

Shouman K, Benarroch EE. Peripheral neuroimmune interactions: Selected review and some clinical implications. *Clin Auton Res. [C].* 2021:31(4):477–489.

Smolin G, O'Connor GR. *Ocular Immunology.* 2nd ed. Boston: Little, Brown; 1986.

Stites DP, Terr Al, ed. *Basic and Clinical Immunology.* 3rd ed. E. Norwalk: Appleton & Lange; 1991.

The basics of the immune system. Innate Immune System. *Immunopedia.org.za*; 2019.

Chapter 3
DIAGNOSES OF THE EYELIDS, LACRIMAL SYSTEM, AND ORBIT

Chapter Outline

DOI: 10.1201/9781003255598-3

Eyelids

Review of Clinical Anatomy

1. Structural characteristics (Figure 3.A)
   a. Skin
      i. Orbital and tarsal horizontal furrows (sulcus)
      ii. Thinnest and spongiest in entire body
      iii. Can swell dramatically
   b. Aperture approximately 12 by 30 mm
   c. Eyebrows
   d. Margins approximately 2 mm thick and 30 mm long
      i. Square edges
      ii. Lacrimal puncta 5 mm from medial angle
      iii. Eyelashes (cilia)
         - None in medial, rounded one-sixth (lacrimal portion)
         - Usually greater superiorly
      iv. Gray line marks anterior edge of tarsal plate
         - Eyelashes anterior to gray line
         - Orifices of meibomian glands posterior to line where non-stratified conjunctival epithelium begins
      v. Glands
         - Anterior glands of Zeiss (sebaceous) and Moll (sweat) open into lash follicle
         - Moll glands also open directly onto anterior lid margins
         - Meibomian (sebaceous) glands in single row (about 50 to 60) open onto posterior lid margin
      vi. Muscles
         - Orbicularis oculi
           - Innervated by cranial nerve VII
           - Sphincter muscle for forced closure (peripheral portion) and involuntary
           - blinking (central portion)
         - Eyelid retractor muscles
           - Levator palpabal superioris (cranial nerve III)
           - Superior and inferior tarsal muscles of Muller (sympathetic)
           - Inferior rectus muscle (cranial nerve III)
      vii. Fibrous tissue
         - Orbital septum
         - Tarsal plates
2. Sensory nerve supply
   a. Ophthalmic division (first) of trigeminal (cranial nerve V) innervates upper lid and small lateral portion of lower
   b. Maxillary division (second) of trigeminal (cranial nerve V) innervates remaining lower lid
3. Vascular supply
   a. Branches of a lacrimal artery and dorsonasal artery from internal carotid
   b. Anastomotic circulation from external carotid through facial, superficial temporal, and intraorbital arteries
   c. Lymphatic vessel drainage into submaxillary and preauricular nodes

I. Irritations and Injuries

A. Burns

Subjective

- History of chemical splash, radiation, or thermal burn
- Pain ranges from mild discomfort to severe

Objective

- First-degree burn (most common)
  1. Superficial chemicals, sunburn, and so forth
  2. Superficial dry erythema
  3. Mild to moderate edema

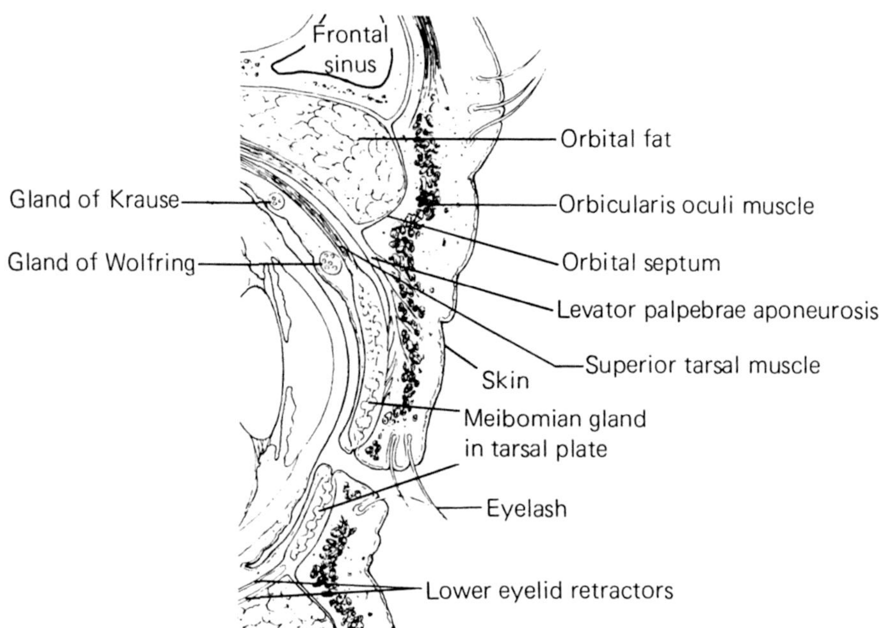

FIGURE 3.A The anatomy of the eyelid.

- Second-degree burn
  1. Thermal burns and so forth
  2. Blistering of skin
  3. Tissue "weeping"
- Third-degree burn
  1. Deeper tissue brown, white, or charred
  2. Extensive erythema and edema

Assessment

- Determine specific causative agent
- Nature of accident
- Duration of contact
- Degree of burn
- Check carefully for eyeball involvement

Plan: Burns

- Refer third-degree burns for secondary (specialist) or tertiary (hospital) care
- For first- and second-degree burns
  1. Mild tissue reactions may require only cleansing of surface with or without topical antibacterial ointment (q4h for 3- to 5-day minimum)
  2. Careful cleansing of area with cold, sterile sponging (e.g., gauze pads) using saline or Burrows solution (e.g., Domeboro)
  3. Debride loose burned tissue
  4. Remove any foreign matter
  5. Open blister formations and let them drain
  6. Frequent cold compress applications
  7. Heavy ointment coverage of area
     a. Antibacterial agents (e.g., Polymyxin B/Bacitracin)
     b. Butesin Picrate ointment as a mild anesthetic (optional)
  8. Loose gauze dressing over ointments
     a. Oral analgesic if necessary (e.g., aspirin or ibuprofen)

Follow-Up

- Dressing should be changed daily (in office or by patient) first 3 to 5 days, depending on degree of burn
- On scab formation, dressing can be discontinued, and thinner layers of antibacterial ointments should be continued for 7 to 10 days

B. Contusion (Blunt) Injuries[1]

Subjective

- History of blunt blow to orbital region
- Variable pain on palpation

Objective

- Variable degree of "pitting type" lid edema
- Ecchymosis ("black eye" or purplish-red blood color; Figure 3.1)
  1. Blood accumulation greater in lower lid
  2. Loose blood may seep across bridge of nose
  3. Blood occasionally forms organized hematoma (firm purplish-black palpable mass, usually lower lid)
- Bony orbital rim tenderness (general or focal)
- Conjunctival hemorrhages may be present as well

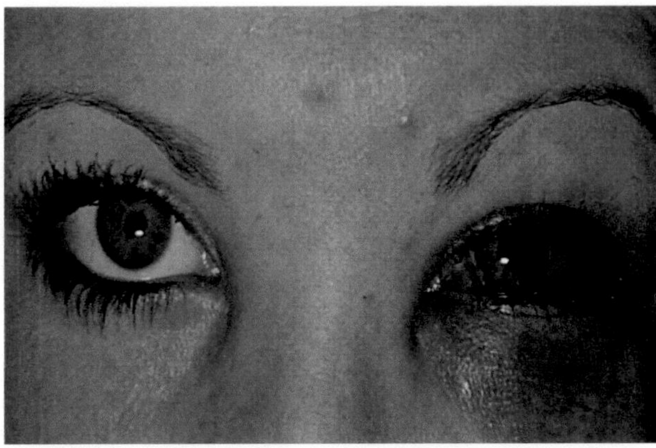

FIGURE 3.1 Ecchymosis with lid edema and subconjunctival hemorrhage secondary to blunt injury (history of snowball). Blowout fracture and crepitus must be ruled out.

Assessment

- Rule out ocular injury
  1. Hyphema
  2. Iridodialysis
  3. Retinal detachment
  4. Anything
- Check inferior rectus for entrapment (blowout fracture; see "Orbit, Injury")
- Examine with careful palpation for "crepitation" (emphysema or air in the tissue)
  1. Means sinus fracture
  2. May be blowout (orbital floor), but much more common is ethmoidal (medial wall) fracture
  3. Refer for radiological evaluation and diagnosis
- Palpate bony tissue for fractures
  1. Simple, comminuted, and so forth
  2. Check associated numbness at nerve distributions

Plan: Contusion (Blunt) Injuries

(See also Appendices 4 and 6)

- For uncomplicated edema secondary to contusion injury
  1. Cold packs for first 24 hours (follow-up heat optional)
  2. Oral decongestants/antihistamine (e.g., Benadryl) if indicated
- For ecchymosis without crepitus or fractures
  1. Cold packs for first 48 hours (to reduce bleeding)
  2. Follow with hot packs for 3 to 5 days
  3. Oral decongestants/antihistamine if desired to reduce edema
- For ecchymosis with crepitus or fractures
  1. Cold packs for first 48 hours
  2. Warm packs for 5 to 7 days
  3. Oral antibiotic for 7 to 10 days (broad spectrum)
  4. Oral decongestant/antihistamine
  5. If substantial fracture or blowout entrapment, refer for ophthalmological consult

Follow-Up

- For ecchymosis without crepitus
  1. Recheck in 3 to 5 days or PRN
- For ecchymosis with crepitus

1. Recheck in 2 to 3 days (rule out cellulitis, and so forth)
2. Return check (RTC) 7 to 10 days (rule out secondary complications)
3. Recheck PRN

C. Foreign Bodies on Tarsus

Subjective

- Contributory history of foreign matter (e.g., sand, fiberglass)
- Foreign-body (corneal) sensation

Objective

- Corneal foreign-body tracking (FBT)
- Localization of embedded material (with slit lamp or loop)
  1. Single or double lid eversion necessary
  2. May be difficult to accomplish due to lid spasms secondary to corneal irritation (use topical anesthetic)

Assessment

- Fiberglass difficult to visualize
- Rule out primary corneal lesions (e.g., dendrite)
- Check corneal epithelium for foreign matter

Plan: Foreign Bodies on Tarsus

- Remove foreign matter (with lid everted)
  1. Lavage (strong irrigation)
  2. Wetted cotton-tipped applicator
  3. Swab tissue with cotton tip (valuable in dislodging poorly visualized materials)
- Use instruments for removal if necessary
  1. Spuds ("golf-club" type)
  2. Forceps (jeweler's type)
- Prophylactic antibiosis (optional) 1×

Follow-Up

- PRN

D. Lacerating Injuries[2]

Subjective

- Contributory history of lacerating injury

Objective

- Consider superficial dermis versus deeper fascia or muscle layer wound
- Parallel (along normal fold) versus vertically oriented wound (probable scar formation)
- Consider wound edges
  a. Straight edges falling together in apposition
  b. Jagged, gaping, irregular (probable scarring)
- Lid lacerations greater than 5 to 10 mm are potential risks for full-thickness penetration

Assessment

- Rule out eyeball involvement
- Evaluate risks of scar formation (keloids)
  1. Depth
  2. Orientation (along folds versus vertical)
  3. Edges
  4. Length
  5. Keloid formation greater in Black patients
- Rule out damage to surrounding or underlying tissues and structures
  1. Lacrimal system
  2. Orbicularis muscle
  3. Lid margin

Plan: Lacerating Injuries

(See also Appendix 6)

- Problem lacerations or secondary tissue damage should be referred for appropriate suturing and surgical care
- For simple lacerations
  1. Clean wound thoroughly (e.g., hydrogen peroxide, Zephiran HCI 1:750)
  2. Remove any foreign matter
  3. Antibacterial ointments (e.g., Polymyxin B/Bacitracin)
  4. NSAIDs for pain management (e.g., Ibuprofen)
  5. Standard dressing

Follow-Up

- Redress wound in 3 days
- Remove dressing in about 1 week
- PRN

E. Subcutaneous Cilia (Ingrown Eyelash)

Subjective

- Occasional localized irritation of lid margin
- May produce corneal foreign-body sensation
- Occasionally cosmetic awareness of irregular lash

Objective

- Eyelash misdirected into epidermis of lid (Figure 3.2)
- May enter lid tissue at one site and exit in close proximity or terminate within tissue

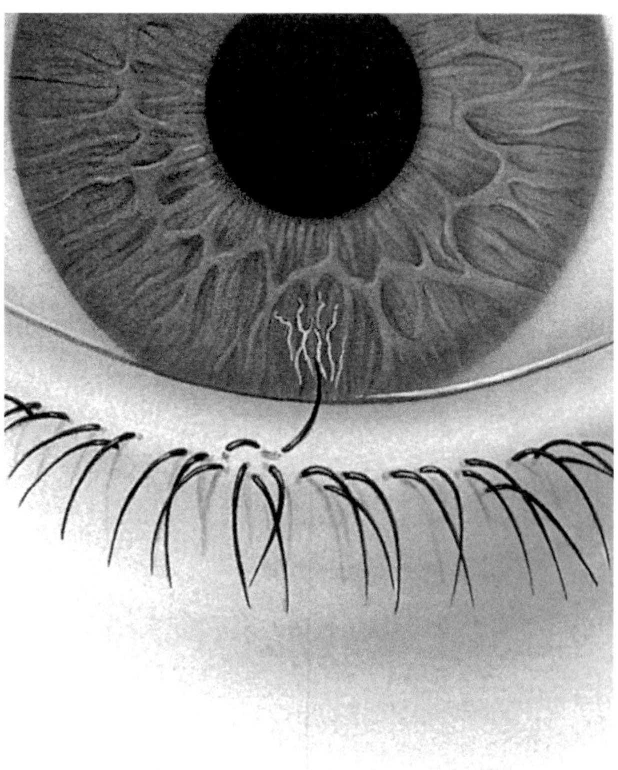

FIGURE 3.2 **Subcutaneous cilia** often redirect into marginal lid tissue and they emerge to create inferior corneal irritation and foreign-body tracking (FBT).

- Occasionally a foreign-body granuloma (small spongy vascularized tissue mass) may develop around ingrown lash
- Infrequently secondary infection or inflammation at site
- Frequently lash will irritate corneal surface

Assessment

- Common cause is chronic toxic Staphylococcus
- Rule out multiple sites
- Rule out cicatricial causes

Plan: Subcutaneous Cilia

(See also Appendix 4)

- Cut loop of lash midway between hair follicle orifice and subcutaneous portion
- Remove distal portion of lash by "threading" it through epithelialized channel
  1. Use cilia or jeweler's forceps
  2. Pull firmly and steadily
- Epilate proximal lash portion from follicle
- Prophylaxis with antibacterial ointment at site

Follow-Up

- PRN

II. Noninflammatory Conditions

A. Basal Cell Carcinoma[3]

Subjective

- Most common malignant tumor (neoplasia) of eyelids
- History of slow-developing, non-resolving lesion
- Usually a positive history of extensive ultraviolet (UV) exposure to sunlight
- Increasing frequency in older patients
- More frequent in fair-complected patients
- Often, previous history of skin cancer
- Previous radiotherapy
- Frequently present as multiple sites

Objective

- More prevalent on the lower lid (Figure 3.3)
- Very early forms look like vascularized nodules, with loss of surrounding skin texture

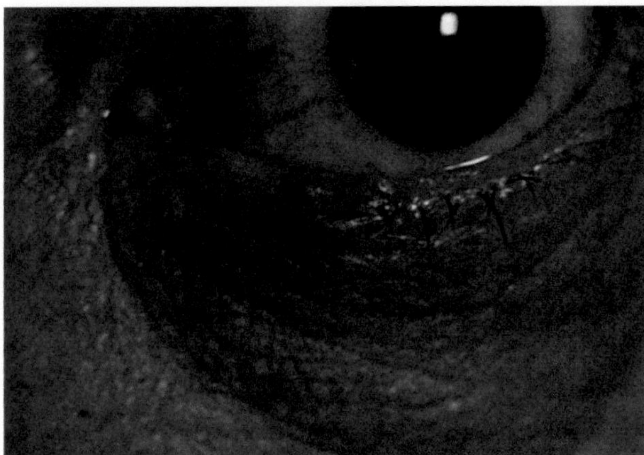

FIGURE 3.3 **Basal cell carcinoma** on the inferior lid margin. Notable objective findings include raised borders with loss of skin texture and umbilicated, central ulceration.

- Varying degrees of central umbilicated ulceration
- Borders tend to be "pearly" or hardened (to both appearance and palpation) and slightly raised
- Variable amounts of pigmentation noted centrally
  1. May be absent in early lesions or amelanotic carcinoma
  2. More prominent in darker races
- Transillumination (with slit-lamp or bright light source) of involved skin surface may reveal a dark periphery and brighter central zone to lesion
- Occasionally, surface of lesions may become secondarily infected, inflamed, or both
  1. Overlying purulent discharge and crustation
  2. Surrounding erythema or ulceration

Assessment

(See also Appendix 2)

- Metastasis almost nonexistent in basal cell
- Inner canthal lesions require more rapid attention due to potential deeper tissue extension
- If lesion secondarily infected or inflamed, run short (1- to 2-week) course of antibiotic-steroid combination
  1. Resolution of lesion indicates no cancer
  2. No response to treatment suggests possible neoplasia
- Most appropriate differential diagnostic test for highly suspicious clinical lesions is tissue biopsy
- High frequency ultrasound and in vivo confocal microscopy are non-invasive imaging techniques
- Aggressive forms (morpheoform) rare
- Basal cell is a slow-growing neoplasia and need not be considered a STAT referral
  1. Referral within weeks to months is adequate
  2. Highly questionable lesions may be monitored

Plan: Basal Cell Carcinoma

- Advise patient of possible nature of lesion, but reassure as to the low-risk nature of this type of cancerous lesion
- Refer for biopsy and pathological diagnosis
- Surgical excision (Mohs procedure) and repair (i.e., skin grafting if indicated) is standard treatment
- Adjunctive therapies include radiotherapy and topical immunotherapy
- Photodocument if possible

Follow-Up

- If surgical referral deferred for any reason (e.g., patient reluctance, fear)
  1. Document (photodocument if possible) and record reasons carefully
  2. Monitor lesion closely (every 3 months)
  3. Recommend biopsy and excision at each visit
- After surgery, recheck patient annually or PRN
- After first positive basal cell diagnosis (biopsy), consider every skin lesion potential basal cell

B. Blepharoptosis (Drooping of Upper Eyelid)[4,5]

Subjective

- Most important consideration in history is to establish congenital versus acquired nature
- If congenital:
  1. Confirm with photos (old, straight-on portrait views)
  2. Check for familial tendencies

- If acquired:
  1. Careful medical history
  2. Evaluate diurnal patterns (for myasthenia gravis)
  3. Check for associated neurological signs
  4. Medications?
  5. Check for mechanical causes (e.g., lid masses)
- Question closely regarding associated diplopia
- Cosmetic concern

Objective

- Varies from subtle difference between lid apertures, to noticeable drooping (unilateral or bilateral), to total unilateral or (less common) bilateral closure
- If congenital
  1. Unilateral or bilateral presentation
  2. Superior tarsal fold usually absent or poorly developed
  3. May show backward torticollis (head tilt)
  4. Brow wrinkling common
- If acquired (Figure 3.4)
  1. Usually unilateral (with exceptions)
  2. Diurnal variations with drooping greater in PM
  3. Increases with stress factors (e.g., fatigue)

Assessment

(See also Appendix 3)

- Congenital versus acquired (most important?)
- Most common possibilities if acquired
  1. Neurological or neuromuscular causes (e.g., third nerve palsy, Bell's palsy, Horner's syndrome, MS)
  2. Myogenic (e.g., Myasthenia gravis)
  3. Aponeurotic (e.g., defective levator aponeurois)
  4. Mechanical (e.g., neoplasm)
  5. Trauma
- Consider anatomical asymmetry in ptosis with normal function
- Photograph, if possible, and monitor aperture sizes

Plan: Blepharoptosis

- For congenital
  1. Reassure
  2. Consider ptosis crutch
  3. Consider conservative cosmetic surgical approach
  4. If vision obscured in newborn, early surgical intervention becomes indicated to reduce risks of amblyopia ex anopsia
  5. Consider botulinum toxin for possible cosmetic effect
     a. Positive effect usually limited (up to 3-month duration)
     b. Can produce neuromuscular toxicities
- For acquired
  1. Establish possible cause at first visit
  2. Refer ASAP to appropriate specialist

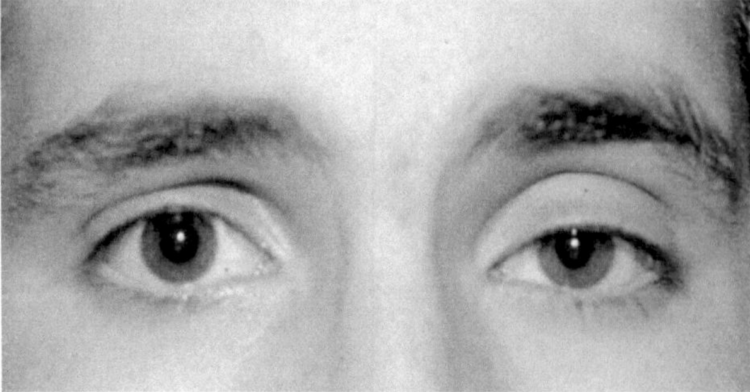

FIGURE 3.4 **Acquired blepharoptosis** of the right lid is secondary to myasthenia gravis. Note prominent superior tarsal fold.

Follow-Up

- Recheck congenital or anatomical cases annually
  1. Compare measurements to previous findings
  2. Recheck neurofunction, and other systems
- Confirm care on referred acquired ptosis patients
- Provide or suggest genetic counseling in severe congenital cases

C. Blepharospasm (Myokymia, Clonus, Essential Blepharospasm)[6]

Subjective

- Unilateral or bilateral
- No pain involved
- Usually "twitching" sensation
- Less common: spastic forced closures (essential)
- Intermittent or constant
- Onset and duration variable

Objective

- Most lid tics not observable
- Check blood pressure
- Palpate lids for masses
- Do glabellar tap (reflex test) for Parkinson's disease
- Examine CV and CVII (cranial nerves V and VII)
- Check refractive error

Assessment

- Rule out disease or foreign-body reactions
  1. Lids (e.g., trichiasis)
  2. Conjunctiva (e.g., foreign matter on tarsus)
  3. Cornea (e.g., keratitis)
- Rule out raised intraocular pressure
- Rule out possible neuromuscular diseases.
  1. Multiple sclerosis (Uhthoff and Lhermitte signs)
     a. Uhthoff's sign: increased neurological signs with increased body temperature
     b. Lhermitte sign: "electrical sensation" down back when bending head forward
  2. Myasthenia (e.g., lid-fatigue test)
- Consider other common etiologies
  1. Emotional status (neurogenic or psychogenic conversion syndrome)
  2. Physical stress and habits
  3. Dietary patterns (when, where, how)
- Consider neurosis or psychosis

Plan: Blepharospasm

- Refer (if appropriate) for cause
- Reassure patient
- With children, instruct parents against negative reinforcement
- Counsel patients on possible causes
- Oral and topical antihistamines and decongestants suggested for relief (questionable: placebo?)
- Quinine reported helpful
- Biofeedback therapy used occasionally
- Botulism toxin used in severe (essential) cases

Follow-Up

- If no diagnosis, call or recheck in 2 to 4 weeks or PRN
- Also nice to call referred patients in 4 to 6 weeks
- Counseled patients should be rechecked in 4 to 6 weeks

D. Chloasma[7] (Large Brown Hyperpigmented Areas)

Subjective

- Cosmetic concern
- Found mostly in pregnant females
- More pronounced in darker pigmented ethnic groups

Objective

- Large brownish spots around lid and brow areas
- Irregular shapes and sizes
- Ill-defined fading borders
- Healthy-looking tissue surfaces

Assessment

- Rule out melanoma (irregular surfaces and changes in tissue characteristics)
- Differentials include nevi or raised lesions

Plan: Chloasma

- No therapy indicated
- Reassure patient
- Sometimes fades
- Treatment options for cosmetic concerns
    - Topical agents such as linoleic acid and ascorbic acid
    - Oral agents such as tranexamic acid
    - Platelet rich plasma injections

E. Coloboma (Notch or Cleft on Eyelid Margin)[8]

Subjective

- Congenital abnormality (nonhereditary)
- Unilateral (more common) or bilateral
- Greater in superior lid
- Patient may report dry eye symptoms
- Frequently detected during routine examination
- Occasionally large enough to produce cosmetic concern
- Associated notching may also occur in eyebrow

Objective

- Most often found in medial portion of superior lid
- Least frequent in lateral aspect of lower lid
- Other congenital deformities frequently associated
    1. Especially with lower lid involvement
    2. Usually cranial boney changes or dermoids
- Notches are usually small, triangular shaped, full thickness in lid margin
- Rounded edges and no lashes
- Occasionally, cleft may be large enough to cause corneal exposure and drying

Assessment

- Examine for associated findings or syndromes, such as dermoids, FLKs ("funny-looking kids")
    1. Facial dermoids (preauricular)
    2. Goldenhar syndrome (oculovertebral dysplasia)
- Check cornea for secondary effects

Plan: Coloboma

- Reassurance
- Patient education
- If cornea involved (i.e., exposure keratitis), lubricate
- In syndrome-related cases, suggest genetic counseling

Follow-Up

- Necessary in complicated cases only
- Photodocument for long-term management

F. Dermatochalasis (Superior Eyelid Overhang)[9]

Subjective

- Middle to older age groups
- Usually bilateral
- Familial tendency
- Often produces cosmetic concerns

Objective

- Draping of superior lid tissue over septum or lid margin (Figure 3.5)
- Loose and redundant tissue fold
- May show puffiness due to fatty tissue herniation
- Produces pseudoptosis

Assessment

- Rule out causes of true blepharoptosis
- Rule out causes of secondary lid edema
- Similar condition (far less common) called blepharochalasis, in younger age ranges caused by edema or inflammatory swelling of unknown etiology

Plan: Dermatochalasis

- Reassurance
- Blepharoplasty if indicated for functional vision (i.e., loss of superior field: uncommon) or cosmetic relief

G. Dermoid (Benign, Developmental Outpocketings of Tissue)

Subjective

- Usually noted at birth or in early years
- Found at numerous sites on body
- More common in syndromes (e.g., Goldenhar, Treacher Collins)
- Most common ocular sites are superior temporal brow region and outer-canthus, usually under lid angle (Figure 3.6)
- Multiple embryological and histological origins
- May change in size through life

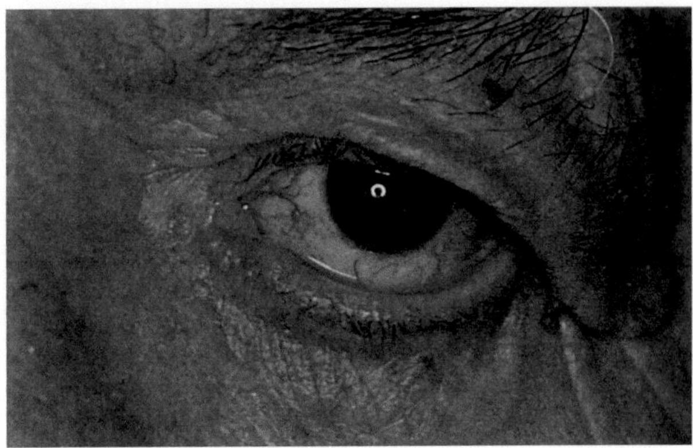

FIGURE 3.5 Dermatochalasis (upper lid) and ectropion (lower lid) in same eye of elderly patient.

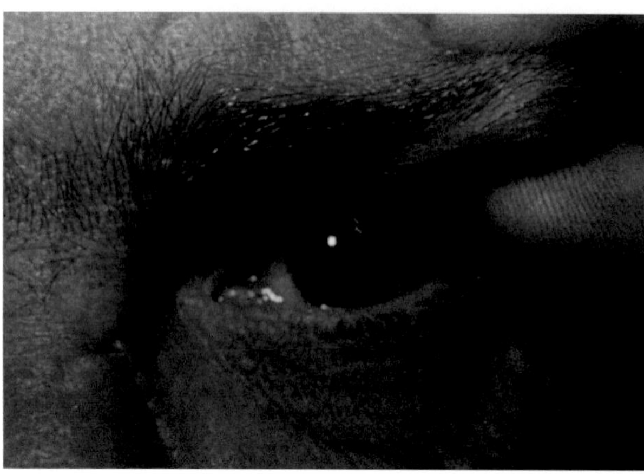

FIGURE 3.6 **Large dermoid** in superior brow region (common site).

  1. Changes frequently produce first awareness (and resulting concern) in later years
  2. Cosmetic concern
- Always painless

Objective
- Solid, firm collagenous-like surfaces
- Smooth surface masses with overlying skin sliding easily over buried surfaces
- Exposed surfaces may contain hair follicles, fatty tissue, sebaceous glands
- Mass usually stationary or slightly movable

Assessment
- Differentiate from very movable subcutaneous sebaceous cyst
- Rule out neoplastic potential
- Check for syndromes (associated stigmata)

Plan: Dermoid
- Reassurance and patient education
- Refer for cosmetic removal if patient desires
- Measure and diagram dermoids reported as "changing"

Follow-Up
- Recheck changing size potential every 6 months
- General recheck annually or PRN

H. Ectropion (Eyelid Turned Outward)

Subjective
- Chronic epiphora (typical "wet eye" presentation)
- May have no complaints

Objective
- Inferior lid margin or lacrimal puncta (punctal ectropion) not in contact with globe or lacrimal lake (Figure 3.5)
- Epiphora
- Usually lid atonia due to aging ("loose lid syndrome")

Assessment
- Rule out cicatricial (scarring) causes
- Rule out mechanical causes

Plan: Ectropion
- Nothing indicated for asymptomatic patients
- Surgical repair necessary for problem cases
- "Taping" methods both temporary and questionable

I. Entropion (Eyelid Turned Inward)

Subjective
- Corneal foreign-body sensation
- Hyperlacrimation or lid spasms
- Infrequently congenital or a problem in children secondary to an epiblepharon (medial lid infolding)

Objective
- Inferior lid and lashes turn inward and rub against corneal surface (Figure 3.7)
- Inferior irregular to vertically oriented foreign-body tracking on cornea
- Commonly caused by spastic response on forced closure of lids (spastic entropion)

Assessment
- Rule out simple trichiasis
- Rule out corneal foreign body
- Check for signs of other infectious and inflammatory lid disorders (e.g., chronic staphylococcal blepharitis)

Plan: Entropion
- Surgical procedure usually indicated
- If surgery contraindicated or refused
  1. Complete epilation (lash removal) indicated
  2. Soft bandage lenses may help
  3. Ongoing lubrication therapy indicated for corneal protection and comfort
- Taping methods may offer temporary relief

Follow-Up
- Manage secondary corneal complications closely

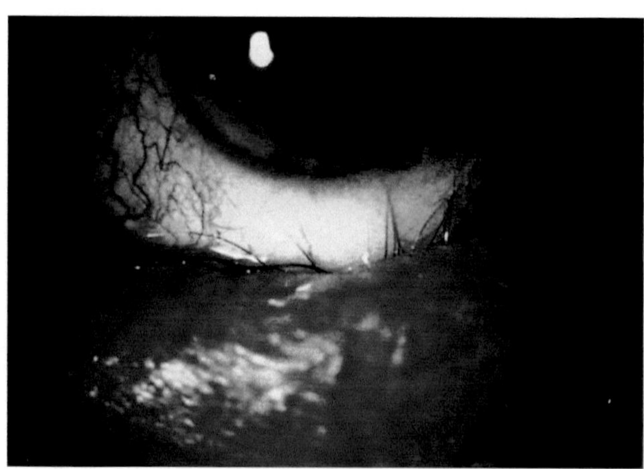

FIGURE 3.7 **Lower eyelid spastic entropion** (inturning after forced blink). Secondary corneal irritation occasionally produces no discomfort due to progressive corneal hypoesthesia.

J. Epicanthus (Inner Canthal Nasal Folds)

Subjective

- Almost always bilateral
- Very common in Asian races
- Common in Caucasian infants
- Associated with flat bridges (e.g., Down's syndrome)
- Pseudostrabismic appearance (frequent pediatric referral)

Objective

- Folds start in upper medial lid and "dissolve" into lower lid (reversed in many syndromes)
- Folds vary in degree (e.g., width, prominence)
- Occasionally may be tight enough to push lashes inward and cause corneal irritation
    1. Especially in cases of dense lashes
    2. With epiblepharon (congenital infolding of lid)
- May present with blepharoptosis (congenital)
    1. Usually hereditary
    2. Greater in males

Assessment

(See also Appendix 3)

- Rule out congenital syndromes (check for stigmata)
- Rule out true strabismus
    1. Cover testing
    2. Hirschberg's reflexes
    3. Motilities (extraocular muscles [EOMs])
    4. Pseudostrabismic "pinch test"

Plan: Epicanthus

- Reassurance and patient (or caretaker) education
- Infrequently, cosmetic surgery (in adults only!)

Follow-Up

- Recheck pseudostrabismus every 3 months for 12 months
- After 12 months, go to every 6 months

K. Hemangioma[10] (Benign Vascular Tumor)

Subjective

- Present congenitally or shortly after birth
- May enlarge during first 6 months, followed by regression
- Sometimes associated with other congenital abnormalities or syndromes
- Painless
- Cosmetic concern

Objective

- Vascular anomalies (tumors) of superficial blood vessels causing flat or slightly elevated, circumscribed, colored lesions on skin surface (Figure 3.8)
- Feel firm and rubbery and difficult to compress
- Varying types
    1. Capillary (strawberry) hemangioma is flat, superficial, and rapidly growing during infancy with usual (but unpredictable) regression by adolescence
    2. Cavernous type is a raised deeper mass
    3. "Spider" angioma (vascular spiders) are non-congenital types that occur during pregnancy, and in other conditions, generally resolving spontaneously
    4. Port-wine stains (nevus flammeus) are deep purple-red skin discolorations (common in Sturge–Weber syndrome; a phakomatotic disease)

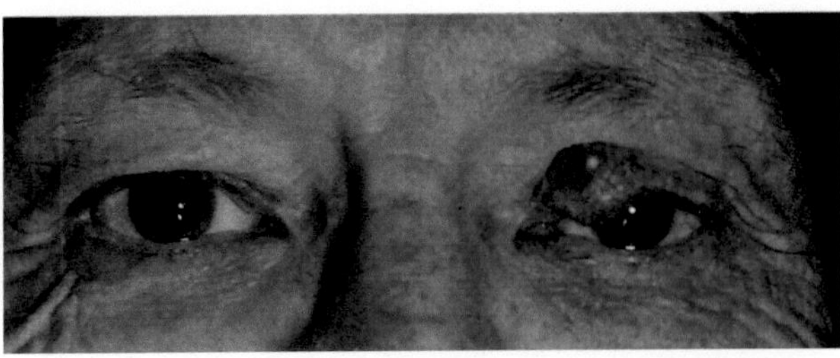

FIGURE 3.8 **Large hemangioma** in the superior eyelid. Elevation and coloration can be viewed on external and internal tarsal surfaces.

    5. Racemose aneurysm is a grapelike vessel cluster
    6. Mixed forms
- Superficial capillary type most common
- Colors vary from faint pink, purple, blue to red
- Straining and crying can cause dramatic changes in size, elevation, and coloration of lesions
- Variable sizes from pinpoint to entire lid (e.g., port-wine stain in Sturge–Weber syndrome)
- When superior lid involved in port-wine stain, glaucoma risk substantially increased
- Increased risk for secondary glaucoma
- Superficial lesions may blanch on pressure (good differential for nevus or melanoma)

Assessment

- Examine the patient carefully for other congenital anomalies
    1. Colobomas
    2. Syndrome stigmata
    3. Choroidal hemangioma
- Determine type of hemangioma and prognosis
- Rule out pigmented lesions
    1. Benign or malignant
    2. Nevus or melanoma

Plan: Hemangioma

- If other congenital abnormalities or signs of any syndromes noted, refer for pediatric or medical workup
- Reassure, educate, and advise patient (or caretaker) as to prognosis
- Therapies include oral steroids, intralesional steroid injection, radiotherapy, systemic propranolol, various laser therapies and surgical removal are used for hemangiomas but should be discouraged during early stages
- Photodocument and measure

Follow-Up

- Recheck children annually and compare photo and measurements
- When likelihood of spontaneous regression unlikely (adolescence or beyond), advise regarding
- cosmetic options

L. Keratoses (Hyperkeratinized Plaques in Elderly)

Subjective

- Most common in adults beyond age 40 to 50
- Distribution over entire body with increased prevalence to exposed skin areas (i.e., face)

- Changes are slow and insidious
- Some forms regarded as precancerous (nonmetastatic)

Objective

- Flat or slightly elevated
- Dry scaly lesions on atrophic patch of skin
- Usually has a light gray-brown coloration
- Well circumscribed lesions with distinct borders
- Appears as plaque "floating" on skin surface

Assessment

- Rule out neoplastic changes
- Rule out keratoacanthoma (rapid-growing, large mass of viral origin)
- Rule out melanomas, nevi, verrucae, papilloma
- Increased suspicion in younger age ranges

Plan: Keratoses

- In early stages, greasy ointment base coverage may abort or arrest advancement
- Chronic erosion of edges, recurrent infection, or inflammation should be biopsied
- Excision for cosmetic reasons or suspicion best accomplished by dermatologist

Follow-Up

- Photodocument if possible
- Ongoing management should include periodic monitoring of any changes
  1. Size, shape, pigmentation
  2. Surface quality and edge erosion
- Recheck large, prominent lesions every 6 to 12 months

M. Nocturnal Lagophthalmos (Incomplete Eyelid Closure)[11]

Subjective

- Exposure keratitis symptoms, that is, foreign-body (FB) sensation
- Chronic AM corneal irritation
- Dry eye syndrome

Objective

- Usually about 2- to 5-mm opening on normal lid closure
- Patient usually able to force complete closure
- Secondary corneal involvement
  1. Superficial punctate keratitis (SPK) in band region (exposed corneal area)
  2. Possible corneal anesthesia
  3. Epithelial erosion (greater in AM)

Assessment

- Rule out tear dysfunction
- Rule out epithelial basement membrane disorder
- Rule out paralytic and cicatricial lagophthalmos
- Check for weak or absent Bell's phenomenon
- Assess closure with head tilted back (chin up)
- Measure lid separation on closure

Plan: Nocturnal Lagophthalmos

- Lubricate cornea (*daytime*: drops; *bedtime*: ointments)
- Overnight soft lenses bandage
- Moisture chamber goggles for sleeping
- Tape lids shut for sleeping
- Consider tarsorrhaphy in cases in which corneal protection is inadequate

Follow-Up

- Manage secondary corneal involvements closely (every 3 months)
- Reassess measurements intermittently

N. Madarosis (Loss of Eyelashes)[12]

Subjective

- Congenital (ocular alopecia) versus acquired
- Unilateral or bilateral
- Usually cosmetic concern

Objective

- Patchy loss or filamentation of lashes (Figure 3.9)
- Occasionally complete loss
- Eyebrows generally not involved (only in congenital alopecia)

Assessment

(See also Appendix 3)

- Most frequent cause is Staphylococcus
  1. Toxic response
  2. May or may not see other signs of lid involvement
- Rule out systemic relationships (e.g., medications, hair loss elsewhere on body, cutaneous lupus erythematosus but not common)
- Rule out trichotillomania (see V. below)

Plan: Madarosis

(See also Appendix 4)

- Antistaphylococcal lid therapy (every 6 to 12 weeks; Table 3.1)
- Photodocument if possible
- Refer for medical evaluation if suspicious

Follow-Up

- Recheck post-antistaphylococcal therapy
- If onset less than 3 months, prognosis guarded to good
- If onset greater than 3 months, prognosis poor

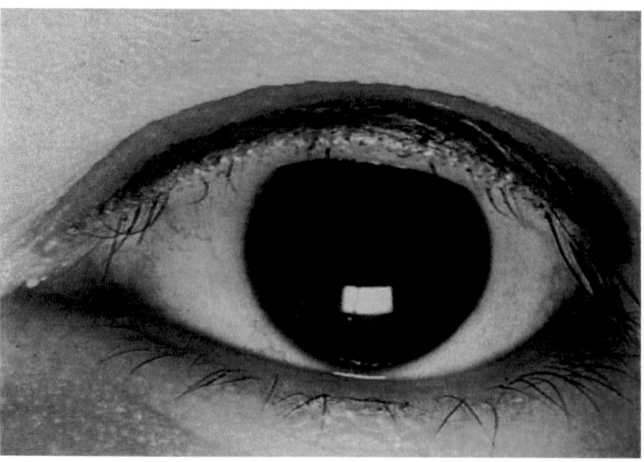

FIGURE 3.9 **Madarosis** with diffuse loss of lashes superiorly and inferiorly.

TABLE 3.1 **Staphylococcal Risk-Reduction Program**

	Dosage/Duration		
Treatment Steps	**Subclinical**	**Chronic**	**Acute**
1. Skin/scalp hygiene	Daily/ongoing	Daily/ongoing	Daily/ongoing
2. Warm compresses	HS/2–4 wk	HS/3–6 wk	q4h/1–2 days
3. Lid massage	Optional	HS/3–6wk	Not indicated
4. Lid scrubs	1–2×/wk/6 mo and RTC	HS/3 mo and RTC	HS/1–2 wk (after pain resolves)
5. Antistaphylococcal lid ointment	Optional	HS/2–4 wk (e.g., Bacitracin)	q4h/5–7 days (e.g., tobramycin)
6. Hypochlorous acid 0.01% lid spray	Optional	qd	bid to tid
7. Steroidal (or combination) ointment or suspension	Optional	bid to tid/1–2 wk	qid for 7–10 days

Abbreviations: tid, 3 times per day; q_____h, every _____ hour(s); HS, at bedtime; RTC, return check; bid, 2 times per day; qid, 4 times per day.

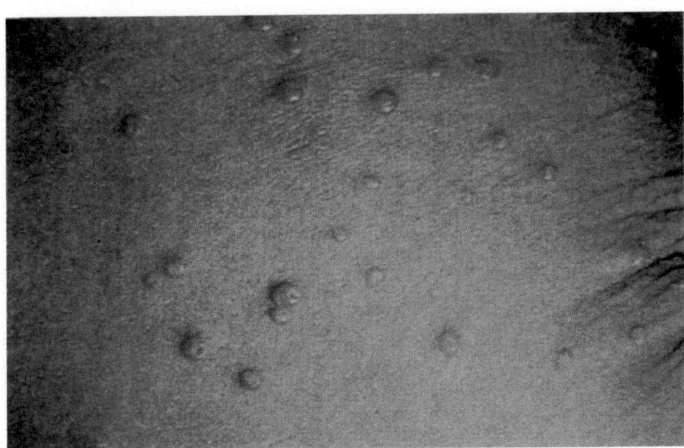

FIGURE 3.10 **Molluscum contagiosum** appearing in a quiescent stage on the temporal/brow region of an infected patient. Lesions usually occur as regional groupings on the skin surface.

O. Molluscum Contagiosum (Viral Wart)[13]

Subjective

- All age groups but most frequent in children
- Occasionally presents as mildly irritating lump on eyelid
- When on lid margin, may cause transient ocular surface irritation (keratoconjunctivitis) of viral etiology
- May be mildly contagious with autoinoculation most common
- Occasional cosmetic concern

Objective

- Small (3- to 6-mm) umbilicated nodule(s) with yellow "cheesy" material (or dry when inactive) central core (Figure 3.10)
- May be multiple on lid and elsewhere on body
- Activity (central discharge) remits and exacerbates spontaneously
- Occasionally lesion may enlarge dramatically but will always resolve without scarring

Assessment

- Rule out basal cell carcinoma
- Differentiate other lumps and bumps
- Consider human immune deficiency virus infection in high-risk patients, highly contagious

Plan: Molluscum Contagiosum

- When lesion quiet (dry central core), leave alone
- When center discharging cheesy or waxy material:
  1. Clean surface with alcohol wipe (other options include phenol and trichloroacetic acid)
  2. Loosen central core material with sharp curetting instrument (e.g., spud, needle)
  3. Squeeze out contents with fingers or cotton swabs (appositional pressure)
  4. Reclean surface with alcohol wipes

Follow-Up

- Recheck in 1 week or PRN
- Same lesion may require multiple treatments (three to five) with eventual resolution

P. Neoplastic Considerations (Beyond Basal Cell)

Subjective

- Lesion does not act or respond as anticipated
- Lesion is not common for patient's age, sex, race, demography
- History of other skin lesions elsewhere on the body
- History of other neoplasias or systemic disease
- Older patients
- Patients with history of excessive UV skin exposure
- Family history of skin cancers
- Fair-complected patients
- Pain and or irritation associated with suspicious lesion
- Acute versus chronic onset and duration
- Rapid or irregular growth patterns

Objective

- Quality of the tissue looks irregular
- Surface integrity and quality questionable
- Changes in lesion not consistent or predictable
- Neovascular patterns around or within lesion
- Recurrent infections or inflammations at site
- Bleeding or ulceration of lesion
- Uncharacteristically large lumps or bumps
- Associated tearing or conjunctival hyperemia
- Erosion of the margins or surface of a lesion

Assessment (Malignant Lesions of the Eyelid and Adnexa)

- Carcinomas
  1. Basal cell epithelioma (most common)
  2. Squamous cell

3. Intraepithelial (Bowen's disease)
4. Adenocarcinoma of the meibomian glands

- Sarcomas
  1. Lymphosarcoma
  2. Reticulum cell
  3. Giant follicular lymphoma
  4. Burkitt lymphoma
  5. Hodgkin's disease
  6. Kaposi's sarcoma, frequently found in acquired immune deficiency syndrome (AIDS)
- Nervous tissue tumors
  1. Neurofibromatosis
  2. Mucosal neuroma
  3. Neurilemoma
  4. Schwannoma of Abrikossoff
  5. Ganglioneuroma
- Pigmented tumors: malignant melanoma
- Metastatic tumors (secondary to primary tumor)

Plan: Neoplasias

- With serious doubt or suspicion regarding any lump or bump of the lid, recommend excision and biopsy
- If referral deferred or refused for any reason, document rationale thoroughly and monitor closely
  1. Photodocument if possible
  2. Diagram and measure accurately

Follow-Up

- Recheck suspicious lesions frequently (every 3 months)
- Photodocument all changes and progressions and remeasure and diagram at each visit
- Continue to advocate for referral and biopsy

Q. Nevus (Pigmented Spot)[14]

Subjective

- Usually congenital or early onset
- Occasionally changes in size or pigmentation
  1. Hormonally related
  2. Pregnancy, puberty
- May be history of other nevi on body
- Cosmetic concern

Objective

- Three types
  1. Dermal
     a. Most common
     b. Deep form
     c. May be raised or flat
     d. Hardly ever becomes malignant
  2. Junctional (Figure 3.11)
     a. Superficial form
     b. Usually flat
     c. May convert to melanoma
  3. Transitional: mixed dermal and junctional form
- Pigmented (usually brownish) or amelanotic (white or clear) spots on skin surface
- Commonly found at lid margins
- Well-defined borders
- Usually less than 8- to 10-mm diameter
- May increase in size with aging (beware of malignant changes, especially in junctional forms)
- May also decrease in size or degree of pigment (usually associated with hormonal changes)
- Occasionally show hairs growing through surface

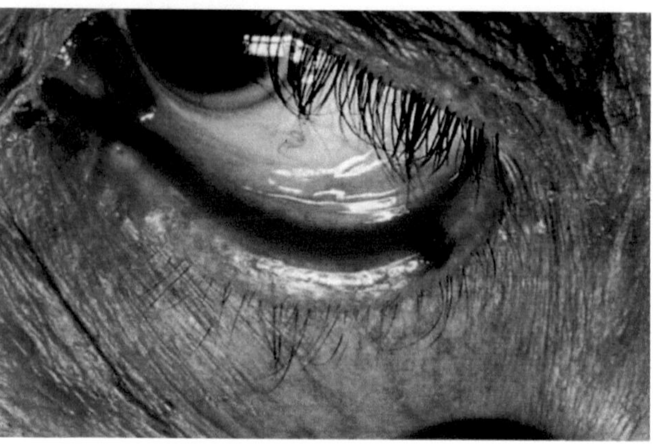

FIGURE 3.11 **Junctional nevus** (flat) on inferior lid margin. Lesion was monitored for 17 years without change in elevation, size, or color.

Assessment

- Rule out other pigment spots
  1. Benign types
  2. Malignant types
- Determine type of nevus
- Examine old photograph if available

Plan: Nevus

- On first presentation, document development of spot and any changes
- Photodocument if possible, or diagram and measure
- Reassure and advise on reporting any changes

Follow-Up

- Monitor every 3 to 6 months if any suspicions
- Recheck annually if normal appearing without change
- Compare photographs, diagrams, and measurements each visit
- If significant changes occur (especially in higher risk types or suspicious lesions), refer for biopsy

R. Papilloma[15] (Benign Epithelial Tumor)

Subjective

- Greater in older patients
- Associated with UV exposure and sun damage
- No symptoms
- Rarely secondarily irritated by infection or inflammation
- Cosmetic concern

Objective

- Epithelial overgrowths (benign tumors)
- Size and shape vary considerably
- Pigmentation ranges from amelanotic to black
- May present singularly or in abundant multiple (Figure 3.12)
- Can be located anywhere but frequently found at mucocutaneous border of the eyelid (Figure 3.13)
- Mass is avascular
- Surface is usually roughened but not eroded
  1. Roughened "granulated" surface is reflection of redundant epithelial cell growth
- Quite different surface texture from normal, surrounding skin

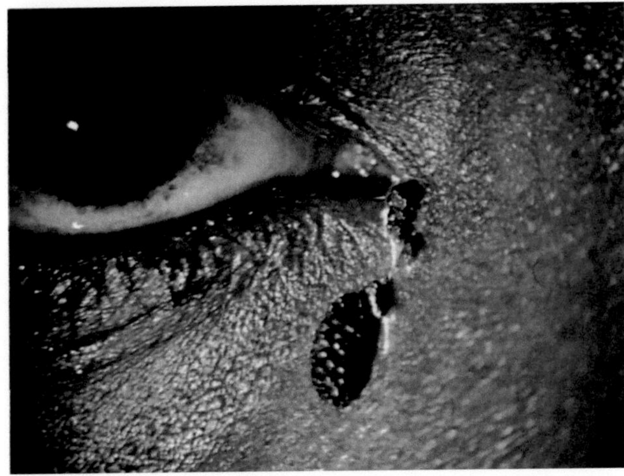

FIGURE 3.12 **Multiple pigmented papillomas** at inner canthal region. Note the redundant cellular surface texture secondary to epithelial reduplication.

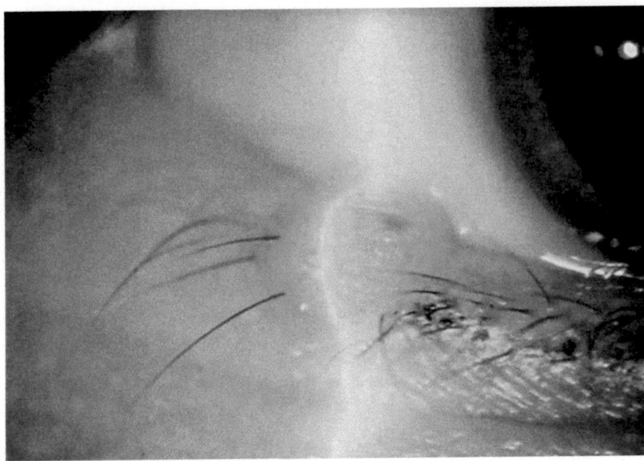

FIGURE 3.13 **Amelanotic papilloma** at the mucocutaneous inferior lid border. Note the eyelashes growing directly through the epithelial overgrowth.

- Little change in growth pattern once developed
- May outgrow underlying blood supply (with increased size, aging) and necrose (blacken and harden)

Assessment

(See also Appendix 3)

- Rule out
  1. Nevus (usually congenital)
  2. Senile solar or actinic keratoses (usually "floating" plaque effect)
  3. Subcutaneous sebaceous cyst (normal overlying skin texture)
  4. Verrucae (umbilicated surface)
  5. Neoplasia
- Consider any history of changes in mass

Plan: Papilloma

- Reassurance and patient education
- Treat any secondary infection or inflammation with standard topical anti-infective or combination drugs
- If patient desires removal for cosmetic reasons:
  1. Grasp with toothed forceps and extend outward
  2. If width of base less than 1 to 2 mm, snip off with sharp (iris-type) scissor
  3. Small bleed controlled by direct pressure
  4. If base greater than 2 mm, refer for excision
- If lesion appears highly suspicious, refer to dermatologist for excision and biopsy

Follow-Up

- If lesion is new or recently reported, photodocument and recheck in 3 to 6 months
- For long-standing lesions, recheck annually
- Any significant changes in mass (any mass) should be referred for excision and biopsy

S. Poliosis (Whitening of Eyelashes)

Subjective

- Congenital (ocular albinism) versus acquired
- May be unilateral or bilateral on upper or lower lids
- Cosmetic concern

Objective

- Patchy or complete whitening (loss of pigmentation) of eyelashes

Assessment

- Most frequent cause is Staphylococcus
  1. Toxic response
  2. May or may not see other signs of lid involvement
- Rule out vitiligo

Plan: Poliosis

(See also Appendix 4)

- Antistaphylococcal lid therapy (for 6 to 12 weeks) (see Table 3.1)
- Photodocument if possible

Follow-Up

- Recheck post-antistaphylococcal therapy
- If onset less than 3 months, prognosis guarded to good
- If onset greater than 3 months, prognosis poor

T. Sebaceous Cyst (Fatty, Pilar Fibrous Cyst of Sebaceous Gland)

Subjective

- No symptoms
- History may include recent onset or long standing
- Two types
  1. Superficial type: very common (Figure 3.14)
  2. Subcutaneous (deep) type: common (Figure 3.15)
- Cosmetic concern

Objective

For Superficial Type

- Range in size from 0.5 to 1 mm, up to 8 to 10 mm (normal range about 2 to 5 mm)
- Caseous ("cheesy"), yellowish material in recently developed cysts (less than 3 to 6 months)
  1. Covered by thin flattened epithelial cell layer
  2. Occasionally, pigmented particles or dirt may be trapped inside cyst (inclusion or retention cyst)

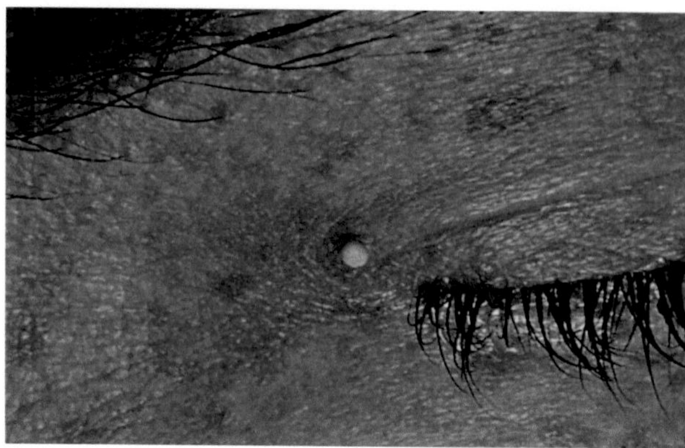

FIGURE 3.14 **Superficial sebaceous cyst** at the outer canthus with hardened, yellowish, caseous material trapped beneath a layer of thin, flattened epithelium.

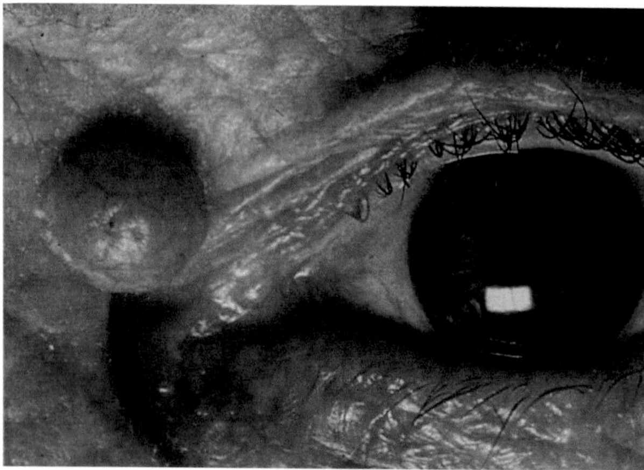

FIGURE 3.15 **Large subcutaneous sebaceous cyst** of long standing (patient history) at the inner canthus of an elderly man. Note the normal skin texture over surface with prominent overlying capillary vessels.

- In older cysts, material becomes fibrotic with a paler yellow-white coloration
- May appear as single cysts or in multiples (milia)
- Common around lids, especially at inner and outer canthal regions

For Subcutaneous (Deep) Type

- Location could be anywhere on body, especially the axillary regions (e.g., armpits, groin)
- Epidermal inclusion cysts
- Slightly movable lump of variable size with normal skin (texture) overlying (skin slides minimally over lump with palpation and "pinching" procedure)
- Extensive range of sizes from 1 to 20 mm or greater
- Sometimes overlying skin may show prominent blood vessels, telangiectasia or venous congestion (blue-red or purplish hue)

Assessment

(See also Appendix 3)

For Superficial Type

- Rule out sudoriferous cyst (clear versus caseous filled)
- Rule out pustules or infectious vesicles (e.g., herpetic, bacterial)
  1. Usually associated erythema and symptoms
  2. Sebaceous cysts are rarely symptomatic or "hot" (inflamed)

For Subcutaneous (Deep) Type

- Rule out papilloma (granulated surface)
- Rule out dermoid (congenital)
- Rule out neoplasia

Plan: Sebaceous Cyst

For Superficial Type

- Reassurance and patient education
- If detected as part of routine examination (common) and patient not concerned, do nothing
- If patient desires removal (for cosmetic purposes):
  1. Consider duration of cyst (from history)
     a. Less than 3 to 6 months, cysts usually soft and easy to drain
     b. Older cysts more fibrous and require considerable forceps manipulation
     c. Do the easier ones initially
  2. Clean surface (e.g., alcohol, Zephiran™) and apply topical anesthetic (on cotton tip) for about 1 minute
  3. Incise epithelial surface (over cyst) with bevel of hypodermic needle or tip of jeweler's forceps
  4. Massage out contents of cyst by opposing two cotton-tip applicators or arms of forceps at base of gland until tinge of blood appears
  5. In older cyst, grasp and pullout fibrotic strands with jeweler's forceps
  6. Prophylax surface of drained cyst with topical antibiotic ointment (e.g., Polymyxin B/Bacitracin) 1×
- Instruct patient on immediate and long-term hygiene

For Subcutaneous (Deep) Type

- Reassurance and patient education
- If patient desires cosmetic removal, refer for surgical excision
- If patient reports abundant axillary sebaceous cysts developing in conjunction with lid cyst(s), consider medical evaluation for possible systemic cause

Follow-Up

- For drained superficial type, recheck 1 week or PRN
- If cyst reoccurs (rarely), redrain and observe
- Advise patient to report any changes in status or characteristics of cyst(s)

U. Sudoriferous Cyst (Serous or Fluid Cyst of Gland of Moll)

Subjective

- No symptoms
- Usually noted during routine external eye exam
- Occasionally cosmetic concern (if cyst observable)

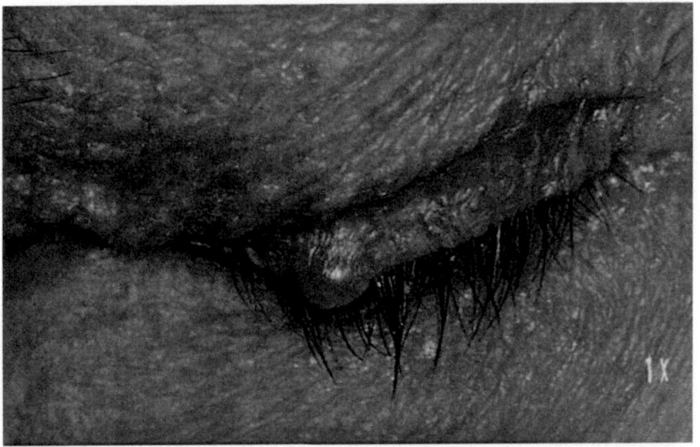

FIGURE 3.16 **Sudoriferous (fluid-filled) cyst** on superior lid margin. Drainage was accomplished with 22-gauge hypodermic needle.

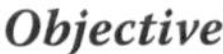

Objective

- Single or multiple cyst(s) on superior or inferior lid margin (Figure 3.16)
- May be fluid or sebum filled (clear or cloudy)
- Usually small (2 to 4 mm) and round
- Can also be inclusion or retention cysts

Assessment

(See also Appendix 3)

- Rule out amelanotic papilloma (solid versus cystic)
- Rule out milia or meibomitis (inflamed lid)

Plan: Sudoriferous Cyst

- Reassurance and patient education
- If patient desires removal:
  a. Lance with 18- to 25-gauge hypodermic needle
  b. Always direct lancing away from globe
  c. Prophylactic antibiotic (1×) optional
- Advise patient on lid hygiene

Follow-Up

- Resolution usually immediate
- PRN

V. Trichiasis (Inturning Lash or Lashes)[16,17]

Subjective

- Congenital (e.g., epiblepharon) versus acquired
- Corneal foreign-body sensation
- Frequently hyperlacrimation and epiphora
- Normal lid position (not entropic)

Objective

- Inferior lid involved more frequently than superior
- Fine filamentary lashes or complete lash(es) turn inward and rub against inferior corneal surface
- Inferior vertical or irregular foreign-body tracking (Figure 3.17)

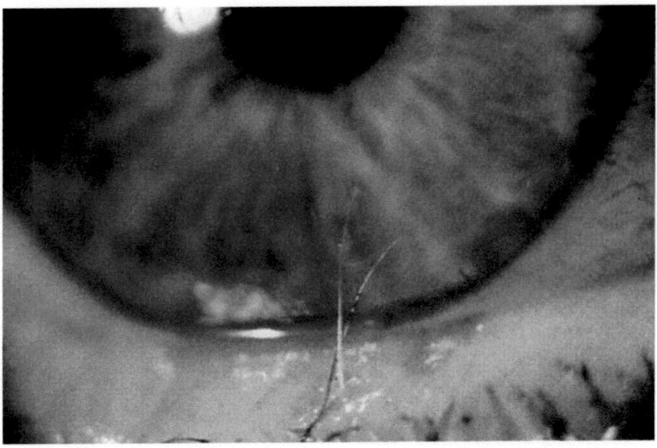

FIGURE 3.17 **Trichiasis** producing inferior, vertical, corneal foreign-body tracking (FBT) with associated corneal irritation.

Assessment

- Frequently caused by chronic staphylococcal reaction
- Rule out cicatricial causes
- Rule out districhiasis (rare): additional row of lashes posterior to the mucocutaneous lid margin

Plan: Trichiasis

(See also Appendix 4)

- Epilation with cilia forceps (or tweezer)
  1. Reemergence very possible
     a. 2 to 4 weeks in youth
     b. 4 to 8 weeks in adults
  2. Repeated epilations not dangerous
- Cauterization of follicle of limited value
- Electrolysis may work, but very uncomfortable
- Radiofrequency treatment and laser ablation of the lash follicle(s) are effective treatments
- Bandage soft lenses of some value
- Treat any active or chronic marginal lid disorders
- Treat secondary corneal involvement with lubrication

Follow-Up

- PRN or recurrence of corneal irritation

W. Trichotillomania (Neurotic Twisting, Twirling of Hairs)[18,19]

Subjective

- Usually perfectly normal-acting person
- May express stressful life conditions
- Associated with anxiety disorders such as obsessive-compulsive disorder (OCD), depression, and substance use disorders
- More common in females than males
- Generally unaware of any neurotic tendencies

Objective

- Unconscious habitual tendency to repeatedly twirl, twist, or pull out a lock of hair

1. Common in males and females with long hair
2. Common in men with beards and mustaches
3. Eyelashes and eyebrows potential sites
- Tendency produces ultimate loss of hair at site
  1. Potential causes of madarosis
  2. Can result in patchy eyebrows with resultant cosmetic concern

Assessment
- Rule out other causes of patchy hair loss
- Check for alternate sites (beyond lashes and brows)
- Confirm habit by asking patient about tendency

Plan: Trichotillomania
- Reassure regarding eyelid involvement
- Advise on tendency
- Recommend a psychiatric consult and possible habit reversal therapy

X. Verrucae (Viral Wart)[20]
Subjective
- History of slow insidious development
- Reported as contagious lesion with autoinoculation tendency
  1. Caused by papillomavirus
  2. Rare
  3. Believed to be transmitted by hands and fingers
- Cosmetic concern

Objective
- Single or multiple, non-secreting papillomatous wart
- Gray-brown to yellowish colorations
- Various shaped (types) presentations
  1. Verruca planar: relatively flat and round
  2. Verruca vulgaris: raised, irregular mass on a broad base (sessile; Figure 3.18)
  3. Verruca digitata: multiple cauliflower-like dentate projections on narrow stalk (pedunculated type; Figure 3.19)

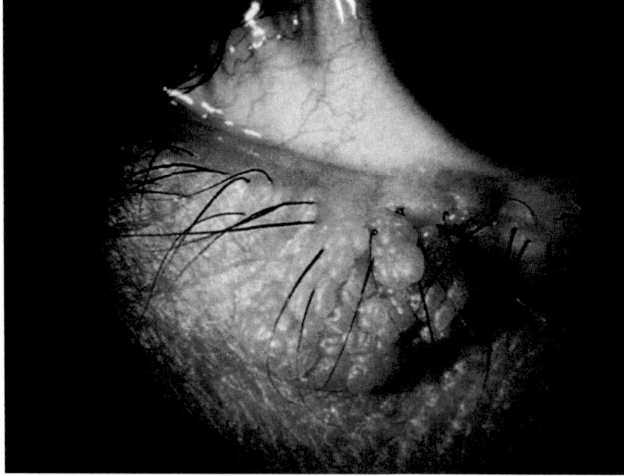

FIGURE 3.18 **Verruca vulgaris** (of yellowish coloration) emanating from inferior lid margin. Proximity to the ocular surface of this viral papillomatous wart is reason for occasional secondary viral keratoconjunctivitis.

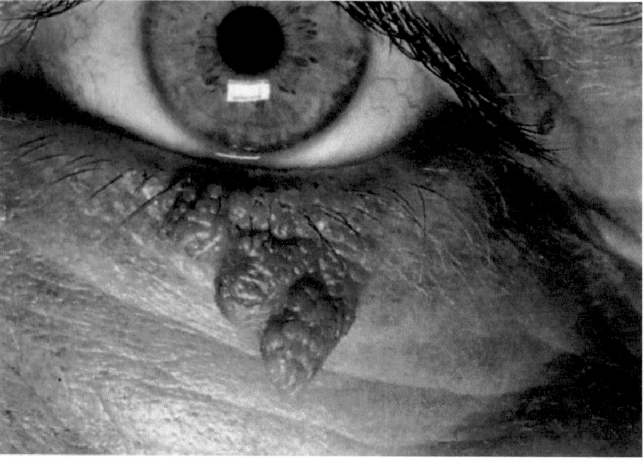

FIGURE 3.19 **Verruca digitata** (of brownish coloration) hanging from the inferior lid margin. Note the cauliflower-like appearance of the surfaces on each pedunculated mass.

- Smooth surfaces with petal-like or cauliflower-like redundant tissue waves
- Infrequently, lesions at lid margin may cause mild secondary viral keratoconjunctivitis

Assessment
(See also Appendix 3)

- Rule out (non-viral) papilloma (roughened surface)
- Rule out molluscum contagiosum (rounded wart with depressed productive central core)
- Rule out neoplasia

Plan: Verrucae
- Reassurance and patient education
- Advise on contagious nature of warts with touching
- If causing no distress (cosmetically or ocularly), do nothing
- If problematic or requested for cosmetic relief, consider removal
  1. First choice should be referral for excision
  2. Occasionally primary practitioners use chemical removal methods (e.g., bichloroacetic acid)
     a. Lengthy process (weeks) versus excision
     b. Produces undue patient discomfort
  3. Laser removal and cryotherapy removal efficient

Follow-Up
- Recheck annually or PRN
- If removed, advise patient on possible recurrences

Y. Vitiligo (Hypopigmentation or Depigmentation)[21]
Subjective
- Usually a bilateral presentation on lids (and any other body surfaces)
- Usually presents before age 20
- Frequent family history (greater than 50% of time)
- Slowly progressive with increasing age (depigmented areas enlarge)
- Condition totally asymptomatic

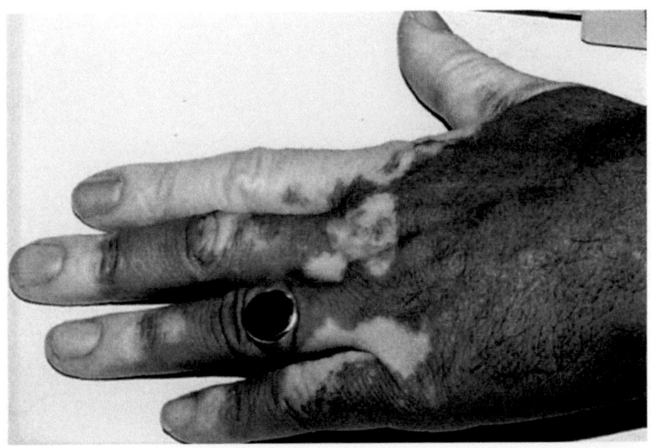

FIGURE 3.20 **Vitiligo** on the hand of a Black patient. These bilateral depigmented patches can be found anywhere on the body, including the face and eyelids.

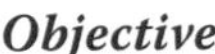

Objective

- Well-defined bilateral patches of depigmented skin (Figure 3.20)
- Generally symmetric appearance
- Any overlying hair (including eyelashes and eye brows) that also loses pigmentation
    1. Cause of secondary poliosis
    2. Partial or complete upper or lower lid, or both
- More prominent (more noticeable) in darkly pigmented ethnic groups and Black patients

Assessment

(See also Appendix 3)

- Determine autosomal-dominant family history (greater than 50% of family carry trait)
- Autoimmune disease
- Rule out associated syndromes (e.g., Vogt–Koyanagi–Harada, albinism)

Plan: Vitiligo

- Education and reassurance
- Cosmetic camouflage (e.g., makeup)
- Skin protection from sun
- Dermatologic referral if patient desires
    1. Non-targeted autoimmune therapies modest efficacy but newer targeted autoimmune therapies being developed
    2. Some topical dermatologic agents have proved effective in certain cases
- Photodocument if possible

Follow-Up

- Reassess ocular (eyelid) involvement annually
- PRN

Z. Xanthelasma[22]

Subjective

- Usually older patients (greater in females)
- Occasionally positive contributory history

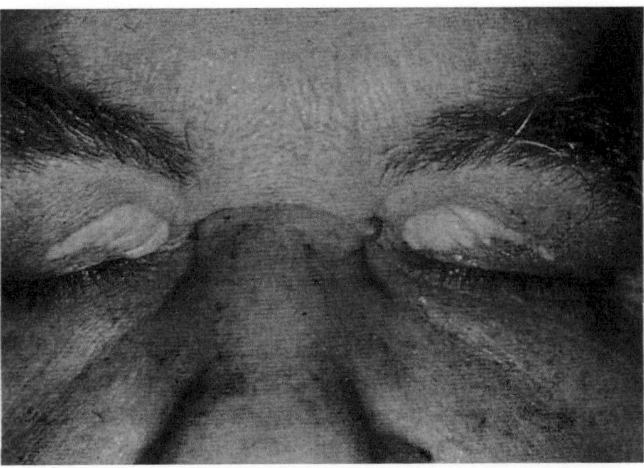

FIGURE 3.21 **Xanthelasma** in the bilateral superior medial sulci of a 58-year-old male with normal serum cholesterol levels. Leading causes are familial tendency or idiopathic nature of these masses.

    1. Hyperlipidemias (e.g., hypercholesterolemia)
    2. Hypothyroid
    3. Diabetes
    4. Diet high in saturated fat
- Family history of xanthelasma most contributory factor
- Cosmetic concern

Objective

- Usually flat triangular masses (base nasalward) at inferior or superior inner canthal lid sulcus (Figure 3.21)
- Light brown to yellowish coloration
- Usually bilateral symmetrical presentation
- May be small patches or moderate to large plaques
- Occasionally can produce a horseshoe-like appearance at the inner canthi within the orbital rims

Assessment

(See also Appendix 3)

- Consider family, systemic, and dietary factors
    1. Family history most common cause
    2. Positive family history with lesions demand careful counseling regarding risk factor control
- Rule out syringomas in younger females (small yellow spots at inner canthi)
- Rule out large superficial sebaceous cysts (usually unilateral and symmetrical)

Plan: Xanthelasma

- Reassurance and patient education
- If high-risk systemic history and not under medical management, refer for workup
- Advise on familial tendency
- Photodocument if possible or diagram and measure
- Cosmetic removal (e.g., laser, chemical peel, excision, etc.) are options but recurrences are likely

Follow-Up

- Recheck annually and remeasure, photodocument or redraw

III. Inflammatory Conditions

A. Allergic Blepharitis[23]

Background Information

(See also Chapter 2)

1. Immediate (type I) allergic response associated with antigen–antibody reaction and histamine release by mast cells
   a. Responsive to oral antihistamines
   b. Most common clinical presentations
      i. Urticaria responses (erythematous patches)
      ii. Hay fever, atopic dermatitis
2. Delayed (type IV) allergic response associated with cell-mediated reactions
   a. Responsive to topical steroids
   b. Contact dermatitis, medicamentosa

Subjective

- Sudden (immediate-type) onset or slowly increasing (delayed type) signs and symptoms
- Personal or family history of allergies or asthma
- History of previous skin eruptions or dermatitis
- Distinct symptom of "itching"
- Constant rubbing or desire to rub eye(s)
- History of allergen (usually difficult to ascertain)
  1. Contactants
     a. Plants
     b. Chemicals
     c. Cosmetics
        i. Associated with recent eyelash extensions (response to acrylate glue), permanent eyelid tattooing, and eyelash dyeing
     d. Soaps
     e. Sprays
  2. Ingestants
     a. Foods
     b. Drugs
- Possible systemic disease relationship
  1. Vascular (angioedema)
  2. Nephritic (kidney disease)

Objective

- Unilateral (contact) or bilateral (contact or endogenous-systemic) presentations (Figure 3.22 and Figure 3.23)
- Localized patches of edema and erythema (with frequent ocular surface involvement)
  1. Variable degrees from mild to dramatic
  2. Variable types
     a. Soft "pitting" edema
     b. Induration (thickening and hardened)
     c. "Brawny" edema (brownish tissue coloration)
- Erythema or eczematoid (dry, scaly) reactions
- Occasional cracking and "weeping" skin folds
  1. Called excoriation
  2. Beware of secondary infection
- Occasional vesicular or pustular formations

Assessment

- Determine offending allergen if possible
- Rule out systemic causes
- Rule out primary or secondary (toxic) infection
  1. Bacterial (especially staph and its exotoxins)
  2. Viral
  3. Any sterile or infectious toxin

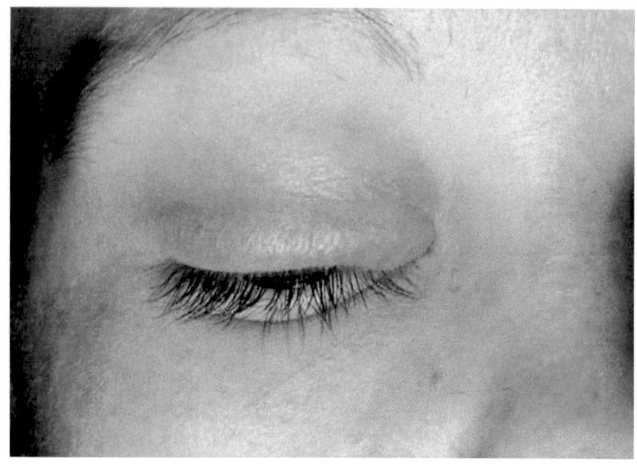

FIGURE 3.22 **Contact-type allergic blepharitis** with moderate lid edema caused by an IgE (immediate type I)-mediated response; responsive to the removal of the allergen, to cold packs, and to antihistamine/decongestants.

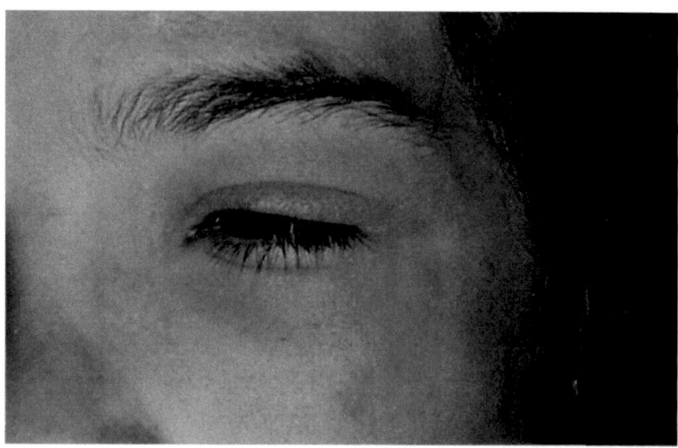

FIGURE 3.23 **Cell-mediated hypersensitive blepharitis** with mild, diffuse lid edema and erythema caused by an adverse reaction to a topical drug. Responsive to discontinuation of the drug, cold packs, and a short course of topical (or oral steroids).

Plan: Allergic Blepharitis

(See also Appendices 4 and 6)

- Remove allergen (only actual cure)
- Frequent cold packs
- Domeboro™ packs (optional)
- Oral antihistamine (e.g., Benadryl, Zyrtec) and decongestants
- If patient has specific prescription for other allergic reactions suffered, institute its use
- Topical astringent or anti-inflammatory creams
  1. Zinc preparations
  2. Hydrocortisone (OTC 1%, Rx 2.5%) qid for 3 to 7 days
  3. Stronger steroids in severe reactions (e.g., Triamcinolone cream 0.1%)
  4. Base topical dosages on degree of presentation
- In very severe conditions, a short course of oral steroids may be indicated (co-manage with physician)

Follow-Up

- Based on degree of initial presentation
  1. Mild: recheck in 3 to 5 days or PRN
  2. Moderate: recheck in 2 to 3 days
  3. Severe: recheck in 24 to 48 hours
- Check intraocular pressure with any steroid use
- Adjust treatment regimen, dosage, duration based on returning signs and symptoms
- If condition is not responsive or worsens in 3 to 5 days, consult patient's primary physician or allergist
- If allergen not determined, advise as to recurrent risk

B. Bacterial Forms of Acute and Chronic Marginal Blepharitis[24,25]

Background Information

1. Generally staphylococcal in origin (especially chronic forms)
   a. Streptococcus and gram-negative bacteria (e.g., *Pseudomonas aeruginosa*) tend to produce hyperacute forms (e.g., heavy discharge, preseptal cellulitis)
   b. Sterile exotoxins from Staphylococcus believed to be toxin-stimulating immune inflammatory response
2. Some general considerations about Staphylococcus
   a. Most common bacteria in and around the eyes
      i. On the lid margin 100% of the time (normal flora)
      ii. On the conjunctiva 75% of the time
   b. Gram-positive noncapsulated spheroidal bacteria
   c. Most common strains associated with eye care
      i. *S. aureus* (hemolytic)
      ii. *S. epidermidis* (nonhemolytic)
   d. Staphylococcus produces 32 exotoxins that can affect the eye
      i. Alpha-toxin (dermonecrotic) significant irritant to ocular membranes
      ii. Produced by *S. aureus*
   e. Leading cause of marginal infiltrative keratitis (inferior cornea)
   f. Can cause central corneal ulceration, but slower proliferating and less inflammatory organism than Streptococcus (gram-positive) and the gram-negative bacteria
   g. Bacteriocidal (cell wall active) antibiotics (or higher concentration bacteriostatic agents) are most effective treatment drugs—ointments are typically used on lids for longer retention time
      i. Bacteriocidals
         - Penicillins (oral use only)
         - Cephalosporins
         - Aminoglycosides
         - Bacitracin (topical ointment)
      ii. Bacteriostatics (in high concentration)
         - Not used often due to better options
         - Erythromycin (ophthalmic and oral forms)
         - Sulfonamides (15% concentration)
   h. About 65% of staphylococci are resistant to 10% sulfonamides
   i. About 85% of staphylococci produce penicillinase or lactamase enzymes, which neutralize penicillin
      i. Penicillinase-resistant penicillins (or cephalosporins) should be used for Staphylococcus
         - Methicillin
         - Oxacillin
         - Dicloxacillin
         - Augmentin
         - Keflex (cephalosporin)
      ii. Rule out penicillin allergies before using any penicillins
         - True penicillin allergy (i.e., clinically significant) is rare
         - 10% cross-sensitivity between penicillin and cephalosporins is probably overestimated
         - Alternative oral agent
           – Azithromycin
           – Doxycycline
3. Frequently combined seborrheic and staphylococcal origin in young adults
4. Most common form is nonpurulent (squamous) type
   a. Increased marginal hyperemia
   b. Marginal telangiectasia (red vascularized sites)
5. Squamous types may have significant nonbacterial immunological (hypersensitivity) etiologic component
6. All types may be caused by noninfectious factors
   a. Makeup
   b. Pollutants
   c. Ametropias
   d. Soaps, preservatives
7. Synonyms
   a. Chronic marginal blepharitis
   b. Staphylococcal blepharitis
   c. Ulcerative blepharitis
   d. Seborrheic blepharitis

Subjective

For Acute Forms

- Moderate to severe pain (especially on palpation: Figure 3.24)
- Rapid onset, worsening over 24- to 48-hour period
- May be associated with prodromal history
  1. Trauma (often streptococcal or gram-negative)
  2. Systemic illness (e.g., sore throat, ear infection)

For Chronic Forms

- History of months to years duration
- No distinct symptoms
- Mild irritation

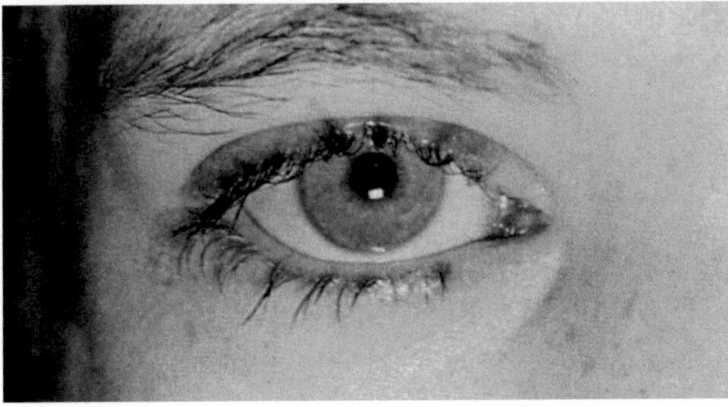

FIGURE 3.24 Subacute marginal blepharitis demonstrating a low-grade chronic inflammation of the eyelid margins generally responsive to standard antistaphylococcal therapy or combination (antibiotic/steroid) ointments.

- Chronicity usually annoyance to patient
- Often reports of "eyes stuck shut on waking"
- May report family history of condition
- History of recurrent hordeola or chalaza
- May show poor hygiene tendencies or problems with chronic dry dermatitis and dandruff (seborrhea)
- Cosmetic concern
- Commonly referred to as "granulated lids"

Objective

For Acute Forms

- Usually unilateral: bilateral forms strongly suggest systemic cause
- Moderate to dramatic lid edema and erythema
- Generally entire lid margin (360°) affected
- Mild to moderate crustations
- Frequently associated with ocular surface involvement (e.g., conjunctivitis, keratitis)
- Frequently presents with (or leads to) preseptal cellulitis
  1. Edema and erythema spread beyond orbital rims
  2. Pain (on palpation) spreads beyond orbital rims

For Chronic Forms

- Almost always bilateral (Figure 3.25)
- Thickened, rounded, ill-defined, hypertrophic lid margins (tylosis)
- Moderate to abundant flat yellowish crustations around base of lashes (rosettes)
- Varying degrees of associated eyelash involvement
  1. Madarosis
  2. Poliosis
  3. Trichiasis
- Hordeolii or chalazia (or residual signs)
- Occasional shallow ulcerations at lid margins
- May produce superficial, cracking, and "weeping" eruptions (eczematoid) at skin fold sites
  1. Particularly at outer canthal lid fold
  2. Any location possible

Assessment

(See also Appendix 3)

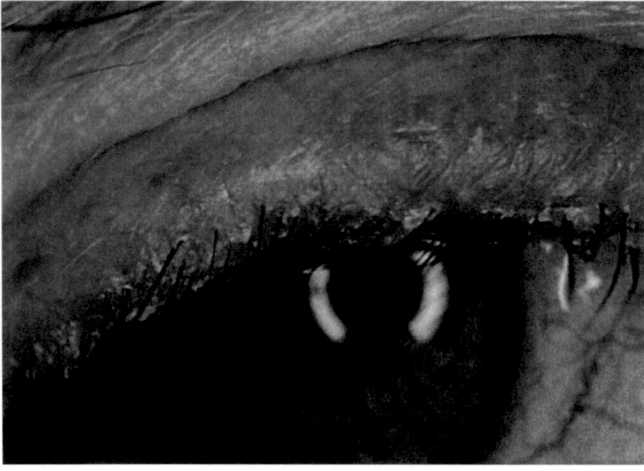

FIGURE 3.25 **Chronic blepharitis** with eyelid margin hypertrophy, flat crustations at base of lashes (rosettes), lid margin induration (thickening and hardening), and small ulcerations. This form of blepharitis is often associated with chronic seborrhea (dry, squamous form) and/or with Staphylococcus.

For Acute Forms

- Consider causative agent
  1. From clinical presentation (history and physical findings) if possible
  2. Culture if hyperacute or nonresponsive
- Rule out impetigo
  1. Staphylococcal or streptococcal infection
  2. Young adults or children with poor hygiene
  3. Usually warm-weather incidence
  4. Soft yellowish pustules
  5. Silvery or gold crustation forms over days to weeks
  6. Vesicle formations found on surrounding skin
  7. Requires broad-spectrum topical and oral agents
- Rule out other causes of blepharitis
  1. Viral
  2. Pediculosis
  3. Allergic
- Rule out preseptal (and orbital) cellulitis
- Rule out acute dacryocystitis
  1. Localized inferior nasal involvement
  2. Associated wet eye syndrome (epiphora)
- Rule out acne rosacea

For Chronic Forms

- Differentiate dry-seborrheic (squamous) type from pure infectious staphylococcal type (with heavy crustations) from combined presentations (common)
- Rule out meibomitis
- Rule out demodicosis
- Rule out lingering acute or subacute forms
  1. Streptococcal and gram-negative bacteria
  2. Impetigo
  3. Viral forms
  4. Pediculosis
- Rule out acne rosacea

Plan: Bacterial Forms of Marginal Blepharitis

- Antistaphylococcal Risk Reduction (see Table 3.1)
- See also Appendices 4 and 6

Follow-Up

For Acute Forms

- Should be stable or improving in 48 to 72 hours
- Continue treatment for at least 5 to 7 days
- If condition is worsening
  1. Reconfirm diagnosis
  2. Check on patient compliance and reinstruct
  3. Reevaluate for preseptal cellulitis development
  4. Consider adding broad-spectrum oral antibiotic
- On resolution, instruct on preventive measures

For Chronic Forms

- Improvement usually significant in 4 to 6 weeks
- Gradually reduce dosages to maintenance levels
- If no improvement
  1. Reconfirm diagnosis
  2. Check on patient compliance and reinstruct
  3. Continue treatment plan
  4. Discontinue ointments in squamous forms
- Advise patient on potential chronicity
- Reduce fatty foods in all seborrheic types
- Instruct on ongoing preventive and maintenance therapy

Prevention and Maintenance

- Refer to Figure 3.26

PREVENTIVE CARE OF THE EYELIDS

PATIENT INSTRUCTION SHEET

Affix professional card or stamp here

Recommended for: ______________________ Date: ____________

Followup appointment: Date______________________ Time____________

Step #	Explanation / Instruction	Initial frequency	Ongoing schedule
1	General hygiene a. Face cleaning (with soap and/or water) b. Scalp cleaning (with anti-dandruff shampoo) c. Lid cleaning (eyelids, eyebrows, etc)		
2	Warm compresses a. Warm reusable eye mask or eye pad (e.g., microwave or electric, multiple brands) b. Apply to closed eyelids for 10–15 minutes c. Perform 1 to 2 times per day		
3	Lid massage a. Place fingertip under margin (edge) of lower lid b. Press fingertip firmly inward against eyelid c. Replace fingertip at inner, middle, and outer lid margins		
4	Lid scrubs a. Use a sterile disposable lid wipe (multiple brands) b. Close eyelids and wipe lid margins (edges) back and forth with lid wipe c. Use a separate lid wipe for each eye d. Rinse lids with warm water		
5	Ointment application (optional) a. Squeeze 1/4 inch of ointment onto fingertip and discard it b. Squeeze 1/2 inch of ointment onto fingertip and wipe it onto the closed lid margins c. Dab extra ointment at the outer corner of the lid margins d. Wait 3 to 5 minutes and gently wipe the closed lids dry		

These eyelid procedures are **NOT A CURE** for your condition. However, done properly as recommended by your doctor, these simple procedures can help control your problem and prevent more serious complications to your eyes.

Your next followup appointment (if indicated):

Date:______________________ Time:__________

FIGURE 3.26 Patient instruction sheet for "preventative care of the eyelids."

C. Chalazion (Granuloma of Meibomian or Zeiss Gland)[26]

Subjective

- Very common lid lump
- External chalazion is granuloma of Zeiss gland
- Internal chalazion is granuloma of meibomian gland
- Acute chalazion is a synonym for hordeolum
- Frequently associated with chronic blepharitis
- Painless unless inflamed (acute chalazion)
- May remain stationary in size or progress (slowly)
- Occasionally present after hordeolum (secondary chalazion)

Objective

- Hard, firm, round or elongated mass inside lid
- External form (Zeiss) extend or evulse outward (frequently located at lid margin; Figure 3.27)
- Internal form (meibomian) remains internalized or points inward toward palpebral conjunctiva (Figure 3.28)
- Both types can become superficially infected or inflamed

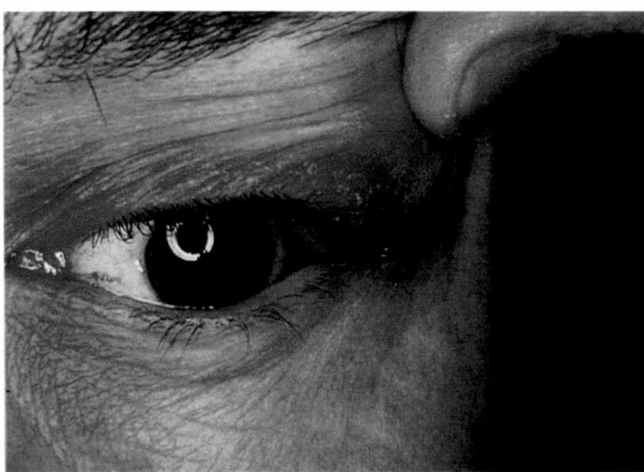

FIGURE 3.27 External chalazion extending through the temporal aspect of the superior lid. Overlying external and internal tissue will often show inflammatory changes and exudate.

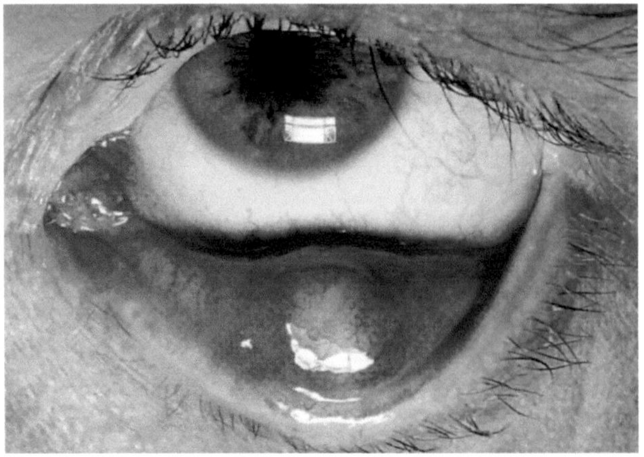

FIGURE 3.28 Internal chalazion in the inferior eyelid. Note the observable granulomatous formation at the site of the involved meibomian gland with diffuse, surrounding inflammatory changes (overlying palpebral conjunctiva).

Assessment

(See also Appendix 3)

- Rule out neoplastic lumps and bumps
- Rule out systemic possibilities in chronic recurring chalazia (i.e., granulomatous diseases)
- Rule out lid infectious causes
- Rule out acute rosacea in recurrent forms

Plan: Chalazion

- If chalazion measures less than 8 to 10 mm
  1. Hot compresses as frequently as possible
  2. No less than qid for additive effect
- If chalazion greater than 8 to 10 mm, surgical excision indicated
- Direct steroidal injections occasionally used
- Treat any superficial infections or inflammations before surgical excision

Follow-Up

- If heat therapy employed, recheck in 2 weeks
  1. If reducing, continue to resolution
  2. If no improvement (and patient compliant), consider additional 2 weeks or surgery
- Advise patient on possible recurrences and instruct on weekly lid palpations for early detection

D. Demodicosis[27,28]

Background Information

1. Two mite species normal part of lid flora
   a. *Demodex folliculorum* (Figure 3.29)
      i. Lives in lash follicle
      ii. Most abundant in hair follicles on tip of nose and eyelid margins
   b. *Demodex brevis*
      i. Found in sebaceous and meibomian glands
2. Demodex increases with age; found in 84% of patients 60 and older
3. Usually subclinical, but if excessive in amount can produce toxic or hypersensitive marginal-type reaction, damage meibomian glands, and cause bacterial contamination

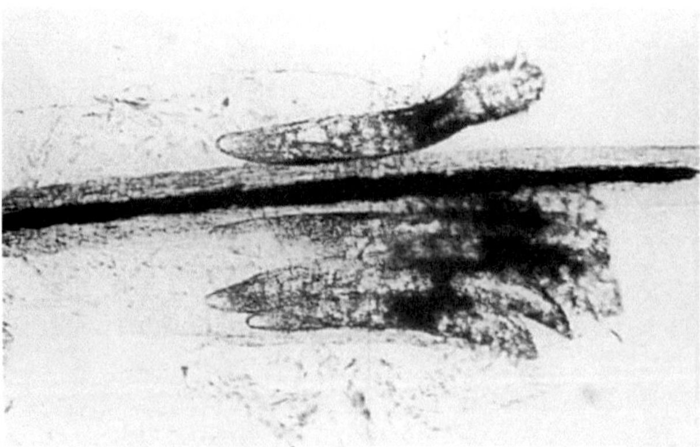

FIGURE 3.29 *Demodex folliculorum* mites adherent to an epilated eyelash observed under oil immersion microscopy. More than 8–10 organisms on 5 to 6 lashes suggests clinical infestation.

Subjective

- Often patient is symptom free (in for routine care)
- Older patients frequently report the "itchy-burnies," foreign-body sensation, lid crusting, and redness

Objective

- Bilateral, indurated (thickened by chronic edema and inflammation) lid margins (Figure 3.30)
- Inflammation ranges from subclinical to moderate
- Collarettes (cylindrical dandruff) attach around base of each lash
  1. Vary in degree from thin rings to full length of cilia
  2. Differ from staphylococcal rosettes (flat crusts at base of lash) in length of lash involvement
- Hair follicle damage causing misalignment, madarosis, and trichiasis
- Meibomian gland dysfunction
- Lid inflammation can affect ocular surface and cause keratoconjunctivitis
- Can be observed in advanced cases by epilation and microscope (oil emersion slide) examination

Assessment

- Rule out other marginal blepharitis (especially staphylococcal)
- Rule out pediculosis

Plan: Demodicosis

- Older treatments such as mercuric oxide ointment or Vaseline™ have been ineffective

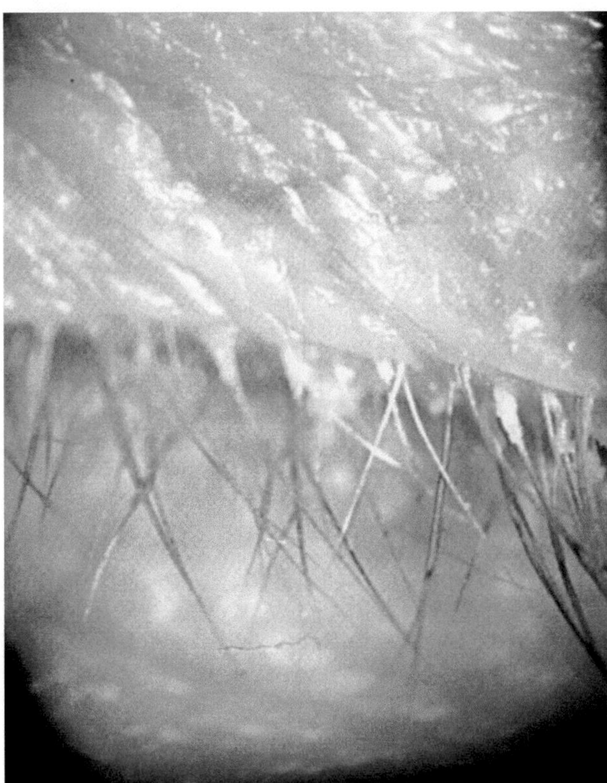

FIGURE 3.30 **Demodicosis** is the clinical manifestation of *Demodex folliculorum* mites producing "collarettes" or crustations around the stalk of lashes as they emanate from the infected hair follicles.

- Goal is to reduce the Demodex overpopulation
- Treatment of choice—Tea Tree Oil (e.g., Cliradex, Ocusoft Oust Demodex Cleanser)
  1. For mild cases BID lid scrub with 5–10% Tea Tree Oil solution for 10 to 14 days
  2. For moderate cases in-office treatment with 50% Tea Tree Oil solution weekly plus at home therapy with 10% solution
- Microblepharoexfoliation (e.g., BlephEx) will mechanically remove attached biofilm

Follow-Up

- Recheck after 10- to 14-day treatment plan
- If no improvement
  1. Recheck diagnosis
  2. Confirm compliance and reinstruct
  3. Reinstitute treatment plan for additional 10-day period
- Advise patient on chronicity
- Ongoing light Tree Tea Oil lid scrubs weekly
- Recheck lids in 6 months or PRN

E. Herpes Simplex Virus (HSV)[29,30]

Background Information

1. Most common virus in humans (only natural host)
2. Two forms of virus: herpes simplex virus type 1 (HSV-l) (oral) and herpes simplex virus type 2 (HSV-2) (genital)
3. Sources of HSV infection
   a. Primary infection
   b. Recurrent infection (after primary attack)
   c. Transmission from symptomatic or asymptomatic carrier
4. Transmission is through direct contact
   a. Mostly saliva and mouth contact
   b. Also contact with active skin lesions (vesicles)
   c. Incubation period approximately 1 week
5. Primary HSV attacks uncommon but dramatic
   a. Mostly in children and young adults
   b. Older age ranges protected by immunity
6. Greatest risk for primary infection from age 6 months to 5 to 10 years old (as immunity begins to develop)
   a. Approximately 70% of children infected by 5 years of age
   b. Approximately 90% of these infections remain subclinical
   c. Approximately 70% immune to HSV by 15 to 25 years of age
   d. Approximately 90% immune to HSV by 60 years of age
7. Recurrence will occur in 25% of HSV infections
8. Aggravating or inciting factors for recurrence
   a. Sunlight (UV)
   b. Trauma (especially localized to ocular area)
   c. Extreme heat or cold
   d. Fever
   e. Steroids
   f. Infectious disease (systemic or ocular)
   g. Surgery
   h. Epilation

Subjective

- Mild to moderate discomfort (moderate to severe in primary attacks)

- Patient frequently reports history of recurrence and fever blisters at mucocutaneous border of lip
- Rule out genital HSV infection by history

Objective

- Usually unilateral but could spread across midline (Figure 3.31)
- Lower lid involved more frequently than upper
- Diffuse patches of small, sometimes pinpoint size vesicles on a mild to moderately edematous (swollen) erythematous base
- Clear fluid vesicles change to yellowish pustules within a 3- to 5-day period
- Yellowish pustules harden into crusts over a 7- to 10-day period and shed without scar formation
- Occasionally vesicles or pustules may break down into shallow ulcers that heal within about 2 weeks
- Mild to moderate lymphadenopathy may be present (can be severe in primary infection)

Assessment

(See also Appendix 3)

- Differentiate primary from recurrent attack
- Rule out herpes zoster virus
- Rule out bacterial infection
- Rule out other eyelid dermatoses
- Rule out AIDS

Plan: Herpes Simplex Blepharitis

(See also Appendices 4 and 6)

- Treatment optional in mild cases (HSV blepharitis is a self-limiting condition)
- Dermatological Acyclovir topical cream (tid to q4h)
  1. May be used off label
  2. Other topical antivirals not effective on skin
  3. Add oral acyclovir or valacyclovir in more severe presentations
- Prophylactic topical antibiotics optional
- Supportive therapies
  1. Cold packs
  2. Domeboro packs
  3. Alcohol wipes

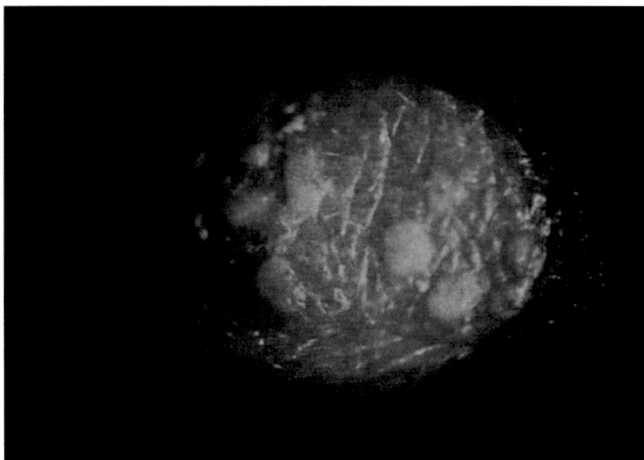

FIGURE 3.31 Herpes simplex blepharitis pustules on lower lid. Clinical presentation usually involves fluid-filled vesicles becoming pustules that dry and resolve over 10–14 days.

- Regarding ocular surface:
  1. Not involved: do not treat
  2. Hyperemia without keratitis (SPK): optional
     a. Lubricants
     b. Prophylactic broad-spectrum antibiotic
  3. Keratitis (SPK): Viroptic tid to qid, Ganciclovir gel 0.15% tid
  4. Dendrite(s): Viroptic q2h, Ganciclovir gel 0.15% q3h

Follow-Up

- Recheck skin and ocular surface at 3- to 5-day intervals
- Consider medical or dermatological referral if lesions not remitting within 7 to 10 days
- Advise patient on recurrent nature of disease and "triggering" factors
- Recheck eyes and lids annually or PRN

F. Herpes Zoster Virus (HZV)[31,32]

Background Information

1. Varicella-type virus infecting dorsal root ganglion
   a. Virus called chickenpox in children
   b. Virus called shingles in adults
2. Highest incidence in elderly and immunocompromised
3. Usually affects the ophthalmic division of trigeminal nerve
4. When HZV affects the nasociliary branch
   a. Vesicle at tip of nose (Hutchinson's sign)
   b. Approximately 60% risk of ocular involvement (ophthalmicus)
   c. Approximately 40% risk of ophthalmicus without Hutchinson's sign

Subjective

- Acute attack usually preceded by a tingling sensation in the scalp region on affected side
  1. Often noted early with hair combing or brushing
  2. Precedes observable clinical signs
- Prodomal itching and mild irritation around eye
- May report history of shingles elsewhere on body
- On clinical manifestation, pain becomes quite severe

Objective

- Always unilateral with lesions up to midline
- Diffuse inflammatory erythema spreads from forehead down to upper (and sometimes lower) lid
- Fluid-filled vesicles form first on erythematous base
  1. Follow nerve fiber linear patterns (dermatomes)
  2. Varying levels of surrounding edema
- Within 3 to 5 days, vesicles erupt into ulcerations
  1. HZV ulcers will produce permanent scarring
  2. Scars may produce ectropion, ptosis
  3. Certainly, scarring remains cosmetically apparent
- Lymphadenopathy may be present during acute phase
- Postherpetic neuralgia results in chronic ongoing pain of moderate to severe degree

Assessment

(See also Appendix 3)

- Rule out herpes simplex virus
- Rule out bacterial infection
- Rule out other eyelid dermatoses
- Rule out systemic neoplastic disease (especially lymphoma)

1. Often associated with HZV infections in adults
2. Medical evaluation indicated in primary attacks

- Rule out eyeball involvement (common)
- Rule out AIDS, especially in atypical presentations (e.g., no pain and/or variable objective signs)

Plan: Herpes Zoster Virus

(See also Appendix 6)

- Medical or dermatological consultation sometimes indicated
- Oral antivirals available
    1. Acyclovir (Zovirax) (Figure 3.32)
        a. 800 mg, 5 times daily (4 g/day) for 7 to 10 days
    2. Famcyclovir (Famvir)
        a. 500 mg tid for 7 to 10 days
    3. Valacyclovir (Valtrex)
        a. 1000 mg tid for 7 to 10 days
    4. Brivudine (Zerpex)—available in some European countries
        a. qd dosing
        b. Reduces pain sooner than Valacyclovir
    5. Amenamevir—available in Japan
- Oral steroids valuable to manage pain
- Start medication within 72 hours of rash appearance to minimize postherpetic neuralgia
- Supportive therapies
    1. Warm and cold packs
    2. Domeboro packs
    3. Alcohol wipes
    4. Nonnarcotic and if necessary narcotic analgesics
- Topical prophylactic antibiotic ointments (and steroid combinations) often used in healing phase
- Regarding ocular involvement (common and variable):
    1. No involvement: do not treat
    2. Variable findings: treat accordingly

Follow-Up

- Advise patient carefully
    1. Regarding postherpetic neuralgia
    2. Regarding permanent scarring
    3. Regarding ongoing ocular risks (highly variable)
    4. On recurrent attacks
- Recheck eyeball annually or PRN

G. Hordeolum (Staphylococcal Infection of Zeiss, Moll, or Meibomian Glands)[33,34]

Subjective

- Staphylococcal infection to single or multiple glands
    1. External type involves Zeiss or Moll glands
    2. Internal type involves meibomian gland(s)
- Acute presentation, usually within 24 to 48 hours
- Moderate to dramatic generalized lid tenderness with distinct tenderness on focal palpation of affected gland
- Frequently associated with chronic blepharitis

Objective

- External type (often called "stye") most common (Figure 3.33)
    1. Presents at lid margin
    2. External suppuration (exudate points outward)
    3. May suppurate through gland orifice or break through skin surface
    4. Mild to moderate edema and erythematous ring limited to immediate surrounding area

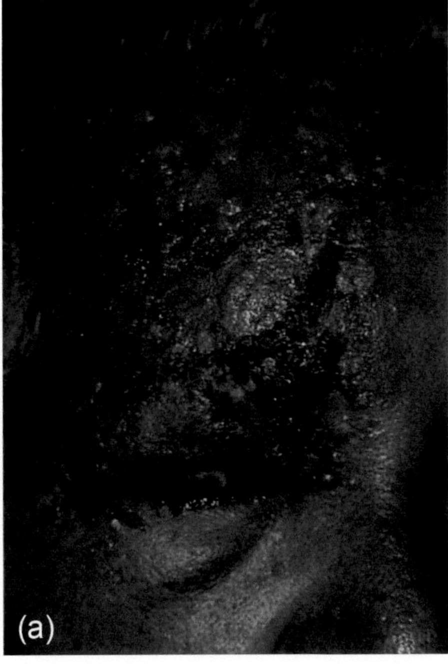

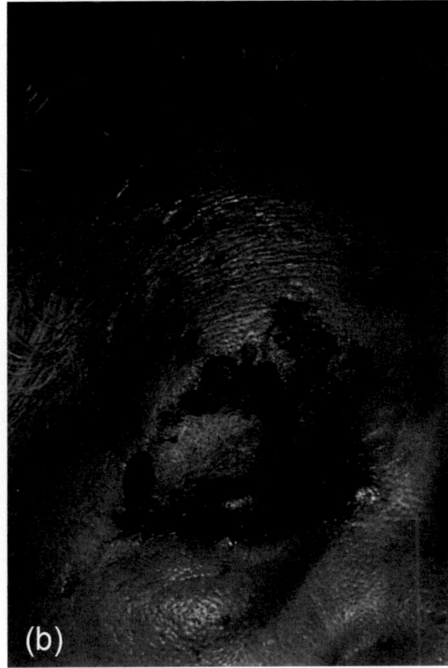

FIGURE 3.32 **(a) Severe herpes zoster ophthalmicus** demonstrate acute dermatologic and blepharitic vesicles, ulcerations, and exudative lesions 4–5 days after initial symptoms. **(b)** Patient responds within 72 hours to oral and topical acyclovir and corticosteroid therapy. Therapeutic efforts must be initiated within the first 3–5 days for maximum potential, immediate and long-term benefits.

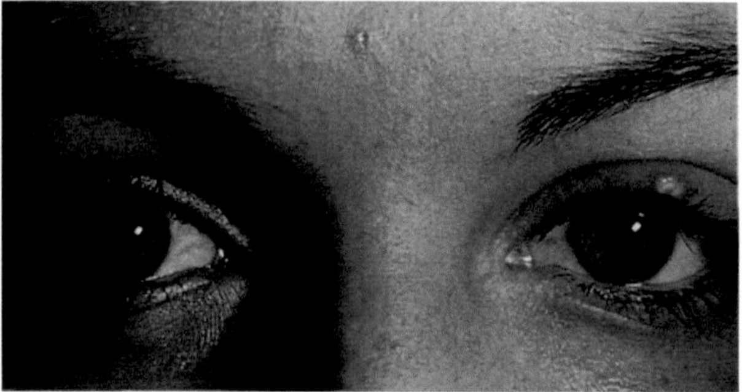

FIGURE 3.33 **External hordeolum** (also referred to as a "stye") presents as a self-limiting, superficial suppuration of a Zeiss or Moll gland with mild lid irritation and edema secondary to staphylococcal infection.

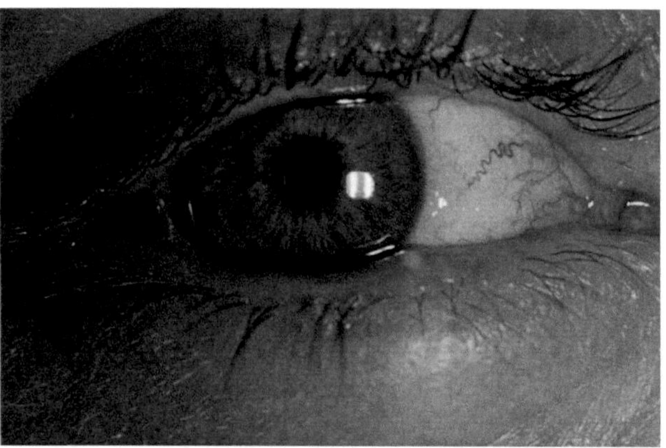

FIGURE 3.34 **Internal hordeolum** (also referred to as an "acute chalazion") with a staphylococcal infected, inspissated meibomian gland producing secondary edema and erythema of the lower lid. Direct palpation at the site of lesion produces severe pain.

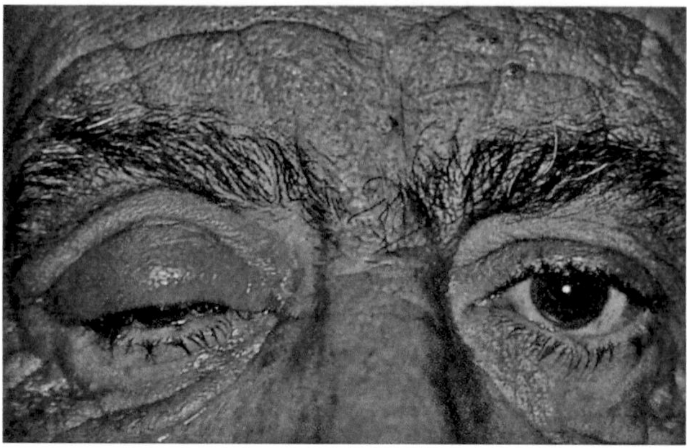

FIGURE 3.35 **Preseptal cellulitis** secondary to a hordeolum in the superior eyelid. Edema, erythema, and palpable pain (inflammatory cascade) can spread superiorly and inferiorly, through loosely connected lid tissue as far as orbital rims, brow region, and temporal region.

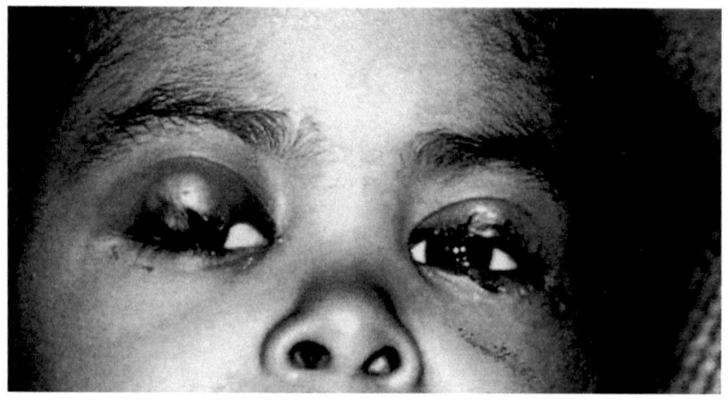

FIGURE 3.36 **Lid abscess** resulting from an untreated internal hordeolum. Encapsulated infected meibomian gland will not respond to topical or oral antibiotics and will require surgical incision and drainage.

- Internal type (also known as acute chalazion) less common but more frequently seen in the office setting due to increased pain and clinical signs (Figure 3.34)
  1. Deeper response (internal lid tissue; Figure 3.35)
  2. Sometimes lump may point inward toward palpebral conjunctiva or out meibomian orifice
  3. Lid edema and erythema is moderate to severe, often diffusing throughout the involved (upper or lower) lid causing a preseptal cellulitis sometimes burying the localized swollen gland
- Occasionally, a virulent organism (with or without treatment) may progress, enlarge, and encapsulate into a lid abscess (Figure 3.36)

Assessment

(See also Appendix 3)

- Carefully palpate edematous and erythematous lids for area of focal tenderness
- Rule out other causes of painful lid edema
  1. Acute blepharitis (diffuse)
  2. Acute dacryocystitis (inferior nasal tenderness with secondary hyperlacrimation)
- Beware of secondary preseptal cellulitis
  1. Common complication with internal hordeolum
  2. May be present on first visit or within 48 hours after initiating topical therapies
  3. Cellulitis will not respond to topical therapy
- Differentiate clinical degree to determine appropriate therapeutic approach
  1. External type (therapeutics optional)
  2. Internal without preseptal cellulitis (topicals)
  3. Internal with preseptal cellulitis (topicals and orals)
  4. Lid abscess (surgical drainage plus orals)

Plan: Hordeolum

(See also Appendix 4)

- For external hordeolum
  1. Warm packs qid
  2. Topical bacitracin ointment bid to qid (optional)
- For internal hordeolum
  1. Warm packs qid
  2. Topical bacitracin ointment bid to qid
  3. With preseptal cellulitis, add oral agents, for 7 to 10 days

   a. Penicillinase-resistant penicillin (i.e., Augmentin), 500 to 875 mg bid
   b. Cephalosporin (e.g., Keflex), 250 mg up to qid or 500 mg bid
   c. Sulfamethoxazole-trimethoprim (e.g., Bactrim) 400 mg/80 mg or 800 mg/160 mg bid Doxycycline 100 mg bid for MRSA suspected infections
- For lid abscess (encapsulated infection)
   1. Surgical incision and drainage
   2. Oral antistaphylococcal drug
- Significant pointing or suppuration of external or internal type may be optionally drained by superficial needling and gentle milking of gland (it will be painful)

Follow-Up
- Recheck all internal hordeolii within 48 to 72 hours
   1. If stable or improving, continue treatment for 5 to 7 days (minimum) and recheck
   2. If worsening, consider preseptal cellulitis or abscess and adjust treatment accordingly
- On resolution, instruct patient on ongoing staphylococcal preventive-maintenance program (see Figure 3.36)

H. Insect Bites or Stings
Subjective
- Contributory history (e.g., mosquito, bee, small carnivores!)
- Itching
- Stinging sensation
- Occasionally throbbing pain
- Rarely (but very possibly) systemic reactions

Objective
- Pinpoint lesion (with stinger possibly embedded)
- Usually focal edema around site (may be diffuse)
   1. Erythema possible
   2. Bleeding possible

Assessment
- Rule out any severe allergic, asthmatic, or atopic history
- Do not worry about identifying (or catching) the culprit

Plan: Insect Bites or Stings
- If stinger in situ, "flick" it out with fingers
   1. Do not use grasping instruments producing pressure
   2. Do not pinch or grasp stinger with fingers; at risk of injecting additional toxin
- Cold packs
- Oral decongestant/antihistamine (e.g., Benadryl) if indicated
- Topical hydrocortisone (0.5 to 1%) ointments or creams if needed for subjective relief
- If severe systemic reaction developing or history of significant allergic tendencies, consult physician

Follow-Up
- PRN

I. Meibomian Gland Dysfunction (MGD, Meibomianitis)[35–45]
Background Information
1. Leading cause of evaporative dry eye disease
2. Two types:
   a. Hyposecretion (more common)
   b. Hypersecretion
3. Hyposecretion
   a. Gland obstruction → lipid quality and quantity reduced
   b. Meibum stasis caused by gland obstruction, drop out, or inflammation
   c. Meibum stasis results in bacterial contamination and release of lipid degrading enzymes that further increases meibum viscosity and free fatty acids that increase inflammation, and the cycle continues
4. Hypersecretion associated with seborrheic dermatitis, atopic disease, and acne rosacea
5. Tear film changes result in irritation, inflammation, and ocular surface disease
6. Gland function affected by many factors
   a. Hormonal disturbances
      i. Androgens stimulate meibum production
      ii. Estrogens increase inflammation
   b. Aging
   c. Systemic medications (e.g., Accutane)
   d. Topical medications (e.g., topical beta-blockers, prostaglandin analogs, carbonic anhydrase inhibitors
   e. Diet
      i. Omega-3 fatty acids → increase improves MG function

Subjective
- Early stages may be asymptomatic
- Symptoms include irritation, burning, dryness, foreign-body sensation, photophobia, pain, redness, fluctuating vision
   1. Can be exacerbated by activities requiring concentration (e.g., computer, TV, driving, etc.)
- Signs and symptoms do not necessarily correlate
- Non-specific irritation (greater in morning)
- Commonly presents with ocular surface involvement and associated corneal symptoms (i.e., FB sensation)

Objective
- Usually bilateral (Figure 3.37)
- Meibomian gland orifices plugged (inspissation; Figure 3.38)
   1. A line of whitish-yellow plugs along lid margin (milia)
   2. Usually greater on inferior lid margin
   3. Meibum thick and difficult to express from glands
      a. Express glands (e.g., Meibomian Gland Evaluator) to visualize meibum
      b. Clear, easily expressed (normal lipids) to viscous and not easily expressed (severe gland disease)
   4. Gland structure and loss (i.e., dropout) can be evaluated with infrared meibography
- Lid margin hyperemia and telangiectasis
- Eyelid margin frothing
- Chronic forms produce thickened, rounded lid margins (induration)
- Frequent ocular surface involvements
   1. Sodium fluorescein and lissamine green staining of the cornea and conjunctiva
   2. Blepharoconjunctivitis (greater inferiorly)
   3. Blepharokeratoconjunctivitis (inferior to diffuse)
   4. Tear film disturbances, including quick tear breakup time (BUT) and "frothy" tear meniscus

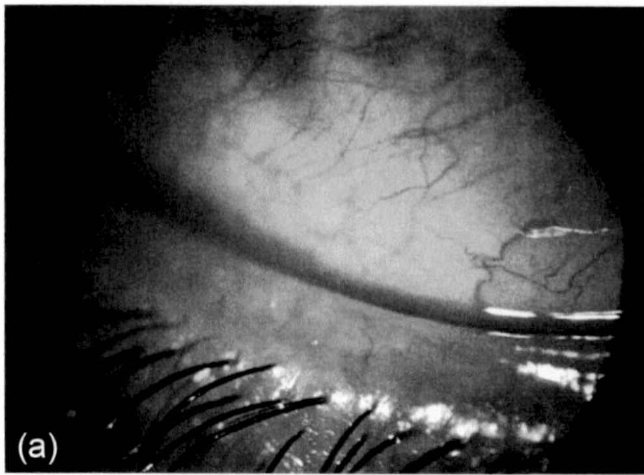

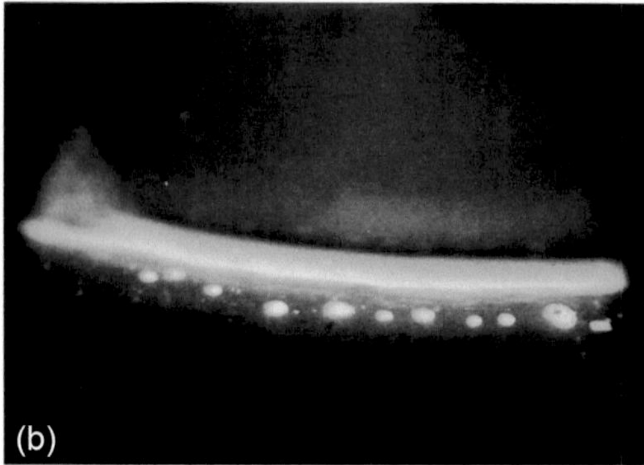

FIGURE 3.37 **(a) Meibomian gland congestion** producing mild to moderate inspissation of meibomian glands' tubules and orifices at the lid margins. **(b) Congested meibomian gland orifices** highlighted by sodium fluorescein dye.

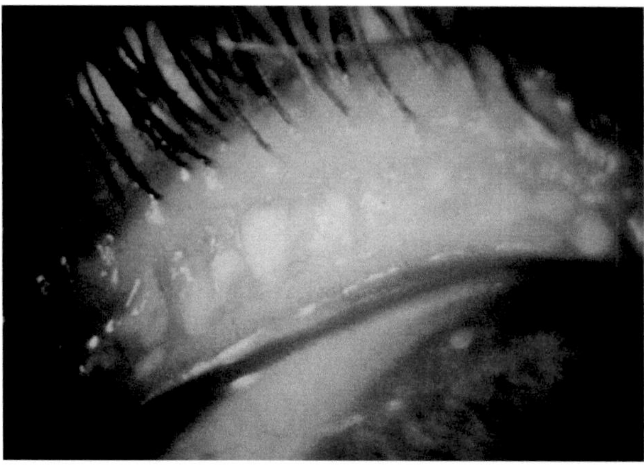

FIGURE 3.38 **Severe meibomian gland dysfunction** of the superior lid caused by chronic inflammation of the meibomian glands producing caseation of the glands sebum (meibum). Caseous material must be expressed by vigorous, repeated eyelid/meibomian gland massage and heat application.

Assessment

(See also Appendix 3)

- Rule out aqueous deficient dry eye (see Chapter 5, I. D.)
- Rule out marginal blepharitis types including Demodex infestation
- Rule out acne rosacea
- Often associated with chronic alcoholism
- Rule out nutritional factors

Plan: Meibomian Gland Dysfunction (MGD, Meibomianitis)

(See also Appendix 6)

- Treatment depends on severity of symptoms and signs
- Treatment options below listed in order of asymptomatic/mild to moderate/severe disease
    1. Review impact of diet, work/home environment (e.g., humidity, computer usage, etc.), medications
    2. Recommend increased omega-3 fatty (triglyceride form) acid via diet or supplements
        a. The author prefers an EPA to DHA ratio of 3:1 (e.g., Nordic Natural EPA Xtra)
    3. Warm compresses to closed eyes for minimum 4 minutes qd to bid
    4. Lipid-containing artificial tears, preservative free for frequent use
    5. Topical azithromycin
    6. Lower lid debridement at Line of Marx with golf club spud
    7. Eyelid thermal pulsation devices apply heat followed by mechanical pressure to empty the obstructed gland
        a. Lipiflow applies a 10-minute warming period to internal superior and inferior lid followed by automated meibomian gland expression
        b. iLUX applies a 40-second warming period to internal superior and inferior lid followed by manual expression
        c. TearCare applies adjustable heat externally to superior and inferior lids followed by manual expression
    8. Intense pulsed light (IPL)
        a. Developed for dermatology but has been used "off-label" for MGD
        b. Light emitting system (visible to infrared wavelengths) pulsed at various durations
        c. Evidence from clinical trials to date have not been conclusive
    9. Anti-inflammatory ophthalmic drops (steroids if ocular surface inflammation exacerbated)
    10. Orals are prescribed at sub-antimicrobial levels for anti-inflammatory and bacterial lipase reduction
        a. Doxycycline and Minocycline 50 mg qd to bid
        b. Tetracycline 250 mg qd to qid
        c. Azithromycin (e.g., Z-Pak)
- Topical combination antibiotic and steroid suspension, qid for anterior blepharitis associated
    1. Administer after lid massage
    2. Do not use ointments in meibomianitis
    3. Drop suspension on fingertip and apply to lid
    4. If ocular surface involved, drop 1 gtt on eye
- Bandage soft lenses or scleral lenses for significant superficial punctate keratitis

Follow-Up

- Should be stable or improving in 1 to 2 weeks
- Reduce medications slowly (2 to 4 weeks) or prescribe maintenance medications as needed
- If condition not responding to maximal therapy
  1. Reconfirm diagnosis
  2. Check for compliance and reinstruct patient
  3. Recheck history for alcoholism or acne rosacea
- Advise patient on potential chronicity

J. Pediculosis[46]

Background Information

1. Infrequent (fortunately!) infestation of eyelid margins by body lice (*Pediculus corporis*), head lice (*Pediculus capitis*), or pubic lice (*Phthirus pubis*)
2. Transmitted by contact with carrier, heavy scalp infestation, contaminated garments, bedsheets, or by sexual contact
3. Most common in children and young adults through school contacts, play, clothing

Subjective

- Usually, a subacute presentation with symptoms of mild to moderate itching and irritation of eyelids (usually bilateral)
- History may include exposure to known carrier(s) (as in a classroom situation)

Objective

- Gross observation of lids reveals crusty marginal appearance, sometimes with brownish discoloration
- Slit-lamp examination reveals nits (eggs) and actual organisms adherent to lashes and skin of lid (Figure 3.39)

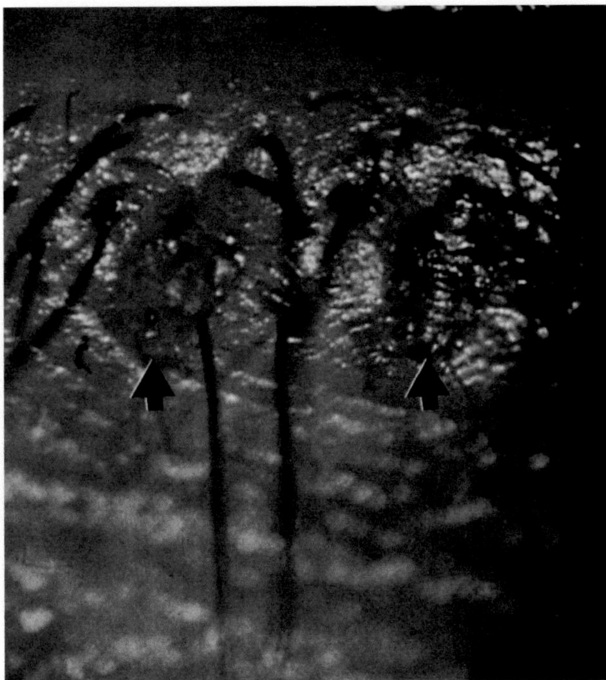

FIGURE 3.39 **Pediculosis** of infestation of the lid margin by pubic lice demonstrated nits (eggs) attached to eyelashes and the organism itself (arrow) straddling two lashes.

- In more severe infestation, shallow ulcerations may develop, as well as secondary keratoconjunctivitis

Assessment

- Rule out other forms of marginal blepharitis
- Attempt to determine source of infestation

Plan: Pediculosis

- Coordinate appropriate management of source of infestation
- Remove (as best as possible) nits and lice from lid
  1. Toothed or jeweler's forceps work well
  2. Careful debridement with alcohol-saturated cotton-tip applicator may be effective
- Numerous agents are recommended for treatment at a bid to tid frequency for approximately 5 to 7 days. However, some must be used very carefully on the lid margins due to potential irritative (toxic) effects of pediculicides to the ocular surface
  1. One percent mercuric oxide ointment
  2. Eserine ointment (not recommended due to miosis)
  3. Plain petroleum jelly or any bland ointment base
  4. Pyrethrin ointments (pediculicide and toxic)
  5. Kwell shampoo (pediculicide and toxic)
  6. RID shampoo (pediculicide and toxic)
- Advise patient to wash pillowcases, bed sheets, towels, and hats in hot water
- If nits persist after 1-week treatment
  1. Recheck diagnosis
  2. Confirm compliance and reinstruct
  3. Retreat for additional week
  4. Consider reinfestation from untreated primary source

Lacrimal System

Review of Clinical Anatomy

1. Secretory Portion
   a. Accessory glands of Krause and Wolfring
   b. Lacrimal gland in the anterior lateral portion of the orbit in the lacrimal fossa
      i. Large orbital portion and smaller palpebral portion
      ii. 3 to 5 ducts (orbital) and 5 to 7 ducts (palpebral) open into superior temporal fornix of lids
   c. Lacrimal (aqueous) secretions controlled by complex multiple nerve innervations
      i. Lacrimal nucleus of facial nerve (cranial nerve VII)
      ii. Postganglionic fiber from cranial nerve VII with zygomatic branch of maxillary branch of trigeminal (cranial nerve V)
      iii. Postganglionic sympathetic fibers from superior cervical ganglion to sphenopalatine ganglion also supply blood vessels to the gland
         - No effect on lacrimal secretions
         - Gland drains through lymphatics to preauricular lymph nodes
2. Excretory Portion
   a. Lacrimal puncta is an opening leading to canaliculi about 3 mm in size on lid margins surrounded by avascular connective tissue

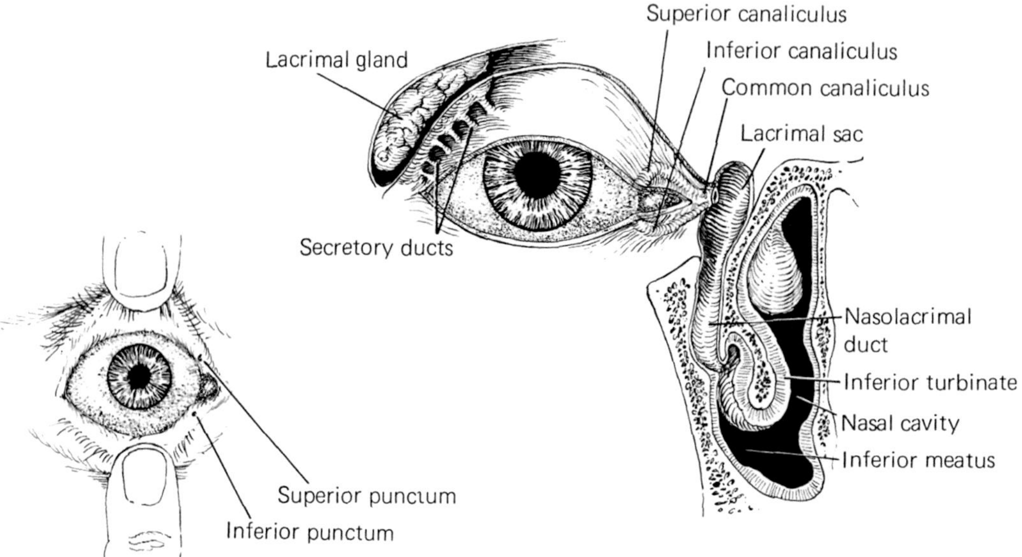

FIGURE 3.B The lacrimal drainage system.

b. Canaliculi (upper and lower) drain tears to lacrimal sac
   i. Vertical portion = 2 to 3.5 mm
   ii. Horizontal portion = 8 mm
   iii. Join to common canaliculi
c. Lacrimal sac located in medial portion of orbit in lacrimal fossa continues interiorly as nasolacrimal duct
d. Nasolacrimal duct is downward extension of sac into inferior nasal meatus on lateral wall and possesses numerous folds functioning as valves (Figure 3.B)

I. Irritations and Injuries

A. Foreign Bodies

See Obstructions.

B. Laceration[47]

Subjective

- Most common injury to lacrimal system
- Caused by penetrating or ripping wounds to eyelids
- Does not need emergency repair

Objective

- Usually extensive swelling and bleeding
- Puncta or canaliculi may be torn or cut

Assessment

- Differentiate lid laceration from canaliculi involvement
- If possible, differentiate puncta from canaliculi involvement
- Rule out presence of foreign matter in the wound

Plan: Laceration

- Better to wait for 24 to 48 hours to permit swelling and bleeding to subside
- Frequent cold packs and mild pressure
- Refer to oculoplastics for surgical repair and possible conjunctivodacryocystorhinostomy (that's the longest word in the book!)

Follow-Up

- Lacrimal surgical procedures often take 2 months or more to heal and thus require diligent compliance
- Prognosis usually guarded regarding complete repair (i.e., often resolves with chronic residual tearing)

II. Noninflammatory Conditions

A. Dacryostenosis

See Obstructions.

B. Obstructions[48]

Subjective

- Most common congenital abnormality of the system
  1. Up to 30% of newborns (delayed opening of valve of Hasner)
  2. Most open spontaneously within weeks to months
- Not uncommon in adults, especially elderly (Figure 3.40)

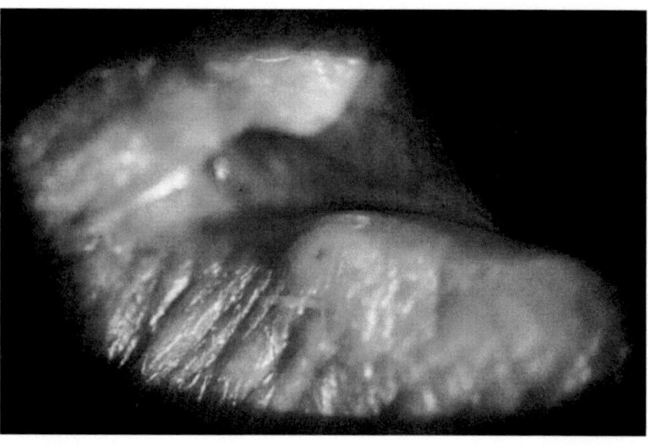

FIGURE 3.40 **Punctal atresia, stenosis, and ectropion** all demonstrated in the lacrimal puncta of a 94-year-old woman presenting with chronic epiphora. Conservative management included intermittent punctal probing, secondary infection prevention, and patient reassurance.

1. Usually idiopathic (no established cause)
2. Narrowing of canaliculi (dacryostenosis)
   a. Sometimes caused by eyedrops
      i. Phospholine iodide
      ii. Antiviral agents, especially idoxuridine (IDU)
      iii. Epinephrines
      iv. Systemic 5-fluorouracil and docetaxel (anticancer drugs)
   b. Sometimes disease (e.g., ocular pemphigoid)
   c. Sometimes trauma (e.g., repeated probing)
3. Occasionally obstruction is mechanical (Figure 3.41)
   i. Trauma and resulting cicatrix (scarring)
   ii. Tumors (benign or malignant)
   iii. Localized strictures in system
   iv. Occult matter (e.g., punctal and canicular plugs, makeup, dirt particles, lashes)
   v. Dacryoliths (calcium deposits in tubules)

- Common complication of inflammation or infection
  a. Congenital or acquired dacryocystitis
  b. Mucous plugs
  c. Secondary strictures
- Infrequently, nasal or sinus disease or surgery may cause secondary obstruction

Objective

- Epiphora, usually from inner canthal region
- Punctal integrity, position usually normal
- Drainage tests (e.g., Jones, Saccharin) positive
- Dilation and irrigation difficult or impossible
- Dacryocystorhinogram (x-ray) (done only in serious or suspicious cases, usually definitive)

Assessment

- Congenital versus acquired
- Rule out inflammation or infection (pain, discharge)
- Rule out signs of tumor
- Rule out punctal anomalies

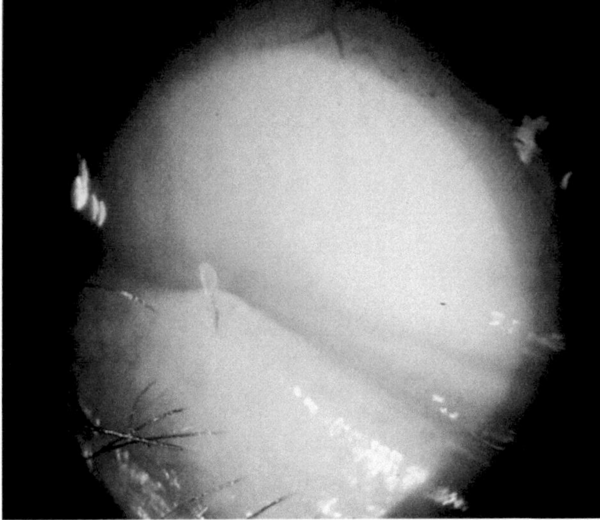

FIGURE 3.41 **Lacrimal punctal obstruction** caused by a loose, migratory lash coming to rest in the inferior puncta. A complaint of epiphora is usually the presenting sign, and untreated conditions could result in internal obstruction from developing dacryoliths (calcium salts in canaliculi).

- Rule out nasal or sinus disease
- Do diagnostic tests if clinical picture is confusing
  1. Drainage tests (e.g., dyes)
  2. Dilation and irrigation (D&I) of lacrimal drainage system
  3. X-ray studies if indicated

Plan: Obstructions

- Manage congenital and acquired dacryostenosis same as chronic dacryocystitis
- Treat primary cause of obstruction appropriately
- Often frequent heat and firm massage (hot cloth wrapped around massaging finger) with or without other therapies may have positive effect
- D&I procedure
  1. Usually effective for following causes
     a. Discrete obstructions (e.g., mechanical)
     b. Subacute inflammation or infection
  2. Usually ineffective for following causes
     a. Dacryostenosis (primary or secondary), especially in elderly patients
     b. Strictures
     c. Disease causes (e.g., tumors, nasal or sinus)
- Probing (Bowman's) often required in resistant cases with limited success and risk of aggravation
- Referral for surgical repair should be limited to absolute necessity and serious requests only
  1. Reason is difficulty and guarded prognosis of lacrimal repair procedure (dacryocystorhinostomy)
  2. Refer to oculoplastics specialist
- Carefully advise and educate patients on condition, chronicity (if applicable), compliance to therapies, and prognosis of treatment, management, and surgical repair

Follow-Up

- Follow-up on treatment of primary conditions as indicated
- Monitor untreated conditions at 3- to 6-month intervals
  1. For spontaneous resolution
  2. For deterioration
  3. For complications
- Recheck D&I procedures in 1 week (for resolution or retreatment)
  a. Occasionally sequential or periodic D&Is prove successful versus single procedure
  b. Non-invasive approach versus repeated probing
  c. Usually no hope after 3 to 5 unsuccessful attempts
- Stress compliance with any treatment regimen

C. Punctal Anomalies[49]

Subjective

- May be congenital or acquired
- Lower punctual problems usually most clinically significant
- Most often associated with signs and symptoms of associated (usually primary) disorder

Objective

- Epiphora, usually at inner canthus
- Examination of lower puncta area demonstrates
  1. Absent (imperforate) puncta (usually congenital)
  2. Atresia, stenosis, or closure (usually in elderly)
  3. Duplication or double puncta

4. Punctal ectropion (puncta turning outward and not communicating with lacrimal lake)
   a. Rarely congenital (e.g., blepharophimosis)
   b. Commonly acquired (e.g., eyelid laxity in elderly)
   c. May also follow injury or burns (scarring)
- Simple blockage by foreign matter, lashes
  1. Dacryoliths (calcium salts)
  2. May cause secondary acute or chronic dacryoscystitis
- Tumors of the inner canthus (benign or malignant)
- Secondary to advanced ocular surface diseases, such as keratitis sicca-type syndromes, inflammation

Assessment

- Congenital versus acquired
- Determine primary cause
- Rule out canalicular involvement by dilation and irrigation (D&I)
- Rule out other causes of wet eye presentations

Plan: Punctal Anomalies

- Treat the primary cause as indicated
- Attempt gentle opening of closed puncta with sharp punctal dilator (e.g., Katena) or needle
- Dilate puncta with progressive-diameter dilators
- Warm pack surrounding tissue tid to qid for 1 week
- Refer serious cases or requests for surgical repair

Follow-Up

- Outcome of any nonsurgical approaches usually unrewarding
- Surgical approaches such as Three-snip punctoplasty and stent cannulation have guarded prognosis

D. Tumors of the Canaliculi (Excretory) System

Subjective

- May be benign or malignant
- Fortunately very uncommon
- Can mimic chronic dacryocystitis or stenosis and thus can go undiagnosed for extended period
- Can appear as painless swelling (or mucocele)
- Frequently associated nasal or sinus symptoms

Objective

- May be external or internal (usually lacrimal sac)
- Mimic common signs of obstructed system
  1. Epiphora
  2. Same response to dilation and irrigation
- Frequently produces "bloody tears"
- Usually some degree of palpable or observable mass in region of drainage system

Assessment

- Rule out dacryocystitis and dacryostenosis by lack of response to standard therapies
- Rule out other causes of obstruction
- If suspicious, refer for dacryocystography (x-rays)
- Refer suspicious masses in region for biopsy

Plan: Tumors of the Canaliculi System

- Refer for surgical excision (dacryocystectomy)
- Patient refusal for immediate care should be carefully documented in records
- Postoperative radiation therapy frequently applied

Follow-Up

- Recheck after referral to confirm care
- Due to wide range of tumor types in the area (and attendant risks), prompt care and careful follow-up monitoring is essential

E. Tumors of the Lacrimal Gland[50]

Subjective

- Considered rare (but "it ain't rare if it's in your chair!")
- May be benign or malignant
- Adenoid cystic carcinoma most common form
- Onset may be insidious (slow) or fast
- Pain on palpation possible
- Patient may report diplopia

Objective

- Lid swelling may be moderate to severe
- Pseudoptosis common
- Variable degrees of proptosis (exophthalmos)
- Displacement of eyeball (down and in), causing diplopia

Assessment

- Rule out dacryoadenitis
- Slow progression usually implies benign nature
- Fast progression implies malignant mass

Plan: Tumors of the Lacrimal Gland

- Refer for surgical excision
  1. Exenteration has historically been first treatment option
  2. Eye sparing tumor excision with adjuvant therapy has become a better alternative if possible
- Usually extensive radiation therapy also required

Follow-Up

- Malignant forms require close follow-up monitoring for metastasis or recurrence

III. Inflammatory Conditions

A. Dacryoadenitis[51]

Subjective

- Relatively rare condition
- More common in children/adolescents and third- to fourth-decade women
- Sometimes referred to as Mikulicz's syndrome or lymphoepithelial lesion
- Acute or chronic onset
- Usually tenderness on superior temporal palpation
  1. Anatomical site of gland
  2. Tenderness usually spreads beyond gland alone
- Frequent history of mononucleosis

Objective

- Unilateral or bilateral
- Eyelid shows variable degree of edema and erythema
- Produces "S"-shaped lid (Figure 3.42)
- Discharge may be associated
- Nonocular-related signs:
  1. Salivary gland involvement
  2. Preauricular lymphadenopathy
  3. Mononucleosis-related symptoms

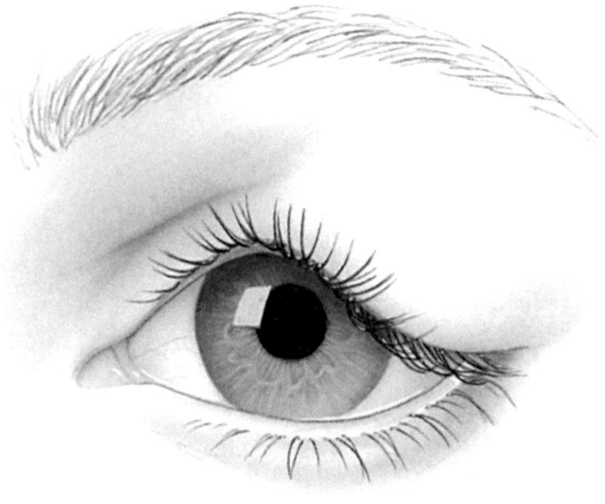

FIGURE 3.42 **S-shaped lid** produced by an inflammatory swelling of the lacrimal gland (superior temporal aspect) from dacryoadenitis.

Assessment
- Rule out lacrimal gland tumor (biopsy may be required)
- Rule out preseptal cellulitis and orbital cellulitis
- Rule out bacterial (mucopurulence) vs. viral (painless swelling and bilateral) etiology
- Chronic usually inflammatory and associated with autoimmune diseases
  1. Take careful medical history
  2. Sjögren's syndrome, Crohn's, sarcoid, and granulomatosis with polyangiitis frequently associated

Plan: Dacryoadenitis
- Refer to internist for medical evaluation and laboratory evaluation
- Treatment usually includes systemic antibiotics if bacterial
- Viral self-limiting and resolve in 4 to 6 weeks
- Treatment for underlying systemic causes, if any, such as autoimmune diseases

Follow-Up
- Syndrome often includes degeneration of gland
- May produce long-term dry eye problems

B. Dacryocystitis (Congenital and Acquired)[52]

Background Information
1. Infection or inflammation of lacrimal sac
2. Usually secondary to obstruction in the system
3. Most common infectors:
   a. Streptococcus
   b. Staphylococcus
   c. Gram-negative bacteria
   d. Streptothrix and fungi (canaliculitis)

Subjective

Congenital (or Infantile) Form
- Frequent complication of congenital dacryostenosis
- Subacute (mild to moderate tenderness on palpation) or chronic (painless) presentation for weeks to months
- Occasionally a family history of condition
- May be unilateral or bilateral

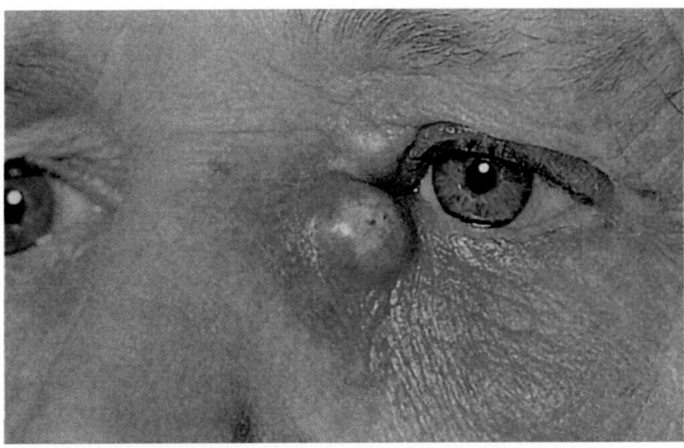

FIGURE 3.43 **Acute dacryocystitis** of the right lacrimal drainage apparatus producing severe pain, epiphora, diffuse inflammation (preseptal cellulitis), and pronounced distention of the lacrimal sac.

Acquired (Adult) Form
- Patients typically >40 years old
- Most frequently a unilateral presentation
- Usually acute onset with moderate to severe pain
  1. Dramatic tenderness at inferior inner canthus
  2. Pain generally diffuse around eye and orbit
  3. Often patient reports associated headache
- May present as chronic low-grade insidious infection with pain only on firm palpation of inner canthus

Objective

Congenital and Acquired Forms
- Almost always epiphora (wet eye presentation)
- Acute presentations (Figure 3.43)
  1. Usually moderate swelling of sac
  2. Mild to moderate localized edema and erythema throughout inferior nasal region
  3. Occasionally a hardened distention of the sac (mucocele) will produce a focal enlargement in the swollen area
  4. Purulent discharge is usually present in varying degree (depending on nasal congestion)
  5. Frequently a secondary conjunctivitis
  6. Secondary preseptal cellulitis in most acute cases
- Chronic presentation
  1. Similar to acute presentations but less severe
  2. More common congenital presentation
     a. Common pediatric referral
     b. Chronic epiphora and infection
  3. Purulent discharge often exaggerated by massage of the lacrimal sac area (toward puncta)
  4. Condition can persist for up to 9 to 12 months in congenital form with spontaneous remission (opening of the valve of Hasner)
  5. In adults consider autoimmune diseases

Assessment

(See also Appendix 3)

Congenital and Acquired Forms
- Attempt to determine cause of obstruction
  1. In congenital form, usually valve of Hasner
  2. In adult forms, rule out tumor (bloody tears)

- Determine presence or absence of mucocele
- Rule out preseptal cellulitis
- Rule out streptothrix (solid regurgitate on massage)
- In severe or nonresponsive cases, culture discharge

Plan: Dacryocystitis

(See also Appendices 4 and 6)

Congenital and Acquired Forms

- Reassure and educate parents or patient
- Acute presentations
  1. Warm pack (wrapped around finger) qid
  2. Topical antibiotic drops (e.g., Polymyxin B/Trimethoprim) qid in mild cases without preseptal cellulitis.
  3. In moderate to severe cases or in patients with preseptal cellulitis, use broad-spectrum oral antibiotic (co-manage children on oral agents with pediatrician)
  4. If patient has fever, refer for IV antibiotics
  5. Never D&I an acute case
  6. On resolution of symptoms (reduced tenderness), D&I (adults) and introduce gentle massage over sac (children and adults) qid
  7. Mucoceles must be surgically incised and drained
- Chronic presentations
  1. Introduce more vigorous (firm) massage on first presentation qid
  2. D&I adult patients
  3. Warm packs can be combined with massage by using rapped finger technique for both
  4. Medication is optional in chronic cases, if no infection (discharge) is noted
- Advise patients or parents on chronicity and need for ongoing care and compliance

Follow-Up

Congenital Form

- Recheck acute presentations in 3 to 5 days
  1. If stable or improving, continue treatment for 10 to 14 days and taper over following week to warm packs and massage bid to tid for 3 months
  2. If condition worsening:
     a. Culture (and sensitivities)
     b. Adjust medications based on laboratory work
  3. If condition not resolving within 3 to 4 weeks, refer to pediatric ophthalmologist for D&I or nasolacrimal duct probing (Bowman's)
- Recheck chronic forms every 6 to 12 weeks until resolution or until child reaches 1 year of age
  1. Reassure parents continually and stress need for compliance in spite of apparent lack of progress
  2. Explain nature of problem (valve-opening delay) and likelihood of spontaneous opening by 12 months
  3. Treat secondary complications appropriately
  4. If no resolution by 9 to 12 months (or total noncompliance or resistance of parents or child), refer for nasolacrimal probing

Acquired Form

- Manage acute presentations as for congenital form
- D&I procedure will frequently be unsuccessful if older patients with primary unresolved obstructions (e.g., dacryostenosis, strictures)
- Nonresponsive chronic conditions may require ongoing therapy or referral for reconstructive surgery of the lacrimal system (recommend oculoplastic: specialist due to complexity of procedures and high failure rate)

Orbit

Review of Clinical Anatomy

1. Margins
   a. Lateral: zygomatic bone and zygomatic process of frontal bone
   b. Superior: frontal bone
   c. Medial: angular process of frontal bone and frontal process of the maxilla (with lacrimal fossa)
   d. Inferior: zygoma and body of maxilla
2. Lateral Wall
   a. Anterior: zygoma
   b. Posterior: greater wing of the sphenoid
3. Roof
   a. Lateral: zygoma (anteriorly) and greater wing of the sphenoid (posteriorly)
   b. Medial: lacrimal bone (anteriorly) and ethmoid bone (posteriorly)
   c. Trochlear (pulley for tendon of superior oblique rectus muscle) near anterior margin
4. Floor
   a. Anterior orbital plate of maxilla
   b. Medial: orbital process of palatine bone
   c. Lateral: orbital surface of zygoma
   d. Posterior: infraorbital sulcus from infraorbital fissure
5. Medial Wall
   a. Anterior: lacrimal bone
   b. Medial: orbital plate of ethmoid bone (main structure)
   c. Posterior: body of the sphenoid bone
6. Foramen and Fissures
   a. Inferior margin: infraorbital foramen
   b. Posterior
      i. Infraorbital fissure
      ii. Superior orbital fissure
      iii. Optic foramen (Figure 3.C)

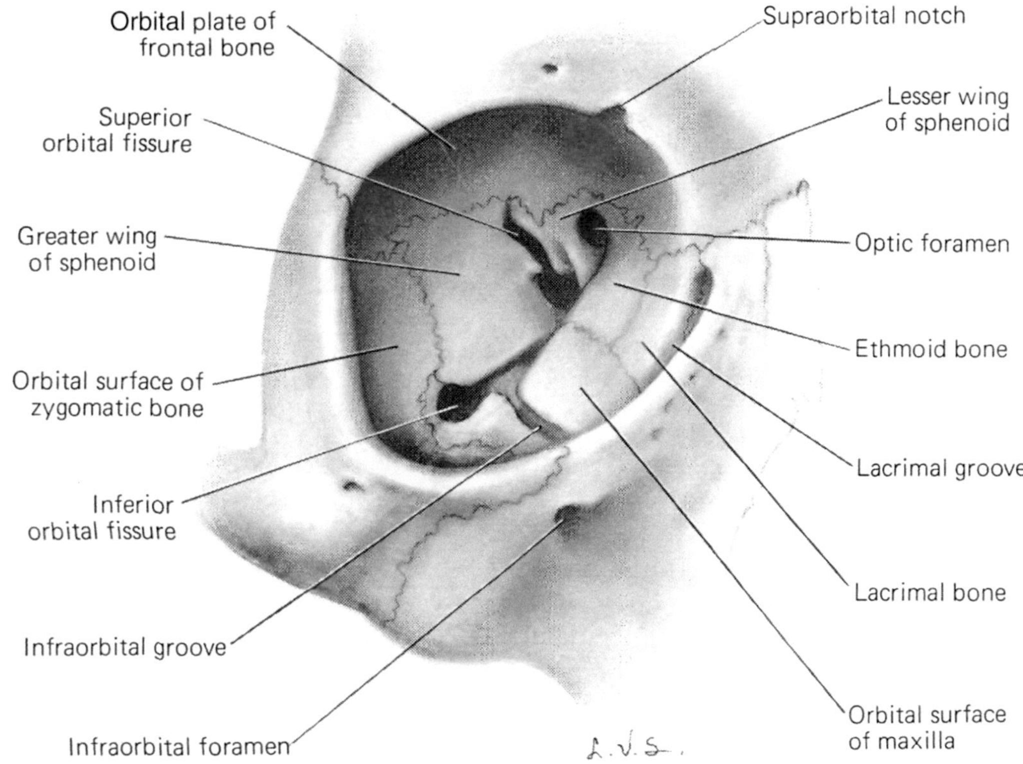

FIGURE 3.C Anterior view of the bones of the right orbit.

I. Irritations and Injuries

Contusion (Blunt) Injury

Subjective

- Contusion injuries most frequent
- Can also be caused by head and facial injury
- Consider foreign-body history as well
- Eyeball usually damaged from injury
- Pain on palpation, especially at fracture sites

Objective

- Surrounding soft tissue usually swollen and traumatized
- Rim may be spared or involved in any type of injury
- Orbit may fracture at numerous sites
  1. Roof
  2. Medial wall
  3. Apex (optic canal)
  4. Floor (blowout fracture: may be complicated by entrapment of inferior rectus muscle and resultant restriction of upward eye movement)

Assessment

- Measure visual acuity to determine damage to either the eye or optic nerve, or both
- Assess damage to eyeball (anterior and posterior)
- Rule out blowout fracture (restricted movement)
- Rule out foreign body (by history and x-ray)

Plan: Contusion Injury

- Treat damage to eye and other soft tissue
- Consider x-ray studies in seriously injured orbits
- Refer blowout fractures to oculoplastic surgeon if resultant diplopia on upward gaze problematic

Follow-Up

- Monitor nonsurgical blowout fractures for 3 to 6 weeks for possible spontaneous release

II. Noninflammatory Conditions

A. Congenital Abnormalities

Subjective

- Very uncommon
- Most are cosmetically very obvious

Objective

- Anophthalmos: globe absent and orbit reduced
- Craniostenosis: prominent orbits and globes
- Hypertelorism: laterally displaced orbits
- Microphthalmos: small orbit(s) and globe(s)

Assessment

- Rule out developmental syndromes (e.g., Crouzon's)
- Rule out intracranial abnormalities

Plan: Congenital Abnormalities

- Refer for pediatric "funny-looking kid" (FLK) syndrome workup
- Assess potential visual function

Follow-Up

- If pediatric diagnosis established, monitor eyes and associated structures for changes every 6 months
- Advice and counsel parents on visual prognosis

B. Exophthalmos[53]

Subjective

- May be congenital or acquired
  1. Congenital forms usually associated with syndromes
  2. Acquired forms usually associated with potentially serious progressive disease
- Most common presentation of orbital disorders

Objective

- May be unilateral or bilateral
- Exophthalmometry (Hertel-type) readings
  1. Greater than 21 mm in either eye (bilaterally)
  2. Greater than 3 mm difference between eyes in unilateral conditions
- Resistance on repositing (pushing in) globe
- May show increased intraocular pressure

Assessment

(See also Appendix 3)

- Most common cause in adults (unilateral or bilateral) is Graves' disease (hyperthyroidism)
  1. Ballet's sign: extraocular muscles palsies (especially superior rectus)
  2. Cowen's sign: jerky consensual pupil reflex
  3. Dalrymples's sign: lid retraction
  4. Grove's sign: lid resistance on downward gaze
  5. Jellinek's sign: increased lid pigmentation
  6. Joffroy's sign: weak forehead wrinkling on upward gaze
  7. Knie's sign: unequal pupil dilation
  8. Mobius' sign: poor convergence
  9. Riesman's sign: bruit over closed eye
  10. Rosenback's sign: tremor of closed lids
  11. Stellwag's sign: infrequent blink rate
  12. Suker's sign: weak lateral-gaze fixation
  13. Von Graefe's sign: lid lag on downward gaze
- Rule out other causes
  1. Space-occupying lesions
  2. Orbital cellulitis (most common cause of unilateral exophthalmos in children)
  3. Leukemia
  4. Pseudotumor
  5. Glaucoma
  6. High myopia (unilateral or bilateral)
- Rule out contralateral size reduction disorders or enophthalmos (retracted globe)
- Rule out anatomical asymmetry

Plan: Exophthalmos

- Do exophthalmometry (unilateral and bilateral comparisons) with Hertel type or Luedde type (unilateral readings only)
- Refer Graves' disease suspects for thyroid screen
- If space-occupying lesion suspected
  1. B-scan ultrasonography
  2. Orbital x-rays (e.g., Caldwell, Waters)
  3. Computed tomography (CT) scan
  4. Magnetic resonance imaging (MRI) studies
- Congenital forms should be monitored (by exophthalmometry) annually or upon apparent cosmetic change in appearance
- Treat secondary complications appropriately (e.g., corneal exposure from Graves' disease)

Follow-Up

- Instruct patients on monitoring appearance
- Confirm diagnostic studies and care of referred patients

C. Tumors[54]

Subjective

- May be congenital or developmental
- Benign and malignant types

Objective

- Usually manifest as proptosis or exophthalmos
- Reduce ocular motility causes diplopia sometimes only in certain fields of gaze
- May present as inflammatory conditions
- Usually unilateral

Assessment

- Common orbital tumors in children
  1. Capillary hemangioma
  2. Dermoid (e.g., epidermoids, choristomas)
  3. Lymphangioma
  4. Metastatic neuroblastoma
  5. Neurofibroma
  6. Optic nerve glioma
  7. Pseudotumor
  8. Rhabdomyosarcoma
- Common orbital tumors in adults
  1. Cavernous hemangioma
  2. Lymphangioma
  3. Lymphoma
  4. Meningioma
  5. Metastatic neoplasia
  6. Primary neoplasia
  7. Pseudotumor

Plan: Tumors

- Refer all acquired space-occupying lesions
  1. B-scan ultrasonography
  2. X-ray evaluation
  3. CT scan
  4. MRI studies
- Monitor congenital, benign tumors every 6 months

Follow-Up

- Discuss cosmetic removal of benign tumors if indicated
- Co-manage (e.g., alternate visits) metastatic and sight or life-threatening tumors with specialists

III. Inflammatory Conditions

Orbital Cellulitis[55]

Subjective

- Acute or subacute presentation
- Diplopia
- Pain ranges from moderate to severe
- Occasionally patient suffering general malaise (i.e., fever, chills, vomiting)
- Most common in children (secondary to sinusitis)

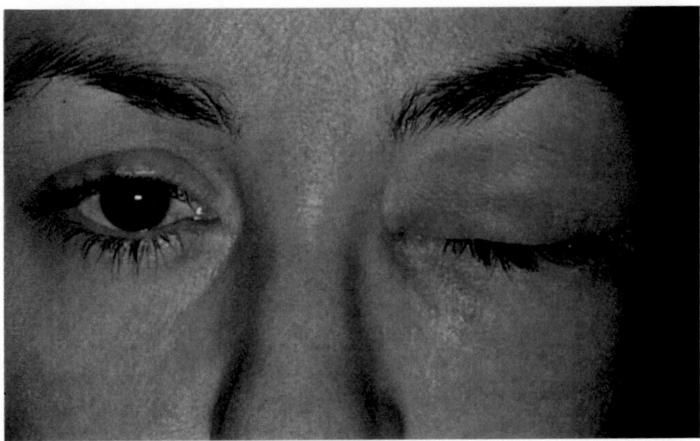

FIGURE 3.44 **Orbital cellulitis** of the left orbit in a 28-year-old female with an acute ipsilateral sinus infection. Lid edema and erythema is usually accompanied by varying degrees of proptosis, conjunctival chemosis, and extraocular restrictions in positions of secondary gaze resulting in diplopia.

Objective

- Most commonly unilateral (in children)
- Progressive lid edema and erythema (Figure 3.44)
  1. Usually deep, dark purple-red coloration
  2. Tender and warm on palpation
- Proptosis
- Conjunctival hyperemia and moderate to severe chemosis
  1. Most diagnostic sign in early presentations
  2. Frequently precedes proptosis and diplopia
- Restriction of ocular motility (painful)
- Diplopia
- Vision often not significantly reduced

Assessment

(See also Appendix 3)

- Differentiate possible causes (Figure 3.45)
  1. Sinusitis (especially in children)
  2. Infection
     a. Staphylococcus
     b. Streptococcus
     c. *Haemophilus influenzae*
     d. Fungal
  3. Cavernous sinus thrombosis (especially bilateral)
  4. Trauma
  5. Neoplasia (primary or metastatic)
- Differentiate preseptal cellulitis
  1. Similar infectious causes
  2. Similar lid signs and symptoms
  3. Following signs essential to preseptal cellulitis diagnosis
     a. No diplopia
     b. No restrictions in ocular motility
     c. No proptosis
     d. No conjunctival chemosis
     e. Usually preceding lid or adnexal (especially lacrimal) infection or inflammation

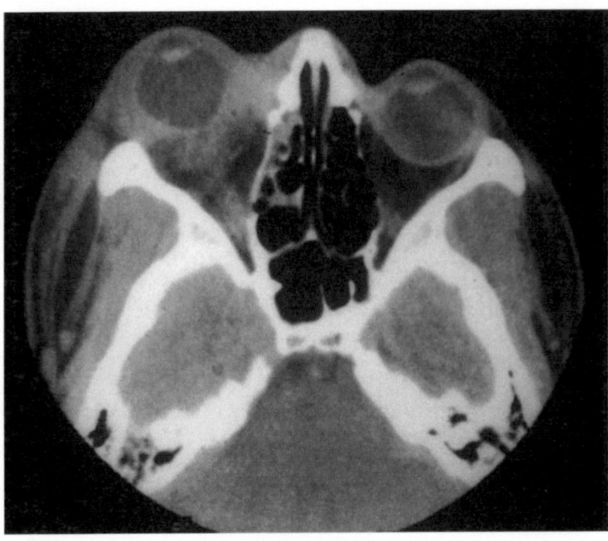

FIGURE 3.45 **Computerized tomography scan of orbital cellulitis** demonstrating pronounced proptosis and orbital congestion, which limits extraocular muscle activity leading to restricted ocular movements and diplopia.

Plan: Orbital Cellulitis

(See also Appendix 6)

- Refer emergently to medical practitioner
  1. Pediatrician
  2. Pediatric ophthalmologist
  3. Primary care physician
  4. Internist
- Usually requires hospitalization, IV antibiotics, and drainage (for abscesses)
- Condition is life-threatening, so act quickly

Follow-Up

- Same-day verification of referral and care
- Verify resolution of cause before administering routine follow-up management or vision care

References

1. Classé JG, Semes LP. The initial asof ocular contusion injury. *Optom Clin.* 1993;3(2):115–45. PMID: 8268691.
2. Cochran ML, Czyz CN. Eyelid laceration. 2021 Feb 28. In: *StatPearls* [Internet]. Treasure Island: StatPearls Publishing; 2021 Jan–. PMID: 29261910.
3. Furdova A, Kapitanova K, Kollarova A, Sekac J. Periocular basal cell carcinoma: clinical perspectives. *Oncol Rev.* 2020;14(1):420. Published 2020 Apr 30. doi:10.4081/oncol.2020.420
4. Shahzad B, Siccardi MA. Ptosis. 2020 Aug 10. In: *StatPearls* [Internet]. Treasure Island StatPearls Publishing; 2021 Jan–. PMID: 31536311.
5. Bacharach J, Lee WW, Harrison AR, Freddo TF. A review of acquired blepharoptosis: prevalence, diagnosis, and current treatment options. *Eye.* 2021;35(9):2468–2481. doi:10.1038/s41433-021-01547-5
6. Defazio G, Hallett M, Jinnah HA, Conte A, Berardelli A. Blepharospasm 40 years later. *Mov Disord.* 2017 Apr;32(4):498–509. doi: 10.1002/mds.26934. Epub 2017 Feb 10. PMID: 28186662; PMCID: PMC5941939.

7. Sarkar R, Bansal A, Ailawadi P. Future therapies in melasma: what lies ahead? *Indian J Dermatol Venereol Leprol.* 2020;86:8–17.
8. Kanukollu VM, Ahmad SS. Eyelid coloboma. 2020 Jun 30. In: *StatPearls* [Internet]. Treasure Island: StatPearls Publishing; 2021 Jan–. PMID: 32644331.
9. Rossi Santos Silva K, Cardoso Rossi D, Petroianu A. A new classification of the lateral dermatochalasis of upper eyelids. *Plast Reconstr. Surg Glob Open.* 2021;9(7):e3711. Published 2021 Jul 23. doi:10.1097/GOX.0000000000003711
10. Amspaugh B, Plager D, Gillig T, Moore D, Risner D. Capillary hemangiomas of the eyelid and orbit: a review of treatment and outcomes. In: ARVO Annual Meeting Abstract, May 2008, Volume 49.
11. Fu L, Patel BC. Lagophthalmos. 2021 Feb 25. In: *StatPearls* [Internet]. Treasure Island: StatPearls Publishing; 2021 Jan–. PMID: 32809496.
12. Arrico L, Abbouda A, Abicca I, Malagola R. Ocular complications in cutaneous lupus erythematosus: a systematic review with a meta-analysis of reported cases. *J Ophthalmol.* 2015;2015:254260. doi:10.1155/2015/254260
13. Biswas J, Sudharshan S. Anterior segment manifestations of human immunodeficiency virus/acquired immune deficiency syndrome. *Indian J Ophthalmol.* 2008;56(5):363–75. doi:10.4103/0301-4738.42412
14. Oellers P, Karp CL. Management of pigmented conjunctival lesions. *Ocul Surf.* 2012 Oct;10(4):251–63. doi: 10.1016/j.jtos.2012.08.002. Epub 2012 Aug 11. PMID: 23084146.
15. Cochran ML, Czyz CN. Eyelid papilloma. 2020 Jul 10. In: *StatPearls* [Internet]. Treasure Island: StatPearls Publishing; 2021 Jan–. PMID: 29262072.
16. Salour H, Rafati N, Falahi MR, Aletaha M. A comparison of argon laser and radiofrequency in trichiasis treatment. *Ophthalmic Plast Reconstr Surg.* 2011 Sep–Oct;27(5):313–6. doi:10.1097/IOP.0b013e31820e59f5. PMID: 21785382.
17. Kirkwood BJ, Kirkwood RA. Trichiasis: characteristics and management options. *Insight.* 2011 Apr–Jun;36(2):5–9. PMID: 21717925.
18. Pereyra AD, Saadabadi A. Trichotillomania. 2020 Jul 3. In: *StatPearls* [Internet]. Treasure Island: StatPearls Publishing; 2021 Jan–. PMID: 29630238.
19. Robson KJ, Cunningham NM, Kruzan KL, Patel DS, Kreiter CD, O'Donnell MJ, Arpey CJ. Pulsed-dye laser versus conventional therapy in the treatment of warts: a prospective randomized trial. *J Am Acad Dermatol.* 2000 Aug;43(2 Pt 1):275–80. doi:10.1067/mjd.2000.106365. PMID: 10906651.
20. Rashighi M, Harris JE. Vitiligo pathogenesis and emerging treatments. *Dermatol Clin.* 2017 Apr;35(2):257–65. doi: 10.1016/j.det.2016.11.014. PMID: 28317534; PMCID: PMC5362109.
21. Nair PA, Singhal R. Xanthelasma palpebrarum: a brief review. *Clin Cosmet Investig Dermatol.* 2017 Dec 18;11:1–5. doi:10.2147/CCID.S130116. PMID: 29296091; PMCID: PMC5739544.
22. Masud M, Moshirfar M, Shah TJ, Gomez AT, Avila MR, Ronquillo YC. Eyelid cosmetic enhancements and their associated ocular adverse effects. *Med Hypothesis Discov Innov Ophthalmol.* 2019 Summer;8(2):96–103. PMID: 31263720; PMCID: PMC6592309.
23. Bertino JS Jr. Impact of antibiotic resistance in the management of ocular infections: the role of current and future antibiotics. *Clin Ophthalmol.* 2009;3:507–21. doi:10.2147/opth.s5778
24. Lindsley K, Matsumura S, Hatef E, Akpek EK. Interventions for chronic blepharitis. *Cochrane Database Syst Rev.* 2012 May 16;2012(5):CD005556. doi:10.1002/14651858.CD005556.pub2. PMID: 22592706; PMCID: PMC4270370.
25. Wu AY, Gervasio KA, Gergoudis KN, Wei C, Oestreicher JH, Harvey JT. Conservative therapy for chalazia: is it really effective? *Acta Ophthalmol.* 2018 Jun;96(4):e503–9. doi:10.1111/aos.13675. Epub 2018 Jan 16. PMID: 29338124; PMCID: PMC6047938.
26. Liu J, Sheha H, Tseng SC. Pathogenic role of demodex mites in blepharitis. *Curr Opin Allergy Clin Immunol.* 2010;10(5):505–10. doi:10.1097/ACI.0b013e32833df9f4
27. Fromstein SR, Harthan JS, Patel J, Opitz DL. Demodex blepharitis: clinical perspectives. *Clin Optom.* 2018;10:57–63. Published 2018 Jul 4. doi:10.2147/OPTO.S142708
28. Kanukollu VM, Patel BC. Herpes simplex ophthalmicus. 2021 Apr 25. In: *StatPearls* [Internet]. Treasure Island: StatPearls Publishing; 2021 Jan–. PMID: 32644620.
29. Wilhelmus KR. Antiviral treatment and other therapeutic interventions for herpes simplex virus epithelial keratitis. *Cochrane Database Syst Rev.* 2015 Jan 9;1:CD002898. doi: 10.1002/14651858.CD002898.pub5. PMID: 25879115; PMCID: PMC4443501.
30. Opstelten W, Eekhof J, Neven AK, Verheij T. Treatment of herpes zoster. *Can Fam Physician.* 2008;54(3):373–7.
31. Andrei G, Snoeck R. Advances and perspectives in the management of varicella-zoster virus infections. *Molecules.* 2021 Feb 20;26(4):1132. doi: 10.3390/molecules26041132. PMID: 33672709; PMCID: PMC7924330.
32. Bragg KJ, Le PH, Le JK. Hordeolum. 2021 Mar 23. In: *StatPearls* [Internet]. Treasure Island: StatPearls Publishing; 2021 Jan–. PMID: 28723014.
33. Bae C, Bourget D. Periorbital cellulitis. 2020 Nov 19. In: *StatPearls* [Internet]. Treasure Island: StatPearls Publishing; 2021 Jan–. PMID: 29261970.
34. Baudouin C, Messmer EM, Aragona P, Geerling G, Akova YA, Benítez-del-Castillo J, Boboridis KG, Merayo-Lloves J, Rolando M, Labetoulle M. Revisiting the vicious circle of dry eye disease: a focus on the pathophysiology of meibomian gland dysfunction. *Br J Ophthalmol.* 2016 Mar;100(3):300–6. doi: 10.1136/bjophthalmol-2015-307415. Epub 2016 Jan 18. PMID: 26781133; PMCID: PMC4789719.
35. Nelson JD, Shimazaki J, Benitez-del-Castillo JM, et al. The international workshop on meibomian gland dysfunction: report of the definition and classification subcommittee. *Invest Ophthalmol Vis Sci.* 2011;52(4):1930–7. Published 2011 Mar 30. doi:10.1167/iovs.10-6997b
36. Nattis A, Perry HD, Rosenberg ED, Donnenfeld ED. Influence of bacterial burden on meibomian gland dysfunction and ocular surface disease. *Clin Ophthalmol.* 2019 Jul 12;13:1225–34. doi: 10.2147/OPTH.S215071. PMID: 31371918; PMCID: PMC6635833.
37. Chhadva P, Goldhardt R, Galor A. Meibomian gland disease: The role of gland dysfunction in dry eye disease. *Ophthalmology.* 2017 Nov;124(11S):S20–6. doi: 10.1016/j.ophtha.2017.05.031. PMID: 29055358; PMCID: PMC5685175.
38. Nichols KK, Foulks GN, Bron AJ, Glasgow BJ, Dogru M, Tsubota K, Lemp MA, Sullivan DA. The international workshop on meibomian gland dysfunction: executive summary. *Invest Ophthalmol Vis Sci.* 2011 Mar 30;52(4):1922–9. doi: 10.1167/iovs.10-6997a. PMID: 21450913; PMCID: PMC3072157.
39. Tao T, Tao L. Systematic review and meta-analysis of treating meibomian gland dysfunction with azithromycin. *Eye.* 2020 Oct;34(10):1797–808. doi: 10.1038/s41433-020-0876-2. Epub 2020 Apr 28. PMID: 32346111; PMCID: PMC7608442.
40. Fogt JS, Kowalski MJ, King-Smith PE, Epitropolous AT, Hendershot AJ, Lembach C, Maszczak JP, Jones-Jordan LA, Barr JT. Tear lipid layer thickness with eye drops in meibomian gland dysfunction. *Clin Ophthalmol.* 2016 Nov 7;10:2237–43. doi: 10.2147/OPTH.S120158. PMID: 27853352; PMCID: PMC5106234.
41. Korb DR, Blackie CA. Debridement-scaling: a new procedure that increases Meibomian gland function and reduces dry eye symptoms. *Cornea.* 2013 Dec;32(12):1554–7. doi: 10.1097/ICO.0b013e3182a73843. PMID: 24145633.
42. Tauber J, Owen J, Bloomenstein M, Hovanesian J, Bullimore MA. Comparison of the iLUX and the lipiflow for the treatment of meibomian gland dysfunction and symptoms: a randomized clinical trial. *Clin Ophthalmol.* 2020;14:405–18. Published 2020 Feb 12. doi:10.2147/OPTH.S234008
43. Geerling G, Tauber J, Baudouin C, et al. The international workshop on meibomian gland dysfunction: report of the subcommittee on management and treatment of meibomian gland dysfunction. *Invest Ophthalmol Vis Sci.* 2011;52(4):2050–64. Published 2011 Mar 30. doi:10.1167/iovs.10-6997g

44. Cote S, Zhang AC, Ahmadzai V, et al. Intense pulsed light (IPL) therapy for the treatment of meibomian gland dysfunction. *Cochrane Database Syst Rev.* 2020;3(3):CD013559. Published 2020 Mar 18. doi:10.1002/14651858.CD013559
45. Veraldi S, Nazzaro G, Esposito L, Genovese G, Pontini P, Gelmetti C. Pthiriasis of the eyelashes. *G Ital Dermatol Venereol.* 2020 Apr;155(2):198–201. doi: 10.23736/S0392-0488.19.06350-8. Epub 2019 Sep 12. PMID: 31525840.
46. Rishor-Olney CR, Hinson JW. Canalicular laceration. 2020 Dec 2. In: *StatPearls* [Internet]. Treasure Island: StatPearls Publishing; 2021 Jan–. PMID: 32809637.
47. Patel J, Levin A, Patel BC. Epiphora. 2021 Feb 25. In: *StatPearls* [Internet]. Treasure Island: StatPearls Publishing; 2021 Jan–. PMID: 32491381.
48. Nadeem N, Patel BC. Punctal stenosis. 2021 Feb 25. In: *StatPearls* [Internet]. Treasure Island: StatPearls Publishing; 2021 Jan–. PMID: 32809413.
49. Yang J, Zhou C, Wang Y, Fan X, Jia R. Multimodal therapy in the management of lacrimal gland adenoid cystic carcinoma. *BMC Ophthalmol.* 2019;19(1):125. Published 2019 Jun 8. doi:10.1186/s12886-019-1110-5
50. Patel R, Patel BC. Dacryoadenitis. In: *StatPearls.* Treasure Island: StatPearls Publishing; February 25, 2021.
51. Taylor RS, Ashurst JV. Dacryocystitis. In: *StatPearls.* Treasure Island: StatPearls Publishing; June 26, 2020.
52. Topilow NJ, Tran AQ, Koo EB, Alabiad CR. Etiologies of proptosis: a review. *Intern Med Rev.* 2020;6(3):10.18103/imr.v6i3.852. doi:10.18103/imr.v6i3.852
53. Kannan S, Hasegawa M, Yamada Y, Kawase T, Kato Y. Tumors of the orbit: case report and review of surgical corridors and current options. *Asian J Neurosurg.* 2019;14(3):678–85. doi:10.4103/ajns.AJNS_51_19
54. Danishyar A, Sergent SR. Orbital cellulitis. In: *StatPearls.* Treasure Island: StatPearls Publishing; January 17, 2021.

Chapter 4
DIAGNOSES OF THE CONJUNCTIVA, SCLERA, AND EPISCLERA

Chapter Outline

DOI: 10.1201/9781003255598-4

Conjunctiva

Review of Clinical Anatomy

1. Structural characteristics (Figure 4.A)
   a. Thin, transparent mucous membrane lining inner eyelid (palpebral portion) and anterior sclera (bulbar portion)
      i. Fornices (from palpebral to bulbar portions) loosely connected
      ii. Can swell dramatically
   b. Two layers
      i. Stratified nonkeratinized epithelium from two to seven layers thick
      ii. Lamina propria composed of connective tissue, blood vessels, nerves, glands, PMNs, mast cells (greater limbal and superior), macrophages, lymphocytes, and lymphoid follicles (in children)
   c. Epithelium continuous with cornea and lacrimal drainage system
   d. Medial angle structures formed partly by conjunctiva
      i. Plica semilunaries (semilunar vertical folds)
      ii. Lacrimal caruncle is modified piece of skin covered by nonkeratinized stratified epithelium consisting of sebaceous glands and fine hairs
   e. Glands
      i. Goblet cells secret mucous to the tear film
      ii. Accessory lacrimal glands
         – Krause's located in substantia propria secrete aqueous fluid
         – Wolfring and Manz's secrete mucin

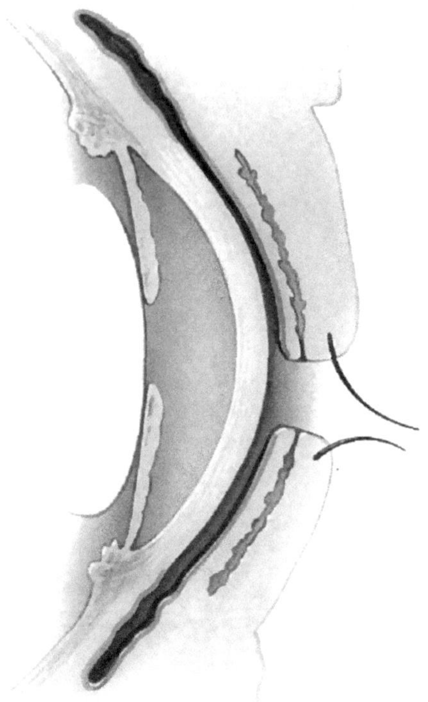

FIGURE 4.A The anatomy of the conjunctiva.

2. Nerve supply
   a. Bulbar portion innervated by ciliary nerves and sympathetic for blood vessels
   b. Palpebral portion innervated by frontal nerve (superior) lacrimal. First division, cranial nerve V (inferior lateral) and infraorbital. Second division, cranial nerve V (inferior medial)
3. Vascular supply
   a. Main supply is from peripheral and marginal arterial arcades
   b. Posterior branches supply peripheral conjunctiva while prominent anterior branches (seven anterior ciliary arteries) move forward towards cornea
      i. Anterior portions called superficial (conjunctival) and deep (episcleral) pericorneal plexus
      ii. Deep (episclerals) make up limbal vasculature and appear dull red to purple in color
      iii. Anterior and posterior branches anastamose

I. Irritations and Injuries

A. Burns

Chemical, thermal, radiation, and other burns to the ocular surface should always be treated as emergency keratoconjunctival conditions (i.e., assume corneal involvement) and are covered in detail in Chapter 5.

B. Foreign Bodies

Subjective

- History of foreign material in eye
- Mild to moderate irritation (especially if cornea is secondarily involved)

Objective

- Palpebral conjunctival foreign bodies on tarsus observed with superior and inferior lid inversion
- Bulbar conjunctival foreign bodies imbed in the superficial conjunctival tissue (usually in areas of palpebral fissures)
- Immediate surrounding and diffuse hyperemia develops rapidly
- Occasionally an associated subconjunctival hemorrhage will appear
- If foreign body present for a prolonged period, a spongy vascularized mass (foreign-body granuloma) may develop

Assessment

- Rule out corneal involvement
- Rule out penetrating or perforating intraocular involvement
  1. Nature of entry (e.g., high-velocity projectile)
  2. Perform careful external and internal ocular examination
- Consider soft tissue (globe) x-ray or ultrasound evaluation

Plan: Foreign Bodies

- Topical anesthesia for examination
- Remove foreign material from conjunctival tissue
  1. Lavage (irrigate) vigorously
  2. Swab with moistened cotton-tip applicator

3. Remove embedded particles with sharp instrument (e.g., needle, jeweler's forceps, spud)

- Irrigate copiously after removal
- Prophylax with broad spectrum antibiotic ointment 1 x optional
- Reassure regarding secondary subconjunctival blood (iatrogenic if removed by sharp instrument)

Follow-Up

- Recheck in 3 to 5 days or PRN
- If irritation persists, recheck for additional foreign material (frequent with granular or particulate material or fiberglass)

C. Laceration

Subjective

- History of lacerating or abrading injury
- Usually mild irritation
- Patient gravely concerned by "bloody" appearance

Objective

- Relatively dramatic hemorrhagic response on bulbar conjunctival surface (Figure 4.1)
- Conjunctiva becomes edematous and usually folds upon itself under traction exerted toward the outer canthus
- Full-thickness lacerations produce pure white (bare sclera) appearance at site of wound with excess surrounding tissue edema and blood
- Occasionally, associated laceration of episclera will produce a thickened white loose flap

Assessment

- Rule out corneal involvement
- Rule out penetration or perforation
- Check carefully for any foreign material

Plan: Laceration

(See also Appendix 4)

- Topical anesthesia for examination
- Lavage (irrigate) tissue copiously

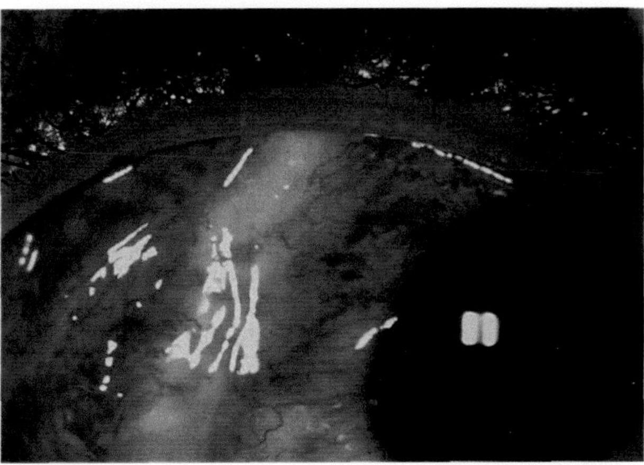

FIGURE 4.1 **Conjunctival/tenon capsule laceration,** accompanied by subconjunctival hemorrhages, surrounding an area of exposed, bare (white) sclera. Redundant, edematous conjunctival tissue will respond and regenerate normally within 2 to 4 weeks with nonsurgical topical lavage, antibiosis, and warm compress therapy.

- Topical antibiotic (e.g., Polymyxin B/Bacitracin) q4–6h for minimum 5 to 7 days or until significant healing begins
- Sutures not needed for conjunctival laceration alone
- If episclera also involved (white flap), consider lid effect during blink
  1. If flap reduced and flattened during blink, no sutures indicated
  2. If flap elevated and rolled with each blink, may need suture repair
- Warm packs and continued irrigation (tid) will promote healing and insure asepsis

Follow-Up

- Recheck in 48 to 72 hours to rule out complications and measure progress (probably minimal)
- Recheck in 5 to 7 days and subsequently every 5 to 7 days until completely healed (usually about 2 to 4 weeks)
- Monitor for any secondary infection or adverse ocular tissue effects: rare (e.g., fibrosis)

II. Noninflammatory Conditions

A. Calcium Concretions (Lithiasis)

Subjective

- Asymptomatic finding (usually during general examination)
- Occasional reports of very large concretions producing corneal irritation (rare)
- Common finding in elderly patients

Objective

- Small, white to yellowish hard spots on palpebral conjunctiva (Figure 4.2)
  1. Usually about 1 to 3 mm in size
  2. Rarely larger than 5 mm
- May be single or multiple
- Common to both inferior and superior conjunctiva
- Usually flat, but may be slightly raised if large

Assessment

- Differentiate from inclusion (lymphatic) cysts
  1. Cysts are clear or translucent to light or slit-lamp examination
  2. Solid masses are opaque to light examination

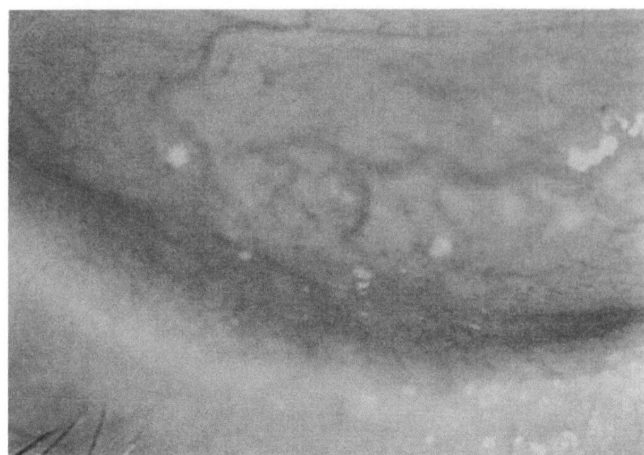

FIGURE 4.2 **Conjunctival concretions (lithiasis)** on the inferior palpebral conjunctiva.

- Rule out other ocular surface lesions
- Rule out infectious or inflammatory causes (rare)

Plan: Calcium Concretions

- If asymptomatic, no treatment indicated (usually)
- If irritating or disconcerting to patient, remove
    1. "Tease" out with jeweler's forceps or other instrument sharp enough to pry and lift
    2. Probable small conjunctival bleed will respond to direct pressure and self-resolve

Follow-Up

- With no treatment: PRN
- With removal: 5 to 7 days or PRN

B. Dermolipoma

Subjective

- Asymptomatic presentation
- Present congenitally, but may be too small for cosmetic awareness
    1. Tend to increase in size slowly
    2. First awareness or cosmetic distress may not occur until second or third decade of life
- Occasionally, infant's parent, caretaker, or pediatrician may note it initially in early childhood and report it as acquired lesion (with concern)

Objective

- Firm, elevated, distinctly yellow mass present at outer canthal (lateral) angle (Figure 4.3)
    1. May be obscured (buried behind lid) in primary gaze position
    2. When eye turns inward, mass becomes visible
- Exposed surface may be perfectly smooth and clear or may contain surface appendages, including fatty tissue, glands, and hair follicles
- Mass is slightly movable, hard to palpation, and painless
- If displaced superiorly, may be mistaken for lacrimal gland (superior temporal position); lacrimal gland usually larger and softer

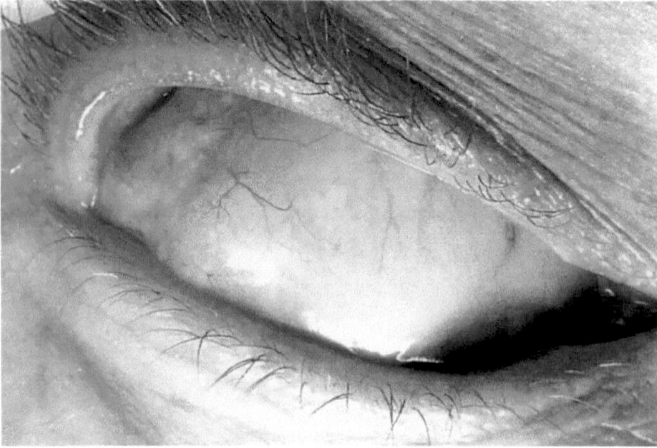

FIGURE 4.3 **Dermolipoma** under the superior lid in the outer canthus, observable only on retraction of the superior lid and downward left abduction.

Plan: Dermolipoma

- Reassure patient and explain nature and course
- If patient desires cosmetic removal, refer to experienced ophthalmic surgeon

Assessment

- Rule out other ocular surface lesions
- Rule out neoplasia
- Rule out cyst (versus mass)
- Reassure patient and explain nature and course
- If patient desires cosmetic removal, refer to experienced ophthalmic surgeon

Follow-Up

- Without treatment, recheck annually or PRN
- With removal, routine follow-up evaluation

C. Granuloma[1]

Subjective

- Painless mass
- Usually insidious development (chronic inflammation)
- Patient may be unaware or mildly concerned
- May have granulomas elsewhere on body

Objective

- Variable position, size, shape, and reddish color (Figures 4.4, 4.5)
- Most common presentation on palpebral conjunctiva
- Spongy vascularized tissue mass
- Occasional secondary surface inflammation or infection or ulceration with loose blood elements
- May be pedunculated (stalk-like projection)
    1. Often overgrows lid margin and appears as lid papilloma
        a. Differentiate by smooth (contoured to the ocular surface) posterior surface of the granuloma versus irregular contour of lid margin papilloma
        b. Also differentiate from neoplasia which would have irregular posterior surface and other neoplastic signs

Assessment

(See also Appendix 3)

- Rule out systemic history of inflammatory or granulomatous disease (e.g., sarcoidosis)
- Frequently cause goes undiagnosed
    1. Ruptured chalazion
    2. Allergic reaction
    3. Infection (subclinical)
    4. Acne rosacea
- Rule out mechanical causes of granuloma formation
    1. Foreign body
    2. Chronic irritant

Plan: Granuloma

- Usually self-limiting, self-resolving mass
- Refer for causes (e.g., systemic)
- Treat secondary superficial involvement (e.g., infection, inflammation)
- Heat therapy (compresses) useful for granuloma
- Photodocument if possible for follow-up purposes
- Consider surgical excision for cause or cosmesis

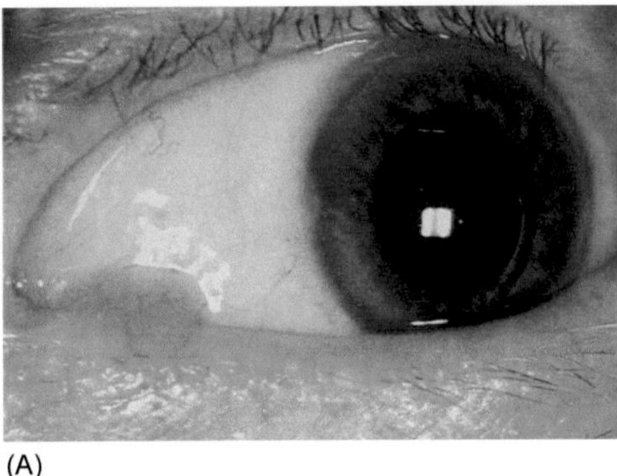

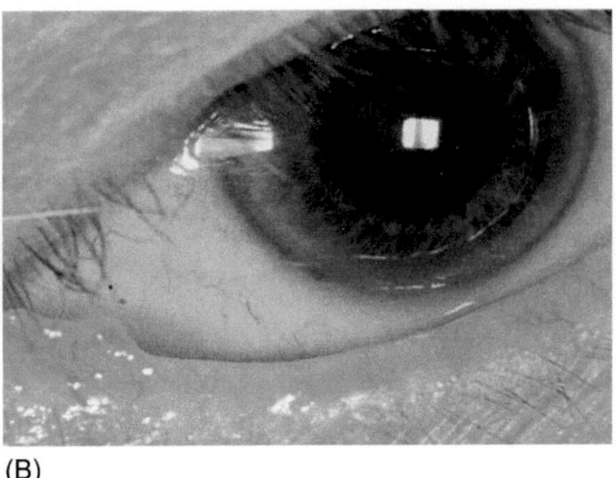

FIGURE 4.4 (A) **Palpebral conjunctival granuloma** "climbing" over the lid margin into prominent view. The anterior side of the mass is characterized by the typical spongy, vascularized appearance of granulomatous tissue, whereas the posterior side (facing the eyeball) assumes the smooth, continuous contour of the ocular surface. **(B) Lid margin epithelioma** varies from the palpebral conjunctival granuloma in its irregular surface and neovascular appearing anterior surface, which is present on its posterior side as well.

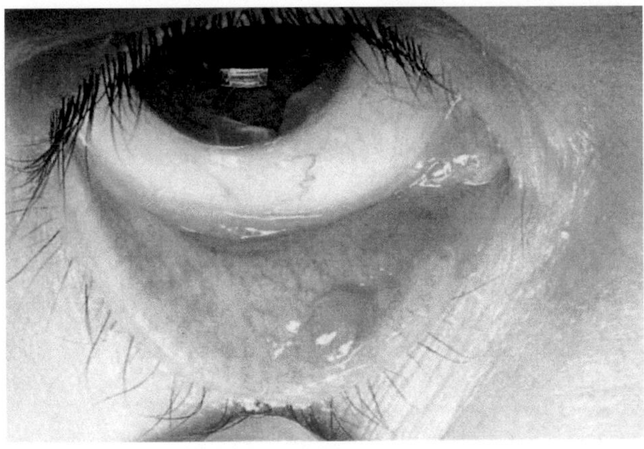

FIGURE 4.5 **Palpebral conjunctival granuloma** beneath the inferior lid margin in the right eye of an asymptomatic patient.

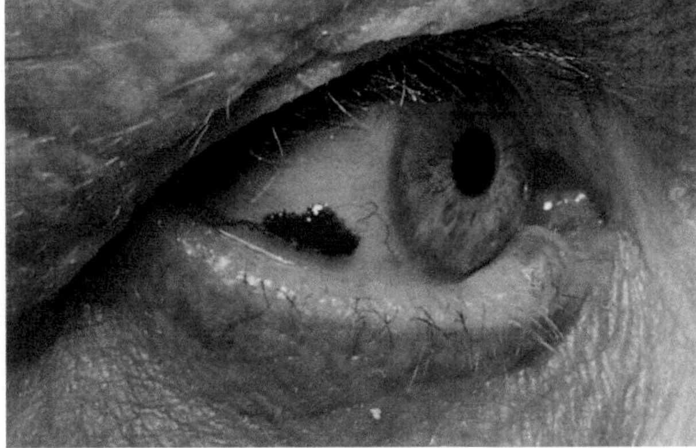

FIGURE 4.6 **Conjunctival hemangioma** in the temporal aspect of a right eye. The slightly raised, broad-based nature often creates patient/cosmetic concern, but may be removed by laser.

Follow-Up
- Without referral and excision, recheck first presentations in 3 to 6 months
- Chronic masses should be rechecked every 6 months
- With significant changes, refer for excision

Note: **Pyogenic granuloma** is a misnomer. It is neither pyogenic (i.e., pus producing) or granulomatous (by histology). It is a vascular hemangioma that is red and typically attached to the palpebral conjunctiva. Etiology usually involves recent history of ocular inflammation or trauma (e.g., surgery, burns, chronic foreign body such as exposed punctal plug). Treatment includes topical or injectable steroids or surgical excision.

D. Hemangioma

Subjective
- Usually present congenitally or in early years
- May enlarge with age
- Cosmetically apparent and often disconcerting

Objective
- Raised broad-based bulbar conjunctival vascular tumor masses (benign; Figure 4.6)
- More frequently toward inner canthus or deep in fornices
- Reddish to darker purplish tortuous vessel masses

Assessment
- Differentiate lymphangioma (lighter color) or lymphoma (with history of lymphosarcoma)
- Rule out other red(dish) ocular surface masses

Plan: Hemangioma
- Reassure and educate patient
- If requested (for cosmetic concern), refer to ophthalmology
  1. Excision
  2. Cautery
  3. Laser

Follow-Up
- If no referral, check annually
- Advise on any changes PRN

E. Inclusion (Lymphatic or Retention) Cyst

Subjective

- Asymptomatic presentation
- Depending on position and size, may produce patient distress or cosmetic concern

Objective

- Small to moderate size (2 to 5 mm) cystic formations producing a clear to white to yellow color (Figure 4.7)
- Locations are variable (in order of frequency)
  1. Deep fornices (inferior or superior)
  2. Inferior or superior palpebral conjunctiva
  3. Inner canthal caruncle and plica area
  4. Bulbar conjunctiva (greater nasalward)
- May be fluid filled (clear) or casseous (yellow)
- Frequently multiple in one or both eyes

Assessment

- Rule out other cystic ocular surface lesions
- Rule out infection, inflammation, or trauma

Plan: Inclusion Cyst

- Treatment neither essential nor indicated
- If patient requests removal (usually cosmetic), primary drainage procedure may be attempted
  1. If fluid filled, simply lance with needle
  2. With caseous cysts, lance, and massage
  3. Prophylactic antibiotic (1×) optional
  4. Generally, lancing puncture will close and cyst will refill within days
- Permanent removal best achieved by referral for surgical excision of entire cyst at its base
- Cysts are frequently recurrent (even with surgical excision), so advise and monitor postoperative patients (with surgeon)
- Advise patients on possibility of recurrent lancing or excision

Follow-Up

- Follow-up patient based on degree of presentation or within 1 week of any procedural approach

F. Keratinization (Xerosis or Bitot's Spot)[2]

Subjective

- History of poor nutrition specifically Vitamin A deficiency especially children in developing countries
- May be due to defects in Vitamin A absorption and storage with chronic liver diseases (alcoholism), upper GI surgery, irritable bowel syndrome (IBS), and pancreatitis
- Often a history of excessive exposure to UV light and dry, arid climate

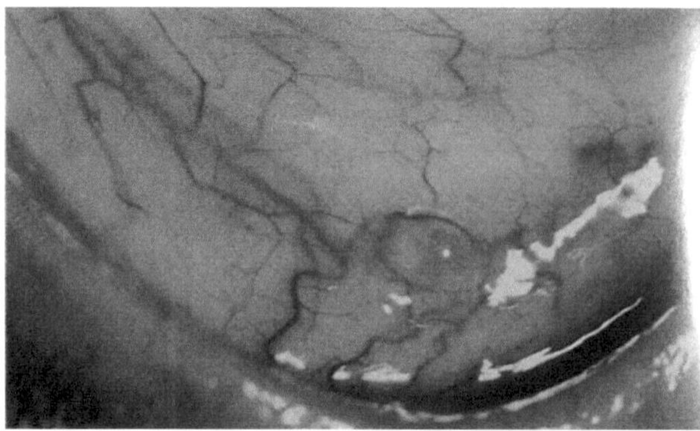

FIGURE 4.7 Lymphatic (inclusion or retention) cyst on the inferior palpebral conjunctiva. Lancing, massage, and drainage proved unsuccessful with cyst refilling within 1 week.

Objective

- Dry, hardened, rough patch(es) on exposed areas of bulbar conjunctiva
- Granular, keratinized epithelial surface
- Rarely, a wet, frothy appearance may develop over roughened area (called "Bitot's spot")

Assessment

- Vitamin A deficiency (avitaminosis A)
- Most often secondary to drying effects
  1. Environmental
  2. Exposure
  3. Radiation (especially UV sunlight)
- Retinoid dermatologic agents (Accutane) have been cited as aggravants

Plan: Keratinization

- Heavy lubrication therapy (drops or ointments every hour for relief of symptoms and reduction in tissue keratinization)
  1. Mucomimetic agents helpful
- Attempt to remove any aggravants or allergens
- Vitamin A supplementation via vitamin supplements or diet sources
- Bitot's spot(s) can be swabbed to reduce frothing effect (but without therapy, will recur)

Follow-Up

- During active treatment plan, recheck every 2 to 4 weeks
- If condition worsens (with or without therapy), pursue cause aggressively and treat specifically
- On resolution of acute (or subacute) phase, continue artificial tears tid indefinitely unless primary cause completely removed (Vitamin A deficiency)
  1. Recheck regularly (every 3 months) for complication

G. Lymphangiectasia

Subjective

- Common ocular surface involvement
- Asymptomatic or (rarely) mildly uncomfortable
- Usually noted during general examination
- Occasionally patient may express concern or cosmetic distress over "bubble on white of eye"

Objective

- Variable-size and -shaped clear fluid-filled cyst on bulbar conjunctiva (greater temporal ward; Figure 4.8)
  1. Usual size range from 2 to 10 mm
  2. Round or linear
- Focal or segmental dilations of fine thin-walled conjunctival lymphatic vessel(s)
- May be single or multiple sites and dilations
- Single cyst may be multilobulated
- Always clear and transparent (with slit-lamp examination)

Assessment

(See also Appendix 3)

- Rule out other cystic ocular surface lesions
- Differentiate from inclusion (lymphatic) cyst
  1. Inclusion cyst has thicker walls, hence appears translucent (or yellowish)

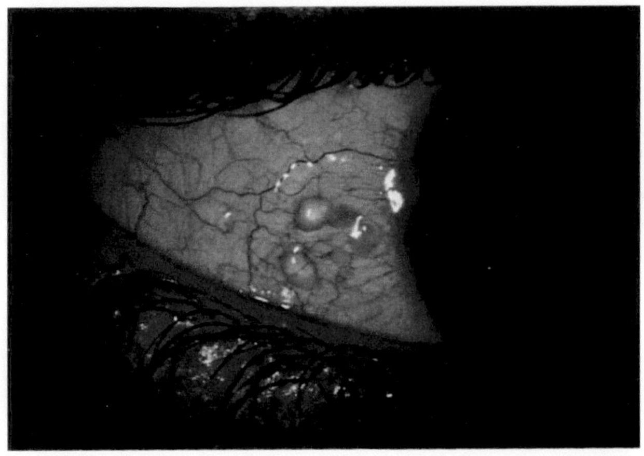

FIGURE 4.8 **Lymphangiectasia** presenting as multiple small cysts. They can also present as elongated, clear, tubular cyst formations.

2. Positioning of inclusion cysts more common nasalward and on palpebral conjunctiva

Plan: Lymphangiectasia

- For small asymptomatic cysts, no treatment
- For larger cysts or to allay patient concern or request
  1. Drain cyst by simple 25-gauge needle puncture (angled away from ocular surface)
  2. Gentle massage through closed lid to flatten
  3. No medication necessary (tears do the job)
- Occasionally cyst(s) may drain spontaneously

Follow-Up

- Best to advise, explain, and reassure patients, even those unaware of presence (they will notice it eventually and wonder whether you missed it, or worse, did not want to tell them!)
- With no treatment, follow routinely or PRN
- If drained, follow-up optional (1 week) and again in 3 to 6 months for possible recurrence (rare)

H. Melanosis (Congenital Form)

1. Conjunctival

Subjective

- Present at birth or shortly thereafter
- Greater in darker pigmented ethnic groups
- May increase with age

Objective

- Flat pigmented patches, usually at limbus (Figure 4.9)
- Variable size and shape
- Grayish brown to black coloration

Assessment

(See also Appendix 3)

- Differentiate from deeper, blueish, diffuse congenital scleral melanosis
- Rule out choroidal involvement (internal)

Plan: Conjunctival Melanosis

- Reassure patient or parent
- No treatment indicated

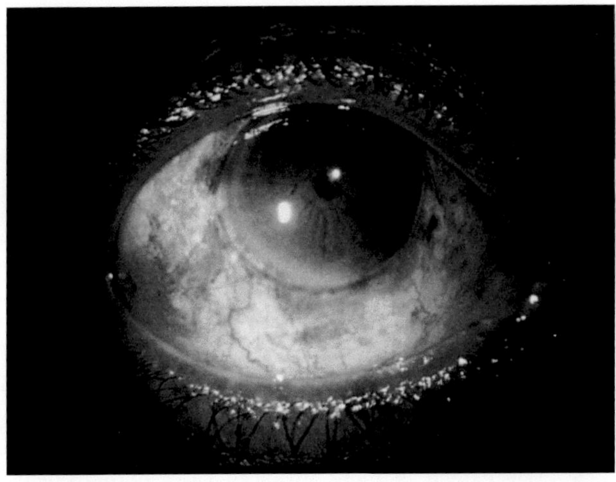

FIGURE 4.9 **Conjunctival/scleral melanosis** of long standing (by history) presenting in a Black male. History, avascular nature, and flat configurations of variable size and shape generally suggest benign conjunctival and scleral melanosis.

Follow-Up

- Recheck annually during childhood or PRN
- Advise patient on slight long-range risk of melanoma (instruct on reporting changes in any pigmented lesions on body)

2. Scleral (Congenital Melanosis Oculi)

Subjective

- Unilateral congenital presentation
- Possible autosomal-dominant trait (if 50% or more of immediate family shows signs)

Objective

- Deep (scleral or episcleral) blueish coloration
- Associated dark brown iris (unilateral)
- Increase choroidal pigmentation producing darker appearance to ipsilateral fundus
- Periorbital skin on affected side usually darker than opposite side
- If pigment distribution over C-V (cranial nerve 5) areas (forehead through cheek region), condition is called nevus of Ota or oculodermomelanocytosis (much greater among Asian patients)

Assessment

(See also Appendix 3)

- Differentiate from congenital conjunctival melanosis
- Rule out blue scleral causes

Plan: Scleral Melanosis

- No treatment indicated
- Careful counseling necessary (especially in Caucasian presentations) regarding risks
  1. For malignant melanoma (choroid or body)
  2. For secondary glaucomas

Follow-Up
- Annually or PRN
- Always be conscious of associated risks

I. Melanosis (Primary Acquired Form)[3]
Benign or precancerous melanosis.

Subjective
- Most common >60 years of age
- Asymptomatic presentation
- Greater in males than females
- Patient generally concerned and apprehensive

Objective
- Spontaneous development of irregular, diffuse, flat patches of grayish-black bulbar conjunctival pigmentation
- May extend in more advanced cases onto palpebral conjunctiva
- Intensity and geography of pigmentation increase and diminish over 1 to 3 years, occasionally with complete disappearance
- The more clock hours of conjunctival coverage significantly increase risk of melanoma

Assessment
- Differentiate from cancerous melanoma
- Rule out history of melanoma (or suspicious pigmented lesions, i.e., nevi) elsewhere on body or choroid
- Appearance can be secondary to dermatologic medications (e.g., monobenzone for vitiligo)

Plan: Acquired Melanosis
- Advise patient and reassure and educate
- Manage closely during active changes in pigmentation: every 3 months or PRN
- If any suspicious changes occur (e.g., erosion, elevation) refer for biopsy

Follow-Up
- 75% of all conjunctival melanomas arise from acquired melanosis
- 15% to 17% of benign or precancerous melanosis converts to cancer (melanoma) within 30 years
- Higher percentage converts to choroidal melanoma than to melanoma elsewhere on body
- Mortality of choroidal melanoma is much less than melanoma elsewhere, but is still a threat!

J. Neoplasia
Subjective
Refer to "Neoplastic Considerations" in Chapter 3.

Objective
Refer to "Neoplastic Considerations" in Chapter 3.

Assessment
- More common reddish conjunctival neoplasia (Figure 4.10)
  1. Carcinomas
  2. Sarcomas
- Kaposi's sarcoma frequently associated with AIDS
  1. Hemorrhagic sarcoma
  2. Red papules and nodules on palpebral (less frequently bulbar) conjunctiva

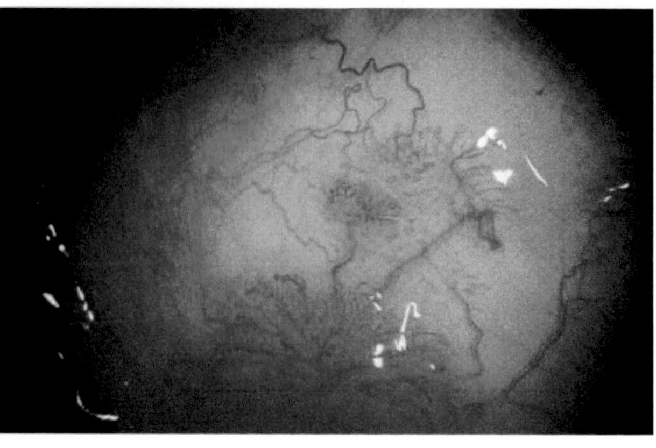

FIGURE 4.10 **Conjunctival epithelioma** on the bulbar conjunctival surface. Fine, radiating vessels associated with raised, irregular, vascularized lesions are highly suggestive of neoplasia.

- Rule out nevus
- Melanoma is a rare but high morbidity and mortality cancer

Plan: Neoplasia
- Suspect lesion should be referred for excision and biopsy
- Follow-up on referral to confirm care
- Refusal to accept referral advice should be carefully documented in records

Follow-Up
- Excised patients with positive biopsy should be carefully instructed on possible recurrent signs
- Recheck every 6 months for 1 to 2 years (with surgeon), then annually or PRN

K. Nevus
Subjective
- Usually congenital or develop early in life
- Fairly common pigmented lesion
- Always asymptomatic, except for cosmetic distress
- Greater frequency at inner canthus

Objective
- Smooth, flat surface lesion with well-demarcated pigmented edges
- May have variable degrees and intensity of pigment ranging from negligible (amelanotic) to deep and dark
- Pigmentation may increase significantly during puberty and other hormonal changes
- Usually superficial (junctional) type on bulbar or palpebral conjunctiva with or without slight elevation
- Occasionally may show cystic type changes

Assessment
- Rule out other pigmented ocular surface lesions
- Rule out neoplastic changes

Plan: Nevus
- If suspicious enough, refer for excisional biopsy
- Reassure and advise patient
- If referral not indicated, photodocument if possible or diagram and measure carefully

Follow-Up

- Recall schedule
  1. Three months for first presentations
  2. Every 6 to 12 months routinely
  3. PRN
- Compare for qualitative and quantitative change, each follow-up visit
- If suspicious changes, obtain oculodermatologic consultation

L. Papilloma[4]

Subjective

- Occurs most frequently in 21–40-year-olds but can be seen in children
- Asymptomatic
- Development and growth can be rapid (weeks)
- Occasionally develops in multiple sites
- Usually fear or cosmetic concern

Objective

- Elevated, variable size and shape, benign epithelial tumor
- Most common at limbal juncture (transitional tissue site)
- Deeper vasculature may appear through surface
- Variable pigmentation
  1. Amelanotic (pinkish)
  2. Translucent (with vessels showing through)
  3. Moderately to heavily pigmented
- Frequently lobated or pedunculated
- When at limbus, may give appearance of corneal involvement

Assessment

(See also Appendix 3)

- Rule out neoplasia
- Papilloma versus nevus or melanosis
- Rule out infectious or inflammatory associations
- Associated with herpes papilloma virus (HPV)

Plan: Papilloma

- Reassure and educate patient
- If suspicious or cosmetically requested, refer for excision and biopsy

Follow-Up

- Without surgical referral, monitor qualitative and quantitative changes
  1. Papillomatous changes in size and shape are considered within normal limits
  2. Watch for neoplastic changes
- With surgery, continue to monitor patient every 3 to 6 months for recurrences (rather common)

M. Pigmentations[5–7]

Subjective

- Positive history of contributory cause
  1. Exogenous (e.g., metal particles, eyedrops)
  2. Endogenous (e.g., disease, genetics)
  3. Medicamentosa
  4. Makeup
- Quiet, non-inflamed, painless presentations

Objective

- Argyrosis (caused by silver), most common
  1. Greatest effect in fornices as back line(s) or generalized graying of tissues
  2. May show pigment spot(s) on bulbar conjunctiva (greater at inner canthus)
- Medicines (topical and systemic)
  1. Adrenalin: brownish conjunctival cysts
  2. Epinephrine (topical ophthalmic forms) and oral tetracyclines: blackish particles
  3. Mercury: blueish gray (lids and conjunctiva)
  4. Other offending metals: gold, iron
- Makeup, primarily mascara (carbon black)
- Ochronosis is an acquired pigmentation (blueish or black deposits and tissue discoloration) secondary to recessive traits associated with metabolic involvement (alkaptonuria)
  1. Scleral pigmentation earliest sign of alkaptonuria seen as young as mid 20s
  2. Also diffuse changes
  3. Patient may be suffering advanced osteoarthritis
  4. Pigment changes also seen on skin, ears
  5. May see “oil drop” like brown pigmentation at the limbus

Assessment

(See also Appendix 2)

- Attempt to determine cause by careful history
- Rule out other pigmented lesions

Plan: Pigmentations

- Remove cause, if established
- Reassure, educate, and advise patient

Follow-Up

- If cause not determined, monitor for any changes
- Counsel patient on possible causes
- Routine follow-up or PRN

N. Pinguecula[8]

Pinguecula is not a contraindication to soft contact lens wear

Subjective

- Common
- Frequent history of outdoor and UV exposure
- Usually asymptomatic and stable history
- Occasionally, patient will report acute onset
  1. More likely a first awareness
  2. Secondary inflammation often creates first awareness and alarm
  3. Frequent cosmetic concern

Objective

- Yellowish, slightly elevated triangular mass(es) with base toward limbus, adjacent to, but not on corneal surface
- Found at exposed lateral areas on bulbar conjunctiva (greater nasal, but may be temporal)
- Usually bilateral presentation
- Generally free of blood vessels, but occasionally become surrounded by hyperemic injected vessels

Assessment

(See also Appendix 3)

- Rule out other ocular surface lesions
- Differentiate from pterygium
- Differentiate inflamed presentations
    1. From angular conjunctivitis
    2. From episcleritis

Plan: Pinguecula

- No treatment indicated for quiet lesions
- If hyperemic, can be decongested with mild vasoconstrictors or cold packs
- If inflamed and symptoms of irritation and foreign-body sensation, treat with topical steroids (e.g., loteprednol 0.5%) qid for 1 week
- Lubricants may be comforting to symptomatic patients
- Rarely done but can be excised and radiated for cosmetic purposes

Follow-Up

- Because of association with sunlight (UV aggravate), UV tints and regular outdoor sunglasses may help to reduce increasing size, thickness, and color
- Routine follow-up evaluation or PRN

O. Pterygium

Pterygium is not a contraindication to soft contact lens wear. Refer to "Degenerations" in Chapter 5, Section II.

P. Subconjunctival Hemorrhage[9]

Subjective

- One of the most common ocular surface presentations
- Usually seen as an acute or subacute (STAT or ASAP) presentation
- Ominous, rapid-onset appearance of "blood" on the eye leads to dramatic patient concern
- Patient may or may not be able to elicit a positive history
    1. Trauma (e.g., ocular, head) including contact lens wear and ocular surgeries
    2. Valsalva-like maneuvers
        a. Coughing
        b. Sneezing
        c. Vomiting
        d. Strangulation
        e. Constipation
        f. Seizure
    3. Systemic causes (e.g., vascular disease)
- Painless presentation

Objective

- Loose blood in the bulbar subconjunctival spaces (Figure 4.11)
- Usually unilateral but could present bilaterally
- Flat sheaths of uniform red blood without vessel patterns (may show streaks as blood spreads)
- Blood accumulates more toward the limbus, where a clear space (line or ring) is usually visible as a border between the blood and cornea
- Spread of blood may occur in any direction, to any degree during the first few hours or days
- Over an average of 7 to 21 days, bright red color turns to dark red to pink to yellow and back to clear white
- Rarely does permanent blood staining persist

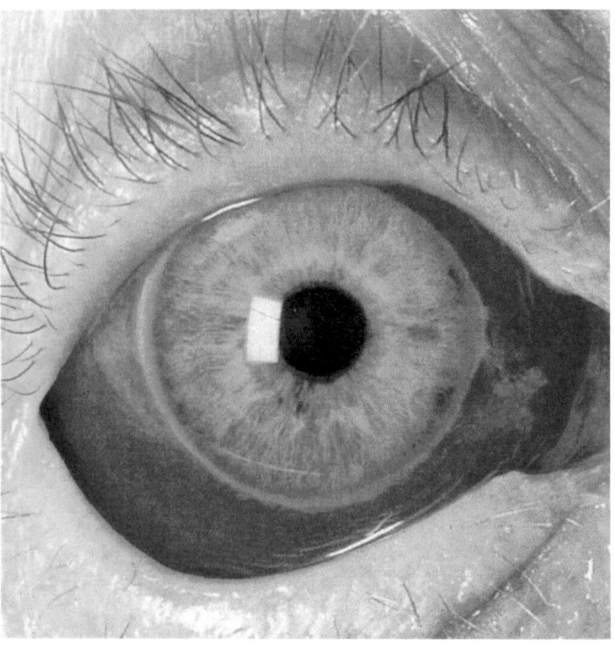

FIGURE 4.11 **Subconjunctival hemorrhage** of 5-day duration in the right eye with a classic clear ring surrounding the limbal border.

Assessment

(See also Appendix 3)

- Rule out history of trauma
    1. Ocular
    2. Head
    3. Remote (to eyes or head)
- Rule out local inflammatory disease
    1. Hyperacute (hemorrhagic) conjunctivitis
    2. Usually produce small multiple hemorrhages
- Rule out associated systemic diseases
    1. Systemic vascular disease (e.g., hypertension) or blood dyscrasias
    2. Anticoagulation meds (e.g., warfarin, Eliquis, aspirin)
    3. Leukemia
    4. Febrile diseases
- Other common causes
    1. Menstruation
    2. Telangiectasia (shows focal elevation within hemorrhagic area)
    3. Valsalva-like maneuvers (common)
    4. Conjunctival vascular tumors
- Idiopathic (probably most common)

Plan: Subconjunctival Hemorrhage

- Attempt to determine cause
    1. Careful history
    2. Blood pressure
    3. Ocular examination (external and internal)
- Refer appropriately for cause, if indicated
- Reassure patient
- Advise on no need for (or effective) treatment
    1. May suggest alternate hot or cold packs to aid in reabsorption of loose blood
    2. Probably more a placebo than therapy

- Explain slow resolution (by color) over 7 to 21 days
  1. Dense blood (thick black sheaths) may take longer (3 to 6 weeks)
  2. Management remains the same

Follow-Up

- Recheck at 1 week if patient (or physician) concerned
- If recurrent presentation, recheck at 3 to 6 months
- More than two recurrences within 1 year, obtain full medical workup by physician

Q. Telangiectasia

Subjective

- Asymptomatic patient (often general-examination patient)
- Patient may be concerned or completely unaware of finding
- Occurs in any age group

Objective

- Isolated, superficial, localized dilated, or convoluted blood vessel (arteriole) on bulbar conjunctival surface (Figures 4.12, 4.13)
- May appear as saccular-like aneurysms, berry-shaped, or simple convolution
- Usually single finding but may be multiple
- More often unilateral (but could be bilateral)
- Rarely, increased prominence (and elevation) could produce secondary superficial irritation

Assessment

- Rule out any chronic superficial irritant
- Possible systemic causes
  1. Vascular disease
  2. Diabetes
  3. Collagen vascular diseases
  4. Acne rosacea
  5. Neoplasias (especially with elongated dilated vessel emanating from posterior eye)
- Idiopathic: most common

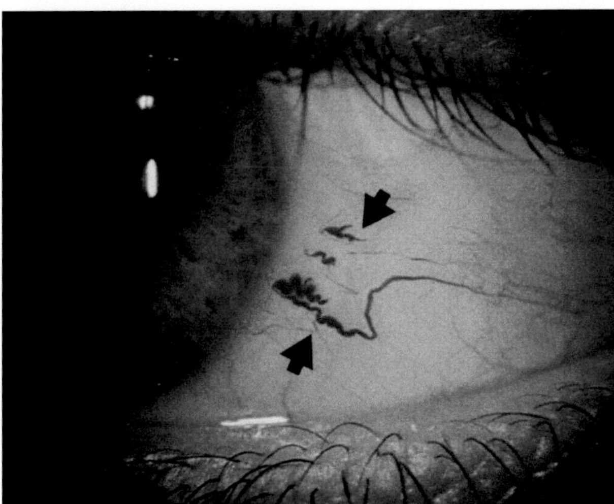

FIGURE 4.12 **Telangiectasia** on the bulbar conjunctiva in the lateral aspect of a left eye. Multiple configurations can be observed, including saccular-like aneurysms (top arrow) and a dilated, convoluted arteriole (bottom arrow).

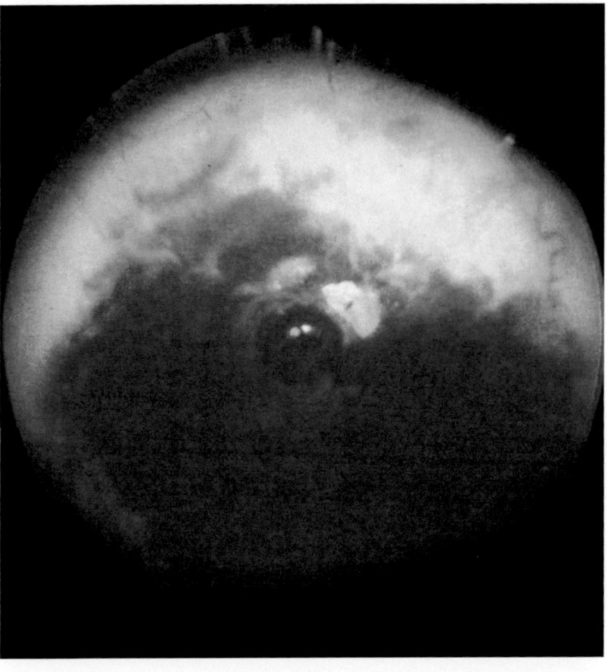

FIGURE 4.13 **Telangiectasia** with subconjunctival hemorrhage reveals a round, circumscribed, focal elevation at superior border of the hemorrhage. Previous documentation of underlying telangiectasia would be reassuring to examiner.

Plan: Telangectasia

- No treatment indicated
- Reassure patient
- Document in patient's record (draw or photograph)

Follow-Up

- Monitor routinely or PRN
- Patient at slightly higher risk for subconjunctival hemorrhage
  1. Produces ominous-appearing focal elevation within hemorrhagic area
  2. Previous documentation will rule out other remote causes for elevation (e.g., foreign body)

III. Inflammatory Conditions

A. Allergic Conjunctivitis[10–15]

1. Atopic Reactions

Subjective

- Immediate (type I) IgE-mediated reaction, within minutes, or delayed (type IV) cell-mediated reaction, within hours to days
- Frequent patient or family history of allergies or asthma (especially type I)
- Often a seasonally related condition (e.g., hay fever) or perennial (e.g., cats, dogs, etc.)
- May or may not report specific allergen (substance)
- Predominant irritation is unrelenting itching
- Other symptoms include tearing, redness, foreign-body sensation, and eyelid swelling

Objective

- May be unilateral (usually contact response) or bilateral (often from endogenous cause)
- Vision may fluctuate or remain unaffected
- Pink to red bulbar hyperemic injection
- "Glassy"-appearing luster to mucous membranes
- Chemosis (subconjunctival infiltration and edema) (Figure 4.14)
  1. Produces mild to dramatic swelling of bulbar conjunctiva
     a. Conjunctival tissue elevates and "rolls over" limbus (obvious with slit beam)
     b. "Watchglass" effect when complete peripheral cornea covered by conjunctiva (Figure 4.15)

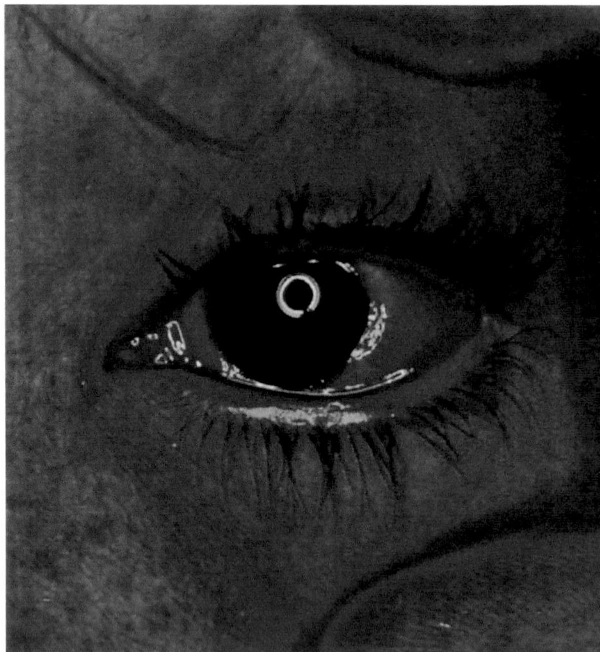

FIGURE 4.14 **Conjunctival chemosis** of a mild to moderate nature associated with an allergic conjunctivitis producing conjunctival infiltrative edema.

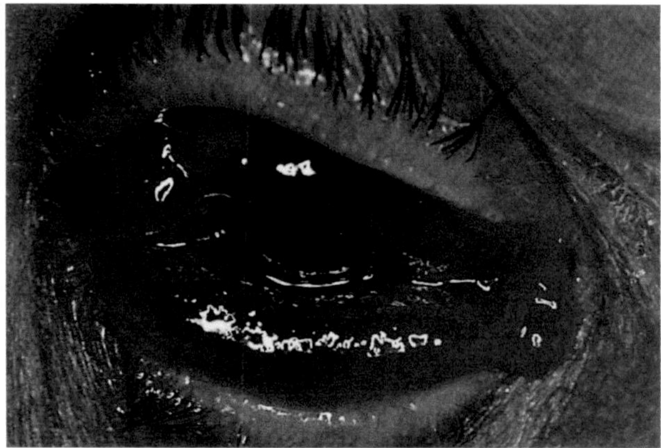

FIGURE 4.15 **Conjunctival "watchglass" effect** produced by severe conjunctival chemosis. Note the clear, "watchglass" of cornea visible in the middle area of the grossly elevated, chemotic, bulbar conjunctiva covering the peripheral cornea.

  2. More common and predominant on temporal conjunctiva due to eye-rubbing pattern at outer canthus (usually same side as dominant hand)
- Mucoid (stringy) whitish discharge
  1. Strands often spread across cornea
  2. Accumulates in fornices and at inner canthus
- Associated mild to severe lid edema and erythema
  1. Inferior lid usually affected more due to gravity
- Small "velvety" to "giant" papillary changes on upper and lower palpebral conjunctiva
  1. Frequently, follicular changes also present
  2. Associated edema often "buries" papillae (and follicles)
- Laboratory workup (if done) usually shows eosinophilia (type I) or basophils (type IV)

Assessment

(See also Appendix 3)

- Rule out other causes of red eyes
- Rule out other types of conjunctivitis (Table 4.1)
- Differentiate (if possible) by history or laboratory workup (optional), immediate versus delayed reaction
- If possible, determine specific causative agent (but don't drive yourself and your patient crazy!)
- Rule out vernal conjunctivitis

Plan: Atopic Reactions

(See also Appendices 4 and 6)

- Prescriptive (Rx) and non-prescriptive considerations
  1. Topical antihistamine/mast cell stabilizers (dual activity agents)
     a. First line of treatment
     b. Antihistamine treats acute symptoms and mast cell stabilizer prevents future reactions
     c. OTC and Rx
     d. Rx 1 drop qd am or bid depending on drug choice (e.g., Olopatadine, Ketotifen, Bepotastine besilate, Alcaftadine)
     e. For contact lens wearers
        i. Acuvue Theravision with Ketotifen (approved in US, Canada, and Japan)
           - Contact lens drug delivery system
           - Clinically significant decreased itching after 15 minutes and 12 hours of lens wear compared to control lens
  2. Topical Steroids
     a. Use for more severe acute or delayed (Type IV) reactions
     b. Loteprednol etabonate 0.25% or 0.5% less likely to have steroid-based side effects compared to ketone-based steroids (Refer to Chapter 1)
     c. Reduces itching and redness
     d. Short term usage
     f. Dosage depends on severity and should be tapered
     g. Combine treatment with duel activity agents
     h. Refer to Table 4.2 for selections
  3. Intracanalicular Dexamethasone Insert (Dextenza)
     a. Insert in place into inferior puncta and canaliculus bilaterally
     b. Releases 0.4 mg dexamethasone for up to 30 days

TABLE 4.1 **Conjunctivitis: Clinical Presentations**

Bacterial	Viral	Allergic	Chronic
Subjective			
All age groups	Unilateral or bilateral	Onset in hours or days	Chronic
Unilateral or bilateral	± systemic history	Unilateral or bilateral	Bilateral
± irritation	3–7 day history	± allergic history	Cosmesis
2–3 day history	Previous conjunctivitis frequently reported	Seasonal	± irritation
No reduced visual acuity	Burning sensation	Itching	Sometimes seasonal
May have URI history	May have URI history	History of allergen	No reduced visual acuity
AM lashing matting	± visual acuity	No reduced visual acuity (fluctuations)	Easily aggravated
Objective			
Meaty red	Pink/purple > toward plica	Pink/purple	Angular injection
> toward fornices	Quick TBUT	Chemosis	Inferior hyperemia
Movable vessels	Tearing	Mucoid	No discharge
Blanch with mild vasoconstrictors	Follicles	± Lid edema	Papillae
Cornea clear	Enlarged preauricular node or lymphadenopathy	Papillae	Variable TBUT
Papillae		Occasional follicles	Occasional xerosis
Mucopurulent			
Assessment (Differential Diagnosis)			
Rule out	*Rule out*	*Rule out*	*Rule out*
Viral	Secondary causes	Early bacterial	Staphylococcal toxins
Allergic	Common (non-specific)	Early viral	Viral
Secondary causes	PCF	Seasonal reaction	Chlamydia
Staphylococcus aureus	EKC	Contact allergen	Exposure
Streptococcus pneumoniae	Herpes simplex and zoster	Endogenous allergen	Ultraviolet radiation
Haemophilus influenzae	Adult inclusion/Chlamydia	Vernal	Tear dysfunction
Chlamydia	Lab: monocytes, inclusion bodies, giant cells	GPC associated with CLs	Moraxella
Gonococcus		Lab: basophils, eosinophils	Allergens (seasonal)
Lab: PMNs			Lab: variable
Plan			
Hygiene	Hygiene/contact	Remove allergen	Lid procedures
Irrigation	Lubrication	Air conditioning (optional)	Ultraviolet tints
Warm compresses	Warm/cold compresses	Cold compresses	Lubricants
Antibiotics (optional)	OTC ocular decongestant	OTC topical decongestant–antihistamine (astringents)	Zinc preparations
Hypertonic saline	Hypertonic saline	Oral OTC or Rx decongestant–antihistamines	Aminoglycosides
Combo steroids (for severe cases)	Educate and counsel	Antihistamine/Mast cell stabilizer	Oral antihistamine–decongestants
Instructions and follow-up	Follow-up	Steroids or NSAIDs	
Self-limiting			

Abbreviations: URI, upper respiratory infection; TBUT, tear breakup time; PMN, polymorphonuclear cell; PCF, pharyngoconjunctival fever; EKC, epidemic keratoconjunctivitis; GPC, giant papillary conjunctivitis; CL, contact lens; OTC, over the counter; Rx, prescription.

   c. Effective against itch and redness
   d. Monitor for IOP increase
4. Mast cell stabilizers (e.g., Cromolyn sodium, Lodoxamide)
   a. No longer prescribed often due to dual combination agents
5. Oral (Rx) medications rarely required for ocular allergic reactions
   a. Oral steroids should be withheld as backup therapy in nonresponsive conditions
   b. Oral antihistamine-decongestant drugs can be administered freely (in lieu of contraindications), especially preparations of known effectivity for patient with allergic history (i.e., previously prescribed agents)
   c. Most oral antihistamine-decongestants available OTC (see Table 4.2)
6. Nonprescriptive (OTC) drug considerations
   a. Decongestant and antihistamine combination drops

TABLE 4.2 Examples of Prescription and Over-the-Counter Medications for Conjunctivitis

Category	Generic Names	Brand Names	Route	Rx/OTC	Source
Antihistamines	Brompheniramine	Dimetapp	Oral	OTC	Foundation Consumer brands
	Chlorpheniramine	Generics	Oral	OTC	generics
	Diphenhydramine	Benadryl	Oral	OTC	J&J, generics
	Dimenhydrinate	Dramamine	Oral	OTC	Prestige Consumer Healthcare, generics
Combinations	Chlorpheniramine and pseudoephedrine	Chlor-Trimeton Allergy D	Oral	OTC	Novartis, generics
Anti-infectives	Bacitracin	Bacitracin	Topical	Rx	generics
	Besifloxacin	Besivance	Topical	Rx	Bausch & Lomb
	Ciprofloxacin	Ciloxan	Topical	Rx	Allergan, generics
	Gatifloxacin	Zymaxid	Topical	Rx	Allergan, generics
	Ofloxacin	Ocuflox	Topical	Rx	Allergan, generics
	Gentamicin	Generic	Topical	Rx	generics
	Moxifloxacin	Vigamox	Topical	Rx	Allergan, generics
	Tobramycin	Tobrex	Topical	Rx	Novartis, generics
Broad-spectrum combinations	Neomycin, polymyxin B, and bacitracin	Generic	Topical	Rx	generics
	Polymyxin B and bacitracin	Generic	Topical	Rx	generics
	Polymyxin B and trimethoprim	Polytrim	Topical	Rx	Allergan, generics
Antivirals	Acyclovir	Generic	Oral	Rx	generics
	Famciclovir	Generic	Oral	Rx	generics
	Ganciclovir	Zirgan	Topical	Rx	Bausch & Lomb
	Trifluridine	Viroptic	Topical	Rx	Pfizer
	Valacyclovir	Valtrex	Oral	Rx	GlaxoSmithKline
Astrigents	Zinc sulfate	ZinoxCare	Topical	OTC	Advacare Pharma
Antihistamine/Mast cell stabilizer	Alcaftadine	Lastacaft	Topical	OTC	Allergan
	Bepotastine besilate	Bepreve	Topical	Rx	Bausch & Lomb
	Ketotifen	Zaditor	Topical	OTC	Novartis
	Olopatadine	Pataday	Topical	OTC	Novartis
Corticosteroids	Dexamethasone	Generic	Topical	Rx	generics
	Difluprednate	Durezol	Topical	Rx	Novartis
	Fluorometholone	FML	Topical	Rx	Allergan, generics
	Hydrocortisone	Cortizone 10	Topical	OTC	Sanofi
	Loteprednol	Lotemax	Topical	Rx	Bausch & Lomb
	Prednisolone	Pred Mild,	Topical	Rx	Allergan, generics
		Pred Forte	Topical		
Anti-infective/steroid combinations	Neomycin	Maxitrol	Topical	Rx	Novartis, generics
	Polymyxin B, dexamethasone				
	Tobramycin/Dexamethasone	Tobradex	Topical	Rx	Novartis, generics
	Tobramycin/ Loteprednol	Zylet	Topical	Rx	Bausch & Lomb
	Neosporin, polymyxin B, bacitracin, hydrocortisone	Generic	Topical	Rx	generics
Decongestants	Brimonidine	Lumify	Topical	OTC	Bausch & Lomb
	Naphazoline	Clear Eyes	Topical	OTC	Prestige Consumer Health
	Phenylephrine	Sudafed PE	Oral	OTC	J&J
	Pseudoephedrine	Sudafed	Oral	OTC	J&J
Combinations	Phenylephedrine and	Sudafed PE	Oral	OTC	J&J
	Diphenhydramine	Sinus Congestion			
	Naphazoline and pheniramine	Naphcon A	Topical	OTC	Alcon
		Opcon-A	Topical	OTC	B&L
Irrigating solutions	Balanced salt solution with BAK	Eye Stream	Topical	OTC	Alcon
	Isotonic solution with boric acid	Advanced Eye Relief Eyewash	Topical	OTC	Bausch & Lomb
Lubricants	Mucomimetics	Refresh, Systane, Soothe	Topical	OTC	Allergan, Alcon, B & L
	Ointments	Systane ointment			Alcon
		Refresh ointment	Topical	OTC	Allergan
		Soothe ointment	Topical	OTC	B & L

Rx, prescription; OTC, over the counter; BAK, benzalkonium chloride.

i. Are slightly more effective as combination because of synergism
ii. Dosing q3h or q4h due to short acting duration
iii. Usage has decreased due to antihistamine/mast cell stabilizers

b. Oral antihistamines
i. Initial dose can effectively begin to reverse histamine release
ii. Diphenhydramine (Benadryl) effective
- Advise on drowsiness and ocular dryness
- Dosage per insert directions

iii. Second generation (Loratadine, Fexofenadine, Cetirizine)
- Ocular dryness may occur
- Dosage per insert directions

c. Refer to Table 4.2
d. Always rule out (by history) patients with potential idiosyncratic responses or contraindications to any drugs (Rx or OTC)

- Nontherapeutic (drugless) considerations
  1. Remove allergen (offending substance), if known
     a. Only complete cure for allergic reactions
     b. Allergen may be determined from careful history
     c. Contactants (e.g., external substances, eyedrops, cosmetics, soaps)
     d. Ingested (e.g., food, medicines)
     e. Injected (e.g., insect bite or sting)
     f. Airborne (e.g., pollen, spores, house dust)
     g. Pollutants (anything!)
  2. Frequent cold compresses (for vasoconstriction)
     a. One of the most valuable therapies for subjective and objective relief
     b. Always include with any combined treatment plan
  3. Air-conditioning for seasonal problems may be helpful
- Preventive measures
  1. Reasonable attempts to determine the allergen should be conducted so as to advise patient
  2. If appropriate (no contraindications or history of significant previous reactions), a "scratch test" may reveal offending substance
     a. Scratch clear skin (e.g., medial forearm) surface gently with needle to create slightly reddened area (approx. 5-mm diameter)
     b. Rub suspect substance (allergen) on area
     c. Wait 24 to 48 hours for mild localized edema or increased diameter (Arthus response)
     d. Positive reaction identifies allergen
  3. Counsel patient on risks of re-exposure
  4. Advise on chronicity and seasonal recurrences
  5. If reactions are severe or frequently recurrent, refer to allergist for complete workup and possible desensitization program

Follow-Up

- In moderate to severe reactions, schedule patient for 24- to 48-hour checkup
- Reschedule beyond second visit only for slowly responding conditions or during steroid management
- Instruct on preventive measures

2. Giant Papillary Conjunctivitis[16–18] (GPC)

Background Information

1. Probably a combined reaction: type I (mast cells and eosinophilia) and type IV (basophils)
2. Much less common in modern soft lens wearers due to frequent lens replacement
3. Immune reaction probably incited by "micro trauma"
4. Reported causes in order of clinical frequency
   a. Soft contact lens wear
   b. Hard contact lens wear
   c. Protruding sutures postoperatively
   d. Prosthetic (artificial) eyes
   e. Other mechanical irritants

Subjective

- Onset varies according to cause
  1. Soft lens wearers vary depending on replacement frequency and lens material
  2. Hard lens wearers usually greater than 3 to 5 years
  3. Protruding sutures within weeks to months
  4. Prosthetic eyes within months to years
- May show no symptoms with distinct physical findings or distinct symptoms with no findings
- Generally mild to moderate non-specific irritation and itching
  1. Present both with and without lens wear
  2. May increase temporarily on removal of lens
- Frequent reports of increased lens awareness and eventual loss of wearing time or inability to continue wear
- Lens movement on blinking becomes excessive
  1. Results in fluctuating vision or constant blur
  2. Frequent decentration of lens
  3. Ultimately dislodging and folding of lens(es)

Objective

- Almost always bilateral (Figure 4.16)
- Mild to moderate conjunctival hyperemia (greater in superior bulbar regions)
- Small to giant diffuse papillae on tarsus
  1. Vary in areas of concentration
     a. Upper tarsus (near fold), sometimes called "zone 3," more common with soft lenses

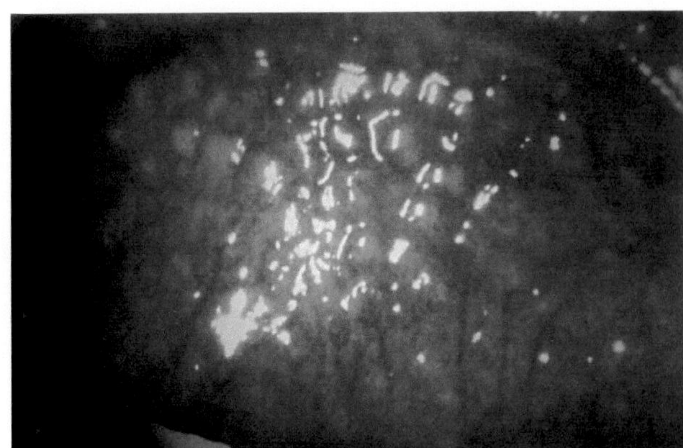

FIGURE 4.16 **Giant papillary conjunctivitis** associated with soft contact lens wear, demonstrating superior palpebral conjunctival papillae with whitish central cores, hyperemia, and infiltrative edema.

   b. Close to lid margin (zone 1) with hard lenses
   c. Diffuse in more severe reactions
2. Often associated with overlying infiltration and edema (which may even obscure papillae)
3. Size range from less than 0.5 mm up to 2 to 3 mm
4. Often tops of large papillae stain with NaFl
5. Larger papillae may show whitish-yellowish central cores
- Lens surfaces usually show light to dense protein buildup on surfaces especially if lenses are not frequently replaced
- Varying degrees of mucoid discharge from absent to dense, stringy accumulations
- Occasionally, superior cornea may be involved
   1. Superficial punctate keratitis (SPK) (greatest at limbus)
   2. Superior mucoid debris or filaments
   3. Limbal infiltrate(s)

Assessment

(See also Appendix 3)

- Rule out other causes of red eye
- Rule out other forms of conjunctivitis
- Rule out vernal conjunctivitis
   1. Usually more dramatic symptoms and signs
   2. Usually flat giant papillae
   3. Frequent corneal component
   4. Seasonal versus specific causative agent (e.g., contact lens)
- Rule out superior limbic keratoconjunctivitis (SLK)
   1. Minimal tarsal reaction
   2. Pronounced corneal involvement
- Determine causative agent (usually obvious)
- Consider immune versus micro trauma versus combined etiology
   1. Increased hyperemia, infiltrates, heavy protein, corneal involvement, or positive response to steroids may suggest primary immune component
   2. Increased papillae (at zone 1 or 3), excessive lens movement (without heavy protein), hard lens materials, sutures, prosthetics, or quick (less than 2 weeks) positive response to temporarily discontinued wear (without therapy) may suggest primary microtrauma component

Plan: Giant Papillary Conjunctivitis

(See also Appendix 4)

- Temporary lens discontinuation for 1–3 weeks if possible depending on severity
- Short-term (e.g., qid for 2 weeks followed by bid for 2 weeks) topical steroid (e.g., Loteprednol etabonate) drops
- Symptoms resolve faster than papillae (can take months)
- Increase soft lens replacement frequency → daily disposable has lowest GPC rate
- Clean rigid lenses and ocular prosthetic more frequently using manufacturer approved solutions (**do not use the following on a hydra-peg treated surface**)
   1. Daily alcohol-based cleaner (e.g., Miraflow, Serine ESC)
   2. Abrasive cleaner (e.g., Boston Cleaner) (**do not use on a plasma treated surface**)
   3. Enzyme treatment
   4. Lens polishing (**do not use on a plasma-treated surface**)
   5. Chemical cleaning (e.g., Progent)
- Remove any exposed sutures
- Manage contact lens wear carefully in conjunction with adjunctive therapies

Follow-Up

- Advise and educate patient on immune, mechanical nature of disorder, and risk of recurrence(s)
- Reschedule patients based on degree of presentation and therapies selected
- If GPC returns, consider
   1. Only use daily disposable hydrogel lens
   2. Refit with different hydrogel material
   3. Refit with rigid gas permeable material
- Recheck patient with GPC history every 6 months on any lens

3. Vernal Conjunctivitis

Refer to "Vernal Keratoconjunctivitis" in Chapter 5.

B. Bacterial Conjunctivitis

1. Acute Forms[19–21]

Subjective

- Found in all age ranges
- Unilateral initially with frequent contralateral autoinoculation reported
- No frank pain or itching (but may report non-specific irritation)
- History of 2 to 3 days with increasing intensity of objective signs
- No associated reduction in vision
- There may be a positive medical history
   1. Especially in children
   2. Upper respiratory infection (URI), otitis media (ear infection) in children
- Frequent reports of "lashes matting" or "eyes stuck shut" on waking
- Frequently associated history of chronic blepharitis
- Patient usually concerned over increasing intensity of redness (main reason for visit)

Objective

- Grossly hyperemic, meaty red bulbar conjunctiva
   1. Hyperemia greater toward fornices
   2. Circumcorneal area relatively clear
   3. Injected vessels easily movable with cotton tip
   4. Injected vessels blanch with mild vasoconstrictors
   5. Vessels show irregular (nonradiating) pattern
   6. Combination of smaller- and larger-diameter vessels
- Cornea clear (always check with slit lamp) but may develop SPK secondary to staphylococcal exotoxins
- Palpebral conjunctival papillae usually present
   1. Papillae present as reddish vascular tufts, varying in diameter from small (velvety appearance when abundant) to large mounds
   2. Often blanched and congested by secondary edema
- Yellowish-greenish mucopurulent discharge
   1. Accumulations usually greater in the morning
   2. Tends to accumulate inferiorly and at inner canthus
   3. Accumulations may also produce hard crustations on lid margins (e.g., staphylococcal rosettes)

Assessment

(See also Appendix 3)

- Rule out other causes of red eyes
- Rule out other causes of conjunctivitis
- Bacteria most prevalent cause of conjunctivitis in children
- Differentiate staphylococcal conjunctivitis (most common form of acute bacterial conjunctivitis) from other organisms
- Possible organisms to consider (limited list)
  1. Staphylococcus gram-positive cocci
     a. *S. epidermidis* (normal flora to lids)
     b. *S. aureus* (normal and pathogenic)
     c. Most common cause of bacterial conjunctivitis mostly through its sterile exotoxins
     d. Present 75% of the time on the ocular surface
        i. Thus, cultures inconclusive
        ii. Clinical signs most valuable
     e. May cause secondary keratitis (SPK, marginal infiltrates, etc.)
  2. Streptococcus gram-positive cocci
     a. *S. pyogenes*
     b. *S. pneumoniae*
     c. Usually cause hyperacute reactions
     d. Frequently bilateral (especially when systemically related)
     e. Petechial hemorrhages common
     f. Occasional pseudomembranous conjunctivitis
  3. Haemophilus gram-negative organism
     a. *H. influenzae* (*H. flu*)
     b. Associated with upper respiratory infections (URI) and otitis media
     c. Common in children
     d. Can also cause hyperacute conjunctivitis
        i. Chemosis
        ii. Bulbar hemorrhages
        iii. Preauricular lymph node enlargement
     e. Has characteristic purplish preseptal flush or cellulitis
     f. Can lead to meningitis if it spreads to the brain but less common due to *H. influenzae* vaccination
  4. Morax–Axenfeld bacillus (*Moraxella*) gram-negative *bacillus*
     a. Causes angular conjunctivitis
     b. Frequent cause of chronic conjunctivitis
     c. Can lead to corneal ulcer in compromised patient
     d. Common in severe alcoholics
  5. *Chlamydia trachomatis* (TRIC organism) gram negative
     a. 2- to 4-week persistent history (true inclusion conjunctivitis usually more insidious)
     b. Mixed bacterial, viral, and immune signs
     c. Positive genitourinary history may or may not be present
     d. Nonresponsive or only temporary with topicals alone
        i. Returns after medications discontinued
        ii. Needs oral antibiotics
           - Single dose 1 gram oral azithromycin
- Rule out other secondary causes
  1. Blepharitis (usually staphylococcal)
  2. Systemic causes (e.g., acne rosacea)

Plan: Acute Forms of Bacterial Conjunctivitis

- Prescriptive considerations
  1. Topical anti-infective agents (ointments or drops)
     a. Broad-spectrum drugs (Table 4.3)
     b. Specific agents (see Tables 4.2 and 4.3)
     c. General dosages (vary with degree of objective presentation)
        i. qid for 5 to 7 days (minimum)
        ii. Duration can be extended safely up to 10 to 14 days if necessary
     d. For resistant organisms
        i. Change anti-infective agent
        ii. Extend course up to 21 days (maximum)
        iii. Consider culture and sensitivity tests
        iv. Oral antibiotics may be indicated
  2. Specific treatment for organisms
     a. Staphylococcus
        i. Topicals
           - Bacitracin
           - Besifloxacin
           - Ciprofloxacin
           - Gatifloxacin
           - Gentamicin
           - Moxifloxacin
           - Neomycin
           - Tobramycin
           - Trimethoprim
        ii. Orals (limited to hyperacute forms only)
           - Penicillinase-resistant penicillins
           - Cephalosporins
           - Doxycycline
           - Tetracycline
     b. Streptococcus
        i. Topicals
           - Bacitracin
           - Besifloxacin
           - Ciprofloxacin
           - Gatifloxacin
           - Gentamicin (+/-)
           - Moxifloxacin
           - Tobramycin
        ii. Orals
           - Cephalosporins
           - Penicillins
     c. Haemophilus
        i. Topicals
           - Besifloxacin
           - Ciprofloxacin
           - Gatifloxacin
           - Gentamicin
           - Moxifloxacin
           - Polymyxin B
           - Tobramycin
        ii. Orals
           - Cephalosporins
     d. Moraxella
        i. Topicals
           - Besifloxacin

TABLE 4.3 Susceptibility of Some Ocular Pathogens to Common Topical Anti-Infective Agents ("The Bugs versus the Drugs")

The "Drugs" → / The "Bugs" ↓	Bacitracin	Polymyxin B	Ciprofloxacin	Gatifloxacin	Moxifloxacin	Besifloxacin	Neomycin	Gentamicin	Tobramycin	Azithromycin	Combination Drugs: Polytrim	Combination Drugs: Ak-Poly-Bac	Combination Drugs: Neosporin
Gram-Positive													
Staphylococcus sp.			X	X	X	X		X	X	X	X		
S. aureus	X		X	X	X	X	X	X	X	X	X	X	X
Streptococcus sp.	X		X	X	X	X			X	X		X	
S. pneumoniae	X		X	X	X	X		X	X	X	X	X	X
S. pyogenes			X					X		X	X		
β-Hemolytic streptococci	X							X	X			X	
Clostridium sp.	X											X	
Gram-Negative													
Escherichia coli		X	X	X	X	X	X	X	X		X	X	X
Haemophilus aepyptius (Koch-Weeks bacillus)			X					X	X		X		
Haemophilus influenzae		X	X	X	X	X	X	X	X	X	X	X	X
Klebsiella sp.							X						X
K. pneumoniae		X	X	X	X	X		X	X		X		
Neisseria sp.			X				X	X	X			X	X
N. gonorrhoeae	X		X	X	X	X		X		X			
Proteus sp.				X	X		X		X		X		
Acinetobacter calcoaceticus									X				
Enterobacter aerogenes		X		X	X	X	X	X	X		X	X	
Enterobacter sp.			X			X	X						X
Moraxella lacunata						X		X	X				
Chlamydia trachomatis			X		X	X				X			
Pseudomonas aeruginosa		X	X	X	X	X		X	X		X	X	X

- Gentamicin
- Neomycin
- Polymyxin B
- Tobramycin

ii. Orals: not indicated

e. Chlamydia[22]
   i. Topicals: not indicated
   ii. Orals
      - Azithromycin single 1 gram dose
      - Doxycycline 100 mg bid × 7 days

3. Topical steroid combination drops or ointments (see Table 4.2)
   a. Avoid use in mild to moderate cases
   b. With severe inflammatory responses or subjective discomfort, use cautiously (in lieu of any contraindications)
   c. Dosage: q2h × 2 days, q4h for 3 to 5 days, then taper
      i. Maximum duration: 7 to 10 days
      ii. Check intraocular pressure for steroid-linked glaucoma

- Nonprescription (OTC) consideration
  1. Topical OTC broad-spectrum anti-infective ointment preparations containing bacitracin and polymyxin B (see Table 4.2)
     a. Readily available
     b. Inexpensive for patient (thus increasing compliance)
     c. Consider if neomycin hypersensitivity risks
     d. Bacitracin component specific for Staphylococcus (most common cause of acute bacterial forms)
     e. Polymyxin B specific against Pseudomonas
     f. Ointment vehicle (in most cases) preferable
        i. Up to 6 hours therapeutic value versus less than 20 minutes with drops
        ii. No risk of corneal entrapment
        iii. No risk of clinical toxicity or systemic absorption (most carried off by mucous threads on the ocular surface) versus drops draining into the lacrimal canals
     g. Ointment most effective when applied on the external lid margins
        i. Site of greatest staphylococcal concentration
        ii. Called reservoir effect (or technique) (Table 4.4)
     h. Some common topical ophthalmic antibacterial ointments have similar components and characteristics as their OTC ointment counterpart (e.g., Polysporin ointments); the following have identical chemistry and formulation

TABLE 4.4 **Reservoir Effect: Step-by-Step Approach and Results**

1. Squeeze out a 1/4-inch ribbon of ointment onto your fingertip and discard (reduces risk of contaminants from tip).
2. Squeeze out a 1/2-inch ribbon of ointment onto your fingertip.
3. Wipe ointment onto the closed external lid margins of the affected eye.
   a. Tell patient to keep eye closed with normal pressure during application.
   b. When treating lid involvements directly, rub ointment in firmly.
4. Apply some extra ointment (dab on) at the inner and outer canthal portions of lid margin (outer canthus more preferable).
5. Body temperature will melt ointment base (white petrolatum) rapidly (30 to 60 seconds), and drug will begin to transport itself actively onto ocular surface (conjunctiva and cornea) by migration of mucous threads as patient is instructed to open eyes and resume normal blinking.
6. Patient will experience minimal blurring effect (versus ointment applied directly into eye in traditional method at inferior cul-de-sac).
7. Any excess ointment base or oils remaining on lid margins may be wiped off (for cosmesis) after 3 to 5 minutes without reducing therapeutic effect due to drug retention behind lid margins and on mucous threads in the fornices (resulting in a continuous reservoir effect for up to 6 hours).

i. Polymyxin B sulfate, 10,000 units
ii. Bacitracin zinc, 500 units
iii. Special white petrolatum qs (best ointment vehicle)
iv. Same concentrations
v. Same pH (7.4), although eyes can tolerate range of 3.5 to 10.5 pH due to tear buffering
vi. Bioequivalent
vii. Equal bioavailability
viii. Identical bioactivity

i. Any prescription versus OTC differences are offset by the "reservoir technique"
   i. Sterile ophthalmic (Rx) requirements negated by fingertip and external eye lid application technique
   ii. Also, consider that components in ointment itself are antibacterial
      - Studies have shown no growth of pathogens in antibacterial ointment
      - Only contaminants found in Polysporin components have been subclinical colonies of molds (e.g., Aspergillus)
      - Bacteria cannot grow well in a non-aqueous media (ointment)
      - Ocular surface itself is not sterile and does not demand sterility due to tear lysozymes, secretory immunoglobin A (slg A), lactoferrin, B-lysin and leukocytes themselves (which increase dramatically with threat of infection)
         1. "Milling" process and any additional filtration (e.g., to reduce ointment base coagulates and particles) of no consequence due to melting effect during reservoir effect
         2. One-eighth ounce "sterile" ophthalmic tubes, originally mandated by Food and Drug Administration (FDA) for one-time use in sterile surgical suites, of no value (and cost-ineffective) once opened and reused in nonsterile environment
         3. Tapered tip on 1/8-oz tubes for intrapalpebral administration unnecessary in fingertip to lid margin application

j. Irreconcilable (nonclinical) differences that must be considered
   i. FDA recommendations on OTC packaging describe external use only and state: "Do not use in the eye"
      - Such recommendations may be reconsidered relative to current research and clinical literature
      - Reservoir technique can be considered external application
   ii. Patients tend to save and reuse larger supplies of medications (e.g., ointments)
      - Carefully instruct against misuse
      - Monitor conditions to resolution

2. Topical astringents and heavy metals, such as zinc and mercuric oxides
   a. Reduce discharge
   b. Some antibacterial qualities (especially zinc against Moraxella angular conjunctivitis and blepharoconjunctivitis)
   c. Silver nitrate is too toxic for general use
3. Antibacterial preservatives found in low, but effective, concentrations in irrigating solutions
   a. Benzalkonium Chloride (BAK)
   b. Chlorobutanol
   c. Disodium edetate (EDTA)
   d. Thimerosol (beware of toxicity)
4. 5% Hypertonic saline may demonstrate anti-inflammatory value
   a. Drops or ointment
   b. Dosage as frequent as q2–4h

- Nontherapeutic (drugless) considerations
   1. Can be used independently or in conjunction with therapeutic approaches
   2. Irrigation with ophthalmic solutions or warm water to clear discharges and dilute or remove bacterial toxins
   3. Warm packs to enhance body's immune-defense system (vasodilation with increased leukocytic action) in vascular tissue
   4. Non-invasive, nontoxic nature of these steps permit ad lib dosages
   5. Instruct with 25–50–100 rule
      a. No worse in 24 ("25") hours
      b. Better in 48 ("50") hours
      c. Gone in 100 hours (about 4 days)

Follow-Up

- Reschedule patient within 3 to 5 days
- Carefully advise (25–50–100 rule) or PRN
- Preventive considerations (for patient and doctor)
   1. Treat both eyes to reduce risk of autoinoculation
   2. Instruct on general lid and skin hygiene
   3. Instruct patient never to touch eyes during acute disease process (infection and reinfection usually originate from bacteria on skin and hands)

4. Never reuse medications beyond 6 to 8 weeks
5. Never patch conjunctivitis
6. Monitor cornea closely during follow-up evaluation
7. Many acute cases "lost to follow-up" probably improve themselves, but call patient to verify resolution

2. Hyperacute Forms[23,24]

Subjective

- Found more frequently in younger age group (children and young adults) and in parents of young children
- Usually bilateral by time of presentation
- Rapidly advancing acute bacterial signs and symptoms
- Patient (or parents) anxious over rapid development

Objective

- Advanced acute bacterial presentation (Figure 4.17)
- Copious mucopurulent discharge accumulating in lower cul-de-sac and overflowing (usually at inner canthus)
- Varying degrees of secondary surrounding tissue involvement
    1. Lid edema and erythema
    2. Dermatoblepharoconjunctivitis
    3. Preseptal cellulitis
    4. Conjunctival chemosis (infiltrative edema)
    5. Toxic corneal epithelial staining (beware of early ulceration)
- Occasional hemorrhagic changes on bulbar conjunctiva ranging from petechiae (small dots) to larger areas of gross subconjunctival blood
- Formations of true or pseudomembranes may develop in fornices and on palpebral conjunctiva
- Frequent follicles and preauricular lymphadenopathy or enlargement present (mimicking viral presentation)
- Laboratory workup indicated (versus optional in acute)
    1. Cultures
        a. Blood agar will grow most organisms
        b. Chocolate agar grows Neisseria and Haemophilus
        c. Thayer-Martin agar grows Neisseria
        d. Technique
            i. Moisten applicator with non-preserved saline
            ii. Roll applicator along lid margins (5 times)
            iii. Don't use anesthetics (reduce organisms)
            iv. Inoculate solid or broth media and label
        e. Cultures must be done prior to any treatment
        f. Order cultures and sensitivities (to specific antibiotics)
    2. Gram stains for morphology of organisms
        a. Gram-positives (violet)
        b. Gram-negatives (red)
        c. Morphologic appearances by shape
            i. Cocci
            ii. Rods
            iii. Bacilli
        d. Morphologic appearance by patterns
            i. Single
            ii. Pairs
            iii. Clusters
            iv. Chairs
        e. Technique
            i. Use dry applicator (swab or spatula)
            ii. Gently scrape inferior palpebral conjunctiva
            iii. Transfer contents of scraping to glass slide
            iv. Fix with 95% methyl alcohol and label
    3. Giemsa stain for cytology of organisms
        a. Polymorphonuclear leukocytes (PMNs) represent
            i. Bacterial infection
            ii. Fungal infection
        b. Mononuclear cells (lymphocytes)
            i. Adenoviral infection
            ii. Viral infection
            iii. Toxic reactions
        c. Eosinophils (PMNs)
            i. Allergic reactions
            ii. Hypersensitivity reactions
        d. Inclusion bodies (difficult to capture or observe) are found with chlamydial infection
        e. Technique is like gram staining
    4. Conditions recommended for laboratory examination
        a. Hyperacute conjunctivitis
        b. Conjunctivitis in newborns
        c. Conjunctivitis resistant to standard or initial therapy
        d. Postoperative conjunctivitis
        e. Corneal ulcers

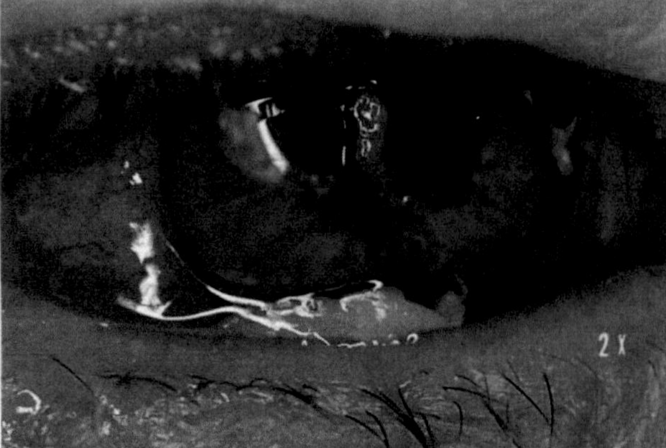

FIGURE 4.17 **Hyperacute bacterial conjunctivitis** with classic findings including gross bulbar conjunctival hyperemia, chemosis, and mucopurulent discharge (floating on the corneal surface).

Assessment

(See also Appendix 3)

- Rule out other causes of red eyes
- Rule out other causes of conjunctivitis
- Possible organisms to consider after Staphylococcus (limited list)
    1. Streptococcus (see "Acute Forms" of conjunctivitis earlier in chapter)
    2. Haemophilus (see "Acute Forms" of conjunctivitis earlier in chapter)
    3. *Corynebacterium diphtheriae* gram-positive club shape

   a. Uncommon, virulent infector
   b. Can lead to corneal ulcer
   c. Causes true membranous conjunctivitis leading to symblepharon and scarring
   d. Secondary trichiasis, entropion, and so forth
   e. Liberates an exotoxin that causes serious systemic disorders (e.g., airway obstruction, cardiac toxicity, paralysis)
4. *Neisseria gonorrhoeae* gram-negative diplococci
   a. Rapid proliferation
   b. Extremely copious discharge ("ballooning" lids)
   c. Positive (or suspicion of) venereal history
   d. Can produce preauricular lymph node enlargement, subconjunctival hemorrhaging, chemosis, and so forth
5. *Pseudomonas aeruginosa* gram-negative rod
   a. Potent secondary infector
   b. Uncommon as a primary conjunctivitis
   c. Rapid proliferation (most rapid organism)
   d. Very high risk of secondary corneal ulcer (if corneal epithelium broken)
   e. May show a phosphorescence with black light
6. Other gram-negative bacteria
   a. Especially common gastrointestinal (GI) organisms (e.g., Serratia, *Escherichia coli*)
   b. Beware of mothers of children in diapers!

- Always consider (and protect against) the risk of corneal invasion of hyperacute bacteria (not including Pseudomonas, surprisingly) through an intact cornea
  1. Streptococcus
  2. Gonococcus
  3. *Haemophilus influenzae*
  4. Corynbacterium (uncommon)
  5. Pseudomonas requires an epithelial defect to enter cornea

Differential consideration for acute and hyperacute bacterial conjunctivitis can be accomplished fairly accurately by age alone (rule of fives).

Age Range	Leading Cause
0 to 5 days	Gonococcus
5 days to 5 weeks	Chlamydia
5 weeks to 5 years	Streptococcus and *Haemophilus influenzae*
5 years and older	Staphylococcus

Plan: Hyperacute Forms of Bacterial Conjunctivitis

(See also Appendix 6)

- Topical therapies (Rx, OTC, and "drugless") same as for acute bacterial conjunctivitis at q2–3h dosages
- Oral antibiotics usually required in hyperacute forms
  1. Penicillins (or penicillinase-resistant penicillin) against Staphylococcus in standard recommended dosages
  2. Cephalosporins (e.g., Keflex)
  3. Children's oral dosages should be determined based on body weight in conjunction with pediatrician
- Refer systemic-related conditions for specific medical care (e.g., URIs, otitis media, sexually transmitted disease)
- Specific treatment for organisms
  1. Staphylococcus (see "Acute Forms" of conjunctivitis earlier in chapter)
  2. Streptococcus (see "Acute Forms" of conjunctivitis earlier in chapter)
  3. Haemophilus (see "Acute Forms" of conjunctivitis earlier in chapter)
  4. Corynebacterium[23]
     a. Topicals
        i. Third generation cephalosporins (e.g., cefmenoxime), Vancomycin, and Arbekacin
        ii. Resistance to fluroquinolones and erythromycin is high
  5. *Neisseria gonorrhoeae*[25]
     a. Considerable antibiotic resistance has been found with topical and oral antibiotics
     b. Refer for intramuscular injection of ceftriaxone
     c. Can cause blindness and penetrate intact cornea

Follow-Up

- Reschedule in 24 to 48 hours based on severity
- Adjust initial broad-spectrum therapy to specific drug, on receipt of laboratory results (if indicated)
- If condition stable or improving within 24 to 48 hours, continue therapy at moderating dosages for minimum of 10 to 14 days
- If condition unstable or worsening within 24 to 48 hours, adjust medications (per laboratory results), increase dosage, add oral medication (if absent), and reconsider diagnosis
- Monitor cornea closely for bacterial keratitis
- On resolution, advise and educate patient on prevention (see Figure 3.25)

C. Toxic and Irritative (Chronic) Conjunctivitis

Subjective

- Common "red eye" presentation easy to diagnose but difficult to establish primary cause as well as effective treatment
- Onset and history are always chronic and insidious
- Frequently "keeps company" with other anterior segment diseases
- Symptoms may be absent or mild to moderate non-specific superficial irritation
- Patient usually most concerned with cosmesis
- Frequently associated with a history of a chronic irritating cause or toxic substance
  1. Some possible irritating causes
     a. Dry, arid conditions
     b. Airborne irritants (e.g., pollutants, pollen, dust)
     c. Allergens (i.e., any substance with the potential to cause a hypersensitive or immune type reaction)
     d. Radiation (e.g., sun, reflectants, UV)
  2. Some possible toxic substances
     a. Chemicals (direct contact or fumes)
     b. Exogenous factors
        i. Bacterial toxins (especially staphylococcal exotoxins)
        ii. Viral toxins (e.g., molluscum, verrucae)
        iii. Chronic use of topical medication (eyedrops or ointments) especially benzalkonium chloride preserved called medicamentosa

            iv. Cosmetics, soaps, perfumes
        c. Endogenous factors
            i. Systemic medications
            ii. Autoimmune responses
        d. *Morax–Axenfeld bacillus* (Moraxella) often reported as persistent (subclinical) cause
            i. Gram-negative bacteria
            ii. Produces scant, transient discharge and angular (palpebral fissure) hyperemia
- Condition reported as easily aggravated by external factors
    1. Wind
    2. Rubbing
    3. Contact lens wear

Objective

- Unilateral or bilateral, depending on primary cause (Figure 4.18)
- Mild to moderate bulbar hyperemia often greater inferior
    1. Inferior pattern usually "4-o'clock/8-o'clock syndrome"
        a. Leashes of vasodilated, superficial bulbar conjunctival vessels pointing to the 4- and 8-o'clock positions on the corneal limbus
        b. Most common sites of lid margin-limbal intersection
        c. Most notorious sites for lid margin and meibomian gland toxic (particularly staphylococcal exotoxins) response
    2. Diffuse inferior hyperemia, usually secondary to "4/8 syndromes"
- Mixed papillary or follicular palpebral conjunctival response usually only mild to moderate in degree
    1. Predominance of one or the other based on primary cause
        a. Bacterial: greater papillary
        b. Viral: follicular
        c. Noninfectious irritants: usually papillary
        d. Noninfectious toxins: usually follicular
    2. Ultimately combined effects over time produce mixed reactions

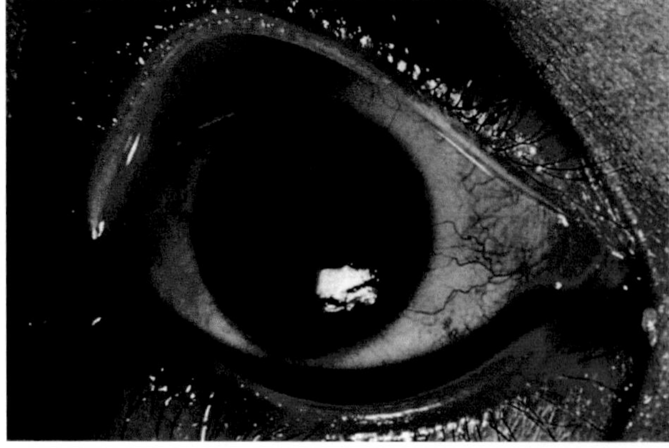

FIGURE 4.18 Chronic/toxic conjunctivitis ("Why are my eyes always red, Doc?") produces a chronic, low-grade redness without discharge or tearing and is caused by numerous toxic antigens.

    3. Superior tarsus often presents greater involvement
- Never a pronounced discharge or exudates
- Frequently an angular, nasal, and temporal hyperemic pattern, most prominent in the exposed palpebral fissure spaces
- Occasionally may demonstrate "phlyctenule" formation(s)
    1. Sometimes called "phlyctenular conjunctivitis"
    2. Pinkish-white epithelial nodule formed as focal reaction to localized toxin
    3. Greater in young children
    4. Sometimes subjectively uncomfortable (if densely infiltrated and secondarily inflamed)
    5. May show mild to moderate surrounding edema
    6. Usually singular lesions close to limbus
        a. May be multiple and located anywhere on bulbar conjunctiva
        b. If translimbal (onto cornea), symptoms increase and termed "phlyctenular keratoconjunctivitis"
- May show rose bengal conjunctival staining
- Infrequently, bulbar conjunctiva may keratinize (harden) producing yellow patches (e.g., xerosis)

Assessment

(See also Appendix 3)

- Rule out other causes of red eyes
- Rule out other forms of conjunctivitis (see Table 4.1)
- Try to establish primary cause (e.g., irritant, toxin) through history and physical findings
- If no obvious primary cause from history or physical, consider non-specific treatment plan(s) according to the following order of classic "non-specific" diagnoses
    1. Staphylococcal toxins (look for other classic staphylococcal signs, e.g., lid problems, inferior patterns)
        a. 4/8 syndrome
        b. Frequently aggravated by soft contact lens wear
    2. Chronic viral infection and/or viral toxins
        a. Generally produces a diffuse hyperemia
        b. Dormant virus may be undiagnosable
    3. Chronic chlamydial infection
        a. Frequently associated with follicles
        b. Usually some form of associated corneal findings
    4. Non-specific allergic response
    5. Dry eye effects (with quick breakup time, positive rose bengal/lissamine green stain: frequent corneal component)
    6. UV sensitivity (outdoor: sunlight irritant; exposure: palpebral aperture hyperemic pattern)
    7. Moraxella "angular conjunctivitis" (sometimes an associated angular blepharitis and scant discharge)

Plan: Toxic and Irritative Conjunctivitis

(See also Appendix 4)

- Treat primary cause if established
    1. Treatment plans should be appropriate for cause and should be modified based on chronicity of response
    2. Adjunctive topical steroids (in combination with primary therapeutic agents) often helpful in reducing secondary toxic, inflammatory response

3. Avoid aggravating chronic condition or precipitating an acute response through introduction of additional toxic medications, eyedrops
- If primary cause is not established, introduce step-by-step treatment plan according to "classic causes"
  1. Explain to patient nature of "non-specific" plan and establish understanding of "no guarantees!"
  2. Step-by-step plan
     a. Antistaphylococcal procedures (see Table 3.25) for 2 weeks
        i. Use all procedures (i.e., hygiene, warm packs, massage, scrubs, hypochlorous acid 0.01%, and bacitracin ointment) with or without clinical staphylococcal signs
        ii. Dosage: bid (minimum)
     b. Frequent cold packs (e.g., q3–4 h) for 2 weeks
     c. Oral doxycycline or azithromycin (one time daily for 3 to 5 days)
     d. Oral (not topical) antihistamine-decongestant for 2 weeks
     e. Lubricants 6 to 10 times daily for 2 weeks
        i. Mucomimetic agents useful
     f. Constant UV protection for 2 weeks
        i. Sunglasses outdoors (with or without bright sunlight)
        ii. UV tints or nonprescription UV protection for constant wear
     g. Ophthalmic zinc preparation for 2 weeks
        i. OTC agents effective against Moraxella
        ii. Dosage: qid with ointment at bedtime
     h. Tobramycin (Tobrex) or gentamicin for 2 weeks
  3. Rx agents most effective against Moraxella
     a. Consider these therapies to rule out chronic chlamydial infection if history is suggestive or positive
     b. Rule out contraindications to oral doxycycline
  4. Steps may be combined, but positive results would not provide definitive diagnosis of primary cause
- Treatment plans on contact lens patients may be conducted with or without continued wear, depending on type of care

Follow-Up

- Follow-up considerations should be based on nature of treatment plan for diagnosed primary causes
- In non-specific step-by-step approach, recheck at 2-week intervals and add next step, when and if indicated
- Overall advice and education to patients
  1. Explain primary cause if established
  2. Counsel on measures to reduce associated aggravants
  3. Advise on potential chronicity, especially in cases of unknown cause(s)
     a. Suggest methods of effective self-care and maintenance
     b. Recommend brief periodic rechecks (should be advised for all chronic conditions) of ocular surface tissues at least once a year or PRN (see Table 4.1)

D. Trachoma[26,27]

Background Information

a. Caused by TRIC organisms (*Chlamydial trachomatis* species)
b. Part of series of oculogenital diseases
   i. Trachoma
   ii. Inclusion blennorrhea (neonatal chlamydial disease)
   iii. Adult inclusion conjunctivitis
c. Tends to be endemic in poor countries that are overcrowded with poor sanitation and among certain ethnic groups
   i. Africa
   ii. South America
   iii. American Indians
d. Leading cause of infectious blindness worldwide
e. Spread by direct contact (hands, sexual, cervical)
f. Associated genitourinary involvement often mild
g. Laboratory workup usually less reliable than clinical diagnosis
h. Severe (corneal scarring) forms far more sight threatening than milder conjunctival forms

Subjective

- Chronic insidious onset
- 2 phases
  1. Active disease more common in children
  2. Repeated infections can lead to second phase with conjunctival scarring, entropion, and corneal scarring
- Measure epidemiological risk factors in patient
- Symptoms are usually absent in noncorneal forms
- Most cases seen in industrialized urban and suburban populations are usually old (and usually scarred)

Objective

- Moderate to severe upper tarsal follicles
- Papillary hypertrophy and moderate to severe inflammation and infiltration of superior palpebral conjunctiva
- Standard classification (MacCallan) based on conjunctival (not corneal) changes
  1. Follicles without scarring or papillae
  2. Follicles with papillary hypertrophy
  3. Papillary hypertrophy obscures follicles
  4. Scarring develops with follicles
  5. Cicatricial scarring replaces follicles
- Superior half of cornea and upper lid secondarily involved and scarred (cicatrix) in numerous ways
  1. Trichiasis and entropion
  2. Superficial epithelial keratitis
  3. Superior pannus (frequently very dense)
  4. Ulceration and corneal scarring leading to blindness
  5. Limbal follicles, swelling, and subsequent depressed scarring (Herbert's pits)
  6. Linear scarring (fine in milder forms and broad lines in advanced cases) on tarsus (called Arlt's lines)

Assessment

(See also Appendix 3)

- Consider patient's ethnic background and country of origin (especially in old, scarred cases)
- Rule out active venereal (chlamydial) disease

Plan: Trachoma

- Treat all cases, mild to severe, with a single oral dose 1G Azithromycin
- Topical tetracycline ointment (Achromycin) bid for 2 to 3 months may or may not help

- Treat family members, intimate associates with a single oral dose 1G Azithromycin
- Refer any suggestive venereal signs or symptoms for medical evaluation
- Active corneal involvement may require topical steroids (with guarded prognosis for response)

Follow-Up

- Most cases usually result in some degree of conjunctival and corneal scarring (cicatrix) with or without treatment
- Active disease usually takes about 3 to 6 months to run its course (with or without treatment)
- Careful instructions to patients under care and to patients at high risk (exposed, endemic, or ethnic populations) should include hygiene and monitoring for early signs

E. Viral and Other Follicular Conjunctivitis

1. Adenoviral Types

Background Information

1. Viruses are single-cell organisms smaller than bacteria
2. Made up of single nucleic acid (DNA or RNA) that cannot grow or multiply independently
   a. Require protein synthesis from another source
   b. Host (infected) cells or chemical substances in our body (or on a contact lens surface)
3. Our susceptibility to viruses varies depending on many factors
   a. Age
   b. Chromosomal factors (genetic)
   c. Physiological factors
4. Defense mechanisms against viral infection
   a. Primary infection produces bodily resistance through immune system response (antibodies) (see also Chapter 2)
      i. Interferon
      ii. Immunoglobins (IgG, IgM, IgA)
      iii. Lymphoid system
      iv. Band T lymphocytes
      v. Polymorphonuclear (PMN) leukocytes
      vi. Killer and natural killer (NK) cells
   b. Circulating antibodies persist (lifelong) as protection against reinfection of same virus
   c. Additional defense is physical barrier to viral spread and penetration
      i. Epithelial surface
      ii. Tear film on ocular surface
      iii. Mucin tear layer and mucopolysaccharides
      iv. Phagocytosis (e.g., macrophages)
   d. Factors that reduce immune response and physical barriers enhance viral susceptibility, spread, penetration, and length of acute infection
      i. General health
      ii. Nutrition
      iii. Genetic factors
      iv. Physiological factors
      v. Ocular surface inflammation
      vi. Immunosuppressive drugs (steroids)
      vii. Acquired immune deficiency syndrome (AIDS)
5. For unknown reasons, viruses live in ganglion or host (infected) cells as dormant obligate parasites and are activated by aggravating factors
   a. Physical (e.g., injury, irritation, contact lens)
   b. Mental (e.g., excitement, stress)
   c. Emotional (e.g., aggravation, fear)
   d. Environmental (e.g., wind, air pollution, UV light)
   e. Physiological (e.g., illness, poor diet, lowered resistance)
6. Philosophies of treating virus
   a. No cures available
   b. Prevention before infection
      i. Health maintenance
      ii. Sanitation (personal, environmental)
      iii. Physiological (nutrition, immune system enhancement)
   c. For inactive infection
      i. Reduce aggravating factors
      ii. Enhance immune system function
   d. For active infection
      i. Palliative measures (symptom relief)
      ii. Inhibit or interfere with virus or host cell RNA, DNA, protein synthesis with antiviral or antimetabolite drug
      iii. Trick of antiviral or antimetabolites is to affect virus or host (infected) cells without interfering with normal cells
         - Acyclovir accomplishes this goal with herpes virus family
         - Viroptic interferes with DNA of all cells and thus is toxic to normal (noninfected) cells
7. Some viruses known to affect the eye

DNA Virus

- Adenovirus Coxsackie
- Cytomegalovirus
- Epstein-Barr (mononucleosis)
- Herpes simplex
- Molluscum contagiosum
- Papilloma (verrucae)
- Vaccinia Poliovirus
- Variola (smallpox)
- Varicella (herpes zoster)
- HIV (AIDS virus)

RNA Virus

- Coxsackie
- Enterovirus 70 (*Haemophilus conjunctivitis*)
- Influenza
- Measles (rubeola)
- Mumps
- Newcastle disease
- Poliovirus
- Rabies
- Rhinovirus
- Rubella

Subjective

- Most common form of acute conjunctivitis in adults
- Patient often does not seek care because of frequent mild and short-lived acute phase
- May be unilateral or bilateral (autoinoculation)
- History of onset and development usually 3 to 7 days
- Occasionally a prodromal medical history
  1. Upper respiratory infection (URI) such as cold, flu, sore throat
  2. Low-grade fever
  3. Most common in pharyngoconjunctival fever (PCF)

- Occasionally a previous history of conjunctivitis
- Mild visual fluctuations (transient)
- Usually mild to moderate burning irritation

Objective

- Presents as a purplish-pinkish bulbar hyperemia (Figure 4.19)
- Injection usually begins at inner canthal (caruncle plica area) and slowly spreads laterally to involve entire bulbar conjunctiva (slightly greater inferior)
- Usually unilateral, but may spread to opposite eye
- Vessels may blanch slightly with mild vasoconstrictor
- Usually a quick NaFl tear BUT
    1. Can produce secondary exposure SPK response with associated corneal irritation
    2. Exposure SPK may stain with rose bengal
- Serous (tearing, watery) discharge (hyperlacrimation)
- Follicular changes (follicles)
    1. Pale mounds of infiltrative cellular accumulation on the palpebral conjunctiva of varying diameter
    2. Variable degrees of overlying (low-grade) inflammatory hyperemia with most vessels surrounding base of elevated accumulated areas
    3. When abundant, follicles produce "rugae"-like folds in lower cul-de-sac (see Figure 4.19)
    4. Follicular changes (folliculosis) in lower cul-de-sac of children considered normal in quiet eyes
    5. Follicular changes on superior tarsal plate (in children or adults) usually not normal
- Occasional ipsilateral (same side) preauricular lymphadenopathy (tenderness on palpation) or lymph node enlargement (more common)
- Laboratory workup (usually not done) usually reveals lymphocytes

Assessment

(See also Appendix 3)

- Rule out other causes of red eyes
- Rule out other causes of conjunctivitis
- Rule out PCF
    1. Sometimes referred to as Beal's follicular conjunctivitis, or swimming pool conjunctivitis
    2. Found in children (usually under ages 15 to 18)
    3. Pharyngitis with low-grade fever precedes eye involvement by 1 to 2 weeks
    4. Often history of recent swimming pool exposure or hot tubs (in some adult presentations or precocious kids!)
    5. Rarely, a transient fine SPK or subepithelial infiltrates (usually peripheral)
    6. Associated with adenoviruses 3 and 7
    7. Generally considered contagious for up to 2 weeks
- Rule out epidemic keratoconjunctivitis (EKC) in early stages
    1. Frequently a history of exposure to another case
    2. Unilateral or bilateral
    3. Usually more hyperacute than mild adenoviruses
    4. Highly contagious during incubation (milder) stages (first 7 to 10 days)
    5. Associated with adenoviruses 8, 19, 21, 37 (and others)
    6. Keratitis occurs in 80% of cases
- Rule out herpes simplex virus (HSV)
    1. Almost always has keratitic component
        a. Coarse SPK
        b. Dendriform pattern (75% to 80% of cases)
    2. Always unilateral
    3. Frequently recurrent history
    4. Reduced corneal sensitivity
- Rule out herpes zoster ophthalmicus (mimicker)
    1. Dermatoblepharitis component
    2. Severe pain
- Rule out chlamydia
    1. Mucopurulent discharge
    2. Large follicles on upper and lower palpebral conjunctiva
    3. Prolonged course with possible sexually transmitted disease history
- Rule out other less common follicular forms of conjunctivitis

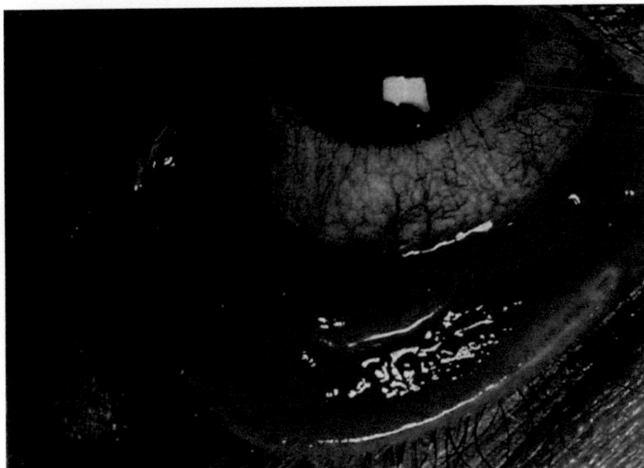

FIGURE 4.19 **Viral conjunctivitis** with diffuse purplish-pinkish bulbar hyperemia. Note the early pseudomembranous formation and the "rugae" folds formed by abundant follicles in the inferior palpebral conjunctiva.

Plan: Adenoviral Types of Conjunctivitis

(See also Appendix 4)

- Prescription (Rx) considerations
    1. No Rx cure for viruses of any kind
    2. Antiviral agents are not effective against adenoviruses
    3. Prophylactic antibacterial use questionable as to value and efficiency
        a. Potential for creating resistant strains of bacteria
        b. Antibacterial agents of no therapeutic value against conjunctival viral infection (as opposed to corneal viruses)
    4. Steroids and steroid combination drugs should be limited (as in bacterial conjunctivitis) to the more severe presentations
- Nonprescription (OTC) drug considerations
    1. Ocular lubricants (mucomimetics) to supplement and protect tear film from desiccation
    2. Topical vasoconstrictors (used limitedly) will improve appearance and may reduce symptoms and inflammation

3. 5% hypertonic saline drops or ointment q2–4h (as anti-inflammatory)

- Nontherapeutic (drugless) considerations
  1. Irrigation with ophthalmic solutions of warm or cold (for symptom relief) water to dilute or remove viral toxins
  2. Warm packs will enhance body's immune (defense) mechanism to fight viral spread (by vasodilation and increased leukocytic action) but will also produce added congestion and discomfort
     a. Suggest course of warm and cold (5 minutes each)
     b. Patient can decide on continuation based on subjective response to either or both
  3. Non-invasive nontoxic nature of these steps permits ad lib dosages
  4. If pseudomembranous fibrin deposits begin to form in fornices (hyperacute forms), remove by means of lavage, wet swabbing, or toothed or jeweler's forceps
     a. May cause discomfort (even with topical anesthetic) and small petechial hemorrhages on removal
     b. True membranes would bleed heavily
- Instruction and preventive measures
  1. Same considerations as described for acute bacterial conjunctivitis
  2. Advise patient, "This may get worse before it gets better"
     a. Explain to patient (at first visit) risk of early presentation of more virulent viral infections (e.g., EKC) versus 7- to 10-day normal course of non-specific adenoviruses
     b. Explain that impossible to tell until recheck visit
  3. State clearly to patient, "You have a virus in your eye and there is no cure for viruses"
     a. Explain any treatment as palliative
     b. Immune system will "treat" and control viral infection over period of time relative to potency of virus and response of system
  4. Carefully instruct on contagious nature of some viruses, especially during early mild stage
     a. Advise on avoiding contact with eye
     b. If hyperacute, eliminate contact with others until reversal of clinical course
     c. School or work may require temporary discontinuance or limited activities

Follow-Up

- Recheck acute presentations approximately 5 to 8 days after reported first signs of infection (or PRN)
  1. If non-specific adenovirus, will improve in 10 to 14 days
  2. If virulent adenovirus (e.g., EKC), will worsen
  3. Cornea usually becomes involved
- Educate patient as to dormant obligate nature of ocular viruses and potential for intermittent mild to moderate exacerbations with varying stress factors

2. Axenfeld's (Chronic) Conjunctivitis

Subjective

- Always a low-grade, insidious, and asymptomatic course
- Only in children (called "orphan's conjunctivitis")

Objective

- Firm palpebral follicles most abundant on tarsal conjunctiva with no corneal involvement
- May produce mild, chronic, serous discharge

Assessment

- Rule out acute or subacute viral forms
- Probably a mild form of trachoma

Plan and Follow-Up

- Usually a self-timing course of months to years
- Monitor every 3 months and stress hygiene

3. Beal's (Swimming Pool) Conjunctivitis

Same as adenoviral types.

4. Chlamydial (Inclusion) Conjunctivitis

Same as chlamydial keratoconjunctivitis. See Chapter 5.

5. Foliculosis

Subjective

- Found mostly in young, healthy children
- May be sparse to florid

Objective

- Palpebral conjunctival follicles with no signs of inflammation (Figure 4.20)
- Usually greatest in inferior cul-de-sac

Assessment

- Rule out causes of inflammatory follicle formation

Plan and Follow-Up: Folliculosis

- No treatment indicated
- Monitor routinely or PRN

6. Hemorrhagic (Acute) Conjunctivitis[28]

Subjective

- Specific cause is Enterovirus 70
- Acute pain, eyelid swelling, redness
- Hyperacute clinical presentation with hemorrhages can be caused by EKC-type adenoviruses or any virulent microorganism (e.g., viral, chlamydial, bacterial)

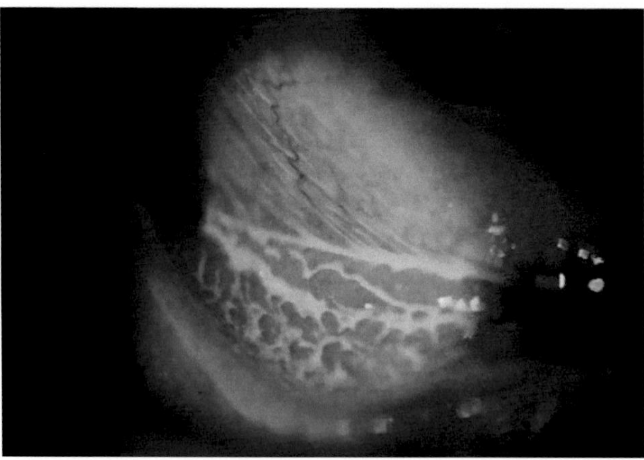

FIGURE 4.20 **Follicles (folliculosis)** or small, pale, discrete accumulations of infiltrative white blood cells (highlighted by sodium fluorescein stain).

Objective

- Rapid unilateral to bilateral presentation
- Dot to diffuse, spreading conjunctival hemorrhage

Assessment

- Rule out EKC syndrome
- Rule out other infectious syndromes

Plan and Follow-Up: Hemorrhagic (Acute) Conjunctivitis

- Treat primary infectious cause
- Instruct on viral syndromes

7. Herpes Simplex Viral (HSV) Conjunctivitis

See Chapter 5.

8. Herpes Zoster Conjunctivitis

See Chapter 5.

9. Molluscum Contagiosum

Same as adenoviral types. See Chapter 3.

10. Newcastle Disease

Subjective

- Virus transmitted by infected bird (especially chicken droppings)
- Likely candidates are poultry workers

Objective

Same as adenoviral types. See Chapter 3.

Assessment

- Determine contact with viral carrier

Plan and Follow-Up

- Remove infectious source and instruct
- Condition will self-limit on removal of source

11. Parinaud's Oculoglandular Fever[29]

Subjective

- Unilateral redness, foreign-body sensation, and tearing
- Ocular analogue of "cat-scratch fever"
- Frequent history of direct exposure to cat(s)
- Occasionally associated with systemic malaise, fever, and headache

Objective

- Always an acute unilateral presentation
- Large follicles with yellowish core associated with diffuse palpebral conjunctival granulomas
- Dramatic ipsilateral preauricular and submandibular lymphadenopathy (tenderness) and enlargement (greater than 1 cm; Figure 4.21)

Assessment

- Determine association with cat(s)
- Consider systemic (cat-scratch fever) involvement

Plan and Follow-Up

- Usually self-limiting but oral antibiotics can speed up resolution
  1. Oral Azithromycin drug of choice → 500 mg day 1, 250 mg qd days 2–5
- Preauricular lymphadenopathy can persist for weeks to months

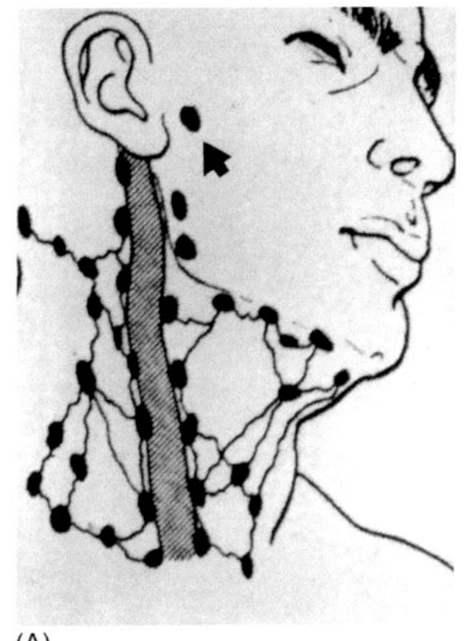
(A)

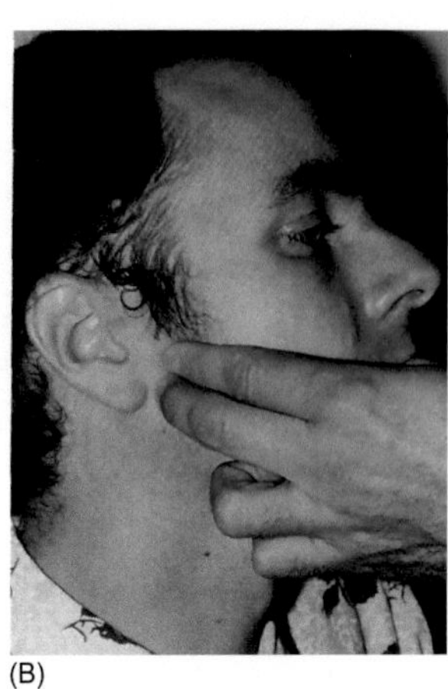
(B)

FIGURE 4.21 **(A) Preauricular lymph node (arrow). (B) Palpating** preauricular lymph nodes.

12. Verrucae

Same as adenoviral types. See also Chapter 3.

Sclera and Episclera

Review of Clinical Anatomy

1. Structural characteristics (Figure 4.B)
   a. Sclera is white, opaque, dense, irregular collagen fibrous tissue serving as outer coat (tunic) of eye, terminating anterior at the corneoscleral limbus (anterior scleral foramen)
   b. Episclera is vascularized cover to sclera connected by fascia bulbi (Tenon's capsule)
   c. Scleral spur (at anterior angle) attaches ciliary muscle to sclera
   d. Thinnest portion (0.3 mm) anterior to recti insertions where anterior ciliary arteries pass through
      i. May be pigmented by uveal pigment
      ii. Ciliary nerve loop may also pass through (Axenfeld loop)

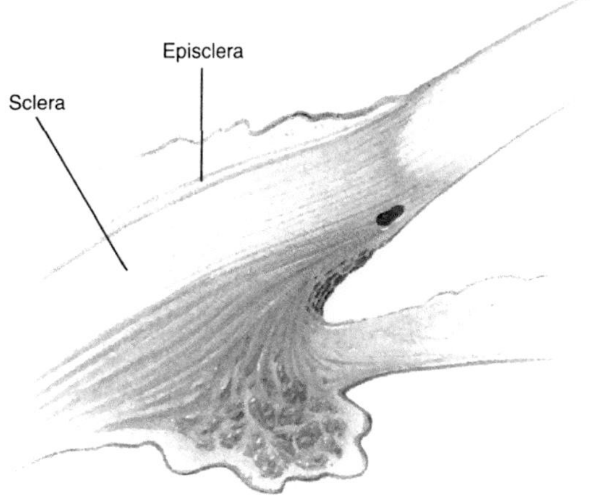

FIGURE 4.B The anatomy of the sclera.

2. Nerve supply
   a. Long ciliary nerves innervate anterior sclera (short for posterior)
   b. Rich innervation yields severe pain on inflammation
3. Vascular supply
   a. Sclera derives nutritional supply from choroid (posteriorly) and episclera (anteriorly)
   b. Episclera supplied by dense plexus of anterior ciliary arteries

I. Irritations and Injuries

A. Episceral Laceration

See Section I. C. of "Conjunctiva."

B. Scleral Perforation

Subjective

- History of high-velocity projectile
  1. Classic example: particle from hammering metal or granite surface
  2. Other common possibilities: BB-gun pellets, fireworks, explosions
- Ocular pain can range from no discomfort, mild or severe pain

Objective

- Site of perforation may or may not be detectable
- Anterior and/or posterior segment inflammation
  1. Conjunctivitis
  2. Keratoconjunctivitis
  3. Uveitis
- Iris transillumination defects may be noted
- Intraocular (choroidal or vitreous) hemorrhage is relatively common
- Intraocular pressure may be dramatically decreased
- Prolonged presence of metallic intraocular foreign body can produce hemosiderosis with induced change in iris coloration (unilateral heterochromia)

Assessment

- Rule out foreign body in anterior angle (with gonioscopy)
- Dilated fundus examination mandatory
- B-scan ultrasound examination of the eyeball and orbit to detect foreign bodies
  1. Computerized tomography (CT) of orbit and cranium to rule out penetration beyond globe
  2. Avoid MRIs with history of metallic foreign bodies

Plan and Follow-Up: Scleral Perforation

(See also Appendix 6)

- Protect eye with Fox shield for transport
- Immediate hospitalization
- Referral to ophthalmic surgeon for foreign-body removal and follow-up IV antibiotic therapy

II. Noninflammatory Conditions

A. Axenfeld's Loops

Subjective

- No symptoms or patient concerns
- Usually noted on general external examination
- More prominent in Black patients

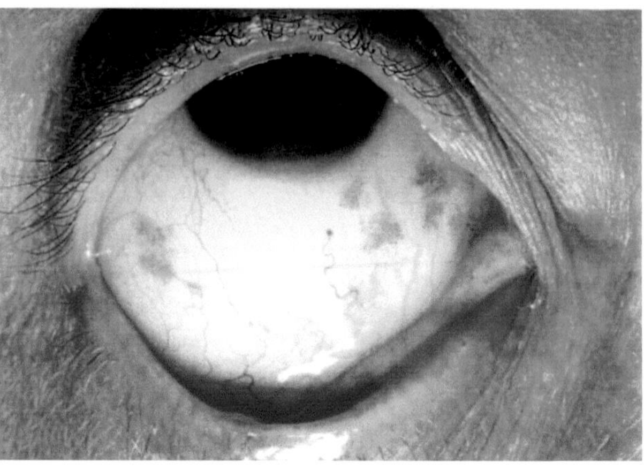

FIGURE 4.22 **Axenfeld's loops** or pale ciliary nerve loops appearing through the scleral surface.

Objective

- Blue to black ciliary nerve loops on the scleral surface (Figure 4.22)
- Usually within a few millimeters of the limbus
- Diffuse on scleral surface (greater nasalward)
- May have small vessel loops (red or blue) adjacent to nerve loop

Assessment

- Rule out other darker-pigmented ocular surface lesions

Plan and Follow-Up: Axenfeld's Loops

- No treatment or special follow-up considerations

B. Blue Sclera

Subjective

- Asymptomatic presentation, usually with no patient awareness of variant
- Take careful history for possible causes in adult or patients with acquired changes
- May be parent concern in obvious presentations in young children and newborns

Objective

- Variable density, intensity, and distribution of pale to dark blue coloration to white of the eyes (Figure 4.23)
- Rather common and generally normal in infants
  1. Relatively large globe size at birth versus thin scleral tunic transmit blue vascular choroid distinctly
  2. Often persists into early childhood
- Unilateral or bilateral (highly diagnostic sign)

Assessment

(See also Appendix 3)

- In children (and elderly) with negative history, presentation usually within normal limits
- In adults and acquired presentations, take careful systemic and developmental history
- Some systemic and developmental causes to consider
  1. Osteogenesis imperfecta
  2. Ehlers–Danlos syndrome
  3. Marfan's syndrome
  4. Paget's disease (pseudoxanthoma elasticum)

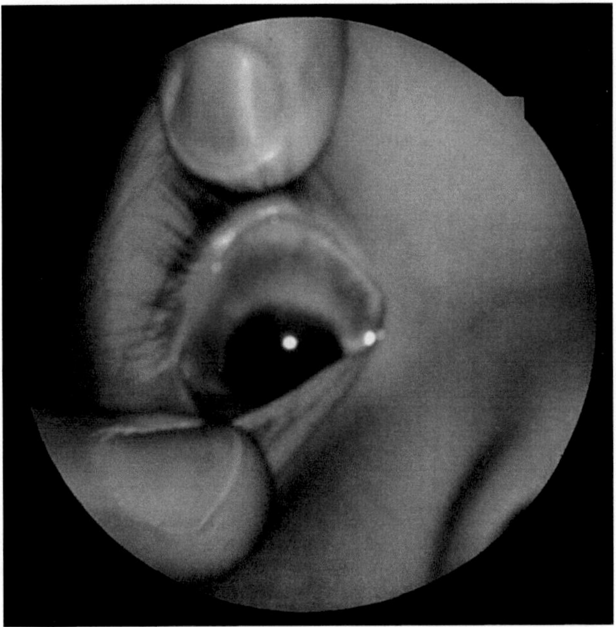

FIGURE 4.23 **Blue sclera** in a 6-year-old Asian child caused by congenital nevus of Ota (oculomelanodermatocystosis).

- Enlargement of globe
  1. Buphthalmos (infantile glaucoma): check IOP
  2. Keratoconus or keratoglobus: check cornea
  3. High myopia (sometimes unilateral): refract
- Pigmentations
  1. Melanosis (usually unilateral)
  2. Nevus of Ota (always unilateral)
  3. Intraocular foreign body (almost always unilateral)
  4. Medicamentosa

Plan: Blue Sclera
- Refer appropriately for cause
- Reassure and explain phenomenon to parents of children and elderly, with thinning sclera effect

Follow-Up
- Routine for normal patients
- For children or suspicious presentations, consider general overall recheck within 6 to 12 months

C. Hyaline Plaques (Focal Scleral Translucent Spots)
Subjective
- Common in older patients
- No associated symptoms or positive history
- Occasionally may produce patient concern

Objective
- Small (approximately 2 to 4 mm) translucent, grayish, flat round spots on the anterior scleral surface (Figure 4.24)
- Multiple, bilateral, and diffusely arranged

Assessment
- Rule out any severe collagen vascular diseases
- Rule out other ocular surface lesions
- Consider scleromalacia perforans

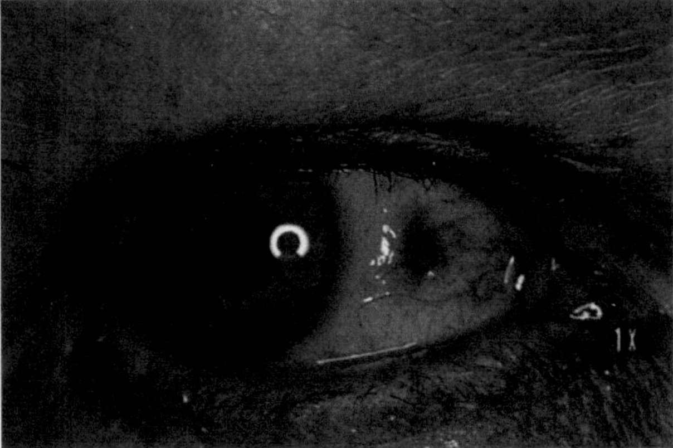

FIGURE 4.24 **Hyaline plaque** or a focal, grayish, translucent spot caused by localized thinning in the sclera of older patients.

  1. Rare scleral melting disease in elderly
  2. Associated with pain and rheumatoid disease

Plan: Hyaline Plaques
- Reassure patient
- No treatment indicated

Follow-Up
- Recheck annually (as part of routine examination) or PRN

D. Icteric Sclera (Jaundice)
Subjective
- No associated ocular history
- Careful medical history (for liver disease)
- Cosmesis may dominate patient's concern

Objective
- Yellowing (rarely, greenish) diffuse discoloration to bilateral sclera (white of the eyes)
- Noninflammatory presentation with no associated ocular findings

Assessment
- Acute or chronic liver disease
- If undiagnosed, take careful medical history

Plan: Icteric Sclera
- Recommend immediate medical examination and care if patient not actively under such care
- No treatment indicated for ocular finding

Follow-Up
- Confirm medical care preferably through phone contact with patient or physician
- Monitor (reversible) ocular finding in concert with medical care

E. Melanosis (Congenital)
See Section II. of this chapter (4 H), "Melanosis."

F. Melanosis (Acquired)
See Section II. of this chapter (4 I), "Melanosis."

G. Scleromalacia Perforans

Subjective

- Painless anterior scleritis without inflammation (no redness)
- Always elderly patient
- Generally very fragile, female patient in poor health
- Uncommon presentation

Objective

- Noninflamed (unilateral or bilateral) eye(s) insidious presentation
- Develops slowly (over months) as a yellowish to white area of necrotic scleral thinning
- End result is exposure of the underlying choroid with a blue to blackish appearance
- No bulging (staphyloma) occurs in the ectatic (thinned) area

Assessment

- Almost exclusively associated with long-standing, advanced rheumatoid arthritis
- Rarely associated with other systemic inflammatory causes of scleritis

Plan: Scleromalacia Perforans

- Consultation and co-management with a medical specialist are most important
- Resolution and healing may be spontaneous
- High-dose systemic steroids indicated
  1. Topical steroids are useless
  2. Subconjunctival steroids are highly contraindicated
- Prognosis is guarded with possibility of insidious progression and globe perforation, even with high dose systemic steroids
- Scleral grafting appears to be of some value in large necrotizing defects (greater than one-third of circumference)
- Secondary inflammatory complications common

H. Staphyloma

Subjective

- Relatively uncommon
- Usually developing in older patients with other ocular or systemic problems

Objective

- Bulging of uveal tissue through thinning sclera
- Dark blue (uvea) appearance to raised ectatic area
- May be circumferential (around cornea) or patchy
- Frequently associated with high myopia and posterior staphyloma

Assessment

- Rule out elevated pigmented (blue) lesions
- Carefully assess ocular, visual, and systemic conditions and etiologies

Plan: Staphyloma

- Refer appropriately for cause
- Attempt to ameliorate any associated visual or ocular conditions

Follow-Up

- Monitor closely (every 3 months) for insidious advancement or complications
- Carefully instruct patient on preventive eye care and signs and symptoms of infections, inflammation

III. Inflammatory Conditions

A. Episcleritis[30]

1. Simple Form

Background Information

1. Episclera is connective tissue sheath between sclera and conjunctiva
2. Vascular (venules) plexus has regular, radiating pattern versus irregular, finer, movable overlying bulbar conjunctival vessels
3. Disease etiologies
   a. Approximately 30% due to collagen vascular and autoimmune diseases (e.g., rheumatoid, Crohn's, Lupus, etc.)
   b. Generally, causes remain unknown or idiopathic
   c. Sometimes mild trauma suggested due to common occurrence in exposed palpebral aperture(s)
4. Eighty percent of episcleritis: simple form (20% nodular)

Subjective

- Acute onset of signs and symptoms (sometimes as fast as minutes to hours)
- Greater in women (usually age 20 to 50) than men (age 30 to 60)
- Patient reports mild to moderate symptoms
  1. Non-specific irritation (e.g., hot, uncomfortable)
  2. Tenderness on direct palpation to irritated site
  3. Sector redness
- Frequent recurrent history of similar problem
- Vision never affected significantly
- Photophobia may be mild to moderate

Objective

- Wedge (sector) of deep injection and inflammation (Figure 4.25)
  1. Usually apex of wedge toward limbus, base away

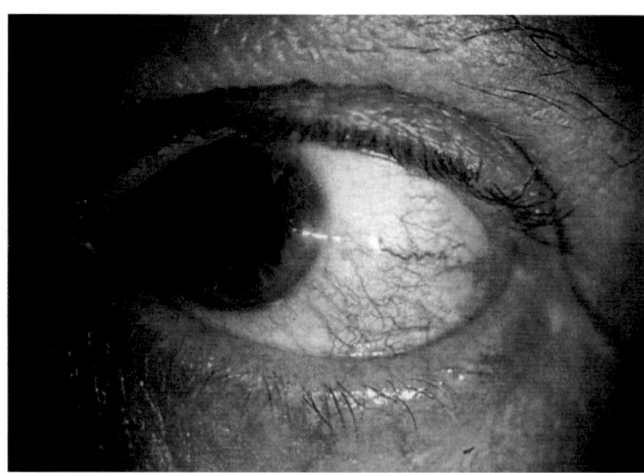

FIGURE 4.25 **Simple episcleritis** in the left eye of a 38-year-old woman reporting tenderness over the inferior temporal region of superficial and deep vessel, wedge-shaped hyperemia.

2. Usually in interpalpebral areas (greater temporal)
3. Deeper vessels show radiating pattern with net of irregular, overlying, finer conjunctival vessels

- Deeper injected vessels will not blanch with pressure (on palpation) or with mild vasoconstrictors
- Deeper (episcleral vessels) are immovable, while overlying conjunctival vessels move freely
- Usually unilateral but occasionally will present with bilateral inflammatory wedges
- Possible hyperlacrimation but never frank discharge
- Inflamed wedge may demonstrate diffuse infiltration or edema causing mild elevation of conjunctiva
- Deeper injection usually pinkish-purple coloration
- Anterior chamber reaction absent
- Palpebral conjunctiva and cornea remain clear

Assessment

(See also Appendix 3)

- Rule out other causes of "red eyes" (Table 4.5)
- Rule out common forms of conjunctivitis (Table 4.1)
- Also rule out inflamed pingueculas (painless) and phlyctenules associated with toxic conjunctivitis
- Rule out scleritis (Table 4.6)
  1. Entirely separate disease category more severe and far less frequent than episcleritis
  2. Usually associated with systemic diseases
  3. Require immediate referral for medical or ophthalmologic management
- Rule out (by history) reported systemic disease causes reported in literature but rarely established in case presentations
  1. Rheumatoid arthritis
  2. Systemic lupus erythematosus (SLE)
  3. Giant-cell arteritis
  4. Polyarteritis nodosa
  5. Sarcoidosis
  6. Herpes zoster
  7. Tuberculosis
  8. Syphilis
  9. Gout
  10. Thyrotoxicosis
- Rule out (from history) direct or indirect trauma
  1. Mechanical injury to ocular surface
  2. Chemical injury
  3. Radiation exposure
- Generally no cause will be established

Plan: Simple Form of Episcleritis

(See also Appendix 4)

- For mild cases, any treatment is optional
  1. Frequent cold packs (q3–4h for 3 to 5 days)
  2. Patient may prefer symptomatic and cosmetic relief
     a. Topical vasoconstrictor (decongestant) drops
     b. Mild steroid (e.g., FML 0.1%, Loteprednol 0.5%)
  3. Oral NSAIDs (aspirin, ibuprofen) for analgesia and therapeusis (?)

TABLE 4.5 Differential Diagnosis of Episcleritis from Conjunctivitis

	Subjective Symptom	Injection	Discharge	Papillae or Bulbar Conjunctiva	Other Identifying Features
Episcleritis	Hot, gritty Mild-moderate pain on palpation and lateral gaze	Salmon pink	Waters occasionally	Bulbar focal hyperemia and infiltration	Wedge-shaped sectoral injection
Conjunctivitis					
Viral	Burn	Pink/purple toward plica	Tearing	Palpebral follicles	Periauricular lymph node
Allergic	Itch	Pink/purple	White stringy mucoid	Chemosis	Allergic history, seasonal
Bacterial	Irritation, foreign-body sensation	Bright red	Purulent mucopurulent	Papillae	Lids and lashes matted in AM
Phlyctenular keratoconjunctivitis	Corneal irritation	Localized pannus	Waters occasionally	Leash of vessels at phlycten	Phlycten invades cornea
Acne rosacea	Chronic recurring corneal irritation	Diffuse bulbar and circumcorneal	Occasional tearing or purulence	Chronic blepharoconjunctivitis	Skin lesions

TABLE 4.6 Comparison of Episcleritis and Scleritis

	Subjective Symptom	Injection	Hyperemic Pattern	Cornea	Anterior Chamber	Associated with Systemic Condition
Episcleritis	Irritation, mild pain	Salmon pink	Sectoral wedge-shaped	No corneal involvement	No reaction (or minimal)	Low correlation with systemic tissue disease
Scleritis	Severe pain	Blue or purple	Diffuse involvement	Decreased corneal sensitivity, sclerosing stromal keratitis	Probable uveitic response with cells or flare	High correlation with systemic connective tissue disease (>50%)

- For moderate to severe (rare) simple episcleritis
  1. Same steps as for mild (above)
  2. If indicated, use 1% prednisolone as steroid
  3. Topical dosages from q2h to qid based on degree
  4. Oral ibuprofen 400 to 600 mg tid or naproxen 250 to 500 mg bid for 1–2 weeks
- Episcleritis is one disease that occasionally will not respond to topical steroids as quickly as most
  1. Masking (eye whitening) effect may even be absent
  2. Always monitor such idiosyncratic cases closely

Follow-Up

- Normal course (with or without treatment) is usually about 10 to 21 days (acute to subacute to resolution)
- Recheck patient on a weekly basis until resolved
- Advise patient at first visit of potential protracted (i.e., 10- to 21-day) course
- Advise on possible recurrences from 3-month to 3-year period
- Reschedule for annual recheck or PRN
- If more than three recurrences, recommend systemic medical workup

2. Nodular Form

Subjective

- Far less common than simple form (20% versus 80%)
- Symptoms all similar to simple form, except more severe
- Pain present without palpation and tenderness on palpation (at site) usually greater than simple form
- Recurrent history not as frequent with nodular form
- Vision remains normal despite increased intensity of clinical presentation
- Photophobic response may be moderate to severe
- Systemic associations continue to be rare (as with simple form)

Objective

- All physical signs same as simple form except for increased intensity and development of a nodule (Figure 4.26)
  1. Nodule is an organized area of cellular infiltrate at the center of the sectorial inflamed wedge
  2. Usually a single site but may be multiple
  3. Frequently associated with increased edema in the immediate area and increased diffuse edema and infiltration throughout the inflamed sector
- Because of increased degree of inflammation, anterior chamber may begin to show mild secondary reaction in the form of trace cells and flare
- Cornea usually remains completely uninvolved
- Rarely, hyperemic sector may expand to involve up to 180° area and resist standard treatment for additional weeks or months
  1. Called episcleritis periodosis fugax
  2. Tends to reoccur more frequently than simple or standard nodular forms

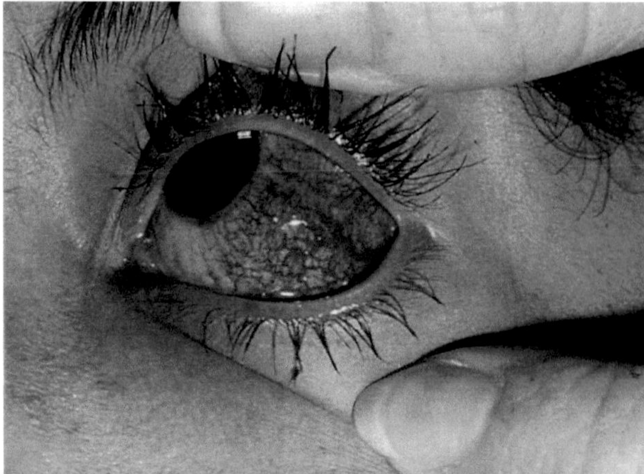

FIGURE 4.26 **Nodular episcleritis** demonstrating a large sector of deep episcleral vessel injection with a central infiltrative nodule (slightly obscured by overlying inflammatory edema).

Assessment

(See also Appendix 3)

- Differentiate nodular episcleritis from simple form
  1. Increased subjective and objective intensity
  2. Presence of nodule
- Remaining differential considerations same as for simple episcleritis

Plan: Nodular Form of Episcleritis

(See also Appendices 4 and 6)

- Same as for moderate to severe simple episcleritis
- Topical steroid dosages should be increased to range of q2–4h based on degree of presentation
- Rarely, in severe presentations, prolonged nonresponsive cases or periodosis fugax cases, a short course of oral steroids (prednisone) may be helpful
  1. Co-manage with internist
  2. Sometimes even with oral agents, response is slow

Follow-Up

- Same as for moderate to severe simple episcleritis
- Course of nodule regression (melting) and sometimes associated signs and symptoms as well may extend into months (usually no more than 2 to 3 months) with or without continued treatment

B. Scleritis[31,32]

Subjective

- Very severe, intolerable pain
- Usually gradual onset with increasing pain radiating to the brow and jaw
- There is often a history of recurrences

Objective

- Vision is reduced with severe photophobia
- Eye (usually unilateral) is red and deeply inflamed (Figure 4.27)
  1. Usually diffuse with 360° involvement
  2. Large diameter, deep scleral (and episcleral vessels) produce a blueish to purplish coloration
  3. Vessels cannot be blanched with phenylephrine
- Profuse tearing
- Sclera appears edematous and thinned
- Inflammatory nodules may be apparent on anterior sclera
- Corneal involvements frequently associated (sclerokeratitis)
  1. Peripheral thinning or guttering (keratolysis)

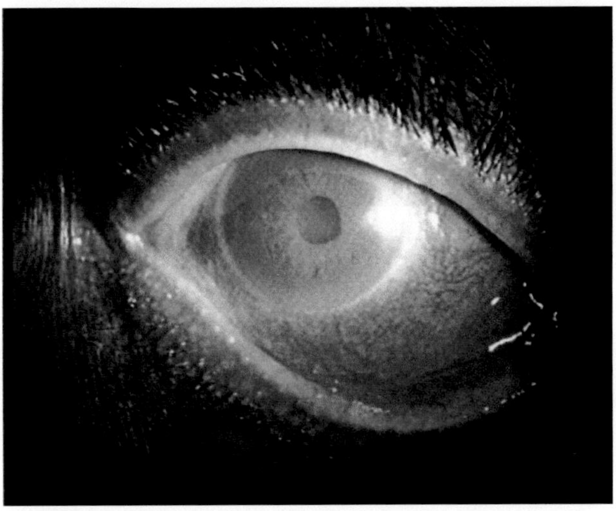

FIGURE 4.27 **Scleritis** producing diffuse inflammation of the entire anterior segment in the left eye of a 68-year-old male with a long-standing history of rheumatoid arthritis.

   2. Deep stromal and endothelial disruption
- Chronic or recurrent anterior uveitis almost always present (sclerouveitis)
- Other ocular findings usually associated
   1. Posterior involvement
   2. Glaucoma
   3. Cataracts
   4. Refractive shifts (towards hyperopia in posterior scleritis)

Assessment

- Rule out episcleritis (see Table 4.5)
- Anterior versus posterior versus diffuse scleritis
   1. Rule out retinal, choroidal, nerve head inflammatory changes
   2. Most posterior scleritis becomes anterior and diffuse
- Consider etiology → High association with systemic disease
   1. >50% Autoimmune disease
      a. Rheumatoid arthritis
      b. Ankylosing spondylitis
      c. Systemic lupus erythematosus (SLE)
      d. Systemic vasculitis
   2. Ocular malignancy
   3. Ocular surgery induced
   4. Infectious
      a. Bacteria (e.g., syphilis)
      b. Virus
      c. Fungi
   5. Idiopathic

Plan: Scleritis

(See also Appendix 6)

- Severity of subjective and objective presentation requires urgent care
- Complete physical examination by a medical consultant (e.g., internist) and lab work is essential
- Referral to an ophthalmic consultant advisable
   1. Uveitic specialist for anterior scleritis
   2. Retinal specialist for posterior scleritis
- Symptomatic relief may require narcotic analgesia
- Intensive inflammatory control critical to reduce anterior and posterior complications
   1. Mild presentations: 600 mg of oral ibuprofen tid, 500 mg Naproxen bid or 50 mg oral indomethacin tid for 1 to 2 weeks
   2. Moderate: 60 to 80 mg oral prednisone for 3 to 5 days, then taper
   3. Severe and posterior involvement: immunosuppressive therapies (e.g., cyclophosphamide, methotrexate) (by internist)
- Topical therapies (questionable value) should include standard uveitic regimes at high dosages and durations (see Chapter 6)
- Subconjunctival or subtenon steroidal injection are controversial

Follow-Up

- Based on severity of presentation and/or consultants (medical and ophthalmic) advice
- Underlying systemic condition should be managed by medical specialist
- Patient must be advised on ocular recurrences and should be closely monitored

References

1. Shields CL, Shields JA. Tumors of the Conjunctiva and Cornea. *Indian J Ophthalmol.* 2019;67(12):1930–1948. doi:10.4103/ijo.IJO_2040_19
2. Feroze KB, Kaufman EJ. Xerophthalmia. In: *StatPearls*. Treasure Island: StatPearls Publishing; April 25, 2021.
3. Cohen VML, O'Day RF. Management Issues in Conjunctival Tumours: Conjunctival Melanoma and Primary Acquired Melanosis. *Ophthalmol Ther.* 2019;8(4):501–510. doi:10.1007/s40123-019-00219-8
4. Theotoka D, Morkin MI, Galor A, Karp CL. Update on Diagnosis and Management of Conjunctival Papilloma. *Eye Vis.* 2019;6:18. Published 2019 Jun 18. doi:10.1186/s40662-019-0142-5
5. Kudrna JJ, Eisenbeisz HC, Huot C. Bilateral Tarsal Conjunctival Pigmentation After Eight Months of Minocycline Therapy. *S D Med.* 2020;73(8):360–365.
6. Tendler I, Pulitzer MP, Roggli V, Abramson DH, Marr BP. Ocular Argyrosis Mimicking Conjunctival Melanoma. *Cornea.* 2017;36(6):747–748. doi:10.1097/ICO.0000000000001191
7. Lindner M, Bertelmann T. On the Ocular Findings in Ochronosis: A Systematic Review of Literature. *BMC Ophthalmol.* 2014;14:12. Published 2014 Jan 30. doi:10.1186/1471-2415-14-12
8. Somnath A, Tripathy K. Pinguecula. 2021 Feb 14. In: *StatPearls* [Internet]. Treasure Island: StatPearls Publishing; 2021 Jan. PMID: 32644391.
9. Tarlan B, Kiratli H. Subconjunctival Hemorrhage: Risk Factors and Potential Indicators. *Clin Ophthalmol.* 2013;7:1163–1170. doi:10.2147/OPTH.S35062
10. Dupuis P, Prokopich CL, Hynes A, Kim H. A Contemporary Look at Allergic Conjunctivitis. *Allergy Asthma Clin Immunol.* 2020 Jan 21;16:5. doi: 10.1186/s13223-020-0403-9. PMID: 31993069; PMCID: PMC6975089.
11. Ackerman S, Smith LM, Gomes PJ. Ocular Itch Associated with Allergic Conjunctivitis: Latest Evidence and Clinical Management. *Ther Adv Chronic Dis.* 2016;7(1):52–67. doi:10.1177/2040622315612745

12. Dudeja L, Janakiraman A, Dudeja I, Sane K, Babu M. Observer-masked Trial Comparing Efficacy of Topical Olopatadine (0.1%), Bepotastine (1.5%), and Alcaftadine (0.25%) in Mild to Moderate Allergic Conjunctivitis. *Indian J Ophthalmol.* 2019;67(9):1400–1404. doi:10.4103/ijo.IJO_2112_18
13. DEXTENZA [prescribing information]. Ocular Therapeutix, Inc.; 2019.
14. McLaurin EB, Evans D, Repke CS, et al. Phase 3 Randomized Study of Efficacy and Safety of a Dexamethasone Intracanalicular Insert in Patients with Allergic Conjunctivitis. *Am J Ophthalmol.* 2021;229:288–300. doi:10.1016/j.ajo.2021.03.017
15. Pall B, Gomes P, Yi F, Torkildsen G. Management of Ocular Allergy Itch With an Antihistamine-Releasing Contact Lens. *Cornea.* 2019;38(6):713–717. doi:10.1097/ICO.0000000000001911
16. Sankaridurg P, Chen X, Naduvilath T, et al. Adverse Events During 2 Years of Daily Wear of Silicone Hydrogels in Children. *Optom Vis Sci.* 2013;90(9):961–969. doi:10.1097/OPX.0000000000000017
17. Maldonado-Codina C, Morgan PB, Efron N, Efron S. Comparative Clinical Performance of Rigid versus Soft Hyper Dk Contact Lenses Used for Continuous Wear. *Optom Vis Sci.* 2005 Jun;82(6):536–48. doi: 10.1097/00006324-200506000-00018. PMID: 15976592.
18. Azari AA, Arabi A. Conjunctivitis: A Systematic Review. *J Ophthalmic Vis Res.* 2020;15(3):372–395. Published 2020 Aug 6. doi:10.18502/jovr.v15i3.7456
19. Kodjikian L, Lafuma A, Khoshnood B, Laurendeau C, Berdeaux G. Efficacité de la moxifloxacine dans le traitement de la conjonctivite bactérienne aiguë : une méta-analyse [Efficacy of Moxifloxacin in Treating Bacterial Conjunctivitis: A Meta-analysis]. *J Fr Ophtalmol.* 2010 Apr;33(4):227–33. French. doi: 10.1016/j.jfo.2010.02.001. Epub 2010 Mar 11. PMID: 20223557.
20. Bremond-Gignac D, Chiambaretta F, Milazzo S. A European Perspective on Topical Ophthalmic Antibiotics: Current and Evolving Options. *Ophthalmol Eye Dis.* 2011;3:29–43. Published 2011 Oct 24. doi:10.4137/OED.S4866
21. Epling J. Bacterial Conjunctivitis. *BMJ Clin Evid.* 2012;2012:0704. Published 2012 Feb 20.
22. Linton E, Hardman L, Welburn L, Rahman I, Chidambaram JD. Adult Conjunctivitis Secondary to Dual Infection with *Chlamydia trachomatis* and *Neisseria gonorrhoeae*: A Case Report. *Am J Ophthalmol Case Rep.* 2018;13:6–8. Published 2018 Nov 14. doi:10.1016/j.ajoc.2018.11.009
23. Aoki T, Kitazawa K, Deguchi H, Sotozono C. Current Evidence for Corynebacterium on the Ocular Surface. *Microorganisms.* 2021;9(2):254. Published 2021 Jan 27. doi:10.3390/microorganisms9020254
24. Churchward CP, Al-Kinani AA, Abdelkader H, et al. Monocaprin Eye Drop Formulation to Combat Antibiotic Resistant Gonococcal Blindness. *Sci Rep.* 2020;10(1):12010. Published 2020 Jul 21. doi:10.1038/s41598-020-68722-8
25. Haimovici R, Roussel TJ. Treatment of gonococcal conjunctivitis with single-dose intramuscular ceftriaxone. *Am J Ophthalmol.* 1989;107(5):511–514. doi:10.1016/0002-9394(89)90495-9
26. Lansingh VC. Trachoma. *BMJ Clin Evid.* 2016;2016:0706. Published 2016 Feb 9.
27. Evans JR, Solomon AW, Kumar R, et al. Antibiotics for Trachoma. *Cochrane Database Syst Rev.* 2019;9(9):CD001860. Published 2019 Sep 26. doi:10.1002/14651858.CD001860.pub4
28. Liu X, Qiu S, Liu Z, Chen D, Liu H, Ding G. Effects of Floods on the Incidence of Acute Hemorrhagic Conjunctivitis in Mengshan, China, from 2005 to 2012. *Am J Trop Med Hyg.* 2020;102(6):1263–1268. doi:10.4269/ajtmh.19-0164
29. Dixon MK, Dayton CL, Anstead GM. Parinaud's Oculoglandular Syndrome: A Case in an Adult with Flea-Borne Typhus and a Review. *Trop Med Infect Dis.* 2020;5(3):126. Published 2020 Jul 29. doi:10.3390/tropicalmed5030126
30. Schonberg S, Stokkermans TJ. Episcleritis. 2021 Feb 13. In: *StatPearls* [Internet]. Treasure Island: StatPearls Publishing; 2021 Jan. PMID: 30521217.
31. Lagina A, Ramphul K. Scleritis. 2021 Mar 7. In: *StatPearls* [Internet]. Treasure Island: StatPearls Publishing; 2021 Jan. PMID: 29763119.
32. Ahmed A, Foster CS. Cyclophosphamide or Rituximab Treatment of Scleritis and Uveitis for Patients with Granulomatosis with Polyangiitis. *Ophthalmic Res.* 2019;61(1): 44–50. doi:10.1159/000486791

Chapter 5
DIAGNOSES OF THE CORNEA

Chapter Outline

DOI: 10.1201/9781003255598-5

Review of Clinical Anatomy

1. Structural characteristics (Figure 5.A)
   a. Transparent tissue measuring approximately 10.6 mm vertically and 11.7 mm horizontally (fully formed by 6 years of age)
   b. Center thickness is 0.52 mm, thickening to 1 mm at periphery
   c. Approximate radii for anterior surface = 7.8 mm; posterior surface = 6.2 mm to 6.8 mm
2. Biochemical and metabolic processes (limited list)
   a. Glycosylation (for energy)
   b. Hydroxylation (for stromal stability)
   c. Translation (for protein synthesis)
   d. Enzymes (for growth)
      i. Plasminogen
      ii. Fibronectin
3. Layers (anterior to posterior)
   a. Mucin layer attached to epithelium
   b. Epithelium (stratified, non-keratinized)
      i. Cellular epithelium serves as the major protective barrier against penetration of pathogens into deeper stroma
      ii. Cellular epithelial layers regenerate every 7 to 10 days
      iii. Anterior-most, superficial squamous cells with microvilli and tight junctures
         - Heal by sliding of surrounding cells
         - Healing rate within hours to days
      iv. Cuboidal/wing cells in single layer
         - Heal by mitotic regeneration and conjunctival transdifferentiation
         - Healing rate from days (mitosis) to weeks (conjunctival transdifferentiaion)
      v. Columnar/basal cells with hemidesmosomes
         - Heal similarly to cuboidal/wing layer
         - Secretes new basement membrane every 8 to 12 weeks

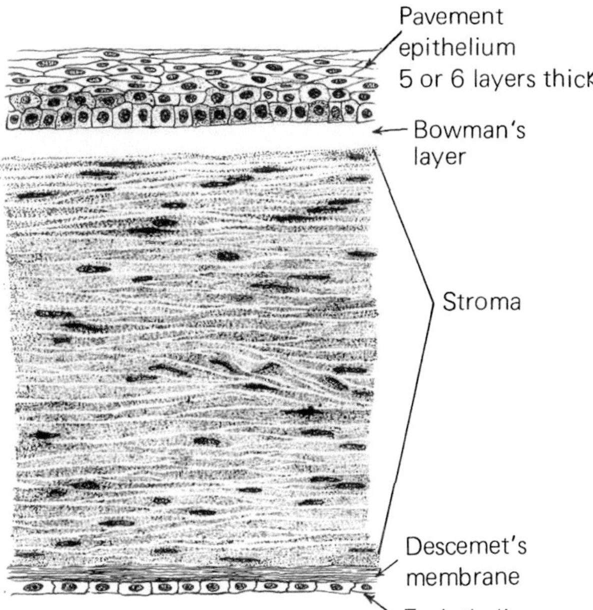

FIGURE 5.A Transverse section of the cornea.

      vi. Basement membrane with hemidesmosomes anteriorly and collagen-anchoring fibrils (type VII) posteriorly
         - Mucoproteinous, non-cellular layer
         - Serves to anchor and stabilize cellular epithelium
   c. Stroma (90% of corneal thickness)
      i. A structure of 70% collagen fibrils, 25% glycoprotein ground substances, and 5% cellular elements arranged in an exquisitely precise pattern (lamellar matrix) permitting transparency to light
         - Disturbance of any single element of this matrix (e.g., positioning, types, or interrelationships of fibrils, inter fibrillary distances, amount of ground substances) will alter transparency (reversible with one element involvement)
         - Simultaneous involvement of two or more elements results in irreversible loss of transparency (scar)
         - Insult to matrix activates keratocyte cells to accumulate at site of insult to synthesize new collagen and glycoprotein
      ii. Anterior-most Bowman's layer made up of acellular randomly ordered collagen fibrils (type IV) in a honeycomb reticular pattern
      iii. Deeper stroma (anterior and posterior) contains
         - Collagen fibrils (seven types) = 70%
            - Type I: basic structural fibril found in linear fibrillar pattern in Bowman's layer and throughout lamellar matrix
            - Type II: not present in human cornea
            - Type III: small reticular fibrils found in fetal (developmental) stages and in stromal scar formation
            - Type IV: basement membrane in honeycomb reticular pattern
            - Type V: Bowman's layer and lamellar matrix
            - Type VI: fibrillar elements found interspersed in proteoglycan (ground) substance
            - Type VII: anchoring fibrils
         - Glycosaminoglycans (ground substance) = 25%
            - Chondroitin sulfate proteoglycan
            - Keratan sulfate proteoglycan
         - Keratocytes (cellular element) = <5%
            - Function to resynthesize stromal proteins
            - Respond to, and accumulate at site of stromal insult
            - Action initiated by intracorneal leukocytes (part of inflammatory response)
         - Leukocytes (inflammatory mediators) = <1%, which activate keratocytes on stromal insult
   d. Descemet's membrane is amorphous collagen serving as basement membrane (posterior limiting membrane) between stroma and endothelial cell
   e. Endothelium is single layer of tightly bound cells
      i. Responsible for relative corneal dehydration
      ii. Non-mitotic means inability to regenerate if destroyed, degenerated, or lost (e.g., surgery)

4. Limbus (corneoscleral juncture) is a 1- to 2-mm transitional zone covered by conjunctiva
   a. Corneal epithelium loses its regular structure and becomes continuous with conjunctival epithelium
   b. Bowman's layer ends in a loose collagen fibril arrangement and amorphous material
   c. Corneal lamellae matrix is lost and fibrils begin to vary in organization and diameter
   d. Descemet's membrane splits into narrow bands on the surface of the trabecular meshwork
   e. Endothelium loses continuity and continues as covering for bands on trabeculum
   f. Blood supply (see conjunctiva) gives off small radial branches that end in deep corneal plexus or as superficial anastomosing plexus with conjunctival arteries
5. Nerve supply
   a. All supply is sensory
   b. Branches of ophthalmic division (third) of trigeminal cranial nerve V demyelinate beyond limbal juncture
   c. Greatest concentration in anterior stroma just beneath Bowman's layer, with branches penetrating Bowman's layer into epithelium
   d. Descemet's membrane and endothelium are not innervated

I. Irritations and Injuries

A. Abrasions

1. Superficial Epithelial Abrasions[1]

Subjective

- Usually a direct history of an acute nature
  1. Trauma to ocular surface
  2. Transient foreign body (with patient reporting it "still in the eye")
     a. Usually particulate matter
     b. Frequently fiberglass history (trouble)
- History and symptoms may be insidious (indirect)
  1. Mechanical factors
     a. Embedded lid (tarsus) foreign matter
     b. Trichiasis or entropion
     c. Contact lens edge (soft or hard), trapped foreign matter, surface problem
  2. Physiological factors (usually delayed reactions)
     a. Epithelial basement membrane disorder (greater in AM)
     b. Other epitheliopathies, dystrophies, degenerations
- One eye generally moderately to severely uncomfortable and occasionally mildly photophobic
- Classic corneal symptoms reported
  1. "Sandy, gritty" feeling
  2. Foreign-body sensation (thinking foreign body still present in eye)
  3. "Something under my upper lid" (sensation resulting from transferred pain during blink)
- In non-acute presentations, always pursue other historical data
  1. Ocular and medical history (including oral medications)
  2. Dry eye syndromes

Objective

- Visual acuity often reduced slightly owing to diffuse corneal edema and staining
- Examine lid margins and eyelashes
  1. Trichiasis or entropion
  2. Infectious (toxic) conditions (e.g., Staphylococcus)
  3. Cicatrix (scarring), colobomas, lid position
- Usually moderate bulbar conjunctival hyperemia
- May show mild circumcorneal flush (with or without anterior chamber reaction)
- Corneal (squamous) epithelium will stain with NaFl
  1. Superficial punctate keratitis (SPK) or foreign body tracking (FBT; Figure 5.1)
  2. Staining usually light, diffuse, and of variable pattern
  3. No pooling or deep staining (basement membrane)
- Based on history, discrete particles may be found
  1. On corneal surface
  2. In cul-de-sac or at inner canthus
  3. Embedded on inferior or superior (more common) palpebral conjunctiva and tarsus
- Topical anesthetic relieves pain entirely
  1. Effective within seconds
  2. Lasts for about 15 to 20 minutes
  3. Continued "dull aching" pain is sign of secondary uveitic reaction
- In physiological edematous reactions
  1. Corneal may show diffuse epithelial edema with squamous epithelial breakdown (SPK)
  2. In dense conditions, patchy staining or entire corneal staining may occur

Assessment

- Determine definitive cause from direct and indirect history
- Rule out risk of secondary (or primary) corneal infection, ulceration
- Examine palpebral conjunctiva (especially superior tarsus) for embedded foreign matter
  1. Single-evert superior lid and examine tarsus under slit lamp or loupe
  2. Double-evert superior lid and examine superior cul-de-sac

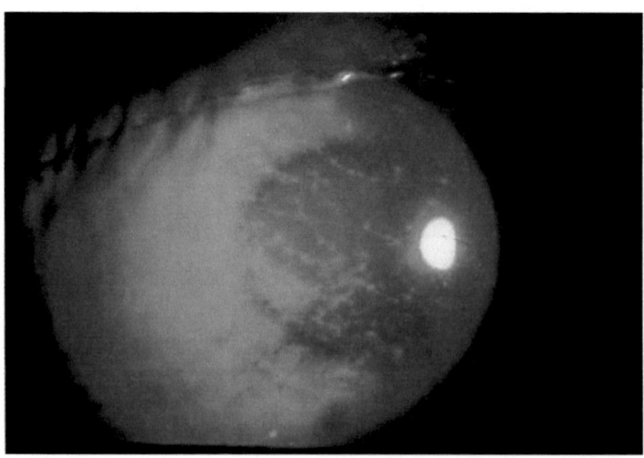

FIGURE 5.1 Foreign-body tracking (FBT) highlighted by superficial sodium fluorescein staining under direct slit-lamp biomicroscopic illumination with black light.

3. Lavage tissue while lid double-everted
4. Swab all non-corneal tissues gently with wet cotton tip and reirrigate superior and inferior cul-de-sacs and inner canthus

- Embedded fiberglass may not be visible and may require "blind" swabbing, possibly for multiple days if foreign-body sensation persists
- Evaluate contact lens materials, fit, design
- Examine corneal tissue (bilaterally) for map, dot, fingerprint changes, and other epithelial or endothelial involvements
- Rule out secondary anterior uveitis

Plan: Superficial Epithelial Abrasions

(See also Appendix 4)

- Eliminate, modify, or treat direct or indirect cause(s) of abrasion
  1. Remove any foreign matter by irrigation or swabbing
  2. Epilate offending lashes in trichiasis or refer entropion for surgical repair (seek oculoplastic surgeon if possible)
  3. Modify or redesign hard or soft contact lenses
  4. Manage epitheliopathies accordingly
- Prophylax corneal surface once in office with aminoglycoside ointment (e.g., gentamicin or tobramycin) after irrigation, swabbing, and reirrigation (if administered)
  1. In mild to moderate involvement, continued use of antibiotic is optional
  2. In moderate to severe involvement (dense SPKs), aminoglycoside drops, or ointments may be continued qid for 48 to 72 hours or until complete corneal resolution
- Give patient (or prescribe) mucomimetic lubricating drops (or ointment) q3–4h starting 2 hours after office visit
- Warm packs should be used q2–4h during first 6 to 12 hours after injury
- With epithelial edema (alone or with mechanical or physiological squamous abrasions)
  1. Hypertonic saline drops q3–4h for 2 to 3 days
     a. 2% or 5% drops (e.g., Muro 128)
     b. Refrigerate during use to reduce sting
  2. 5% hypertonic ointment at bedtime (e.g., Muro 128)
- Aspirin or ibuprofen (in lieu of contraindications) for pain relief during the first 12 to 24 hours; narcotic analgesic for severe pain
- Squamous epithelium heals within 6 to 12 hours with no risk of re-erosion
  1. Thus, no pressure patching, or soft lens bandage is necessary
  2. Advise patient to relax, keep eyes closed, and try to sleep following superficial abrasive (mechanical or physiological) injury or irritation
- Advise patient that discomfort "will probably get worse before it gets better" over the first 12 to 24 hours (especially after topical anesthetic wears off)

Follow-Up

- Recheck cornea or contact patient within 18- to 24- hour period following initial examination
- With or without compliance, squamous epithelial defects should be well healed within that period
- If FBT still present, foreign body (or other cause) is still present and requires retreatment
- If retreatment required for any reason, check corneas every 24 hours until complete subjective and objective resolution
- Reschedule patient PRN or for routine care

2. Deep Epithelial Abrasions (Non-Penetrating)[2,3]

Subjective

- Usually a distinct history of a "gouging" or lacerating-type traumatic incident tangential (versus perpendicular or blunt) to the ocular surface (Figure 5.2)
  1. Fingernail in eye
  2. Flying leaves or other firm materials
  3. Springing tree branches or twigs
  4. Paper cuts to eye
  5. Mascara brushes
- Patient reports moderate to severe pain and photophobia
- Subjective symptoms may be disproportionate to objective findings
  1. Sometimes severe injury yields moderate ("stoical") subjective response
  2. Sometimes mild to moderate injury yields severe response with associated nausea, vomiting, psychogenic reactions

Objective

- Lid spasms ipsilateral (or bilateral) are usually dramatic
- Lid edema and erythema vary from mild to moderate
- Vision is reduced, sometimes significantly (20/200 or less) due to epithelial disruption and edema
- Bulbar conjunctiva is moderate to severely hyperemic with segmental or circumferential limbal flush (from secondary anterior uveitis?)
  1. Cells and flare may not be visible through disrupted corneal surface
  2. Usually reduced intraocular pressure (IOP) in abraded eye (by 3 to 6 mm compared with uninjured eye) confirms secondary uveitic reaction
- Corneal and other ocular signs vary with degree of epithelial involvement, individual patient reactions and duration of abrasion
- Generally abrasion can be evaluated (and managed) based on four basic abrasion criteria

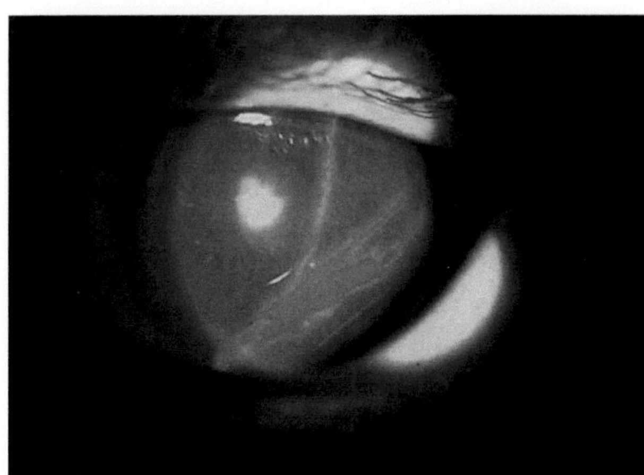

FIGURE 5.2 Superficial corneal epithelial abrasion caused by a tree branch scraping across the corneal surface.

1. Geography: determine and diagram approximate location and percentage of corneal surface and pupillary zone involvement (Figures 5.3 and 5.4)
2. Depth
   a. Determine and diagram (roughly) the layer(s) of corneal epithelial involvement and approximate diameter of each of three layers
      i. Squamous
      ii. Basal cells
      iii. Basement membrane

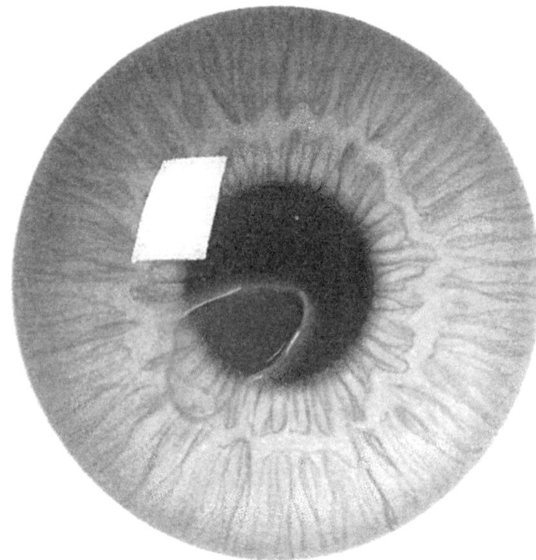

FIGURE 5.3 Geography of small corneal epithelial abrasion. Approximately 20% of inferonasal cornea (4 × 2 mm); approximately 25% of pupillary zone (2 × 2 mm).

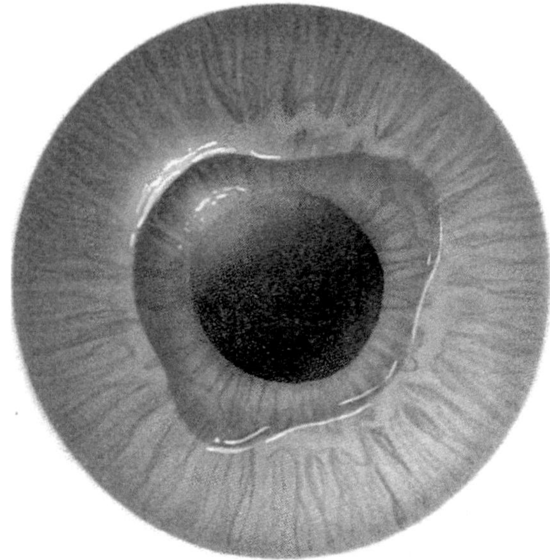

FIGURE 5.4 Geography of large corneal epithelial abrasion. Approximately 35% to 40% of central cornea (6 × 5 mm); 100% of pupillary zone.

   b. Basal epithelial cells tend to produce a hazy, grainy, more irregular NaFl pattern than the deeper, smoother, more continuous basement membrane (EBM) pattern (Figures 5.5 and 5.6)
   c. EBM also appears brighter (in fluorescence) due to pooling and pH differential between basal cells and basement membrane itself (Figure 5.7)
3. Edge quality: determine the degree (and approximate dimensions) of loosened squamous epithelial edges and any resulting "epithelial flaps or tags," which should be incorporated into the overall "geography" of the abrasion (Figures 5.8 and 5.9)
   a. Removal of epithelial flaps is optional
   b. Epithelial healing produces sluffing off the dead epithelial tissue without assistance in small to moderate flaps
4. Edema: determine approximate diameter, intensity, and depth of surrounding edematous reaction to epithelium and stroma and record and diagram in overall diagram (including all four abrasion criteria; Figure 5.10)

Assessment

- Rule out penetration or perforation of the cornea (Figure 5.11)
  1. Corneal penetration equals stromal entry
  2. Corneal perforation equals full-thickness entry and puncture
- Subjective indications for penetration or perforation
  1. Sharp or pointed items abrading in a perpendicular (versus tangential) manner (e.g., pencils, pine needles)
  2. Lacerating wounds (e.g., knife, scissors)
  3. High velocity "projectiles" (anything!) (see also scleral perforation, Chapter 4)
- Objective indications for penetration or perforation
  1. Appearance of stromal channel (grayish white at site of entry or maximal abrasion)
  2. Endothelial disruption directly behind abrasion
  3. Foreign material in aqueous, on iris, lens capsule, in lens, vitreous or on fundus
  4. "Wrinkled" cornea or flat anterior chamber
- Seidel's sign (percolation effect)
  1. Instill fluorescein
  2. With patient in slit lamp, ask to squeeze blink tightly and then release
  3. Observe point of maximal abrasion for signs of "oozing" of NaFl dye (indication of aqueous leakage through corneal perforating wound–called Seidel's sign. Also found in post-op surgery: see Chapter 7)
- IOP may be temporarily reduced in corneal perforation due to aqueous loss
- Assessment of risk for penetration or perforation
  1. Good history is most important
  2. Good slit-lamp examination is second most important
  3. Recognition and appreciation for the extraordinary strength and resistance of Bowman's layer (condensed stroma) will help toward accurate assessment of penetration risk

Plan: Corneal Penetration or Perforation

1. Penetration without perforation
   a. Non-surgical treatment is similar to deep epithelial abrasion

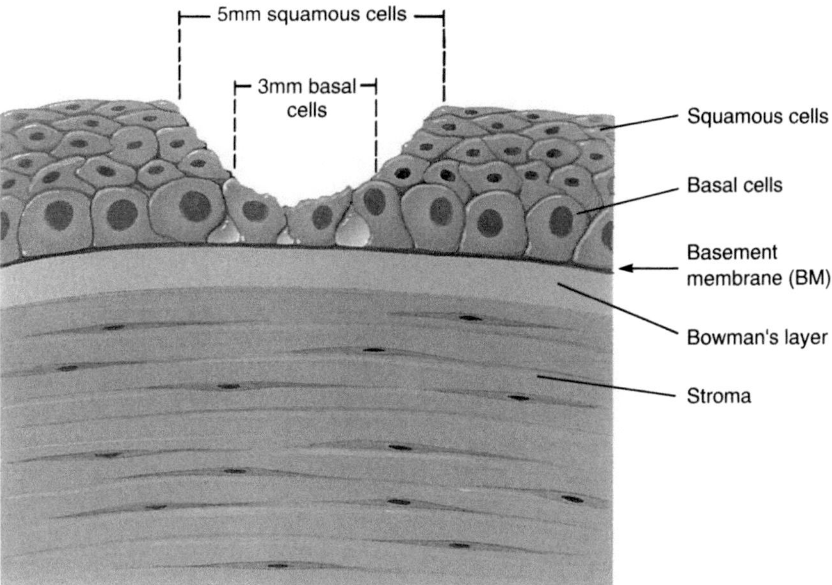

FIGURE 5.5 Corneal epithelial abrasion depth to approximate level of basal epithelial cell layer.

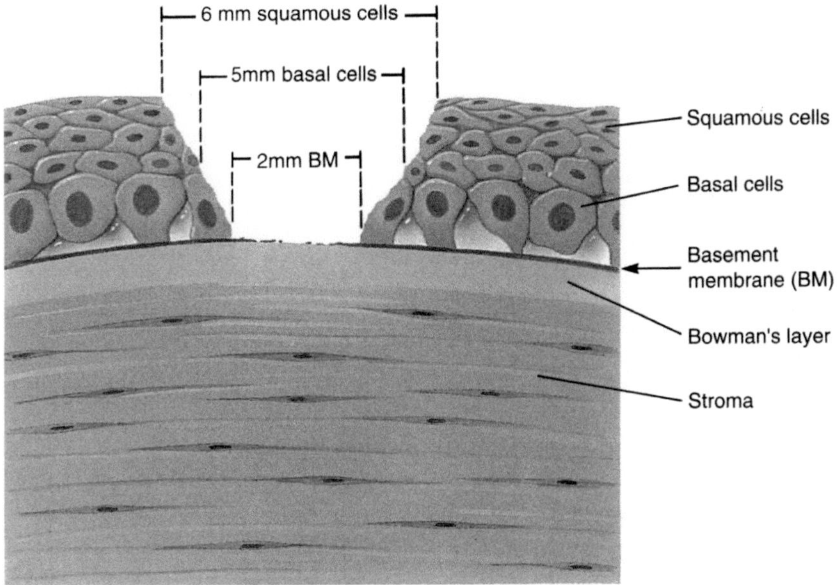

FIGURE 5.6 Corneal epithelial abrasion depth down to epithelial basement membrane level.

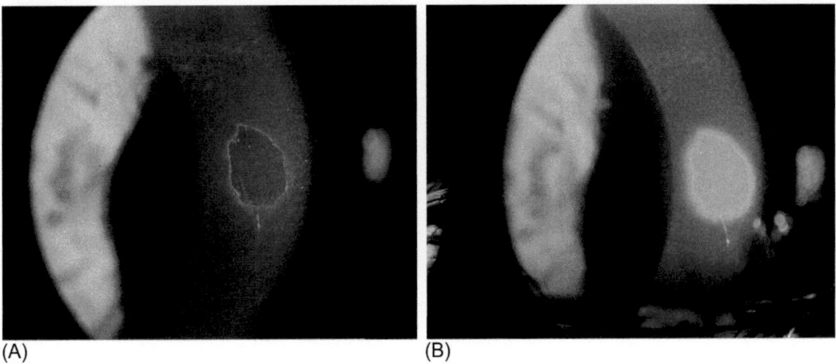

FIGURE 5.7 **(A)** Deep corneal epithelial abrasion without sodium fluorescein stain. Note the epithelial filamentary tag attached to the inferior edge of the abrasion. **(B)** Deep corneal epithelial abrasion with sodium fluorescein stain. Epithelial filament also demonstrates staining in slit-lamp biomicroscopic black light illumination.

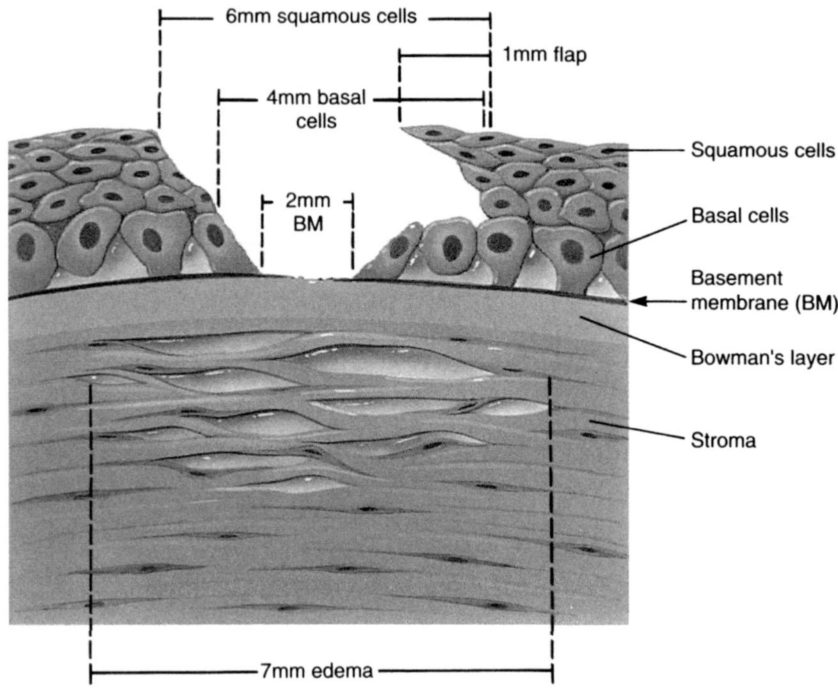

FIGURE 5.8 Deep corneal epithelial abrasion with an epithelial "flap" emanating from the squamous layer.

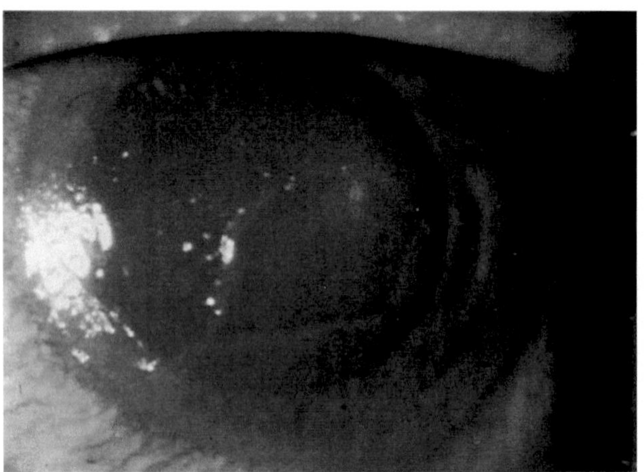

FIGURE 5.9 Deep corneal epithelial abrasion down to basement membrane with loose epithelial edges producing a grayish rim at surrounding borders of the abrasion.

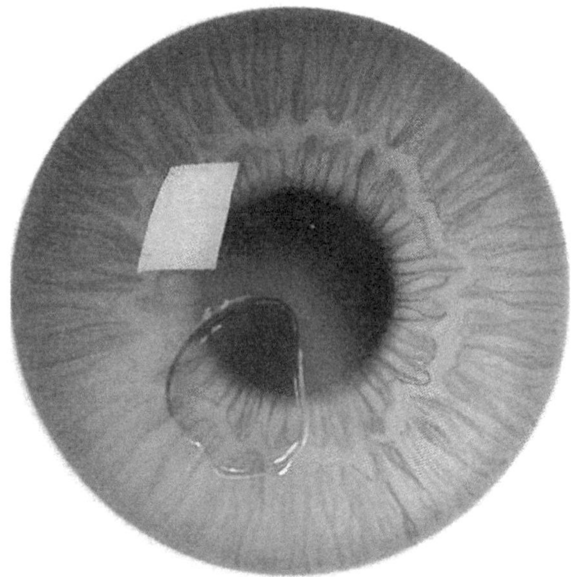

FIGURE 5.10 Overall "epithelial abrasion criteria" diagram. Approximately 15% of inferonasal cornea (3 × 4 mm); approximately 25% to 30% of pupillary zone (3 × 2 mm); approximately 3 × 1 mm superior edge epithelial flap; approximately 7 × 7 mm surrounding epithelial edema.

 b. However, scarring is guaranteed with risk of cosmetic awareness and permanent visual loss
 c. Ophthalmological consultation is indicated (if for only medicolegal considerations)
2. For corneal perforation
 a. Surgical repair should be conducted ASAP by a corneal specialist, if available
 b. Specialty care will include (but may not be limited to) cyanoacrylate glues, bandage soft lenses, topical antibiotic, and systemic antibiosis to reduce risk of intraocular infection
 c. Do not pressure patch perforations for transportation to specialist (use Fox metal shield for protection)

- Use abrasion criteria to evaluate extent, degree, and intensity of deep epithelial abrasions
- Carefully assess associated reactions to deep corneal abrasions (Figure 5.12; see Table 5.2)
  1. Determine variables (usual versus sometimes versus rare)

2. Rule out secondary traumatic anterior uveitis (usual to sometimes)
3. Rule out secondary corneal ulcer (rare)
4. Adjust treatment plan appropriately, per care code for deep corneal abrasion (see Table 5.3), to cover all associated reactions

- Gross assessment of corneal abrasion (when complete instrumentation is not available, such as outside office setting) can be made by simple trans illumination of the cornea with flashlight or collimated light source
- Finally, measure and include in final assessment and advice to patient, a prospective of the expected rate (time) of healing, prognosis, and (notwithstanding the ominous clinical appearance and dramatic subjective discomfort of a deep abrasion) the classic (predictable) physiological occurrences in the normal healing pattern (Figure 5.13)
  1. During first 6 to 24 hours, squamous epithelium slides over wound area
  2. During days 1 to 3, surrounding (remote) basal epithelial cell mitosis pushes new cells into wound site (filling defect)

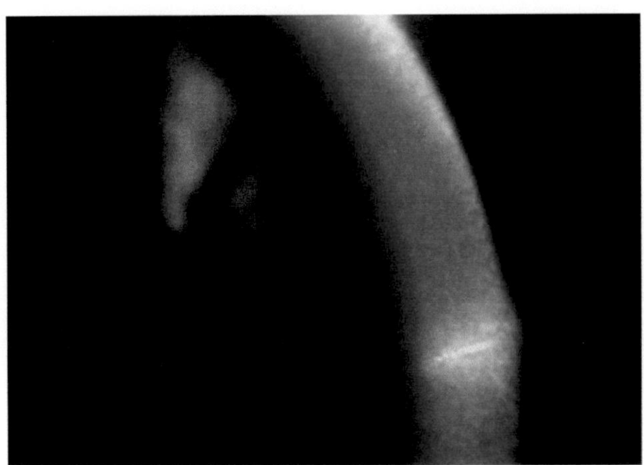

FIGURE 5.11 Stromal penetration caused by a pine needle (removed) producing a thin, opaque channel through the stroma with associated stromal thickening (secondary to edema) and endothelial disruption.

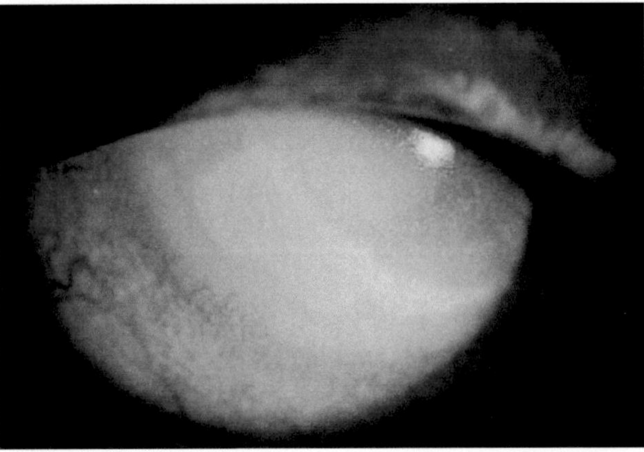

FIGURE 5.12 Deep corneal epithelial abrasion with dense, surrounding epithelial and anterior stromal edema producing deep diffusion of the sodium fluorescein stain.

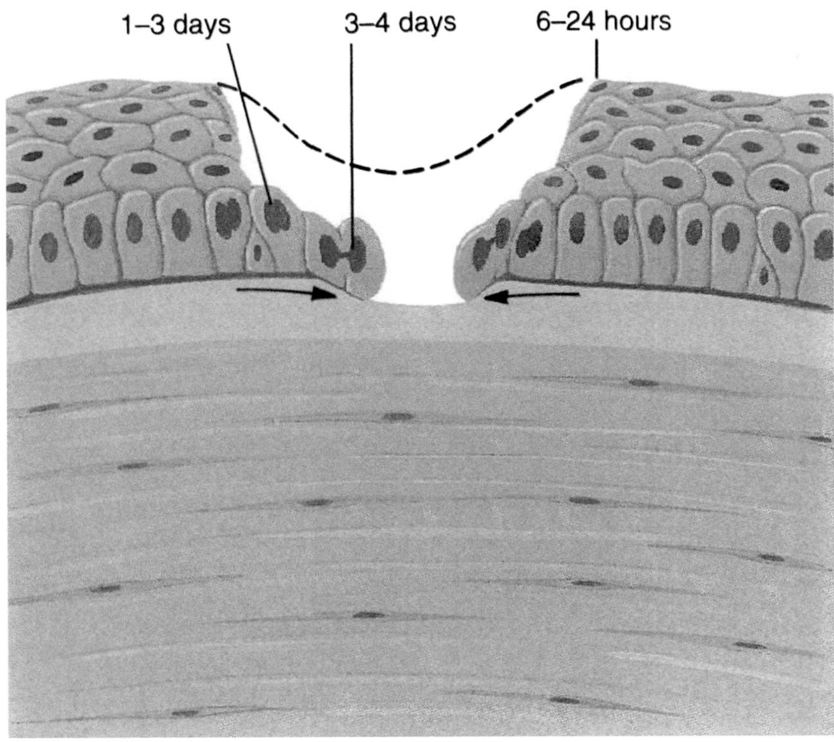

FIGURE 5.13 Deep corneal epithelial abrasions demonstrate cellular healing rates from hours (squamous cells) to days (deeper cells) under normal circumstances.

a. Conjunctival transdifferentiation of migrating conjunctival epithelium may also occur in larger abrasions
b. Usually produces slower healing rate
3. During days 3 and 4, mitosis directly at wound site completes full-thickness healing and, if needed, begins to regenerate new basement membrane (for 8 to 12 weeks)

Plan: Deep Epithelial Abrasions

(See also Appendices 4 and 6)

Follow day-by-day deep corneal epithelial abrasion protocol (Table 5.1)

1. Should be administered only after evaluation of abrasion according to abrasion criteria
2. Consider associated reactions (Table 5.2)
   a. Treat associated reactions according to "care code" (Table 5.3)
   b. Care code may require adjustments or substitutions to following day by day protocol

Day 1 (Day of Initial Presentation)

- Obtain best correctable vision (best visual acuity; BVA) with spectacle lenses or pinhole
- Examine carefully under topical anesthetic
  1. Use "abrasion criteria" to document
  2. Check associated reactions (Table 5.2)

TABLE 5.1 **Healing of Deep Corneal Epithelial Abrasions (Description and Rate of Healing)**

	Subjective	Objective	Assessment	Plan
Day 1	Moderate to severe pain persists Moderate photophobia	Edema may be little improved (or worse) Edges show mild reduction in instability and flapping (≈10%) Depth shows mild to moderate reduction in staining (≈20%) Geography usually shows reduced diameter (≈30%)	For expected norms, follow day 2 "abrasion protocol" For significant variations, refer to Table 5.2	Follow appropriate steps in "abrasion protocol" or "care code" (Table 5.3)
Day 2 or 3	Mild irritation may persist Photophobia reduced or absent	Edema persists (±25% improvement) Edge instability significantly reduced (≈50%) Depth shows significant reduction in deep staining (=75%) Geography dramatically reduced (=80%)	For expected norms, follow day 3 or 4 "abrasion protocol" For significant variations, refer to Table 5.2	Follow appropriate steps in "abrasion protocol" or "care code" (Table 5.3)
Day 3 or 4	Patient comfortable No photophobia or other symptoms	Edema begins significant drying (>60%) Edges stable with resolving infiltrative ring (80–90%) Depth completely filled with no deep staining remaining Geography shows completely covered abrasion area	For expected norms, follow "deep abrasion protocol" For significant variations, refer to Table 5.2	Follow appropriate steps in "abrasion protocol" or "care code" (Table 5.3)

Improvement	Day 1 Abrasion Criteria				Day 2 or 3 Abrasion Criteria				Day 3 or 4 Abrasion Criteria			
(%)	Edema	Edges	Depth	Geography	Edema	Edges	Depth	Geography	Edema	Edges	Depth	Geography
10												
20												
30												
40												
50												
60												
70												
80												
90												
100												

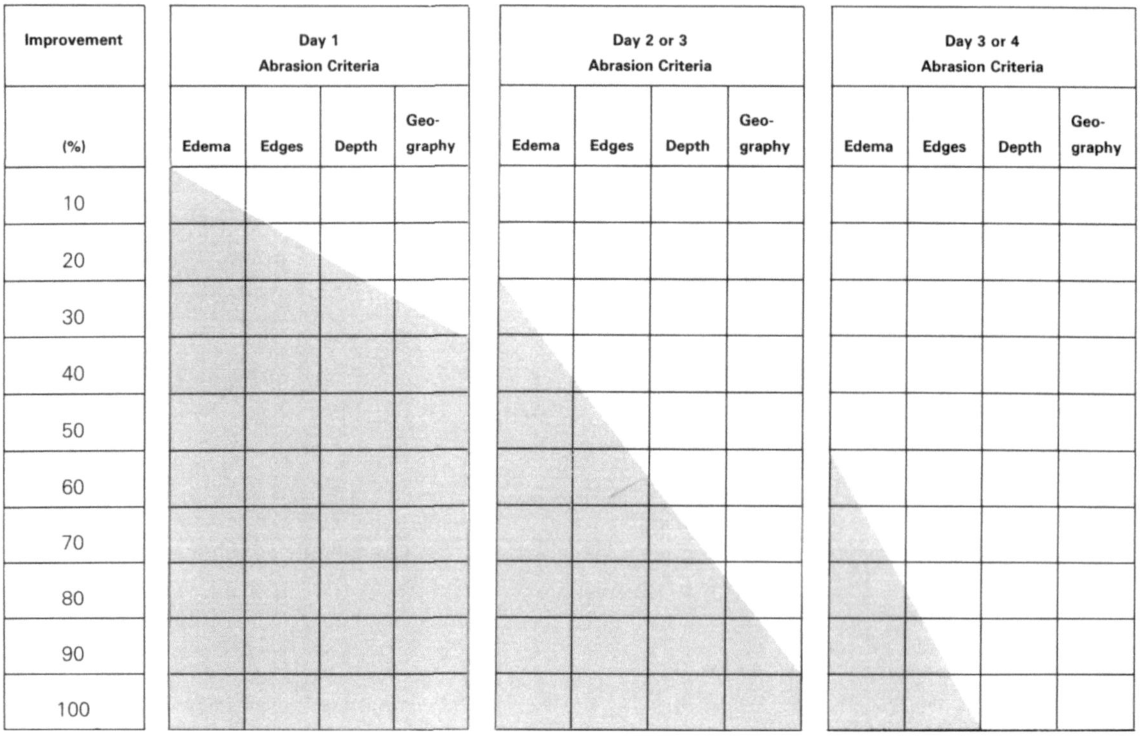

3. Multiple anesthetic drops may be applied (every 15 to 20 minutes, 2 or 3×) if necessary for examination purposes, but *never let patient take topical anesthetic drops for home use!*

- Lavage thoroughly with ophthalmic irrigating solution to reduce risk of secondary fungal infection (especially in vegetative injuries)

TABLE 5.2 Associated Reactions in Deep Corneal Epithelial Abrasion

Clinical Features[a]	Frequency	Care Code[b]
Reduced visual acuity	Usual	8
Discomfort	Usual	1,2,4,8
Photophobia	Usual	3
Lid spasms	Usual	2
Tearing	Usual	8
Exudate	Rare	8,10
Lid edema	Usual	2
Conjunctival edema	Sometimes	2,5
Corneal edema	Usual	2.5
Superficial hyperemia	Usual	2,3,8
Circum corneal flush	Sometimes	2,3,4,6
Anterior stromal infiltration	Sometimes	2,5
Deep stromal infiltration	Rare	2,5,7,(9?),10
Endothelial infiltrates	Rare	2,5,7,(9?),10
Folds in Descemet's	Rare	8,(9?),10
Keratio precipitates	Sometimes	2,3,4,6,7
Cells and flare	Sometimes	2,3,4,6
Fibrin in chamber	Sometimes	2,3,4,6,7,10
Hypopyon	Rare	8,9
Constricted pupil	Sometimes	
Dilated pupil	Sometimes	
Irregular pupil	Rare	8,(9?),10
Elevated intraocular pressure	Rare	(9?).10
Reduced intraocular pressure	Usual	

[a] Intensity will vary on a case-by-case basis.
[b] *See* Table 5.3 for care code explanation.

- Dilate and cycloplege with 5% homatropine or 1% cyclopentolate
  1. To reduce risk of secondary uveitis, observe adequate dilation before patching or discharging patient
  2. Add more dilating drops if necessary
- Instill broad-spectrum antibiotic ointment in eye
  1. Aminoglycoside (e.g., tobramycin) preferable
  2. Non-aminoglycoside (e.g., polymyxin B/bacitracin) acceptable in clean, low (pseudomonal) risk abrasions
  3. Fluoroquinolone (e.g., ciprofloxacin, besifloxacin) valuable in high-risk gram-negative abrasions (e.g., contaminated materials, contact lenses)
- Pressure patch firmly (Tables 5.4 and 5.5)
  1. Not indicated in mild abrasions
  2. Indications in moderate to severe abrasions
     a. Non-compliant patient (rubbing eye)
     b. Loose epithelial edges (e.g., flaps)
     c. Exposed basement membrane
     d. Extremely large (4 to 6 mm) abraded area
- Soft contact lens bandage may be used as an alternative to pressure patching in deep abrasions with mild to moderate basement membrane exposure (less than 3 to 6 mm)
  1. Use thin, large-diameter, disposable, high Dk, silicone hydrogel (e.g., Acuvue Oasys, Air Optix Night & Day Aqua)
  2. Fit plano or minimal power (keeps lens thin)
  3. Demonstrate sufficient movement on the eye
  4. Prophylax with gentamicin or tobramycin drops (over lens) bid to qid
  5. Manage same as with pressure patch
- Advise aspirin (2 tabs 5× daily or 3 g/day) or ibuprofen (400 mg qid) in lieu of contraindications
  1. For analgesia
  2. As anti-inflammatory (prostaglandin inhibitor) against secondary uveitic risk
  3. Contraindications
     a. Gastrointestinal problems
     b. Anticoagulation risks

TABLE 5.3 Care Code for Deep Corneal Epithelial Abrasion

Care Code Number	Drug, Procedure, Advice	Recommended Dosages
1	Four-step pressure patch procedure Lavage with irrigating solution Dilate and cycloplege with 1% cyclopentolate Instill broad-spectrum antibiotic ointment (e.g., gentamicin) in inferior cut-de-sac Apply pressure patch (see Table 5.4) Soft lens bandage alternative (disposable; see Table 5.5)	24-hr duration X PRN
2	Warm compresses	q2–4h
3	Dark glasses	PRN
4	Aspirin or ibuprofen (in lieu of contraindications)	2 tabs q4h × 2–3 ays
5	5% hypertonic saline (ointment and drops) and topical NSAID (optional)	1 qtt q3–4h and ointment at bedtime
6	Cycloplege and dilate (with 1% cyclopentolate)	1 × q2–4h with patch or tid until uveitis resolves
7	1% prednisolone or 0.5% lotemax/fluoromethelone (with family history or diagnosis of glaucoma)	q4h until uveitis resolves
8	Advise and counsel patient (on immediate and long-range prognosis)	At each visit or PRN by phone
9	Refer to ophthalmologist	ASAP
10	Monitor closely	q2–4h

Drugs, procedures, advice, and recommended dosages may vary with the degree and intensity of each presentation.

TABLE 5.4 Application of a Pressure Patch

Materials Needed

Balanced ophthalmic irrigating solution in "squirt" bottle, eg, Eye Wash (B&L), Eye Stream (Alcon)
Broad-spectrum antibiotic ointment, eg, Tobrex (Novartis), Ciloxan (Novartis)
Preshaped gauze eyepads, e.g., Eye Pad Oval, McKesson
Hypoallergenic, one-inch paper, plastic, or cloth adhesive tape, e.g., 3M Micropore (paper), 3M Transpore (plastic), 3M Medipore (cloth) (my preference for adhesion and ease of use is Transpore)

Application of Patch

After conducting all ocular preparatory procedures
 Have patient rest back of head against firm headrest
 Close both eyes with normal pressure and keep closed
 Clean and dry skin of mid-forehead and cheek lateral to ipsilateral eye
 Push back loose hair from forehead and face (Beards are a tough break!)
From side view, assess depth of orbit and prepare two to four pads as single unit (stack)
Fold one pad in half (lengthwise) and place it over closed lid (cotton balls, folded tissues, or gauze pads can also be used) (wet folded pad slightly for improved molding)
Place two to four pads (unit) over folded pad at slight angle (downward temporally) to cover orbit area maximally
Using 6- to 7-inch strips of tape, start first strip at mid-forehead, and angle directly over mid length of pads (on eye)
Pinch skin of cheek upward (toward eye) and pull end strip of tape tightly over cheek (below level of ear); remember to hold strip already applied to mid-forehead
Tape down first strip to cheek skin and release; if strip is tight, it should cause folding of lateral skin toward pads
Starting again at midforehead, apply a second 6- to 7-inch strip at a slightly upward angle from first strip
Contour this second strip over the superior edges of the pads such that all are covered by the strip as it passes over the pads; a slight curve will be necessary (and beneficial) in achieving this coverage
Apply the end of the second strip tightly and firmly onto the skin of the cheek (at a slight downward angle) partially covering the end of the first strip
Apply a third 6- to 7-inch strip in a similar manner as the second strip but in a downward direction to cover the lower edges of the pads
Finally, add one more (fourth) 6- to 7-inch strip over the same course as the first strip (midlength of pads); use this strip to cover the inner edge of strips 2 and 3 as they curve over the surfaces of the pads; apply tightly and firmly to the cheek over ends of other 3 strips

Removal of Patch

Instruct patient ("forcefully") to leave patch in place (no temporary removals) for 24-hr period
Patch should be removed by a practitioner, preferably the same person who applied the patch
Remove tape gently to avoid added irritation to skin (adhesive removers are usually not needed)
 Allergic reactions may appear as mild red erythematous patches under and around taped areas
 Prolonged taping (i.e., retaping for 2 to 3 days straight) often yields mild to moderate skin irritation which will respond to 1.0% hydrocortisone creams or cold packs or will self-limit without care
On ocular examination after removal of a pressure patch, a frequent sequela of the patching (beyond the healing abrasion) may be the development of a mild to moderate striate keratitis secondary to mechanical folding of the cornea and Descemet's membrane; resolution of this normal response is usually rapid (48 to 72 hours) and requires no treatment

TABLE 5.5 Considerations in Pressure Patching versus Soft Lens Bandaging

Consideration	Pressure Patch	Soft Lens Bandage
Indications	Loose epithelial edges Significant basement membrane involvement Chronic patient "eye rubbing"	Any size cellular epithelial abrasion Post foreign-body removal
Contraindications	Active infection or significant risk Severe inflammation Dense edema	Active infection or significant risk Severe inflammation Severe basement membrane involvement
Adverse reactions	Secondary infection Striate keratitis Epithelial mosaic Stromal edema Continued discomfort	Secondary infection Increased inflammation Epithelial mosaic Potential extended lens wear reactions Dislodged or lost
Benefits	Immobilizes lid Warm environment for rapid healing Increases adherence of new cells onto disrupted basement membrane	Increases comfort Rapid healing rate Provides continued binocular visual function Permits continuous topical therapies over bandage lens

  c. Known aspirin toxicity
  d. Advanced kidney disease
  e. Children under 12 years of age
 4. If pain is severe and not managed by a bandage soft lens, consider oral narcotic analgesia
- Counsel patient on immediate and long-range prognosis
 1. Risk of secondary uveitis (25% to 50%), even with prophylactic dilation and nonsteroidal anti-inflammatory agents (NSAIDs)
 2. Stress importance of leaving patch (or soft lens bandage) on to promote proper healing versus recurrent erosion
- Reschedule patient for 24-hour recheck (absolute!)

Day 2 (24–48 Hours after First Presentation)

- Remove pressure patch or soft lens bandage (may be prudent to leave lens in place for 48 hours before removal to ensure lens removal does not adversely impact healing)

   1. Instill 1–2 drops of unit dose non-preserved saline prior to lens removal to moisten contact lens ocular surface
- Obtain BVA
   1. Use same method as day 1
   2. May be worse than day 1 because of increasing edema
- Evaluate patient's subjective discomfort
   1. Without topical anesthetic gives corneal response
   2. With topical anesthetic gives indication of secondary uveitic pain ("dull, aching")
- Compare all objective findings with day 1 findings
- If secondary uveitic signs present
   1. Continue dilation and aspirin or ibuprofen
   2. Introduce topical steroids only in severe (3+) reactions
- Reinstitute day 1 treatment if indicated
   1. Severe discomfort
   2. Minimal healing of basal epithelial cells
- If patch or lens not reapplied
   1. Introduce warm packs q2–4h
   2. Hypertonic saline (drops q2–4h and ointment at bedtime)
   3. NSAID drops may increase patient comfort
   4. Reschedule for 24 to 48 hours

Day 3 or 4

- Obtain BVA
- Reevaluate subjective and objective status versus days 1 and 2
- Reconsider anterior uveitis therapy if indicated
   1. If no worse or better than day 2, reduce or discontinue dilation, aspirin, ibuprofen
   2. If worse, continue dilation, and add 1% prednisolone (or fluorometholone/0.5% loteprednol) q4h

Follow-Up

- All abrasion criteria will improve on a day-to-day basis except edema
   1. Usually increases over first 24 to 48 hours
   2. Will not begin to decrease until patch is discontinued (possibly faster with soft lens)
   3. Often produces stromal hazing and temporary secondary striate keratitis (usually will resolve within 1 week after discontinued patch)
- Continue warm packs for about 1 week
- Continue hypertonic drops for 2 to 3 weeks (tid)
- Continue hypertonic ointment at bedtime for 4 to 6 weeks
- Advise patients on short- and long-term risks of recurrent corneal erosion
   1. Instruct on early symptoms (AM syndrome)
   2. Stress value of 6 weeks of post abrasion hypertonic (5% Muro 128) ointment at bedtime to reduce risk of recurrent abrasion and closed lid edema
   3. Explain importance of therapy to decrease (but not eliminate) risk
- Beware of patients lost to follow-up in early stages of abrasion protocol
   1. Mild to moderate cases may not require aggressive follow-up management
   2. Moderate to severe cases should be followed closely and contacted if non-compliant (see Table 5.1)
- Always follow diabetic patients more closely

B. Blunt (Concussion or Contusion) Injury

Subjective

- A wide variety of causes
   1. Sports injuries (e.g., racket sports, baseball)
   2. Punch in the eye
   3. Blast injuries (to the closed lid)
   4. Industrial, domestic, or automobile accidents
   5. Birth trauma
- Discomfort and general subjective response vary with nature and degree of injury
- Usually associated with decreased vision and pain
   1. Vision loss secondary to edema and uveitis
   2. Pain associated with inflammation and occasional secondary acute glaucoma
- Frequently, presentation is out of concern and fear

Objective

- Many common associated findings
   1. Ecchymosis ("black eye")
   2. Subconjunctival hemorrhage and chemosis
   3. Corneal abrasion (and sometimes laceration)
   4. Corneal edema
   5. Secondary anterior uveitis
   6. Others
- All ocular tissues may be involved
- Caused by birth trauma (forceps delivery or birth canal trauma)
   1. Usually produces vertical folds or tears in Descemet's membrane
   2. Left eye far more frequently involved than right due to typical left occiput birth presentation
   3. Often seen in later life (during general examination) with mild to significant visual reduction
   4. More severe cases show permanent stromal haze
- Cornea (and other tissue) damage varies with nature and degree of injury

Mild Corneal Injury

- Epithelial and anterior stromal edema
- Mild epithelial staining
- Pigment deposits scattered on endothelium

Moderate Corneal Injury (as for Mild, plus:)

- Epithelial rupture (without EBM disruption; Figure 5.14)
- Deep stromal edema
- Folds (or lattice pattern) at Bowman's layer
- Folds in Descemet's membrane (striate keratitis)
- Blood staining on posterior cornea (secondary hyphema)
- Disruption of endothelium
- Substantial reduction in visual acuity (VA)

Severe Corneal Injury (as for Mild and Moderate, plus:)

- Translucent or opaque cornea because of dense, full-thickness edema
- Tears in Descemet's membrane
- Ruptures in corneal stroma (perforation unlikely)
- Hemorrhaging into corneal stroma
- Gross disruption and pigmentation of endothelium

Assessment

- With all blunt (contusive) injury, non-corneal ocular injury must always be ruled out, including (but not limited to) following possibilities

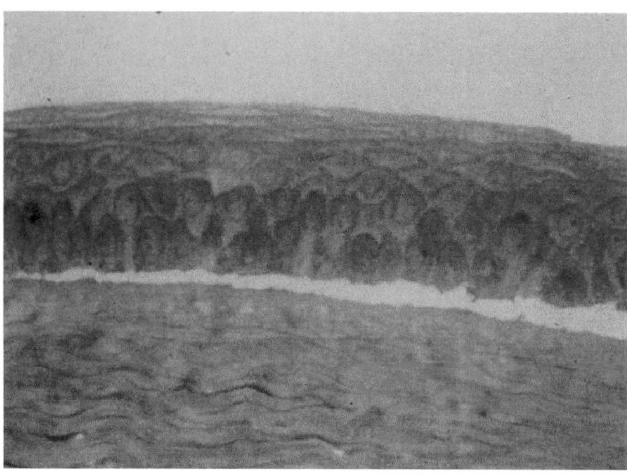

FIGURE 5.14 Cellular epithelial detachment (microgram) separated from epithelial basement membrane. Injury caused by blunt, contusive blow to eye, resulting in a large corneal abrasion with no basement membrane disruption.

1. Anterior segment
   a. Iridoplegia (mydriasis or miosis)
   b. Cycloplegia
   c. Hyphema
   d. Iridodialysis (angle recession)
   e. Traumatic cataract
   f. Luxation or dislocation of crystalline lens
   g. Vossius ring (a complete or incomplete circular pigmented deposit on anterior lens capsule)
2. Posterior segment
   a. Choroidal rupture
   b. Retinal hemorrhage
   c. Preretinal hemorrhage (intravitreous)
   d. Retinal edema (commotio retinae or Berlin's edema)
   e. Macular hole
   f. Retinal tears or detachment
   g. Papillitis
   h. Optic nerve avulsion
   i. Ruptured globe
3. Glaucoma (secondary)

- Determine degree (mild, moderate, or severe) of corneal involvement

Plan: Blunt Injury

- Treat all ocular involved tissues and structures appropriately
- Mild to moderate corneal involvement is usually self-limiting and resolve with or without treatment
  1. Warm packs q2–4h for 3 to 5 days
  2. Hypertonic saline drops q3–4h and ointments
  3. Reassurance of patient
- Severe corneal involvements should be managed by most appropriate available eye care practitioner
- As with mild to moderate involvement, self-limit, and self-resolving nature with or without therapy
- Greater risk of permanent corneal damage (stromal scarring) because of dense edema and ruptured membranes (Descemet's and stromal tissue)
- With significant scarring risk, aggressive medical or surgical therapies may (or may not) be of additional value
  1. Lowering IOP
  2. Cauterization techniques
  3. Penetrating keratoplasty

Follow-Up

- Recheck all blunt trauma cases within 1-week period
  1. Monitor initial damage (resolution or advances)
  2. Recheck all tissues and structures again
     a. If cornea improving, reduce dosages and recheck once again within 1 week
     b. If no improvement, continue treatment and recheck in 2 to 3 days
     c. If patient returns with increased complications, seek corneal consultation (from corneal specialist)

C. Burns[4]

Background Information

1. Lids and associated blink (menace) reflex tends to protect the ocular surface and cornea from many burns
   a. Lid tissue suffers major portion of damage
   b. Measured as first-, second-, and third-degree tissue damage
2. Ocular surface burns classified in three categories
   a. Thermal (or heat related)
   b. Radiation (by tissue absorption)
   c. Chemical (toxic or hypersensitive reactions)
3. Thermal burns to the cornea usually produce an eschar
   a. Focal superficial burn causing "charring" of epithelial cells creating a whitish gray (sometimes raised mass) corneal surface lesion
   b. Underlying stroma usually completely spared
   c. Common causes include heated particles or objects
      i. Cinders
      ii. Match heads
      iii. Heating instruments (e.g., soldering irons)
      iv. Hair "curling" irons
   d. Eschar is removed by standard foreign-body procedures and treated subsequently as a routine deep corneal abrasion
4. Radiation burns to cornea are most commonly related to ultraviolet (UV) light sources (sunlight, sun lamps, and welding arcs)
   a. Photokeratitis can result in severe pain, photophobia, tearing, redness, and decrease vision with significant UV exposure
   b. Onset approximately 6 hours after exposure
   c. Produce focal or diffuse SPKs varying from mild to dense
   d. Treatment and management are similar to standard sterile superficial keratitis care
5. Chemical burns to the eye are considered true ocular emergencies (i.e., care necessary within minutes to save vision)
   a. Three categories should be considered clinically
      i. Aromatic compounds (benzene-ring chemicals)
         - Benzene
         - Turpentine
         - Paint thinners
         - Gasoline
      ii. Acids (pH <7)
         - Battery acid
         - Acids containing heavy metals (far more dangerous than other forms)

   iii. Alkali (pH >7)
      - Ammonia compounds (e.g., cleaning agents, fertilizers)
      - Lye (sodium hydroxide, drain cleaners)
      - Lime (mortar, cement, plaster)
      - Magnesium hydroxide (flares, sparklers, firecrackers)
      - Chlorine (Clorox, pool chlorines)

b. Other agents can also produce toxic or hypersensitive-type chemical reactions to ocular surface
   i. Petroleum products
   ii. Household cleaners
   iii. Detergents, soaps, aerosols
   iv. Tear gas, mace

c. All chemical agents will produce variable degrees of damage to the ocular surface based on the amount of substance entering the eye and its concentration
   i. Amounts will determine localized versus diffuse involvement
   ii. Concentrations will dictate degree and depth of penetration of burn

d. Amounts and concentrations for all chemicals have an effect on their immediate ocular surface reaction, beyond which rapid neutralization begins to occur for all substances, *except alkali*
   i. Besides initial (amount and concentration) reaction, alkali continues to penetrate through its collagenolytic reaction for hours to days after initial contact
   ii. Collagenolytic response can result in unrelenting ulceration, melting, and permanent stromal scarring or perforation
   iii. Reaction is directly proportional to pH (greater pH equals greater tissue damage)

6. Chemical burns to the cornea require accurate assessment, quick action, and careful clinical management to protect the ocular tissue and the visual function

Subjective

- Usually an emergency phone call (hopefully) will be the first encounter with the patient
  1. Patients delaying immediate care to travel to an office or hospital may have allowed additional, irreversible damage to occur
  2. Care is required virtually within minutes to potentiate maximal clinical benefits
- History must include certain facts
  1. When and how accident happened?
  2. What was the substance or chemical?
  3. How much got in the eye?
  4. What specifics are available on the product?
  5. What has been done so far?
- Common causes of ocular (corneal) burns include (but are not limited to)
  1. Accidents in or around the house
  2. Industrial accidents
  3. Agricultural accidents
  4. Car battery explosions
  5. Radiation causes (e.g., arc welding, sun lamps)
  6. Thermal (heat)-related injuries
- Common substances include (but are not limited to)
  1. Chemicals (aromatics, acids, alkali)
  2. Aerosols (e.g., hairsprays, deodorants)
  3. Cleaning compounds and disinfectants
  4. Swimming pool chemicals
  5. Bleaches
  6. Sulfur particles off match heads (when striking)
  7. Cinders or hot ashes from fires
- Patient symptoms include classic corneal irritation
- Discomfort may range from mild to severe

Objective

- Immediate first aid should be administered STAT (emergently) assuming worst possible objective picture (before examination)
  1. Must be based on history alone
  2. Examination should follow first aid and preliminary determinations of nature of substance involved

Mild Involvement

- Lids may be more involved than eye itself
- Conjunctival hyperemia and chemosis about 1 to 2+
  1. May show subconjunctival hemorrhages
  2. Mild circumcorneal flush may be present
  3. No pale ischemic patches should be present
- Corneal epithelium may stain in varying degrees
  1. Iris features clearly visible through cornea
  2. May show diffuse band or inferior SPK pattern
  3. Confluent patches of stain (small or large)
  4. Diffuse, hazy epithelial edema
- Anterior chamber usually quiet or trace cells

Moderate Involvement

- Lid tissue frequently more involved
- Conjunctival tissue is grossly hyperemic and chemotic
  1. Circumcorneal flush more obvious
  2. One (or more) small (less than 3- to 4-mm diameter) patches of ischemia may be noted perilimbally or randomly placed
     a. These patches signify cauterization of superficial conjunctival vessels secondary to focal patch of highly concentrated chemical (e.g., granule, crystal)
     b. Ischemic patches represent partial loss of blood supply (and nutrition) to anterior segment
- Corneal involvement distinct
  1. Iris features are hazy when viewed through cornea
  2. Deep epithelial staining (usually diffuse or greater inferiorly)
  3. From 25% to 50% of epithelium may "melt"
  4. Deep stromal edema producing hazy cornea
- Anterior chamber reaction with or without raised IOP

Severe Involvement

- Dramatic clinical presentation (Figure 5.15)
- Lids (and face) may show extensive involvement
- Diffuse conjunctival chemosis often present
- There may be a paradoxical white eye (with a distinct history of chemical burn and advanced corneal findings)
  1. This paradoxical finding may be a partial or diffuse ischemia (from a high concentration chemical)
  2. Do not be deceived by white eye appearance
  3. Calculate degree of burn by corneal involvement
  4. Diffuse ischemia is a serious risk, potentiating anterior segment necrosis
- Cornea is usually translucent to opaque
  1. Iris features are barely visible or obscured
  2. Dense, deep stromal edema

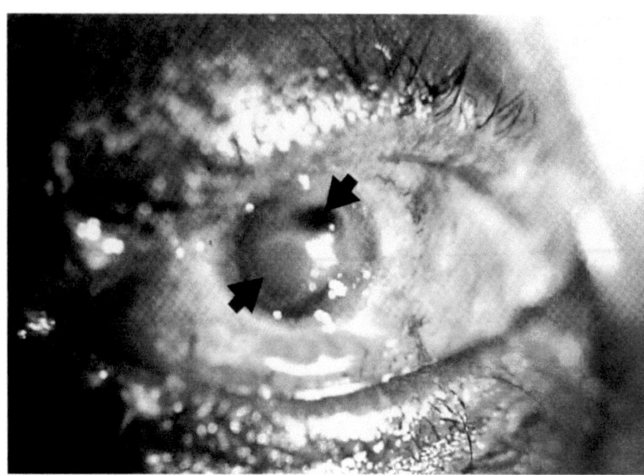

FIGURE 5.15 Alkaline corneal burn untreated for 4 to 5 days, resulting in hyperacute inflammatory response with secondary corneal destruction including formation of a descemetocele (top arrow) and Pseudomonas ulcer (lower arrow).

3. From 50% to 100% of epithelium may "melt" away
4. Occasionally with alkali burns, corneal findings may appear as moderate degree on initial presentation and progress to severe during first 3 to 5 days after injury
   a. Thus, history of alkali burn with even moderate level corneal involvement should be considered severe in clinical approach
   b. Corneal damage by any other chemicals (other than heavy metal acids and alkalis) will demonstrate maximal damage within hours

- Anterior uveitis almost assured (but not visible through dense corneal edematous haze)
- IOP may be significantly raised, especially during the 24 to 48 hours after injury

Assessment

- All differential considerations should be postponed in favor of immediate first aid (refer to "Plan" below)
- Initial assessment begins with careful history
- After proper first aid, objective evaluation will determine mild, moderate, or severe involvement
- A pH evaluation (with standard pH litmus paper applied to the tear meniscus) sometimes helps in determining need for continued irrigation after patient arrives for care

Plan: Corneal Burns

(See also Appendix 4)

- Immediate first aid for all burn patients begins with instruction over the phone as follows
  1. Get name and telephone number
  2. After brief history (as described in "Subjective" above), obtain as much information about chemical involved
     a. Label information (e.g., brand, generic, or chemical name)
     b. Patient's knowledge of substance or chemical
  3. Instruct patient on copious and continuous lavage (irrigation) with ophthalmic irrigator or water
     a. Form lateral trough around eye with paper towels
     b. Anesthetize ocular surface with topical anesthetic drops (optional)
     c. Pull lids away from eyeball and irrigate upper and lower fornices and then inner canthus
  4. Neutralizing agents (acidic or basic) are not indicated
  5. Irrigating bottles or balanced or buffered commercial saline solutions can be used, but are not necessary
  6. Any means of getting copious amounts of readily available neutral solution (i.e., water) in the eye is the best approach
     a. Sink faucets
     b. Shower nozzles (get in the shower)
     c. Hoses (outdoors)
     d. Industrial irrigating apparatus
  7. Delays greater than 3 to 5 minutes or discontinuation sooner than 20 to 30 minutes (minimum) reduce prognosis significantly
  8. Tell patient you will call them back in 20 to 30 minutes and reinforce urgency of irrigation procedure
- If substance or chemical is unknown to patient, immediately contact your local or regional emergency service (e.g., dial 911) or a poison control center
  1. Always keep number available
  2. Identify yourself as a health professional with emergent patient need
  3. If no service available in your area, investigate alternatives (in advance of emergency situation)
- Give emergency service all facts available and ask for assistance with the following information
  1. Nature of substance or chemical (if unknown)
  2. Suggested first aid measures beyond irrigation
- After receiving necessary information, or within 20 to 30 minutes, recontact patient
- Get update on subjective condition
- See patient or have patient seen immediately
- Best to see patient in office
- Avoid hospital emergency rooms unless you are to see patient or unless qualified optometrist or ophthalmologist is on site (or on call) at emergency facility
- On objective evaluation of condition
  1. Consider most appropriately trained eye care practitioner based on level of involvement
  2. Ideally, and when accessible
     a. All severe chemical burns as well as moderate alkali burns should be managed by a corneal specialist
     b. Moderate acid and aromatic burns and mild alkali burns should be managed by properly trained ODs or ophthalmologists
     c. Mild burns are treatable at the primary care level
- Treatment steps for mild to moderate (non-alkaline) chemical burns to the cornea
  1. First aid (as described above)
  2. Direct lavage of corneal epithelium to dislodge and clear any occult particles, granules
  3. Swab superior and inferior cul-de-sacs with wet cotton swab to dislodge and clear any embedded particles (reirrigate after swabbing)

4. Tobramycin (Tobrex) ointment q2h to qid
5. Cycloplege or dilate with 5% homatropine qid or cyclopentolate 1% qid (in moderate cases or when indicated for secondary uveitic reaction)
6. Steroid (1% prednisolone or 0.1% dexamethasone or 0.5% loteprednol) qid for 5 to 7 days and then taper off over 2 days
7. Oral doxycycline 100 mg qd and sodium citrate eyedrops qid to reduce proteolytic enzymes and reduce incidence of corneal melting/perforation
8. Oral or topical (usually painful for patient) potassium ascorbate to reduce risk of ulceration
9. Warm packs qid
10. No pressure patching or therapeutic bandage soft lenses (except UV etiology)
11. Recheck in 24 hours

- Severe chemical burn (including moderate alkali burn) to the cornea usually requires advanced ophthalmic care, often in a hospital setting
  1. All previously described therapies
  2. Oral and intramuscular pain relievers
  3. Oral antiglaucoma medications (e.g., carbonic anhydrase inhibitors) for secondary IOP increases
  4. Collagenase inhibitors (e.g., Mucomyst [acetylcysteine])
  5. Amniotic membrane is preferred over a soft contact lens bandage for epithelial control
  6. Surgical therapies (e.g., keratoplasty, flaps, limbal stem cell transplantation)

Follow-Up

- Singular goal of treatment is to get epithelium to successfully close and cover (non-staining) cornea
- If epithelial healing is delayed, corneal neovascularization and ongoing inflammation, there may limbal stem cells deficiency
- Recheck cornea every 24 hours in moderate to severe cases until epithelium shows pronounced healing
- Recheck mild to moderate cases every 3 to 5 days until complete healing occurs
- Always taper steroids after 5 to 7 days in burns (especially alkali) to minimize ulceration risks
- Continue tobramycin cover (with tapering dosages) until negative staining
- Prognosis
  1. Complete resolution for all mild chemical burns within 1 to 2 weeks
  2. Resolution of moderate (non-alkaline) burns within 2 to 4 weeks (usually)
  3. Moderate alkali burns may take 3 to 6 weeks with risk of mild permanent stromal haze and VA loss
  4. Severe burns frequently run an unrelenting course of corneal decompensation with significant risk of secondary ulceration, infection, scarring, and perforation
  5. Other complications in chemical burns to cornea
     a. Symblepharon (Figure 5.16)
     b. Entropion
     c. Keratitis sicca
     d. Neovascularization and pannus
     e. Chronic anterior uveitis
     f. Chronic glaucoma
     g. Phthisis bulbi

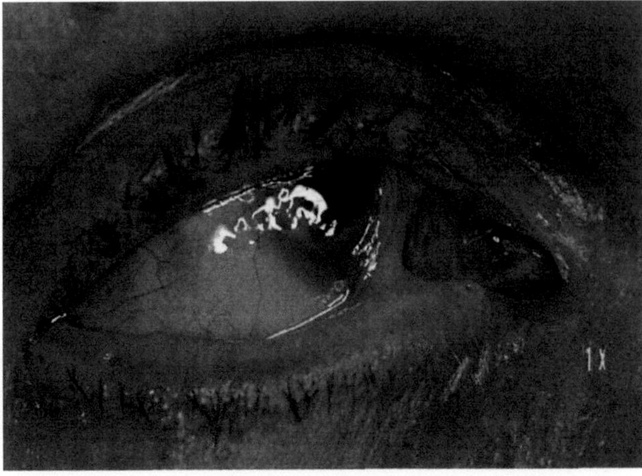

FIGURE 5.16 Symblepharon of the right eye secondary to a severe chemical burn with a broad adhesion extending from the inferior to the superior palpebral conjunctival.

D. Aqueous Deficient Dry Eye or Keratitis Sicca-Type Syndromes[5–21]

1. Clinical Presentation

Subjective

- Age-related dry eye associated with lacrimal insufficiency (reduces basal aqueous tear flow)
- Common syndrome in older (postmenopausal) women
- Almost always bilateral (one eye may be more irritated or more involved than second eye)
- Most common symptom is mild to moderate, mid to late day superficial irritation (corneal type)
- Ocular Surface Disease Index (<33 low symptoms) and DEQ-5 are validated to quantify ocular symptoms
  1. "Sandy, gritty" feeling
  2. Foreign-body sensation
  3. Non-specific ocular surface "dryness," discomfort, or burning irritation
  4. Possible photophobia
  5. Blurred or fluctuating vision
- Patients tend to define times, places, and specific factors that aggravate symptoms
  1. Arid (dry) conditions (especially with wind)
  2. Airborne irritants
     a. Dust
     b. Smoke (e.g., especially cigarettes, cigars)
     c. Fumes (and pollution)
     d. Fine particles (e.g., fabrics, threads, spores)
  3. Air-conditioning (with dehumidification) and heating systems in homes and automobiles
  4. Airplane travel with low air humidity
  5. Bright lights
  6. Extended near work such as electronic device use, reading, television (staring syndrome)
  7. Chlorinated swimming pool water
- Sometimes associated with common medications
  1. Antihistamines (especially non-prescription chlorpheniramine, diphenhydramine)
  2. Tricyclic antidepressants
  3. Antipsychotic agents
  4. Antianxiety selective serotonin reuptake inhibitors (SSRI)

5. Beta-blockers
6. Antiandrogens
7. Decongestants
8. Diuretics
9. Isotretinoin (accutane)
10. Atropine-based compounds
11. Oral steroids
12. Birth control pills (uncertain)
13. Alcohol-based medications (or plain old " booze")

- Dermatological conditions
  1. Seborrhea
  2. Variable dermatites
  3. Eczema
  4. Psoriasis
  5. Rosacea
- History of other ocular conditions
  1. Lagophthalmos
  2. Blepharitis
  3. Meibomian gland dysfunction
  4. Soft or hard contact lenses
  5. Previous corneal refractive surgery (e.g., LASIK)
- General systemic conditions
  1. Primary Sjögren's syndrome based on 4 out of 6 of the following
     a. Positive serum anti-SSA and/or anti-SSB or rheumatoid factor or antinuclear antibody (titer >1:320)
     b. Total ocular staining score >3 and unanesthetized Schrimer's test <5 mm in 5 minutes
     c. Positive labial salivary gland biopsy for lymphocytic infiltration
     d. Unstimulated salivary flow <1.5 mL in 15 minutes
     e. Ocular dry eye symptoms
     f. Dry mouth symptoms
  2. Secondary Sjögren's syndrome
     a. Rheumatoid arthritis
     b. Sarcoid
     c. Lymphoma
     d. Scleroderma
     e. Amyloidosis
     f. Systemic lupus erythematosus
     g. Polymyositis
  3. Neurotropic responses (Bell's palsy)
  4. Autoimmune thyroid (exposure) condition
  5. Hematopoietic stem cell transplantation (Graft versus host disease)
- Patient may report "paradoxical" wet-eye problems
  1. Dry eye stimulates trigeminal reflex
  2. Stimulates excess reflex aqueous tearing

Objective

- Clinical signs and symptoms do not have to correlate
  1. Patient may be asymptomatic with clinical signs
  2. Patient may be very symptomatic with minimal or no clinical signs
- No discharge present
  1. Excess dryness leads to reflexive aqueous tearing ("paradoxical" wet eye)
  2. Occasional mucoid or lipid buildup in inferior cul-de-sac
- Generally a low-grade, angular-type bulbar hyperemia
- Lissamine green staining of bulbar conjunctiva
- Lid margin and inferior fornix tear menisci may be reduced (<0.5 mm) or absent
- Mucoid debris (lipids, desiccated epithelial cells) may accumulate on the ocular surface or in the aqueous tear film or meniscus
  1. Meniscus may demonstrate "frothy" appearance
  2. Not uncommon to have both frothing and debris
- Most typical clinical sign in dry eye or keratitis sicca syndromes is SPK staining greatest in the band region of cornea and conjunctiva (exposed area of cornea and conjunctiva in palpebral fissure region)
  1. Cause of cellular disruption in mild to moderate dry eye is drying and mechanical breakdown of cell wall integrity
  2. Cause of cellular disruption in severe dry eye is a process called squamous cell metaplasia (cell differentiation)
  3. In both forms of disruption area stains with NaFl (disrupted cell junctures) and rose bengal/lissamine green (dead and devitalized cells)
  4. Rose bengal/lissamine green stain is specific for keratitis sicca drying and dead and devitalized cells (drying; Figure 5.17)
- On corneal surface, debris can form filaments producing a condition called filamentary keratitis
  1. Helix of mucin and dead epithelial cells
  2. Lengths range from 0.5 mm to 4 mm to 5 mm
  3. Proximally adherent to corneal epithelium with distal end moving with each blink
  4. Blink causes pull on corneal epithelium with resultant foreign-body sensation (moderate to severe)
  5. Some other causes of filamentary keratitis (see Table 5.10)
     a. Atopic keratoconjunctivitis (see Table 5.10)
     b. Epithelial basement membrane disorders (EBMDs)
     c. Herpes zoster ophthalmicus
     d. Post-cataract and post-penetrating keratoplasty
     e. Recurrent corneal erosions
     f. Staphylococcal keratitis
     g. Superior limbic keratoconjunctivitis (SLK)
     h. SPK of Thygeson

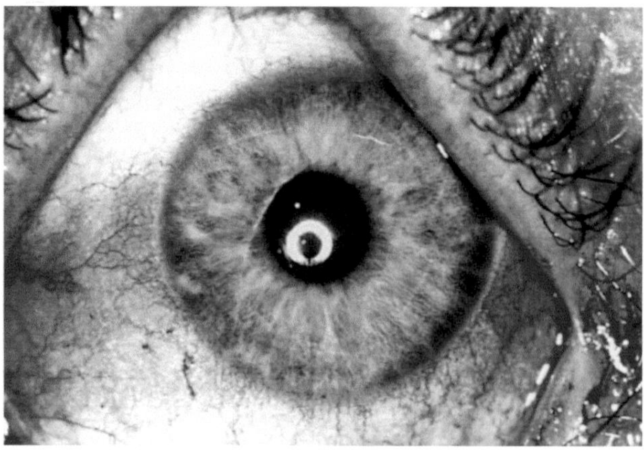

FIGURE 5.17 Rose bengal staining of the nasal and temporal bulbar conjunctiva in the palpebral aperture zones and on the inferior cornea. Staining pattern is typical of dry eye/keratoconjunctivitis sicca syndromes.

i. Toxic keratitis
j. Vernal keratoconjunctivitis

- Occasional dellen formations (Gaule spots)
- Positive tear breakup time (TBUT) with NaFl may be present but results are variable
  1. Wet NaFl strip with saline
  2. Instill in inferior cul-de-sac or superior bulbar conjunctiva
  3. Do not touch or manipulate lids
  4. Have patient take two to three regular blinks first and then stop blinking
  5. Then evaluate NaFl pattern for breakup points by measuring the seconds until first tear film break (10 seconds maximum)
     a. Instantaneous breakup should be noted as "negative staining"
     b. Negative staining diagnostic for epithelial surface abnormalities (epitheliopathies such as EBMD) versus actual tear film disorders (see Table 5.9 for comparison of negative staining and tear breakup time)
  6. Positive TBUT equals random patterns of breakup points in less than 10 seconds but greater than 1 second
- Non-invasive breakup time (NIBUT) can be measured using videokeratoscopy or thermography
  1. More repeatable than conventional TBUT
- Schirmer testing is quite variable, with a high probability of false-negative results in mild to moderate ("marginal") dry eye syndrome
  1. Strip wetting is usually attributable to reflex tearing (with or without topical anesthetics)
  2. Positives in severe dry eye syndromes are far more accurate
  3. Non-wetting indicates lack of tear production (true secretory dysfunction)
- Phenol red thread test uses similar concept as Schirmer
- Hyperosmolarity of tear film
  1. >308 mOsm/l is thought to be significant for dry eye, >328 mOsm/l severe disease
  2. Clinical measurements with Tearlab osmometer and correlation to dry eye signs and symptoms have been variable
- Biomarker testing
  1. Matrix metalloproteinase 9 (MMP 9) measured with InflammaDry
     a. Positive when MMP 9 >40 ng/mL
     b. Results vary depending on sample volume
  2. TearScan Lactoferrin Diagnostic Test Kit
     a. Semi-quantitative assay
- Other findings to note in dry eye diagnosis
  1. Chronic conjunctivitis
  2. Blepharitis and blepharoconjunctivitis
  3. Meibomian gland dysfunction
  4. Corneal epithelial abnormalities

Assessment

(See also Appendix 3)

- Rule out all stimulating causes of dry eye syndrome (from "Subjective," above)
  1. Aggravants
  2. Medications
  3. Systemic causes
  4. Environmental conditions
  5. Ocular problems
  6. Contact lenses
- Classify based on the following: more than one deficiency may be present in any patient
  1. Lipid layer (prevents evaporation) abnormalities (evaporative)
     a. Caused by infectious blepharitis and meibomian gland dysfunction (see Chapter 3, III, I)
     b. Bacterial toxins cause rupture of tear film and secondary epithelial problems
  2. Aqueous layer (thickest layer) deficiencies (aqueous deficient)
     a. Lacrimal and accessory gland abnormalities
     b. Sjögren's syndrome (dry eye, dry mouth, and arthritis)
     c. Drug related
     d. Neurological
  3. Mucin layer (most important protective layer) deficiencies
     a. Goblet cell (conjunctival) abnormalities
     b. Vitamin A deficiencies
     c. Drug related
     d. Stevens–Johnson syndrome (erythema multiforme)
     e. Conjunctival diseases and disorders
  4. Lid resurfacing (Marangoni effect) disorders
     a. Blepharitis (e.g., tylosis)
     b. Nocturnal lagophthalmos
     c. Colobomas (lid notching)
     d. Keratinized lid margins
     e. Trichiasis
     f. Entropion or ectropion
- Most common differential diagnosis is between dry eye syndromes and epithelial basement membrane disease (see Table 5.9)
  1. Morning syndrome vs late-day symptoms
  2. Map-dot-fingerprint configurations intraepithelial vs. band-region SPK pattern (Figure 5.18)
  3. Negative staining versus positive TBUT

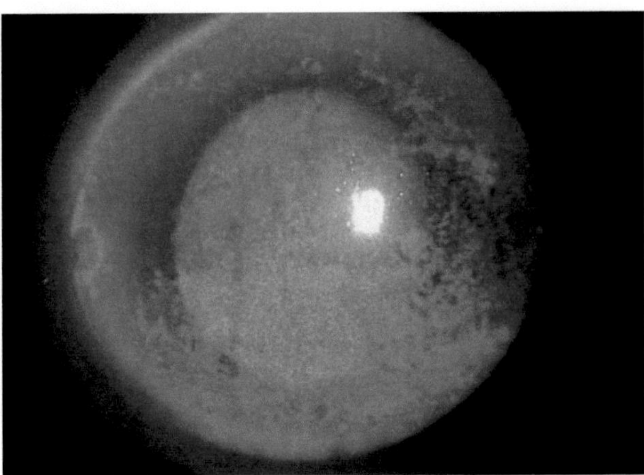

FIGURE 5.18 Band region staining with sodium fluorescein caused by poor wetting of the exposed zone (band region) of the inferior cornea. Commonly referred to as band region SPK (superficial punctate keratitis), this finding is usually a result of superficial epithelial erosion (SEE) secondary to drying and squamous cell dislocation.

- Because of prevalence of both conditions (EBMD and dry eye or keratitis sicca–type syndromes), combined disease conditions (especially in high risk and older age ranges) are very possible
    1. Non-responsiveness to lubrication therapy (for presumed dry eye conditions) should indicate trial of hypertonics (for possible EBMD)
    2. Combined therapies may also be indicated from time to time for symptomatic and physical relief

Plan: Dry Eye Keratitis Sicca–Type

For Mild to Moderate Symptoms (PM or Chronic)

- Lubricating eyedrops and ointments
    1. Palliative care
    2. 5 to 10×/day
    3. Wide range of lubricating agents (see Chapter 1, II. 7.)
    4. Drops to higher viscosity gels and ointments
        a. Increase in viscosity can blur vision making them less patient friendly for daytime use
        b. Patients find ointments difficult to instill
    5. Avoid benzalkonium chloride (BAK) preserved due to epithelial toxicity to avoid toxic medicamentosa
    6. Preservative free drops can be expensive
    7. Dose as needed based on severity
- Anti-inflammatory topical agents
    1. Steroid drops (e.g., 0.5% Loteprednol) used "off label" bid to qid short term (2–4 weeks) for flare ups
        a. EYsuVIS (0.25% Loteprednol) → first topical steroid drop FDA approved for short-term (up to 2 weeks) treatment of signs and symptoms of dry eye
    2. Steroid sparing anti-inflammatory drops
        a. Cyclosporin A 0.5% (Restasis) or 0.9% (Cequa) bid
        b. Lifitegrast 5% (Xiidra) bid
        c. Tacrolimus 0.3% qd to bid used "off label" as alternative to cyclosporin
- Recheck patient in approximately 2 weeks

For Moderate to Severe Conditions

- Same as mild to moderate plus
- Add longer-acting tear substitutes based on degree
    1. Gels (q2h to qid)
    2. Ointments
    3. Lacriserts (Bausch + Lomb)
        a. Hydroxypropyl cellulose, time-released pellets of 12- to 24-hour duration
        b. Insert pellet in inferior cul-de-sac
        c. Procedure difficult for patient and pellet often produces discomfort and dislodges
    4. Possible adverse effects from ointments and Lacriserts, leading to non-compliance
        a. Blurred vision
        b. Irritation (and pellet dislodging)
        c. Difficulty with instillation
        d. SPK
- Autologous serum
    1. Contains epithelial growth and anti-inflammatory factors that inhibit cytokines and MMP-9 inhibitors
    2. Clinical study results have been inconsistent
    3. Pro
        a. Manufactured from patient's own plasma
    4. Con
        a. Non-preserved and has short shelf life
        b. Expensive
- Amniotic membrane extracted eyedrops
    1. Contains growth factors, cell-signaling proteins (cytokines), and anti-inflammatory factors to aid corneal epithelial wound healing
    2. Also used for corneal abrasions, ocular burns
    3. Genesis amniotic membrane extract (Ocular Sciences)
    4. Regener-Eyes ophthalmic solution and ophthalmic lite solution (Regener-Eyes)
    5. Solutions are not FDA approved for ophthalmic treatment
    6. Additional studies are needed
- Recheck patient within 1 week

For Severe Conditions

- All moderate therapies at maximal levels, plus
- Bandage contact lens therapy
    1. Use silicone hydrogel lenses
    2. Daily disposable wear (because of increased risk of infection) is preferred
    3. Monitor patient closely (every 6 weeks or PRN)
    4. Add therapeutic drops over bandage lenses
- Additional therapies
    1. Punctal occlusion (collagen and silicone plugs or laser)
        a. Conflicting data on effectiveness
    2. Scleral contact lenses
    3. Varenicline solution (e.g., Tyrvaya) (see Chapter 1, specialty drugs)
        a. Rx nasal spray
    4. Electrical stimulation of nasal mucosa activates anterior ethmoid branch of trigeminal nerve stimulates lacrimal functional unit to increase basal tear flow
        a. TrueTear (Allergan) has been discontinued
        b. iTear (Olympic Ophthalmics) applies unit externally to nose and mechanically oscillates to stimulate nerve externally
            i. Increase in Schirmer scores and decrease in symptoms
            ii. New technology
    5. Tarsorrhaphy
        a. Used to treat persistent epithelial defects secondary to dry eye
        b. Temporary or permanent
    6. Lacrimal gland stimulating drugs
        a. Cholinergic-parasympathomimetics
            i. Oral pilocarpine and cevimeline used "off label"
- Other therapies to reduce tear loss
    1. Moisture chamber goggles
    2. "Saran wrap" coverings
    3. Lid taping procedures

Follow-Up

For Mild to Moderate Conditions

- If no improvement after 2 weeks
    1. Question patient on compliance and retreat for 2 to 3 weeks if non-compliant
    2. If patient compliant, upgrade treatment
- If improvement (subjective and objective)
    1. Advise patient carefully
    2. Taper therapy to minimal maintenance dosages
    3. Recheck every 4 to 6 months or PRN

For Moderate to Severe Conditions

- If no improvement after 1 week
  1. Reconfirm compliance and continue therapy for additional week if necessary
  2. If compliant, add additional or alternative therapies (primary or secondary level procedures)
- If improvement noted
  1. Taper therapies (slowly) to maintenance level
  2. Advise patient carefully
  3. Monitor closely (every 3 months) or PRN

Patient Advice

- Have any ocular abnormality checked immediately due to increased risk for secondary infection
- Explain chronic (non-curative) nature of underlying disease (if applicable) and primary care treatment goals of protection and prevention of complications
- Therapy must be continued
- Overuse of drops may produce preservative reactions
- Avoid irritating or "triggering" causes of symptoms and physical changes
- Diligently comply with all professional instructions

2. *Stages and "Conversions"*

Background

In 2007 the Tear Film and Ocular Surface Society defined dry eye as the following:

> Dry eye is a multifactorial disease of the ocular surface characterized by a loss of homeostasis of the tear film, and accompanied by ocular symptoms, in which tear film instability and hyperosmolarity, ocular surface inflammation and damage, and neurosensory abnormalities play etiological roles.

a. It is a progressive disease which can lead to a chronic inflammatory condition with reduced tear flow and increased tear evaporation
   i. Historically dry eye has been classified as evaporative or aqueous deficient
      - However, realty is that typically it is not caused by a single-producing gland
      - Multiple factors affect this disease
   ii. The more common, milder ("marginal") forms of dry eye do not demonstrate definite histopathological changes or reproduceable clinical testing, but do manifest clinical signs (generally to a lesser degree) similar to the severe dry eye syndrome
      - Subjective corneal irritation increasing through late day
      - Increased mucoid debris in the tears
      - Conjunctival hyperemia and lissamine green staining
      - SPK (greater in the band region)
      - NaFl and rose bengal/lissamine green corneal staining
      - Reduced tear meniscus
      - Positive TBUT (less than 10 seconds)

b. The greatest diagnostic indicators in mild to moderate dry eye syndromes are non-tear film conditions that have a direct or indirect effect on the quality-not-quantity of the tear film
   i. Medications
   ii. Systemic disease
   iii. Environmental factors (e.g., humidity, air flow, electronic device use)
   iv. Contact lens wear (especially soft lenses)
   v. Eyelid conditions

c. Among the relatively common conditions that have a direct and indirect effect on the tear film, conditions of the eyelids play a role
   i. Because of the intimate, proximal relationship with the ocular surface
   ii. Because of the frequency of the lid conditions
      - Positional abnormalities
        - Ectropion
        - Entropion/trichiasis
        - Lagophthalmos
      - Blinking abnormalities (e.g., Stellwag's sign, infrequent or incomplete blinking, in hyperthyroid Graves' disease)
      - Lid margin abnormalities
        - Keratinized lid margins
        - Notches
        - Scarring
   iii. The most frequent, most common lid conditions are the various forms of blepharitis
      - Meibomian gland dysfunction
      - Staphylococcal
      - Seborrheic
      - Demodicosis
      - Ocular rosacea

d. Rather than consider marginal dry eye as a disease or disorder of the tear film, it can be viewed as a sequence of "effects" caused by associated (non-tear film) conditions (especially blepharitis) that produce four clinical "stages"
   i. Prevention or treatment of the causes, in conjunction with palliative therapies for the effects, will result in improved therapeutic outcomes

e. Stages of marginal dry eye syndrome (Figure 5.19)
   i. *Stage 1*: *Pre-tear film disruption*
      - Lacrimal gland changes or eyelid conditions, through insidious mechanical and/or toxic reactions, begin to compromise the dynamics, chemistry, and overall integrity of the tear film
      - Often, subjective patient reports of discomfort (dryness, burning) are not accompanied by objective, ocular surface signs (subclinical presentation)
      - Evaluate external (e.g., environment, electronic device use) and internal (e.g., medications, systemic health) factors as contributors
      - Examination for symptoms without signs should focus on potential lid problems
      - Treatment options should include aggressive preventive therapies, with or without objective signs (see Chapter 3 and Table 3.1)
   ii. *Stage 2*: *Tear film disruption*
      - This is the only one of the four clinical stages of the marginal dry eye syndrome that involves the tear film directly
      - Accumulating (often untreated) effects of the previous stage begin to disrupt the quality of the tear film, producing chronic and increasing symptomatology, with or without objective signs

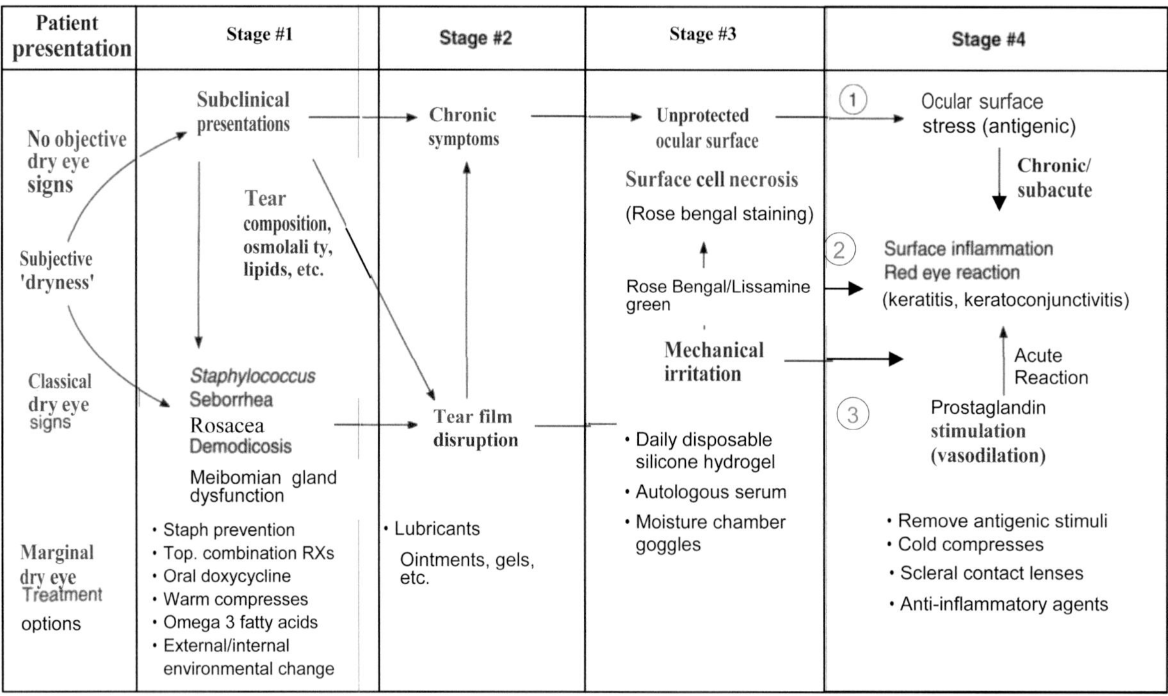

FIGURE 5.19 Marginal dry eye stages and conversion (flow diagram).

- Tear film instability
  - Produce hyperosmolarity that activates osmotic/mechanical stress mechanisms
  - Inflammatory cells are produced
  - Ongoing inflammation initiates ocular surface disease
- Usually a positive TBUT will develop during this stage as well as early corneal changes (erosion, fluorescein staining), especially with contact lens wear
- Management considerations must now focus on protection of the ocular surface (e.g., lubrication therapy) and immediate introduction of treatment of the primary cause (lids or lacrimal gland) if such treatment has not already been initiated

iii. *Stage 3: Corneal exposure*
- Without therapies through the earlier two stages, the cornea has now lost its protective lubricating effects from the tear film
- Subjectively, the patient will begin to experience considerable increase in corneal irritation
- Objectively, exposure and mechanical irritation to the corneal epithelium will begin to produce coalescing fluorescein staining (band region to diffuse) and rose bengal/lissamine staining (on conjunctiva as well) secondary to increasing epithelial erosion and death and devitalization of surface cells
- Treatment steps must be aimed at protecting the corneal surface from further damage

iv. *Stage 4: Inflammatory "conversion"*
- The viscous cycle has started
- The third stage has placed considerable stress on the corneal surface in numerous ways
  - The unprotected ocular surface has begun to disrupt the "homeostatic" balance (physiological, biochemical, and so forth) of the cornea, producing a chronic, insidious infla mmogenic/immunogenic/antigenic/auto antigenic stimulus on the ocular surface tissue converting the unprotected stressful tissue environment into a surface inflammatory response (keratitis)
  - Necrotic debris accumulating on the ocular surface from the devitalized and dying cornea and conjunctival epithelial cells, begins to serve as toxic, autoantigenic material, resulting in a chronic to subacute stimulus converting the unprotected ocular surface into an inflamed tissue (keratoconjunctivitis)
  - The mechanical irritation to the cornea initiates the release of prostaglandins (strong vasodilators), which potentiates rapid vasodilation and an acute red eye reaction
  - This stage of the marginal dry eye syndrome has "fully converted" the noninflammatory causes and effects described in the first three stages into a classic clinical inflammatory response, which will now require standard anti-inflammatory/immunosuppressive therapies

E. Foreign Bodies[22]

Subjective

- Usually obvious history of foreign body (FB) entering eye
- Patient's discomfort ranges from mild to very severe
- History should confirm "when, how, how much (multiple particles), and where" accident occurred

1. Also, careful determination of what kind of matter entered eye
2. Was entry of a "high-velocity" (penetrating) nature or a "soft entry" (embedded superficially)
3. Industrial versus domestic accident?

- Common histories
  1. Objects falling into eye (e.g., rust off muffler while working under car, or fiberglass from ceiling tile)
  2. Windblown particle(s)
  3. Grinding wheel projectile or particle(s) from a hammered surface ("high velocity projectiles")
  4. Discrete matter rubbed in and embedded
- Frequently history of entry is 24 to 72 hours earlier
  1. Symptoms tend to increase or become annoying
  2. Metallic FBs (with resultant rust ring and basement membrane or anterior stromal staining) are most common delayed presentations

Objective

- Distinct appearance of immovable, embedded particle (or multiple particles) on corneal epithelium (with and without slit lamp)
- Frequently a whitish-gray surrounding area of edema or dense infiltrates (Coat's white ring; Figure 5.20) or hemosiderosis (rust ring; Figure 5.21)
- Associated foreign-body tracking (FBT) may be present
- Lid spasms and hyperlacrimation (common) usually make initial assessment difficult (before topical anesthetic)
- FB may be raised above epithelial surface or flush (and often covered) with epithelium
- Other ocular signs like those "associated reactions in deep corneal epithelial abrasion" (see Table 5.2) are usually present relative to degree of involvement
- Occasionally, endothelium may show a faint to pronounced infiltrative ring directly behind site of FB (called annular keratopathy of Payreau)
  1. Secondary immune or infiltrative response to trauma (including FB, abrasion, or contusion injury)
  2. Will resolve within days after FB removal or may "convert" into continuing inflammation

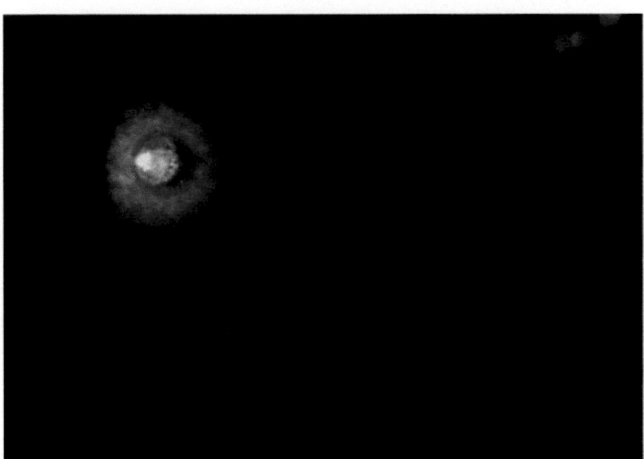

FIGURE 5.20 Coat's white ring or an infiltrative, edematous ring surrounding a non-metallic foreign body (granite). Easily observable with direct and indirect illumination. This ring will self-limit within 1 to 2 weeks of removal of the foreign body.

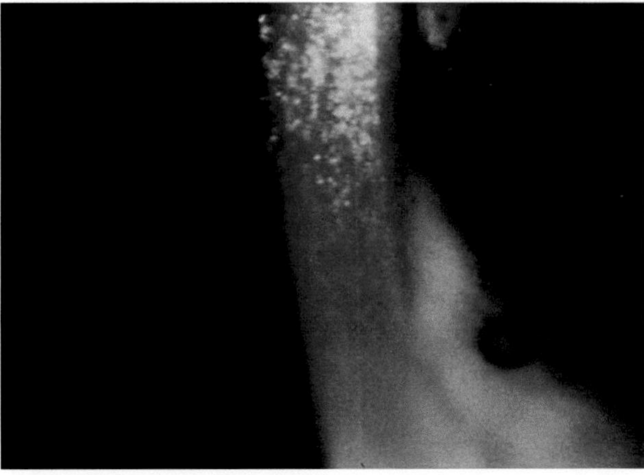

FIGURE 5.21 Rust ring (hemosiderosis) caused by a metallic foreign body of 4-day duration.

Assessment

- Most important to rule out penetration or perforation (see also Corneal Abrasion, above)
- Determine epithelial depth of FB
  1. By history
  2. By slit-lamp optic section (parallelepiped)
  3. By preliminary removal techniques (irrigation)
- Rule out (by history and physical exam) multiple particles
  1. On cornea
  2. On conjunctiva, cul-de-sacs, and lids
  3. Evert and double-evert eyelids
- Evaluate associated reactions and risks
  1. Anterior uveitis
  2. Infectious keratitis (bacterial, fungal ulcer)
  3. Check associated reactions in deep corneal abrasion (see Table 5.2)

Plan and Follow-Up: Foreign Bodies

(See also Appendix 4)

- Stromal (penetrating) FBs should be assessed and treated as penetrating or perforating abrasion or laceration
  1. Probability of permanent scarring and visual loss
  2. Specialty consultation indicated
- Superficially embedded epithelial foreign matter amenable to non-invasive (non-surgical) removal is best treated by properly trained, accessible primary level practitioners
  1. All foreign matter must be removed completely from the corneal epithelium to relieve symptoms and protect eye from potential risks of infection or scarring
  2. All secondary associated reactions should also be treated to relieve and protect patient
- Topical anesthetic drops should be administered in-office (*only*) every 30 to 60 seconds for 1 to 2 minutes before examination and any removal procedure
  1. Usually provides optimal anesthesia for approximately 15 to 20 minutes
  2. If examination and procedural care exceeds length of effective anesthesia, additional dosage(s) are safe and indicated
- Many time-tested techniques and tools are widely used for non-surgical removal of corneal foreign bodies

1. Non-surgical (non-invasive) being defined as no tissue incision, excision, resection, ablation, or cutting, and closing procedures involved in the techniques
2. Commonly performed by non-surgical primary level practitioners as well as trained non-professional medical personnel (e.g., emergency medical technicians, military medics, athletic trainers)

- "Do's and Don'ts" of a dozen of the most commonly used superficial corneal FB removal procedures
  1. Matchbook technique (Figure 5.22)
     a. For removal of superficial FBs outside an office setting (e.g., at home, outdoors)
     b. Rip a fresh paper match from a matchbook without touching the ripped, serrated end
     c. This untouched end is perfect for lifting (by capillary action) small superficial particles off the corneal surface
     d. No specific follow-up treatment is indicated
  2. Forced irrigation technique (Figure 5.23)
     a. For removal of superficial FBs in or out of office
     b. Use balanced ophthalmic irrigating solution in plastic squeeze (squirt) irrigating bottle (e.g., B&L Eye Wash, Alcon Eye Stream)
     c. Direct a high-powered stream at edge of FB
     d. Treatment may include prophylactic antibiotic ointment 1× (in office) and ad lib lubricants and warm packs for 12 to 24 hours
  3. Sweeping swab technique (Figure 5.24)
     a. For removal of superficial FB when nothing else is available
        i. Not a highly preferable technique because of its secondary disruption of excess epithelium (from oversized tip)
        ii. No harm done
     b. Wet cotton-tipped swab with saline or water and pick (usually "sweep") FB off surface
     c. Treatment is (optional) antibiotic 1× and ad lib lubricants and warm packs for 12 to 24 hours

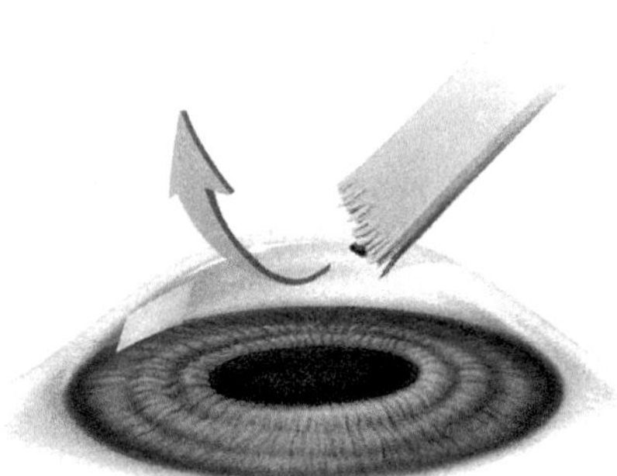

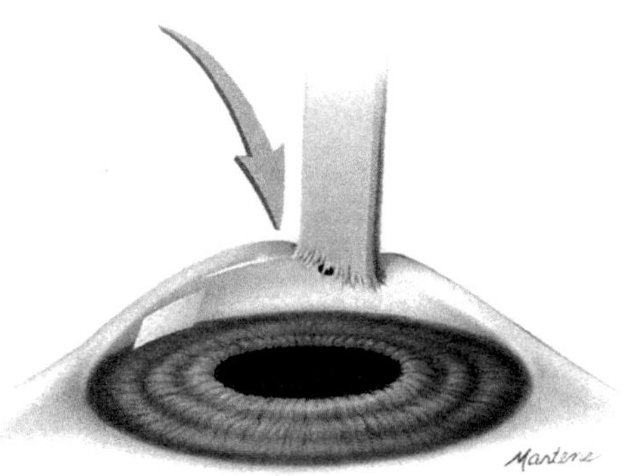

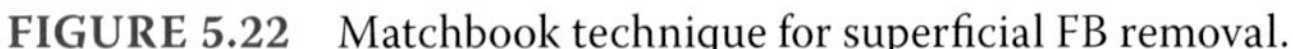
FIGURE 5.22 Matchbook technique for superficial FB removal.

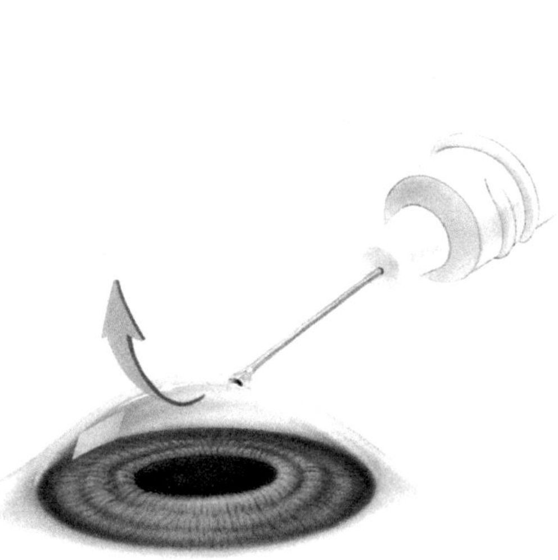

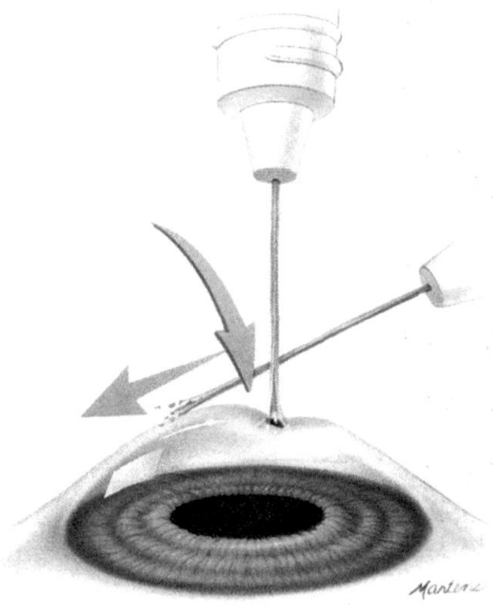

FIGURE 5.23 Forced irrigation technique for superficial FB removal.

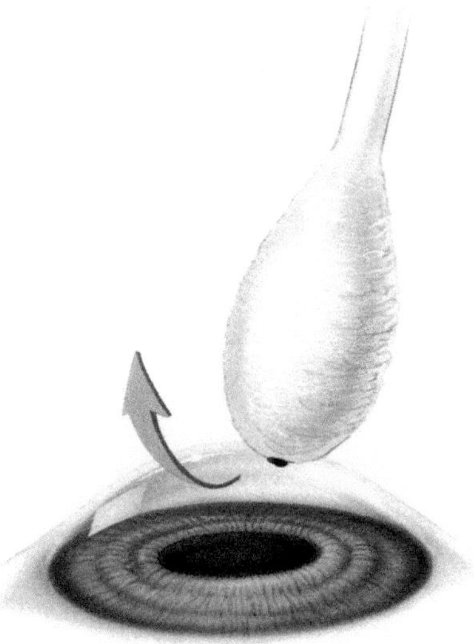

Do sweep directly over small area.

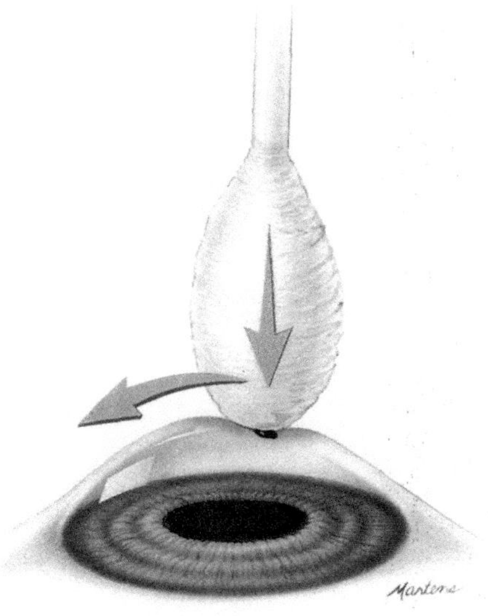

Don't press down on foreign body or sweep over too much corneal surface.

FIGURE 5.24 Sweeping swab technique for superficial FB removal.

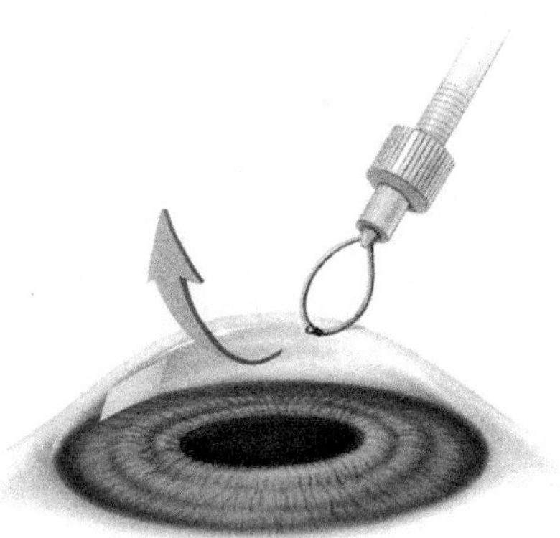

Do tease edges all around until foreign body lifts off completely.

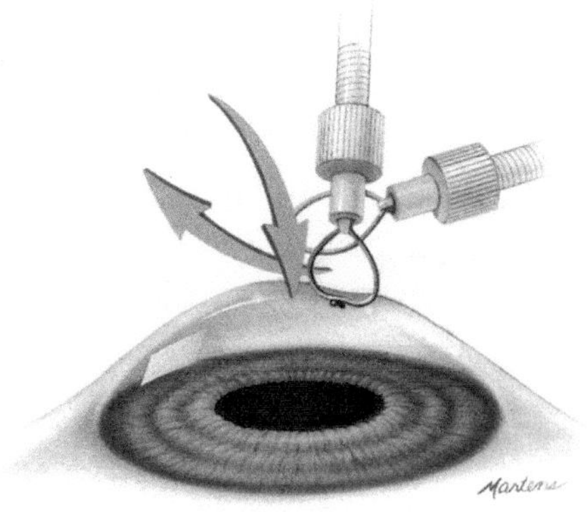

Don't be hesitant and miss cornea completely or press down directly on foreign body.

FIGURE 5.25 Bailey loop technique for partially embedded FB removal.

4. Bailey loop technique (Figure 5.25)
    a. For removal of partially embedded FB partially removed by someone with "heavy hands" or who was concerned with penetrating Bowman's layer with sharp instrument (highly unlikely with proper technique)
    b. Also, good technique for removal of FBs in children who cannot sit still or who may move during procedure
    c. Use Bailey nylon loop in aggressive, teasing movements at edges of FB (penetration virtually impossible with this technique)
    d. Post-procedure treatment per abrasion protocol
5. Needle technique (Figure 5.26)
    a. For removal of partially or deeply embedded FBs
    b. Use common commercially available hypodermic needles (18-, 20-, 22-, or 25-gauge and lengths 5/8, 11/2, or 2 inches)
    c. No syringe needed, although some do use needle without detaching at base
    d. Hold needle directly on shaft or at small plastic or metal flange
    e. Use point of needle to lift edges or loosen overlying cells
    f. Use side of beveled tip to loosen, lift, and lever entire FB for final removal
    g. Avoid snagging basement membrane when using sharp point (usually produces tugging feel, as if snagging canvas and may produce some transient striate lines)
    h. Cellular epithelium usually feels like gelatin consistency with no resistance
    i. Procedure can also be used to remove rust rings (after removal of metallic FB)
    j. Post-procedure treatment per abrasion protocol
6. Cockburn curve technique (Figure 5.27)

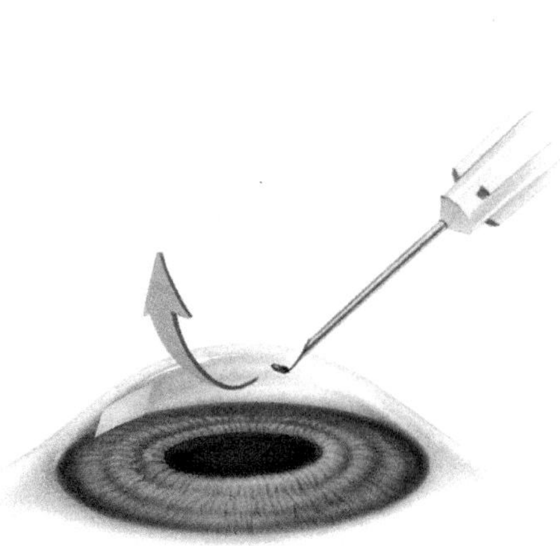

Do approach foreign body edge and then lever and lift edges.

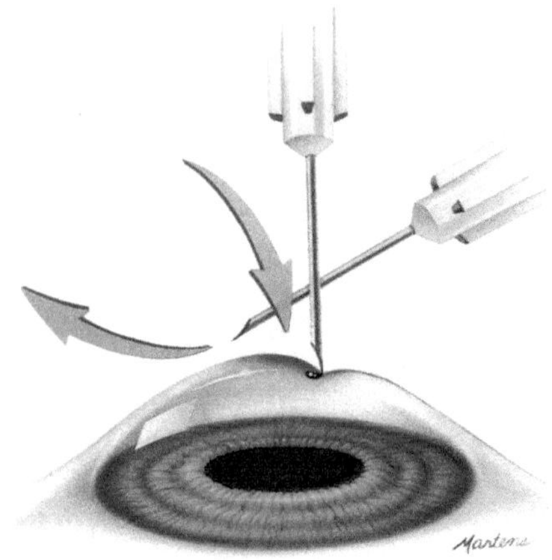

Don't approach cornea with "perpendicular plunge," but conversely, don't be so tentative as to miss foreign body completely.

FIGURE 5.26 Needle technique for embedded FB removal.

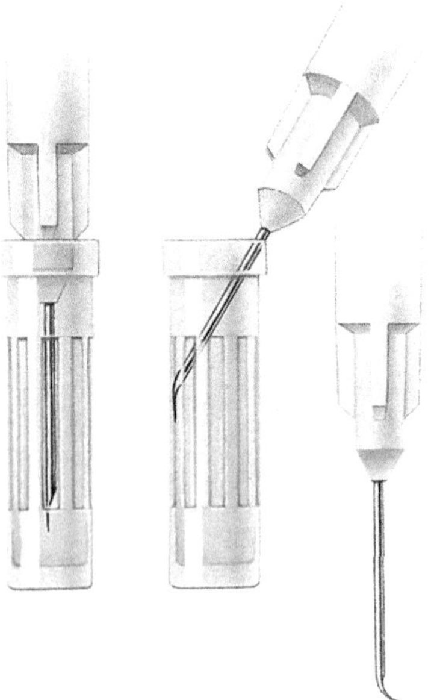

FIGURE 5.27 Cockburn curve technique for embedded FB removal: removing the needle from the jacket.

   a. For removal of partially or deeply embedded FBs
   b. Observe back side of bevel on point of hypodermic needle before removing it from its hard plastic jacket (standard casing for needle)
   c. On removing needle from jacket, drag the back side of the bevel firmly up the side wall causing it to bend in an inward, curved fashion
   d. This curved bend provides a safer method of using a hypodermic needle with minimal risk of snagging basement membrane, and almost no risk of penetration
   e. Procedure is similar to "needle" technique described above (Figure 5.28)
7. Golf club spud technique (Figure 5.29)
   a. For removal of partially or deeply embedded FBs
   b. Commonly used procedure (perhaps more than needles) because of its ease and safety
      i. Curved tip of spud creates a natural lifting and levering effect while protecting against snagging of basement membrane or penetration
      ii. Sharp edges and cupped shape of spud help loosen and lift FB
   c. Limiting factor of spud is relatively large size of head (versus needle tip) for small FBs
   d. May take some extra epithelium because of size
   e. Follow-up per abrasion protocol
8. Jeweler's forceps technique (Figure 5.30)
   a. For removal of partially or deeply embedded FBs
   b. Easy and efficient procedure for large, deep FB that needs a great deal of edge teasing and lift
      i. Often FB remains partially embedded or adherent during edge lifting
      ii. Working on one edge and other edge(s) binds back down into epithelium
   c. Jeweler's forceps can first be used with tip closed (creating sharp, needle-like tip effect) to loosen and lift edge(s)
   d. With edge raised above epithelial surface, forceps are then opened and used to grasp and lift FB off cornea
   e. Follow-up per abrasion protocol
9. Rust ring removal technique (Figure 5.31)
   a. For removal of hemosiderotic cell staining or rust rings with particles embedded in epithelium
   b. Hemosiderosis (oxidizing of metallic FB in epithelium, i.e., rusting) occurs within 2 to 48 hours after embedding
   c. Often, patient is not seen soon enough (frequently, even beyond the 48-hour mark), and significant hemosiderosis occurs

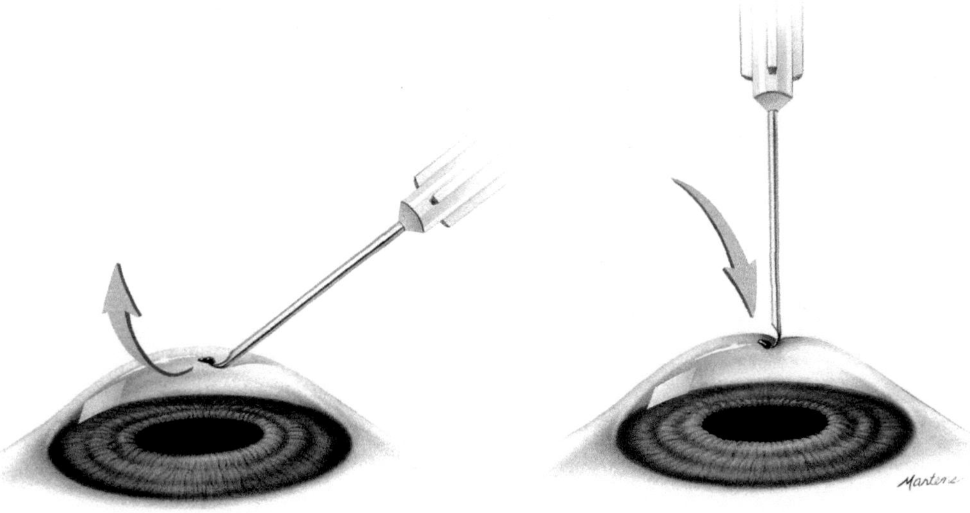

FIGURE 5.28 Cockburn curve technique for embedded FB removal.

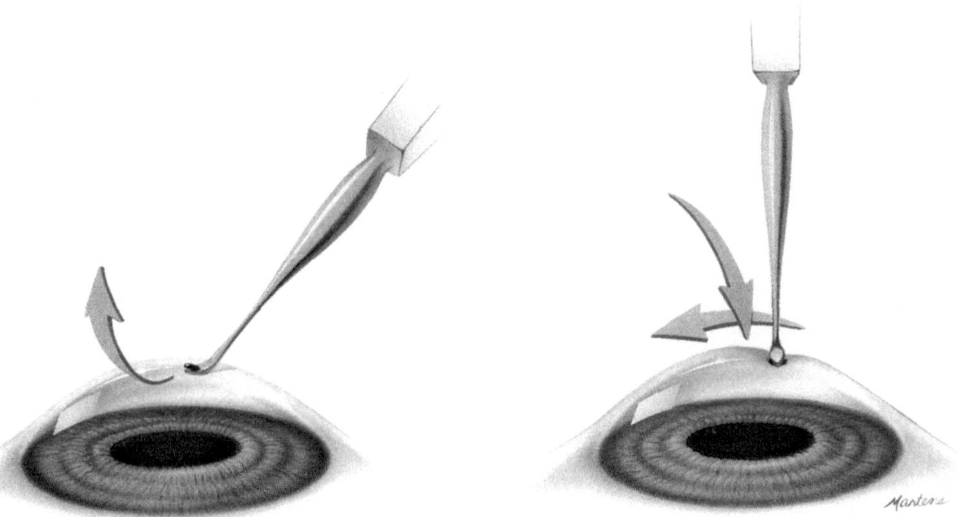

FIGURE 5.29 Golf-club spud technique for embedded FB removal.

   i. Slight benefit in delay is necrosing, softening effect to rust ring permitting easier removal (sluffing off with very gentle manipulation)
   ii. However, care should not be delayed purposely for such effect
   iii. Delays also lead to further staining of basement membrane and potential scar to Bowman' s (stromal) layer
d. All hemosiderotic epithelial cells or oxidized particles (from FB) must be removed to avoid chronic weakening, irritation, re-erosion of epithelium, and risk of infection
e. However, staining of basement membrane and Bowman's layer from prolonged (greater than 48-hour) exposure to oxidation can produce permanent rust ring
   i. Awareness of basement membrane or Bowman's layer involvement usually apparent during procedure as "canvas" texture versus gelatinous (epithelial cell) consistency
   ii. Basement membrane staining need not be removed in lieu of regeneration of new (clear) membrane within 8 to 12 weeks versus "ripping" membrane to remove stain

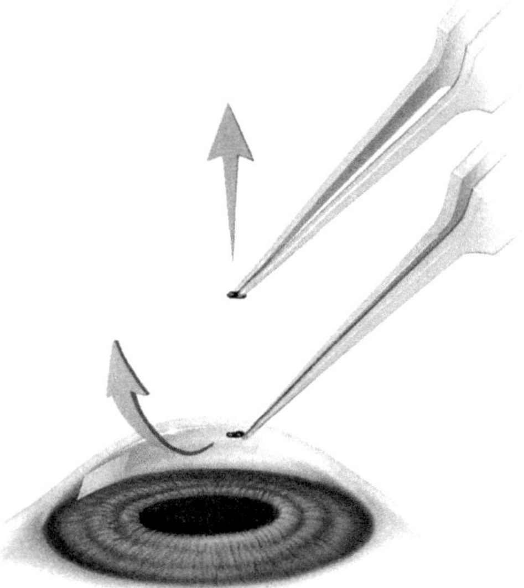

Do loosen edges with closed forceps and lever upwards, then grasp with open forceps and lift off.

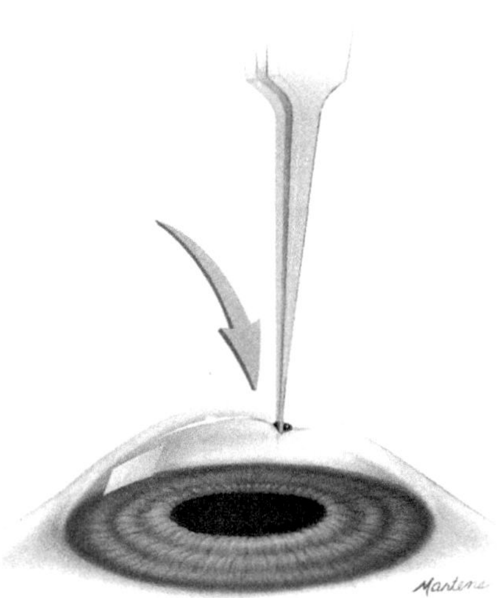

Don't attempt to grasp embedded foreign body with opened forceps without loosening edges first.

FIGURE 5.30 Jeweler's forceps technique for embedded FB removal.

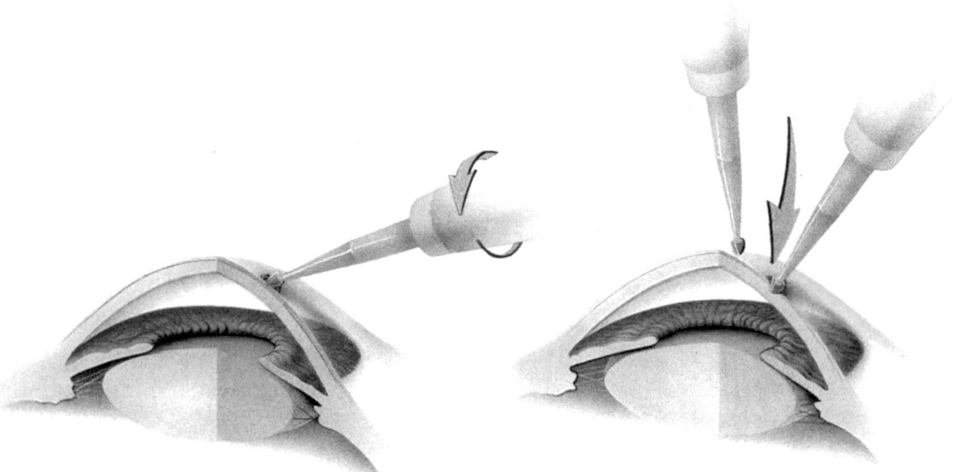

Do lightly drill epithelium down to basement membrane in circular motion.

Don't press down too lightly while drilling, or, conversely, press too firmly, producing snagging or ripping of basement membrane.

FIGURE 5.31 Rust ring removal technique with power drill.

and produce potential of chronic recurrent corneal erosion (RCE) syndrome

iii. Scraping Bowman's layer will result in leucomatous scar usually larger and denser than ring stain

iv. Permanently stained Bowman's (stroma) will not produce adverse effects described for epithelial cells

v. Thus, it is best not to attempt removal of hemosiderotic stains from basement membrane or Bowman's layer

f. Power drill(s) (using fine to coarse burrs) are used to "chew up" stained epithelial cells and oxidizing particles after metallic FB itself is removed from corneal surface

   i. Medium to fine burr preferable

   ii. Coarse burrs (on drill) tend to destroy extra epithelium and may even snag basement membrane or Bowman's layer, with resulting striae or leucoma

g. Limiting factor with power drills (minimized with "Alger brush") is "humming" sound, which tends to alarm an already apprehensive patient

   i. Reassure patient as best as possible

   ii. Certainly, never show the drill (nor any "ominous"-looking instruments)

   h. Follow-up per abrasion protocol
10. Alger brush removal technique (Figure 5.32)
   a. All indications, contraindications, and adverse effects same as with all power drills
   b. Procedure same as with standard power drill
   c. Difference with Alger brush is centrifugal force mechanism, which functions to stop drill if too much downward pressure is exerted onto cornea during procedure
      i. Thus, risk of basement membrane or Bowman's layer snagging or ripping is minimized
      ii. Penetration risk is almost entirely eliminated
   d. Adverse effect continues to be the patient apprehension created by the "drilling" sounds
11. Hand-held burr technique (Figure 5.33)

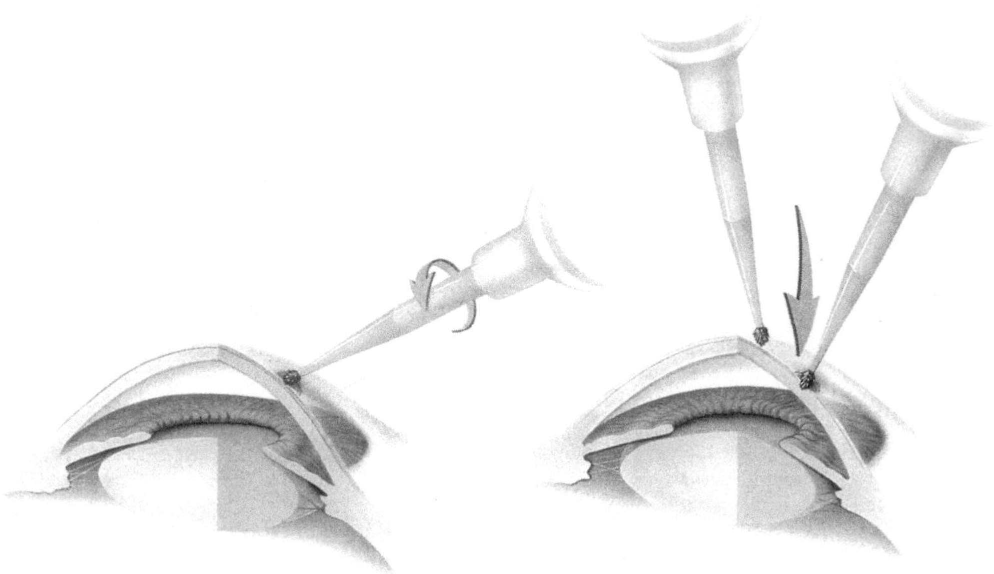

FIGURE 5.32 Alger brush removal technique for rust ring removal.

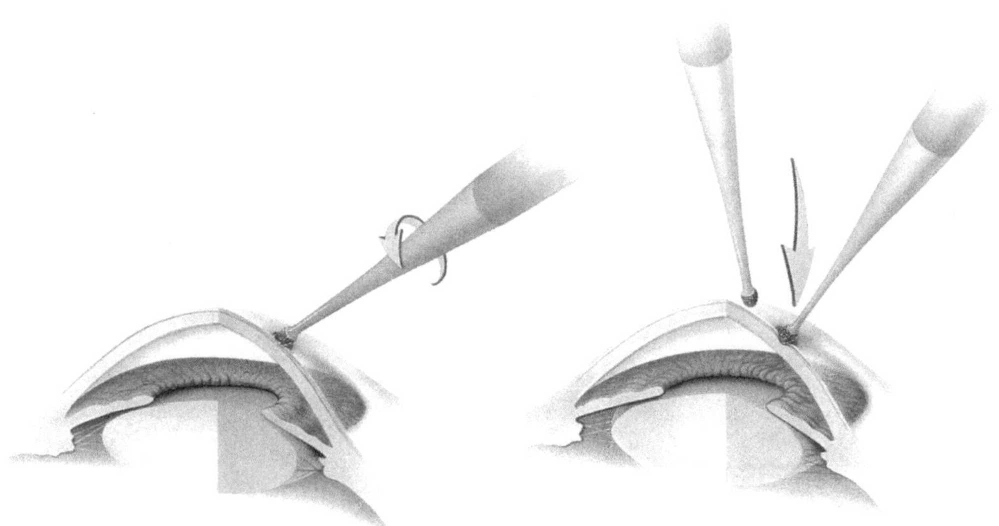

FIGURE 5.33 Hand-held burr technique for rust ring removal.

a. Used to reduce patient apprehension in rust ring removal (with power drills and Alger brush) and associated drill sounds
b. Hold coarse dental burr between tips of fingers, and spin it as it's held directly on rust ring and hemosiderotic epithelium
c. Requires a fairly steady hand but works quite effectively with no drill sounds
d. Principle and procedures remain exactly the same as with power drill or Alger brush use

12. Magnetic technique
a. The use of magnetized instrument to lift metallic FB off corneal surface
b. Hand instruments made with blunt magnetic end for removal of superficial, non-embedded FBs
c. Generally works poorly unless more sophisticated, expensive electromagnets (used surgically for intraocular FBs) are employed
d. For in-office, non-surgical, primary care of superficial FBs, magnetic techniques are not contraindicated, but certainly are inefficient, given the large array of simple highly effective alternative procedures

- Other considerations in corneal removal of FB
1. Use left and right hands for opposite eyes if possible
a. If not, use dominant hand and cross over face when necessary
b. Have patient turn head as much as possible in slit-lamp head rest to minimize interference from patient's nose
2. Slit-lamp hand rests are available to stabilize hand during procedure
a. Head rest can be lowered to point where examiner's elbow can rest (and be stabilized) on instrument table
b. Fingers (on instrument hand) can be stabilized by resting fourth and fifth digits on patient's face
3. Instruments used are readily available through ophthalmic instrument companies and direct from surgical instrument wholesalers
a. Storz: highest quality and very expensive
b. Sklar: high quality and less expensive
c. Wexler: high quality and less expensive
d. Others also available
4. Instrument maintenance and cleaning (Figure 5.34)
a. Keep in a stainless-steel tray of Zephiran HCl 1:750 (benzalkonium chloride) with antirust tablets (change weekly)
b. Instruments can also be stored dry and rinse before use with Zephiran or alcohol
i. Rinse Zephiran or alcohol off thoroughly with water or saline before use
ii. Reclean and dry instruments for storage
c. Heat sterilization (autoclaving) and sterile wrapping for storage is ideal procedure

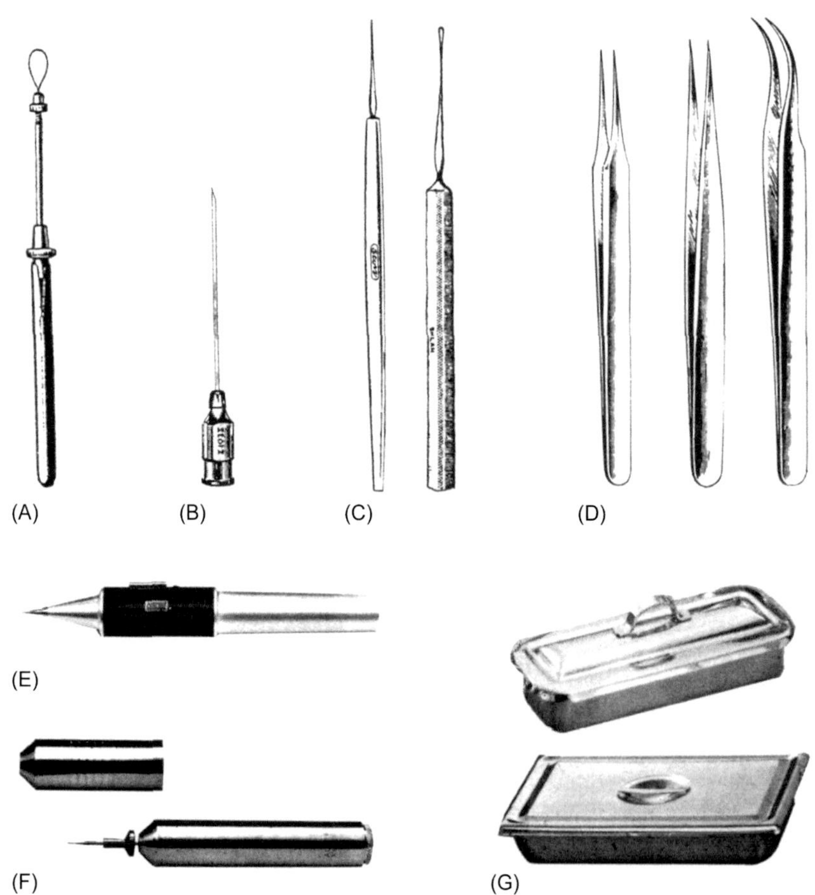

FIGURE 5.34 Common instruments and accessories for FB removal. **(A)** Bailey loop. **(B)** Hypodermic needle. **(C)** Golf club spuds. **(D)** Jeweler's forceps (assorted shapes and sizes). **(E)** Battery-powered drill. **(F)** Alger brush. **(G)** Assorted instrument trays.

F. Recurrent Corneal Erosion (RCE) Syndrome[23]

Background Information

1. Review "Background Information" for epithelial basement membrane (EBM) in Section II. D. of this chapter (Epithelial Basement Membrane Disorders)
2. Any damage to EBM or Bowman's layer causes weakening or loss of adhesions between epithelium and (anterior) stroma
3. These adhesions are produced by a sticky collagen layer on the anterior face of Bowman's layer (collagen type VII) and with finger-like projections (hemidesmosomes) off the basement membrane into the epithelium
4. Basal epithelial cells require at least 8 to 12 weeks to regenerate or repair EBM
5. Persistent, chronic adverse (e.g., dystrophy, diabetes) stimuli with or without acute (or subacute) trauma to cornea can produce prolonged, loose, weak adhesions, resulting in unstable corneal epithelial layer
6. Finally, any injury, irritant, or aggravant to the EBM will leave it unstable, weak, and vulnerable to recurrent breakdown (erosion) and re-erosion for its regenerating period of at least 8 to 12 weeks or more and, if permanently damaged, possibly indefinitely

Subjective

- Two classic histories associated with RCE syndrome
  1. Secondary to corneal injury
  2. Spontaneous (patient denying history of injury)
- Symptoms are typical of corneal irritation and tend to be moderate to severe
  1. "Sandy, gritty" irritation or pain if severe
  2. FB sensation
  3. Lid spasms
  4. Photophobia
- Most presentations occur upon waking (morning or AM syndrome)
  1. Probably secondary to increased edema during sleep (with lids closed and tear evaporation reduced)
  2. Combination of loose epithelial junctures (edema) and disrupted EBM (causing unstable epithelium) aggravated by over dry, unlubricated surface lid opening
- Usually a unilateral presentation (associated with history of recent, or perhaps old, ipsilateral injury)
  1. Occasionally presentation may be bilateral with one eye usually worse than other especially with EBMD
  2. History may or may not reveal underlying associated disease process (e.g., dystrophy, diabetes)
  3. Specific disease or trauma history often lacking making diagnosis exclusively physical and presumptive
- Recurring nature is definitive historical information
  1. Recurrences could be proximal to injury or recurrent after extended (weeks to months) delay
  2. Recurrences may be frequent (e.g., daily) or infrequent (monthly or less)
  3. Acute phase of recurrences may be minor (mildly symptomatic and self-limiting, as in waking) to dramatically acute, painful, and disabling
- When history directly associated with acute injury
  1. Symptom duration may be days to years
  2. Injury is usually of a tangential, cutting nature versus perpendicular (blunt) type (e.g., FB)
     a. Paper cut
     b. Fingernail injury
     c. Sprung tree branch or twig
     d. Glancing type injuries to corneal surface
- When history is spontaneous without associated injury
  1. Careful questioning critical for subtle clues
  2. Usually chronic, low-grade irritation (unilateral or bilateral) with intermittent acute episodes
  3. Medical history significant
  4. Active medication history valuable
  5. Family history of similar problem (dystrophy?)

Objective

- Milder presentations show typical corneal abrasion signs (with associated reactions)
  1. May be as mild as SPK reactions
  2. Often, morning syndrome symptoms may persist longer than observable physical signs
- Re-erosions (abrasions) secondary to injury generally occur in same corneal area as original abrasion
  1. Recurrence may be mild SPK in area
  2. Generally (unfortunately) re-erosion is equal or (more frequently) worse than original abrasion
- Recurrent erosions in the area of Hudson–Stahli's line tend to recur more frequently
- Moderate to severe recurrent erosions tend to show certain classic characteristics (may be diagnostic in absent, vague, or suspicious histories)
  1. Generally, produce inappropriate amounts of associated edema
  2. Edema often produces (immediately or during slow healing) a brownish haze to the involved epithelium (brawny edema)
  3. Abraded area tends to create loose edges with moderate to large epithelial flaps commonly forming
  4. Healing rate is generally slower than the normal rate for a similar abrasion
- Central-ward location and tendency towards dense secondary edema produce substantial visual disturbances
- Physical exam and evaluation should be like abrasion criteria used for deep corneal epithelial abrasions

Assessment

(See also Appendix 3)

- Initial history should determine injury versus spontaneous nature to RCE
- If injury involved, precise nature and time original episode should be documented, especially if original care for initial episode was provided by another practitioner
- If RCE is spontaneous (i.e., no associated injury, proximal or remote), history and examination must differentiate the following possibilities of syndrome
  1. Corneal dystrophy (check for bilateral signs and check other family members)
     a. EBMDs
        i. Most common cause of spontaneous RCE syndrome
        ii. Examine both eyes (and family members) carefully for maps, dots, fingerprints
     b. Other anterior dystrophies (e.g., Reis–Buckler's)
     c. Stromal dystrophies (e.g., lattice, macular, granular)
     d. Endothelial dystrophies (Fuchs')

2. Prior chemical or thermal burns
3. Diabetes mellitus (cause of chronic basement membrane problems)

- RCE syndrome is not uncommon in post-operative patients (e.g., cataracts, retinal detachment surgery, refractive surgical procedures)
  1. May be from secondary epithelial trauma or endothelial disruption and resultant secondary edema
  2. Good reason to evaluate endothelium carefully before referring for elective ocular surgeries
     a. Poor endothelium (e.g., dystrophy, low cell count secondary to age degeneration) significantly increases risk of postoperative RCE
     b. Good ophthalmic surgeon will usually do endothelial count before surgery
  3. Radial keratotomy has shown almost a 20% increase in permanent (greater than 1-year regenerative period) EBM changes, thus increasing risk of RCE syndrome as long-term sequelae of the procedure

Plan: Recurrent Corneal Erosion Syndrome

- Acute presentations of RCE are treated according to normal and customary care for corneal abrasions
  1. Evaluate abrasion criteria
  2. Treat associated reactions (see Table 5.2) according to care code for deep corneal epithelial abrasions (see Table 5.3)
  3. Follow abrasion protocol
- Healing rates for RCE tend to be 1 to 2 days slower than rate charts (see Table 5.1) for non-erosion deep abrasion
- Management for moderate RCE (25% to 50% of cornea or more than one to two recurrences), same as acute presentations (described above), plus
  1. Warm packs (after patch) q4h for 2 to 3 weeks
  2. Hypertonic drops (after patch) q4h for 4 to 6 weeks and optional NSAID drops
  3. Hypertonic ointment (after patch or bandage soft lens) tid for 8 to 12 weeks
  4. Recheck monthly for 4 to 6 months
- Management for severe RCE (greater than 50% of cornea or chronic recurrences) same as moderate (above), plus
  1. Mechanically debride any loose epithelial flaps
     a. Use 1 to 2 drops of topical anesthetic every 15 to 30 seconds for 2 to 3 minutes to soften epithelium and anesthetize cornea
     b. Use wetted cotton swab, spatula, spud, or jeweler's forceps
     c. Remove flaps by pulling or sweeping edges toward center of abraded area
     d. Do not pull flaps directly upward or outward
     e. Remove all flaps down to tight, firm edges
     f. Procedure will increase overall geography of abrasion (possibly by 50% to 100%)
     g. Avoid chemical (toxic) methods of debriding (e.g., chelating agents, EDTA [ethylene diaminetetraacetic acid], alcohol, ether)
  2. Bilaterally patch patient for (maximum) 48 to 72 hours
     a. Bilateral patching will completely immobilize eyes
     b. Follow pressure patching protocol, primarily for eroded eye (see Table 5.4)
     c. Repatch daily for 2 to 3 days (maximum)
        i. Any additional patching beyond 72 hours will probably be non-productive due to advancing edema (secondary to patching)
        ii. If cornea not resolving within 72 hours, bandage soft lens should be considered
     d. Counsel and reassure patient carefully regarding bilateral patching procedure
        i. Patient usually apprehensive and concerned over procedure
        ii. Educate to reasons for bilateral patch
        iii. Should also advise in advance of possible need to retreat (repatch)
  3. An alternative to extended pressure patching or after successful or unsuccessful patching therapy, soft contact lens bandage therapy may be administered (Figure 5.35; see also Table 5.5)
     a. Fit involved eye (both eyes optional) only after resolution of acute inflammatory reaction(s) (i.e., red eye involvement)
     b. In chronically re-eroding corneas (with or without bandage lens wear), an intensive course of hypertonic ointment (q2–3h) for 1 week prior to lens wear (or re-wear) may improve prognosis of soft lens bandaging
     c. Extended wear for at least 8 to 12 weeks
        i. Provides comfort and protection
        ii. Extended wear (7-day max wear and then lens replacement) affords constant protection (especially against AM syndrome)
        iii. 8- to 12-week period permits regeneration of new basement membrane without interference of re-erosions
     d. Fit thin lens design of high Dk, silicone hydrogel disposable lens (e.g., Acuvue Oasys, Air Optix Night & Day Aqua)
     e. Fit plano or low-powered lens
        i. Do not fit high-powered lens with thick center or edge
        ii. Aphakes must be monitored closely
     f. Lens should be stable
     g. Hypertonic drops can be used over lens (if not irritating) tid to qid
     h. Prophylactic gentamicin or tobramycin drops should be used

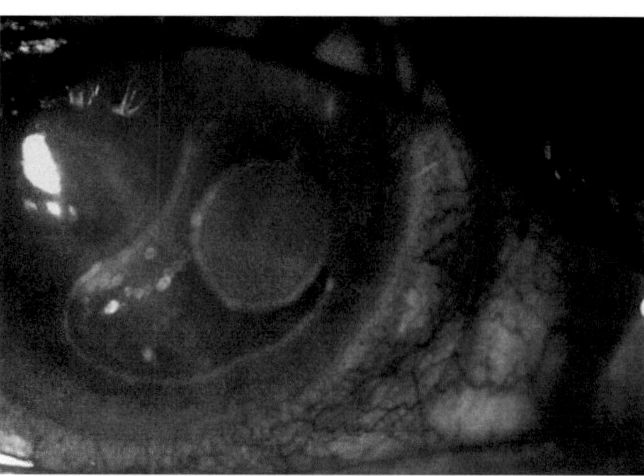

FIGURE 5.35 Recurrent corneal erosion protected by a soft contact lens bandage producing an air and tear vacuole under the lens in the abraded area.

i. qid for first 3 to 4 weeks
ii. tid for second 3 to 4 weeks
iii. hs for duration of extended wear
iv. Maintain qid with any positive staining
i. Patient should be instructed to remove lens on any discomfort or injection and call immediately
j. Recheck patient weekly for first 3 to 4 weeks and then biweekly for duration of bandaging
4. Approximately 75% of all bandaging is successful after first therapy (for 8 to 12 weeks)
   a. Exacerbations or early discontinuations will require additional therapeutic period
   b. Some patients may require multiple periods
   c. Almost all will heal eventually
5. Other options if RCE continues
   a. Autologous serum drops
   b. Amniotic membrane
   c. Doxycycline 50 mg bid (MMP-9 inhibitor)
   d. Topical steroid drops (e.g., loteprednol) bid to qid for 2–3 weeks
6. Anterior stromal puncture, phototherapeutic keratectomy (PTK), and diamond burr polishing for RCEs non-responsive to medical management

Follow-Up

- If standard approaches to acute presentations prove unsuccessful (re-erosions), attempt more intensive therapeutic regimen, or introduce preventive measures, such as protective shields during sleep (for sleep recurrences) and instructions on no rubbing
- After successful intensive therapy (prolonged care, debridement, extended lens bandaging, amniotic membrane, autologous serum, etc.), continue hypertonic drops and ointments (hs) for 3 to 6 months
- RCE syndrome will usually heal if underlying cause is properly diagnosed and remediated (if possible)
  1. If condition is chronic, patient must be instructed on preventive measures and advised of need for indefinite continuation of procedures
  2. Patient can be reassured that preventive measures will reduce and preclude risks of recurrences and permanent visual loss
- Constant patient advocacy and reassurance is critical in the successful long-term management of the RCE syndrome due to multiple factors
  1. Prolonged (chronic) nature of syndrome
  2. Pain and discomfort associated and resultant willingness of patient to comply if properly educated and instructed
  3. Patient's constant fear and apprehensions
     a. About permanent vision loss
     b. About lifelong recurrences of severe pain
- Finally, there is significant value (especially for patients) in a positive attitude towards RCE despite seemingly endless course of syndrome
  1. Explain to patient that most, if not all RCE, eventually heals or is controllable without visual loss
  2. Helps patient feel a little better, gives hope and willingness to cooperate and comply
  3. Helps doctor "stay with" a tough disease and treatment regimen to a usual rewarding conclusion

II. Noninflammatory Conditions

A. Congenital Abnormalities

1. Anterior Chamber (Cleavage) Syndromes

a. Synonyms
   i. Anterior angle syndromes
   ii. Mesodermal dysgenesis syndromes
   iii. Goniodysgenesis syndromes
   iv. Iridogoniodysgenesis syndromes
   v. Iridocorneal (mesodermal) syndromes
   vi. Axenfeld–Rieger (A–R) syndrome
b. Research suggests an arrest in neural crest cell development (rather than mesodermal dysgenesis) in the third trimester of pregnancy
   i. Theory accounts for the dental, facial, systemic manifestations, and increased A–R syndrome glaucoma risks
   ii. Theory creates differential between AR (neural crest) syndromes and iridocorneal endothelial (ICE) syndromes (true mesodermal abnormalities) with decreased glaucoma risk versus cataract
c. A–R syndrome clinical findings follow a graduating or "stepladder" diagnostic approach (Figure 5.36)

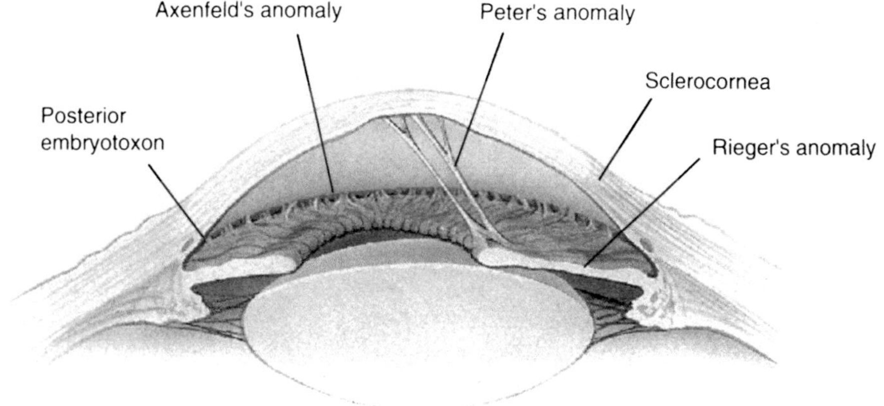

FIGURE 5.36 Composite diagram of A–R and ICE syndromes of the anterior chamber angle and posterior cornea, respectively. The original "stepladder" approach to anterior chamber cleavage syndromes must be reconsidered in light of the varying etiologies (mesodermal or neural crest development) among these clinical entities.

i. Sclerocornea may or may not be an early or mild finding
ii. Posterior embryotoxon
    - Exaggerated, thickened, prominent Schwalbe's line (or ring), usually an invisible demarcation line between trabeculum and posterior cornea
    - Partial or complete bilateral ring
    - Greater at 3- and 9-o'clock positions
    - Frequently visible on gross externals
    - Slit-lamp examination reveals it to be on posterior cornea versus anterior Bowman's layer
    - Best evaluation is by gonioscopy
    - Risk of glaucoma is low, but monitor IOP biannually (even in children with signs)
iii. Axenfeld's anomaly or syndrome (Figure 5.37)
    - Posterior embryotoxon (plus)
    - Prominent iris processes attached to Schwalbe's line (usually abundant)
    - Rarely, pupil abnormalities (e.g., corectopia, dyscoria)
    - Prominent iris sphincter muscle (especially on dilation)

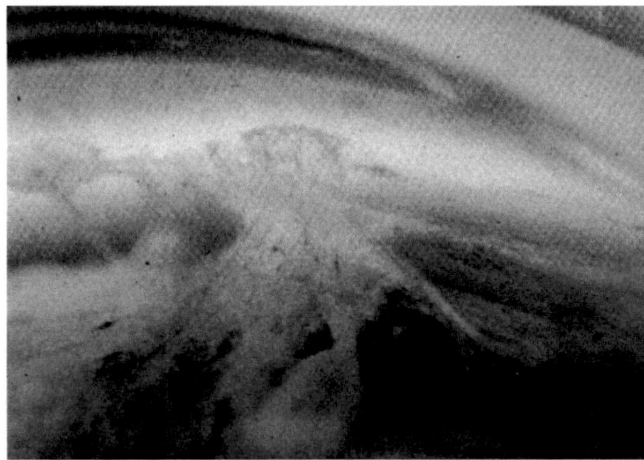

FIGURE 5.37 Axenfeld's anomaly demonstrating a fibrous iris strand adherent to the posterior corneal surface (anterior synechia).

    - Bilateral gonioscopy and diagramming should be done biannually
    - Glaucoma risk from 25% to 50%
    - IOP can rise anytime during life
    - Monitor IOP annually
    - Normal IOP: Axenfeld's anomaly
        - Elevated IOP: Axenfeld's syndrome
        - Associated glaucoma resistant to therapy, so try to refer to a glaucoma specialist
        - Associated with Down syndrome
iv. Rieger's anomaly or syndrome (Figure 5.38)
    - Axenfeld's findings (plus)
    - Iris hypoplasia (i.e., shallow crypts, furrows, and thinned iris stroma)
    - Sphincter muscle prominent with multiple pupillary defects and distortions
    - Often other associated ocular problems (e.g., strabismus, corneal defects)
    - Glaucoma risk from 50% to 75%
    - IOP can rise anytime during life
    - Monitor IOP every 6 to 12 months
    - Anomaly: eye findings only
    - Syndrome: eye findings plus the following:
        - Lower facial abnormalities, including maxillary hypoplasia, flattened nose, and mouth and dental malformations—"funny-looking kids" (FLK) syndromes
        - Other systemic malformations and disorders involving hands, feet, spine, heart, hearing, and occasional mental retardation
v. Peter's anomaly (no longer considered A–R syndrome finding)

d. Differential diagnostic considerations (uncommon mesodermal and other abnormalities) to rule out (Table 5.6)
  i. Peter's anomaly or syndrome
    - Congenital iris hypoplasia
    - Iris strands to posterior cornea, causing posterior keratoconus and leucoma
    - Occasional anterior polar cataract
    - Glaucoma risk about 50% (= syndrome)
    - Child requires early keratoplasty
    - No systemic manifestations

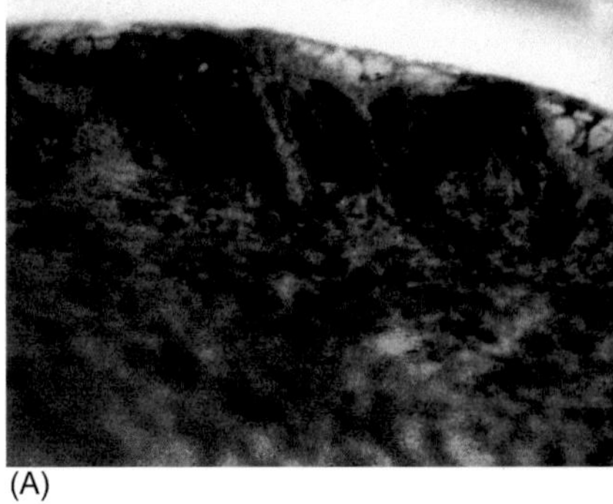

(A)

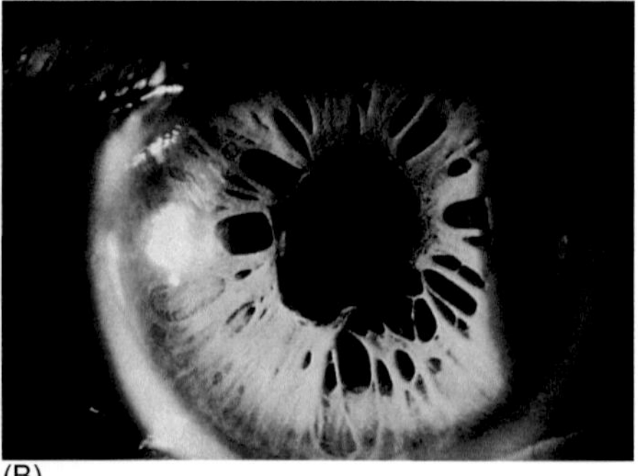

(B)

FIGURE 5.38 **(A)** Rieger's syndrome revealing dense iris processes attached to the posterior cornea at a prominent Swalbe's line (posterior embryotoxon). **(B)** Iris hypoplasia secondary to a thinned iris is most prominent on pupil dilation with distinct radial muscle response and a poor sphincter pupillae reaction.

TABLE 5.6 **Considerations in Anterior Chamber Abnormalities**

	Axenfeld–Rieger Syndromes		Mesodermal Dysgenesis Syndromes		
Considerations	**Axenfeld's**	**Rieger's**	**Peter's**	**PPD**	**ICE**
Age of onset	Congenital	Congenital	Congenital	Congenital or early years	Adolescence
Sex predilection	Equal distribution	Equal distribution	Equal distribution	Equal distribution	Females
Inheritance pattern	Autosomal dominant	Autosomal dominant	Variable	Usually autosomal dominant	Variable
Laterality	Bilateral	Bilateral	80% Bilateral	Bilateral	Unilateral
Posterior embryotoxon	Present	Present	Absent	Absent	Absent
Iris strands (anterior synchiae)	Variable	Prominent	To central cornea	Occasional	Variable
Iris or pupil abnormalities	None	Prominent	Variable	Occasional	Prominent
Corneal involvement	None	None	Central Posterior Keratoconus	Posterior cornea	Edema occasional posterior
Systemic manifestations	Rare	Facial, dental, systemic	None	None	None
Glaucoma risk	25–50%	50–75%	50%	<25%	≈25%

ii. Posterior polymorphous dystrophy (PPD)
   - Occasional iris involvements like A–R syndromes
   - Glaucoma risk less than 25%
   - No systemic manifestations

iii. ICE syndromes
   - Chandler's syndrome (iris atrophy, pupil anomalies, corneal edema, and glaucoma)
   - Progressive (essential) iris atrophy
   - Cogan–Reese syndrome (Chandler's plus iris nevi and ectropion uveae)
   - Posterior embryotoxon never present
   - Glaucoma risk about 25%
   - No systemic manifestations

2. *Megalocornea*[24]

a. A visible horizontal iris diameter of 13 mm or greater
b. 90% in males (X-linked congenital defect)
c. Usually bilateral
d. Often high refractive errors
   i. Especially astigmatism
   ii. May cause reduced best correctable visions
e. Deep anterior chamber with excessive pigmented trabecular meshwork but normal IOP at birth
f. Occasional iridodonesis (tremulous, unstable iris)
g. Adults may experience premature cataract development and glaucoma
h. Most important management consideration is IOP monitoring
   i. Increased risk of elevated IOP
   ii. May occur congenitally or insidiously at any age
   iii. Monitor IOP every 3 to 6 months under 5 to 6 years of age and annually thereafter (for lifetime)
   iv. Increased IOPs (usually difficult to manage) should be referred to glaucoma specialist
i. All other findings can be managed routinely

3. *Microcornea*

a. Visible horizontal iris diameter of 10 mm or less
b. Often associated with systemic or ocular syndrome(s)
   i. May be part of a microphthalmic syndrome
   ii. Consider systemic relationship in FLK syndromes
   iii. If in doubt, refer for pediatric evaluation
c. Associated findings and considerations
   i. High refractive errors

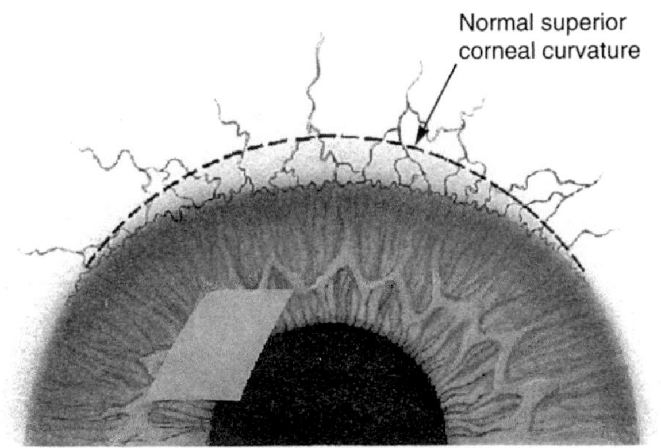

FIGURE 5.39 Sclerocornea reveals a flattened superior corneal dome with prominent limbal vasculature.

   ii. About a 20% risk of increased IOP by adulthood (less than megalocornea risk)
   iii. Anterior chamber syndromes

4. *Sclerocornea*[25]

a. A bilateral, superior prominence of scleral tissue into the corneal zone (Figure 5.39)
   i. Occasionally, inferior involvement produces truncated corneal appearance
   ii. Least likely is 360° involvement, producing the appearance of microcornea
b. Sometimes considered mild stage of anterior chamber syndrome
c. Superficial scleral vessels create prominent limbal arcades, mimicking neovascularization
   i. Arcades anastomose, hence not neovascular
   ii. Also, blood cells usually traceable in and out of corneal zone
d. Other associated findings and considerations
   i. Flat corneas (cornea plana)
   ii. High refractive errors
   iii. Other anterior chamber syndrome signs: monitor IOP annually
   iv. Consider systemic syndromes (e.g., FLK)
e. Always assess and photograph or diagram sclerocornea in general examinations and especially in prefit contact lens evaluations

i. Do not consider it a contraindication for contact lens
ii. Try to avoid chronic edge insult to area by fitting small diameter rigid gas permeable (RGP) or large soft contact lens

5. *Other Congenital Abnormalities*

a. Congenital glaucoma
  i. Central corneal haze
  ii. Descemet's and endothelial folds and tears (Haab's striae)
  iii. Buphthalmos (enlarged globe)
  iv. If present at birth, medical-surgical prognosis poor
  v. If acquired in early months or years (infantile glaucoma), better prognosis
b. Birth trauma
  i. Epithelial edema
  ii. Vertically oriented ruptures in Descemet's
  iii. Findings usually greater in left eye, owing to common left occiput anterior position
c. Numerous other corneal abnormalities related to congenital ocular and systemic syndromes

B. Degenerations

For a diagrammatic summary of corneal degenerations, refer to Figure 5.40 (peripherally oriented) and Figure 5.41 (variable positioning).

1. *Arcus Senilis*[26] *(Figure 5.42)*

Subjective

- Asymptomatic
- More common and pronounced among Black patients due to dark iris background
- 50% by 50 years old and up to 100% by 80 years old

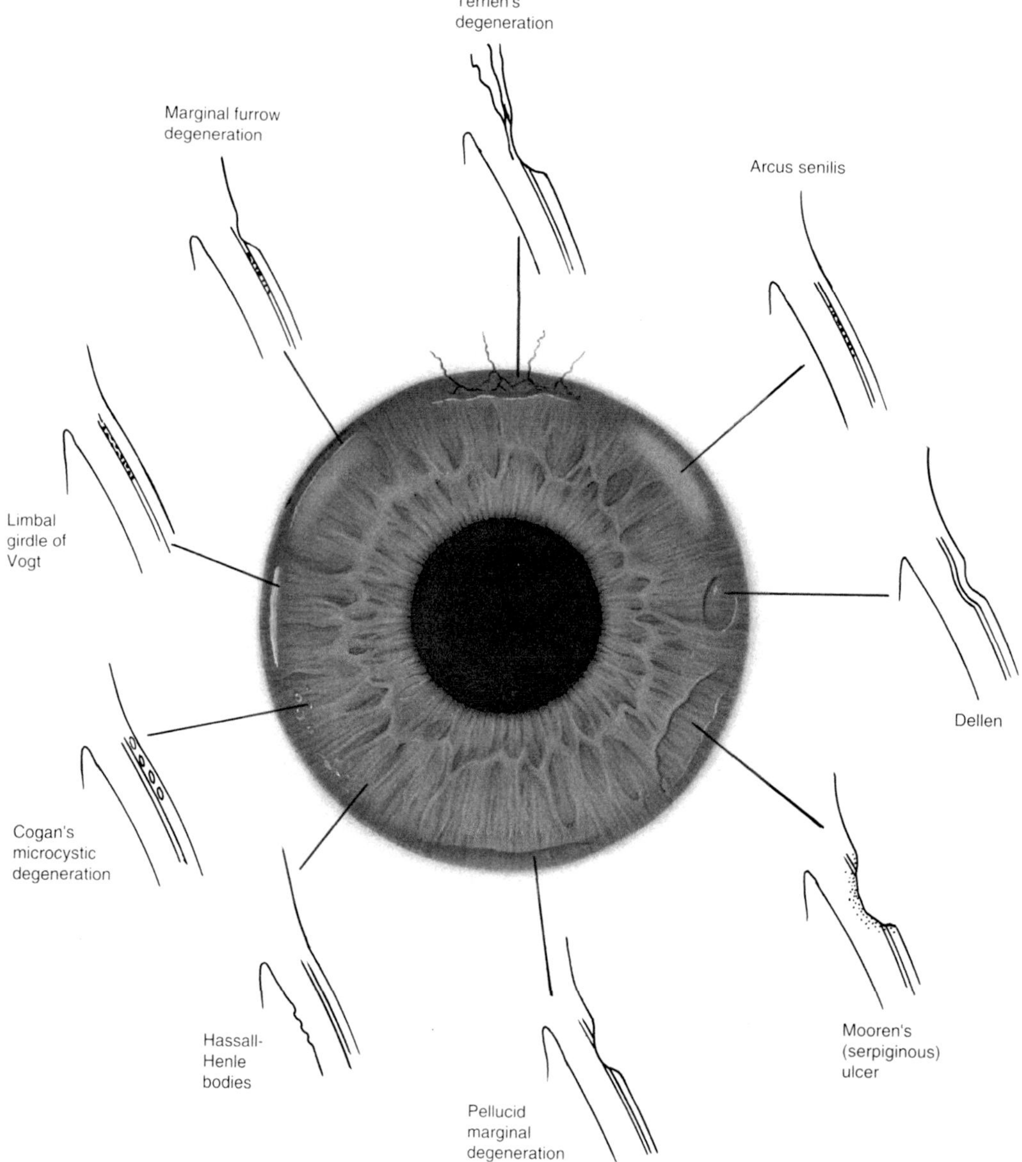

FIGURE 5.40 Peripherally oriented corneal degenerations (diagrammatic summary).

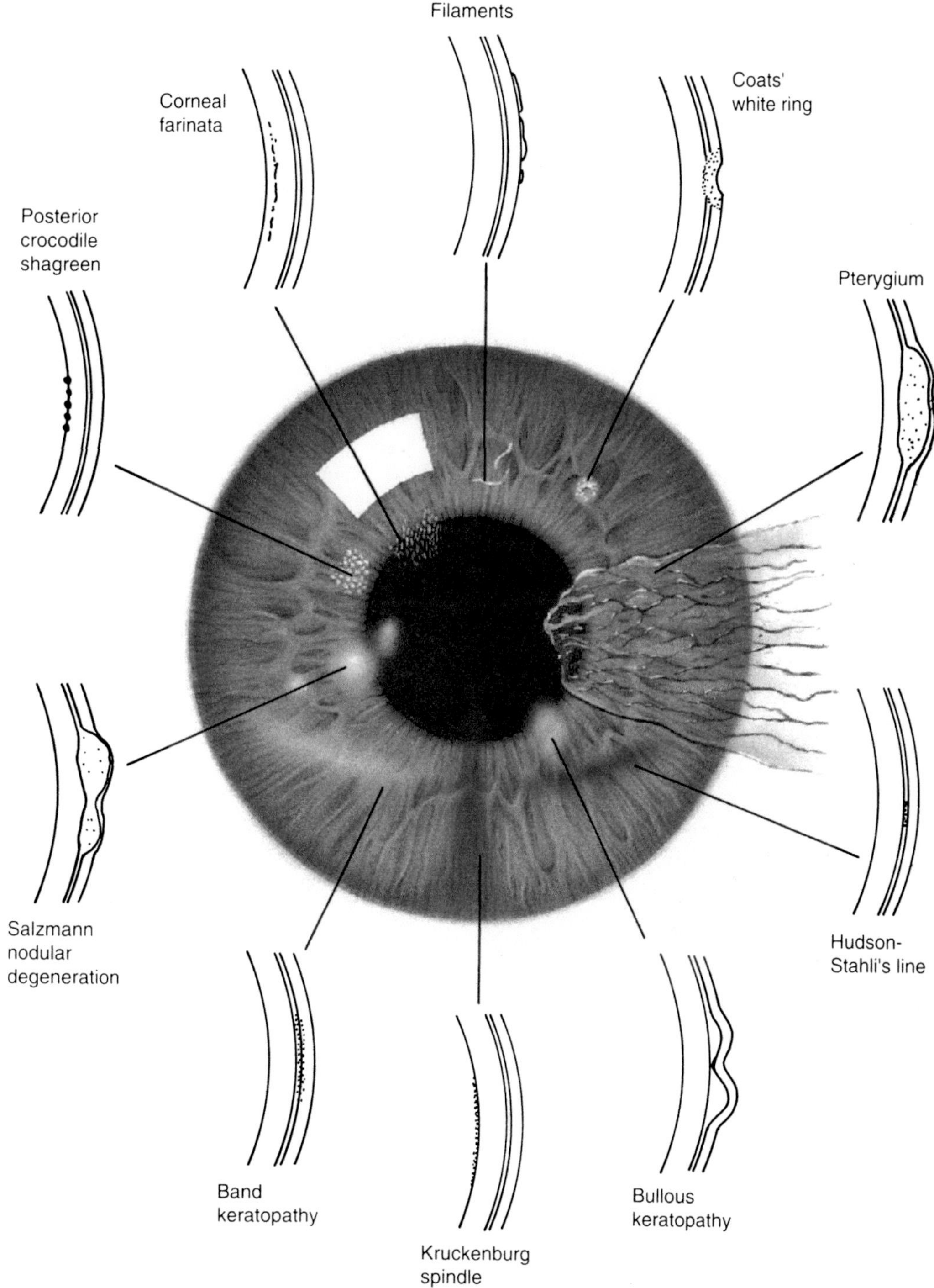

FIGURE 5.41 Variable-positioned corneal degenerations (diagrammatic summary).

Objective

- Usually bilateral
- Broad (1 to 2 mm) whitish midperipheral ring of lipid substances
- Found at level of Bowman's layer
- Gradual development
  1. Inferior first
  2. Superior second
  3. Ultimately a complete ring

Assessment

(See also Appendix 3)

- Most commonly a familial trait
- Rule out risk factors for hyperlipidemias
  1. Usually not a factor after 40 years old
  2. Blood work not indicated without risk factors
- Considered cardiovascular risk factor under 40 years old combined with other classic risk factors

1. Familial history of cardiovascular disease
2. Hypertension
3. Obesity
4. Diets of polyunsaturated fats, high cholesterols, increased salt
5. Stress
6. Smoking
7. No exercise

Plan and Follow-Up: Arcus Senilis

- Advise patients under 40 years old on increased risk and preventative measures
- Refer any patient under 40 years old for medical workup if no medical care for more than 2 to 3 years
- Monitor eye changes routinely

2. Band Keratopathy[27]

Subjective

- Usually asymptomatic in early development
- Late-stage painful epithelial erosions common

Objective

- Calcium accumulation in the palpebral fissure (band) region of cornea (usually bilateral)
- Whitish-yellow haze in epithelium and Bowman's layer
- Occasionally a Swiss cheese–like pattern
- Usually starts at nasal or temporal limbus and spreads centrally over months to years

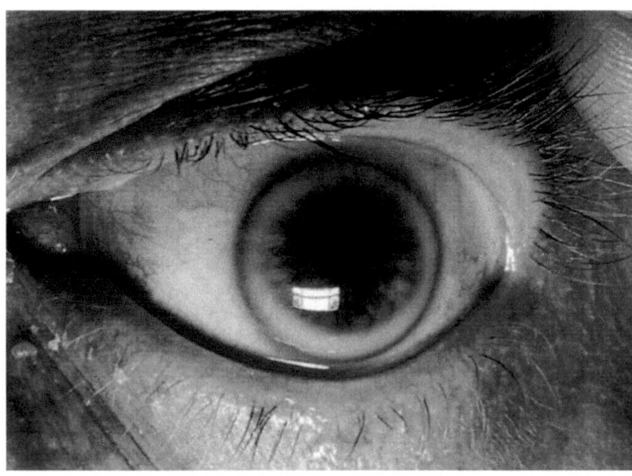

FIGURE 5.42 Arcus senilis presenting 360° accumulations of cholesterol in the peripheral cornea.

Assessment

(See also Appendix 2)

- Rule out Still's triad (juvenile rheumatoid arthritis) in early age presentations
- Rule out hyperparathyroidism

Plan and Follow-Up: Band Keratopathy

- Refer for hyperparathyroidism (hypercalcemic) workup in adult presentations
- Lubrication for mildly symptomatic presentations
- Chelation (usually with EDTA, a preservative) or PTK for severe symptoms
  1. More likely to improve patient comfort than VA
  2. Can reoccur
- Monitor suspicious development every 3 to 4 months

3. Bullous Keratopathy[28]

Subjective

- May present acutely, subacutely, or insidiously
- Often a contributory history of primary cause
- Decrease vision starts in mild cases due to loss of corneal transparency
- Extremely painful, with photophobia and tearing in moderate to severe cases

Objective

(Figure 5.43)

- Result of advanced, prolonged epithelial edema (from any primary cause)
- Formation of epithelial bullae (bubbling effect) which recurrently break down and reform
- Eventually, fibrosis occurs under bullae producing chronically painful and scarred epithelial layer

Assessment

(See also Appendix 3)

- Fundamental cause is reduced endothelial count producing poor corneal dehydration and resultant secondary epithelial edema

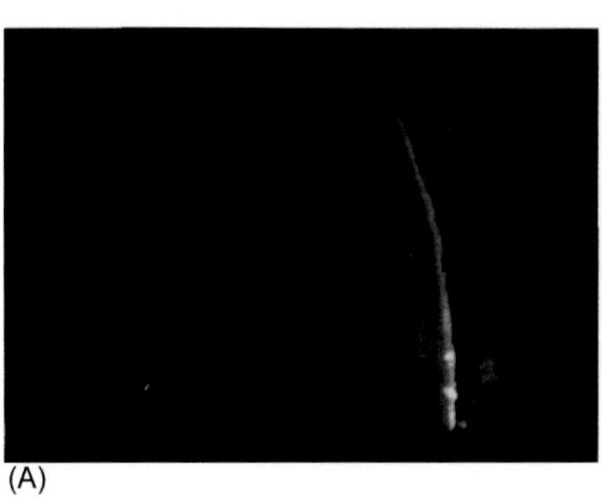

(A)

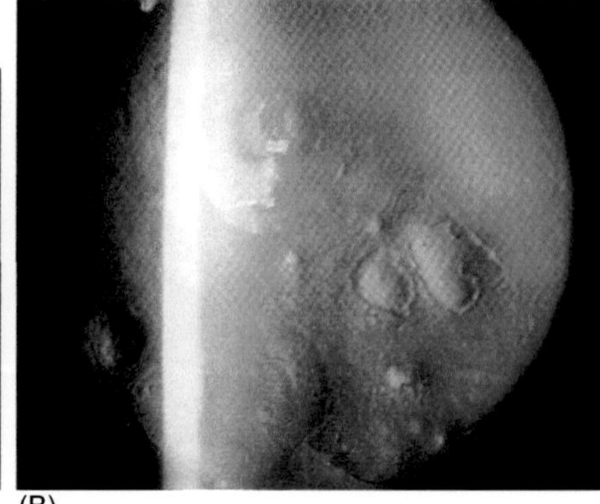

(B)

FIGURE 5.43 **(A)** Bullous keratopathy (slit view) associated with Fuchs' endothelial dystrophy, viewed under slit-lamp biomicroscopy in a slit, optical section. **(B)** Bullous keratopathy viewed by indirect retroillumination.

- Three most common primary causes (in rank order)
  1. Postoperative complication (e.g., cataract surgery)
  2. Fuchs' endothelial dystrophy
  3. Degeneration (from cumulative loss of non-regenerative endothelial cells over lifetime)

Plan and Follow-Up: Bullous Keratopathy

- Consider qualitative and quantitative (cell count) endothelial integrity as indication (or contraindication) for elective intraocular surgery
- Treat advancing epithelial edema aggressively with all antiedema therapies (e.g., hypertonic drops and ointment) before bullae form
- Treat bullae (early) with bandage soft contact lens and prophylactic antibiotics
- With advanced (fibrosed) bullae, treat symptoms but poor prognosis for visual restoration
- Descemet's stripping (automated) endothelial keratoplasty (DSEK or DSAEK) less invasive option than penetrating keratoplasty (PK)
- Penetrating keratoplasty may be necessary in advanced cases

4. Cogan's Microcystic Degeneration

Subjective

- Sometimes considered form of EBM (dot) disorder
- Generally found in older males
- Painful if spontaneous epithelial erosions occur

Objective

- Unilateral or bilateral presentations
- Usually peripheral single or groupings of large (1- to 2-mm) clear or gray intraepithelial microcysts

Assessment

- Differentiate from EBM (dot) dystrophy by following variations
  1. Unilateral presentations
  2. Older age presentation
  3. Male prevalence
  4. Larger cyst formations
  5. Peripheral versus central
- Rule out other causes of spontaneous erosions

Plan and Follow-Up: Cogan's Microcystic Degeneration

- Monitor asymptomatic cases every 6 to 12 months or PRN
- Treat acute erosions same as EBMD

5. Corneal Farinata

Refer to pre-Descemet's dystrophy.

6. Dellen[28] (Gaule Spot)

(See Figure 5.44)

Subjective

- Asymptomatic presentation (usually general exam)
- Any age range

Objective

- Focal, peripheral depressions (thinning) adjacent to the limbus, usually 0.5- to 1-mm diameter (Figure 5.45)
- Borders may slope gently or frequently are sharp and well-defined producing appearance of a "hole"
  1. Hole may approximate one half of the corneal thickness
  2. Tissue remains clear or slight haze
- Eye is never inflamed or hyperemic
- Epithelium remains intact (no staining or symptoms)
- Elongation (along limbal border) may extend 2 to 3 mm
- Most frequent positioning at 3 and 9 o'clock
- Usually associated with an adjacent raised "mass" causing tear film interruption and local corneal dehydration
  1. Conjunctival
     a. Pinguecula (most common)
     b. Chemosis
     c. Subconjunctival hemorrhage (thick)
     d. Other raised lesions
  2. Eyelid
     a. Internal chalazion
     b. Other causes of raised or irregular tarsus

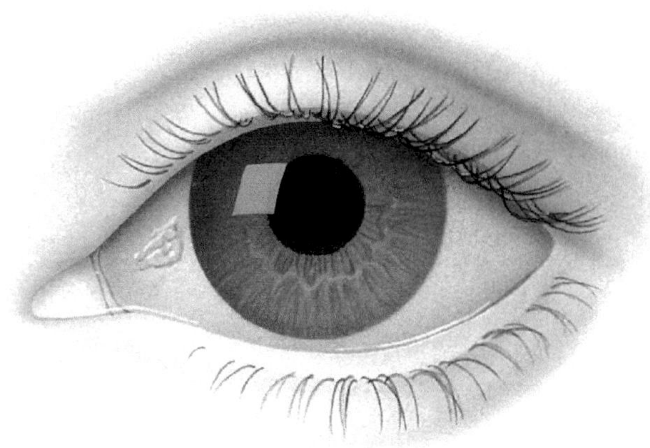

FIGURE 5.44 Dellen or (dellenous) formation created by raised tissue mass (or contact lens edge) disrupting even wetting of corneal periphery on lid closure or blink.

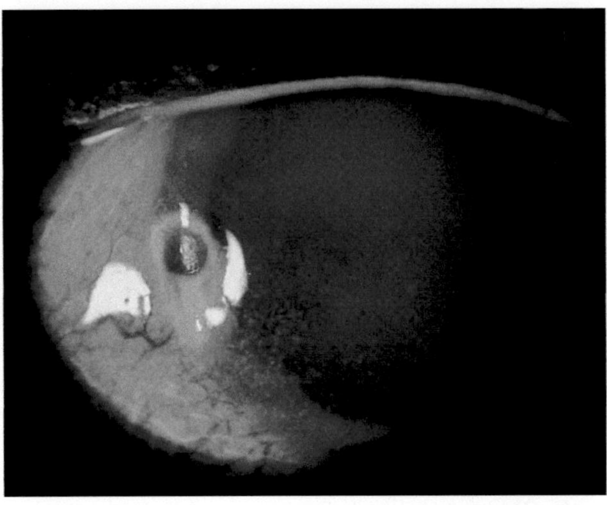

FIGURE 5.45 Dellen formation in the peripheral cornea of a patient with presumed dry eye/keratoconjunctivitis sicca syndrome. Note the associated superficial punctate staining in the band region of the inferior cornea.

c. Also possible with lagophthalmos
3. Thick edge of a firm contact lens

Assessment

(See also Appendix 2)

- Determine cause (raised mass)
- Reason for limited patient risk for dellen unclear
  1. Many people have thick pinguecula, but only small percentage develop dellen
  2. May be associated with a specific human lymphocyte antigen factor
- No risk of perforation (even though it looks it)

Plan and Follow-Up: Dellen

(See also Appendix 4)

- Where possible, remove or reduce cause (mass)
  1. Adjust contact lens (edge)
  2. Remove chalazion
  3. Reduce or control pinguecula
- Removal or protection achieved by lubrication
  1. Eyedrops or ointments q3–4h for 1 week
  2. Bandage soft contact lens coverage
  3. Lid closure (patching) for 24–48 hours
- If no treatment indicated, monitor yearly or PRN

7. Deposits (On or In Cornea)

- Amyloid (systemic manifestation)
- Calcareous (degenerative)
- Coats' white ring (associated with FBs)
- Filaments (epithelial or mucin debris)
- Hyalin (degenerative)
- Keloid (associated with scarring)
- Lipid (degenerative)

8. Hassall–Henle Bodies[29] (Descemet's Warts)

Subjective

- Asymptomatic presentation (usually general exam)
- Associated with aging

Objective

- Small, round, peripheral endothelial indentations produced by thickening of Descemet's membrane
- Appear as corneal guttata (but peripheral)
- Usually associated peripheral edema (may be full thickness)

Assessment

- Rule out Fuchs' endothelial dystrophy (central)
- Peripheral edema sometimes produces appearance of an atypical arcus (diffuse versus defined ring)

Plan: Hassall–Henle Bodies

- No treatment indicated
- Consider (endothelial) risk in elective surgery

9. Marginal Furrow Degeneration[30]

See Figure 5.46.

Subjective

- Asymptomatic presentation (usually general examination)
- Seen in older patients

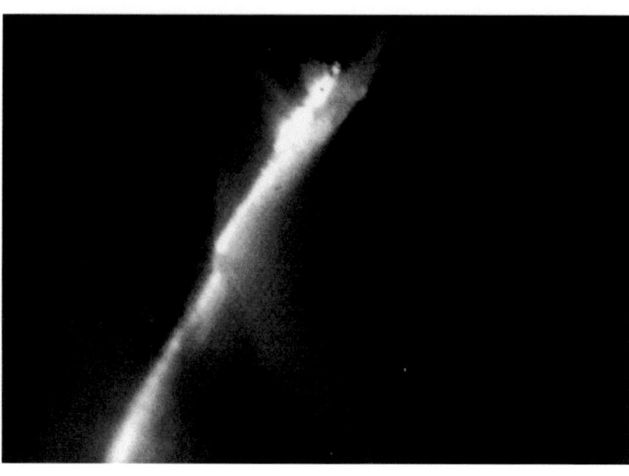

FIGURE 5.46 Marginal furrow degeneration outlined by a slit-lamp biomicroscopic optical section demonstrating the associated peripheral thinning distal to a circumferential, arcus-like corneal ring in an elderly patient.

Objective

- Bilateral thinning (furrowing) of peripheral cornea adjacent to limbus (usually 360°)
- Generally presents with prominent arcus ring
  1. Furrowed trough (thinned cornea) diagnosed by depression of slit between arcus ring and limbal border
  2. NaFl stain may pool in trough area but no positive staining because epithelium intact

Assessment

(See also Appendix 3)

- No risk of perforation
- Rule out Mooren's ulcer (inflamed lesion)
- Rule out rheumatoid disease

Plan: Marginal Furrow Degeneration

- No treatment indicated
- Recheck annually or PRN

10. Posterior Crocodile Shagreen

- Diffuse, grayish polygonal degeneration of posterior corneal stroma
- No associated visual or ocular complications

11. Pterygium[31,32]

See Figure 5.47.

Subjective

- Stable (occasionally advancing) lesion
- More common in outdoor people
  1. Stimulated by UV exposure and arid climate
  2. Probably a tissue response to irritants rather than a true degeneration
- Usually cosmetically unappealing
- May produce subacute symptoms
  1. Irritation and hyperemic appearance
  2. FB sensation
  3. Reduction of vision
     a. Secondary irregular astigmatisms
     b. Obstruction of the visual axis

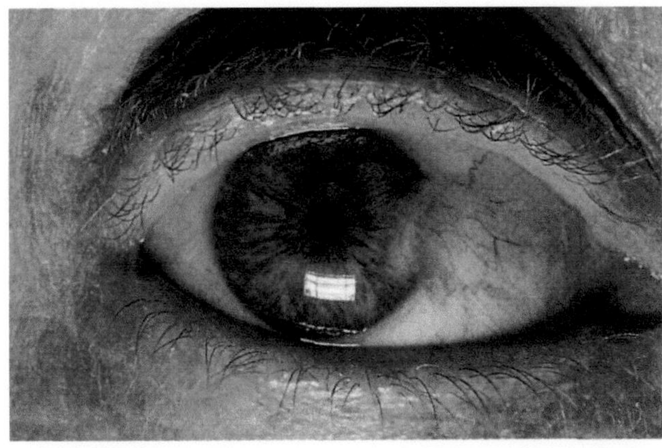

FIGURE 5.47 Pterygium in the nasal aspect of the right eye encroaching approximately 2 to 3 mm onto the corneal surface. Superficial vascularization of the hyperplastic, triangular tissue (apex towards the cornea) produces obvious disturbance to the anterior stromal matrix of the cornea.

Objective

- Thick, fleshy triangular mass of tissue (apex toward cornea) growing (stable or slow, insidious growth) onto nasal corneal surface
- Frequently a bilateral presentation with varying degree of advancement in each eye
- Usually yellowish coloration
- Relatively rich surface vascularization
- Occasionally a ferric line (orange-brown) seen at leading (corneal) edge called Stocker's line

Assessment

(See also Appendix 3)

- Differentiate from pinguecula
  1. Corneal involvement with pterygium
  2. Apex toward cornea with pterygium
  3. Rich vascular supply with pterygium
- Assess stable versus progressive nature
- Rule out other raised ocular surface lesions

Plan and Follow-Up: Pterygium

- Measure and diagram (photodocument if possible)
  1. Recheck first observed lesions in 6 to 12 months
  2. Long-standing lesions usually stable
- If asymptomatic and stable, no treatment; monitor at 1- to 2-year intervals or PRN
- If symptomatic (but stable)
  1. Vasoconstrictors for hyperemia
  2. Lubrication for FB sensations
  3. Topical steroids (e.g., 0.5% loteprednol) qid for 7–10 days when inflamed
  4. Corrective lenses for induced visual astigmatism
     a. Add UV tints to reduce potential cause
     b. Lens also reduces exposure to irritants
- If progressive (towards pupil) or cosmetically unacceptable (patient requesting repair)
  1. Recommend surgical reduction before leading edge approximates border of dilated (dim illumination) pupil
  2. Surgical excision with conjunctival autograph and cyclosporine 0.5% least recurrence rate
  3. Other procedures
     a. Simple excision with bare sclera has high rate of recurrence
     b. Beta radiation has potential serious complications
     c. Mitomycin-C (MMC) used during surgery
     d. 5-fluorouracil (5-FU) less complications than MMC or beta radiation
- Advise patients on guarded post-operative prognosis regarding redevelopment of growth pattern
- Contact lens wear is not contraindicated

12. Salzman's Nodular Degeneration[33,34]

Subjective

- Depending on severity symptoms range from decreased vision, photophobia, foreign-body sensation to asymptomatic
- May present acutely with epithelial breakdown
- Uncommon presentation (more prevalent in females)

Objective

- Bilateral formations of elevated, grayish-blue nodules on corneal surface (anterior to Bowman's membrane)
- More likely to be peripheral than central
- Vision effects depend on location of nodules

Assessment

- Rule out bullous keratopathy (more painful)

Plan: Salzman's Nodular Degeneration

- If asymptomatic, no treatment but monitor closely (every 6 months or PRN)
- If epithelium chronically breaks down over nodules, use bandage soft lenses and prophylactic antibiotics qid or ocular lubricants
- Consider superficial keratectomy, lamellar keratoplasty, or PTK if patient desires (possible) permanent repair

13. White Limbal Girdle of Vogt

a. Common presentation in women over 50 years of age
b. Narrow band of fine crystal-like opacities lined up along nasal or temporal limbal border(s)
c. Usually bilateral and always asymptomatic
d. Old literature related it to band keratopathy and sunlight exposure due to palpebral fissure orientation (both theories unproven)

C. Dystrophies[35–37]

Background Information

1. Most corneal dystrophies are relatively rare and seen infrequently in primary care practice
2. Generally diagnosed during routine (asymptomatic) slit-lamp examination (often first diagnosis in children)
3. Standard clinical characteristics of corneal dystrophy
   a. Autosomal-dominant, autosomal-recessive, or X-linked hereditary pattern
      i. This means that 50% or more of family will show similar findings
      ii. Usually equal sex distribution
      iii. Variable penetration (frequency) and severity (expressivity)
      iv. Good clinical care dictates seeing other family members when evaluating dystrophies

TABLE 5.7 Clinical Highlights of Corneal Dystrophies

		Exceptions to Standard Clinical Characteristics of Dystrophy								Secondary Complications				Management Considerations				General Prognosis			
Primary Layer	**Specific Dystrophy**	**Autosomal Dominant**	**No systemic disease**	**No ocular disease**	**Onset by age 20**	**Bilateral**	**Slowly progressive**	**Central**	**Single layer**	**Visual**	**Epithelial**	**Stromal**	**Other**	**Possible Keratoplasty**	**For symptoms**	**For edema**	**Genetic counseling**	**Excellent**	**Good**	**Guarded**	**Poor**
Epithelium	EBMD (Disorder)				X	X				X	X				X	X			X		
	Lisch									X									X		
	Messman's							X							X			X			
Bowman's	Reis–Buckler									X		X		X	X		X			X	
	Gelatinous drop-like									X				X	X		X				X
	Epithelial recurrent erosion														X				X		
Anterior stromal	Granular (Groenouw's I)(GCD1)									X		X		X	X				X		
	Lattice									X	X			X	X		X			X	
	Granular, type 2 (GCD2)									X				X	X						
	Thiel–Behnke														X				X		
	Schnyder Corneal (Central crystalline)		X					X		X			1						X		
Full stromal	Macular (Groenouw's II)	X						X	X	X	X			X	X	X	X			X	
	Fleck							X					2					X			
Deep Stromal	Central cloudy																	X			
	Posterior-amorphous							X		X									X		
	Pre-Descemet	X			X			X					3					X			
Posterior cornea	Fuchs'	?			X			X	X	X	X	X		X	X	X	X				
	Posterior-polymorphous						X	X		X	X	X	4			X			X		
	X-linked endothelial																				
	Congenital hereditary	X					X	X		X	X	X		X	X	X	X				X

Notes: 1 = cardiovascular complications can result from uncontrolled hypercholesterolemia; 2 = associated with congenital findings (e.g., lens opacities, dermoids); 3 = may appear with other dystrophies; 4 = increased risk of glaucoma (mesodermal dysgenesis?).

b. No associated systemic disease history
   i. Infectious or inflammatory conditions
   ii. Syndromes and congenital abnormalities
c. No primary ocular disease history
   i. Acute or chronic ocular history must be ruled out before definitive diagnosis of dystrophy (e.g., herpetic, uveitis)
   ii. Rule out history of corneal scarring (from old trauma) mimicking dystrophic changes
d. Usual onset of findings by 20 years of age
   i. Dystrophy tends to present during the first or second decade of life
   ii. Mostly a first diagnosis in children
   iii. Major exception: Fuchs' endothelial dystrophy
e. Bilateral condition
   i. No exceptions to this rule
   ii. Findings in second eye may be subtle
   iii. Second eye may advance slower or may arrest sooner than first
f. Slowly progressive changes
   i. Dystrophy never presents suddenly or acutely
      - Complications may cause acute reactions
      - Generally, dystrophic findings are slow and insidious in their progress
   ii. Changes usually start early, develop over years, and stabilize by 20 to 30 years of age
   iii. Changes after 40 years of age are usually degenerations (exception: Fuchs' endothelial dystrophy)
g. Generally centrally located findings
   i. Many exceptions to this rule (see specific dystrophies and Table 5.7)
   ii. Some exceptions start centrally and then spread to periphery
h. Primary involvement of single corneal layer
   i. This is the most important clinical characteristic of dystrophy
      - Used to classify the many types
      - Useful in simplifying diagnostic workup
   ii. Break down cornea to major layers
      - Epithelial
      - Bowman's
      - Stroma (90% thickness of cornea, thus further subdivided)
         – Anterior
         – Full thickness deep (posterior)
         – Posterior (Descemet's and endothelium)

4. Step-by-step diagnostic strategy for corneal dystrophy
   a. Confirm standard clinical characteristics of corneal dystrophy
   b. Determine major layer of involvement
   c. Consider the two to four dystrophies affecting that layer (see Table 5.7)

d. Compare the lesions you're finding to the description of the two to four types
e. One dystrophy will fit the characteristics you are observing more than the others, usually rather obviously (each dystrophy having relatively distinct lesions and patterns)
f. Consider the course and prognosis of the dystrophy you choose and manage patient accordingly
   i. Schedule other family members for slit-lamp examination
   ii. Advise and counsel the patient family
   iii. If prognosis is poor or clinical findings (expressivity) and vision loss are substantial, recommend genetic counseling

1. *Epithelial Layer Dystrophies*

a. EBMD
   i. Also called map-dot-fingerprint dystrophy
   ii. Separate description in Section II. D.
b. Messman's corneal dystrophy (juvenile epithelial corneal dystrophy)
   i. Clinical features
      - Epithelial, gray, round to oval cyst-like opacities
      - Seen best under indirect retroillumination
      - Asymptomatic until middle age
   ii. Exceptions to standard rules for dystrophy: extends to limbus
   iii. Potential complications
      - Irregular astigmatisms
      - Mild epithelial erosions (after 40 years of age)
      - Vision reduction
   iv. Management
      - Routine follow (every 1 to 2 years) or PRN
      - Treat symptoms
      - Epithelial removal but tends to reoccur
   v. Prognosis: excellent
c. Lisch epithelial corneal dystrophy (LECD)
   i. Clinical features
      - Childhood onset
      - Gray opacities whorl-like, feathery, or band shaped
      - Clear epithelium between opacities
   ii. Exceptions to standard rules for dystrophy: none
   iii. Potential complications: reduced vision if opacities increase
   iv. Management: superficial keratectomy
   v. Prognosis: recurrence after keratectomy

2. *Bowman's Layer Dystrophies*

a. Reis–Buckler's (ring-shaped) dystrophy
   i. Clinical features
      - Reticulated opacities that elevate the epithelium
      - Irregular "fishnet" swirls
      - Superficial stromal haze
   ii. Exceptions to standard rules for dystrophy: none
   iii. Potential complications
      - Painful, recurrent epithelial erosions usually decreasing by 30 years of age
      - Anterior stromal opacification
   iv. Management
      - Erosion therapy
      - In advanced cases superficial keratectomy, PTK, or lamellar keratoplasty may improve vision
   v. Prognosis: guarded
b. Gelatinous drop-like corneal dystrophy (GDCD)
   i. Clinical features
      - First decade presentation
      - Sub-epithelial milky-white gelatinous nodules
      - Photophobia, foreign-body sensation, progressive vision loss
   ii. Exceptions to standard rules for dystrophy: none
   iii. Potential complications: reduced vision
   iv. Management: to improve vision
      - Superficial keratoplasty
      - PTK
      - Lamellar keratoplasty
   v. Prognosis: poor due to recurring nodules
c. Epithelial recurrent erosion dystrophy (ERED)
   i. Clinical features
      - First decade presentation
      - Recurrent epithelial erosions due to poor epithelial adherence
      - Spontaneous or minor trauma induced
      - Sub-epithelial haze and opacities
   ii. Exceptions to standard rules for dystrophy: none
   iii. Potential complications: 50% have corneal opacification
   iv. Management
      - Erosion therapy
      - Superficial keratectomy or PTK for opacities
   v. Prognosis: Erosion usually reduce with time and stops by fourth decade

3. *Anterior Stromal Dystrophies*

a. Granular (Groenouw's I) dystrophy (GCD1) (Figure 5.48)
   i. Clinical features
      - First-decade presentation
      - Discrete focal white (translucent) spots
         - Hard white ("cornflake") spots
         - Powdery (small) dots
         - Ring-shaped opacities
      - Glare and photophobia are early symptoms
      - VA reduces gradually (no worse than 20/200)
   ii. Exceptions to standard rules for dystrophy: none
   iii. Potential complications: reduced vision
   iv. Management: penetrating or lamellar keratoplasty

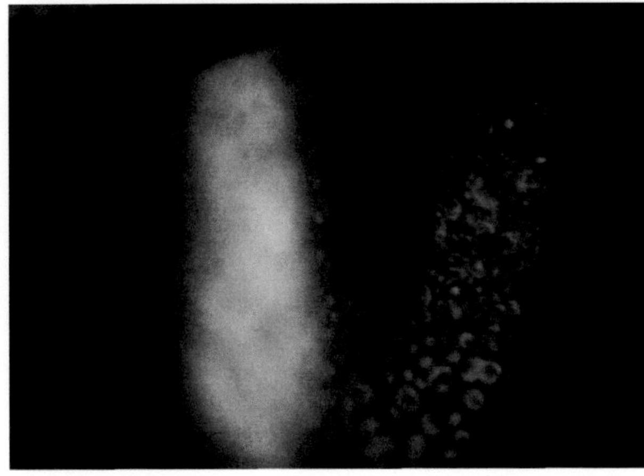

FIGURE 5.48 Granular dystrophy (Greonouw's 1), an anterior stromal dystrophy demonstrating "cornflake-like" spots, small dots, and ring-shaped opacities with variable visual results.

- v. Prognosis: good but recurrence is possible after surgery
- b. Granular corneal dystrophy type 2 (GCD2)
  - i. Clinical features
    - Initial signs of whitish dots (less than GCD1), progressing to thorn- or spoke-like, and can eventually be arranged linearly
    - Epithelial erosions
    - Dense opacities in adulthood
  - ii. Exceptions to standard rules for dystrophy: none
  - iii. Potential complications: reduced vision
  - iv. Management
    - Phototherapeutic keratoplasty (PTK) contraindicated since injury exacerbates dystrophy
    - Penetrating keratoplasty when reduced vision is problematic
  - v. Prognosis: good
- c. Lattice dystrophy (of Biber)
  - i. Clinical features
    - Anterior stromal refractile lines
    - Central haze (after third to fourth decade of life)
    - Lines may thicken or bead
  - ii. Exceptions to standard rules for dystrophy: none
  - iii. Potential complications: epithelial erosions in advanced cases
  - iv. Management
    - Treat erosions
    - Keratoplasty with severe VA reductions
  - v. Prognosis: guarded
- d. Schnyder corneal dystrophy (SCD) (central crystalline dystrophy of Schnyder; Figure 5.49)
  - i. Clinical features
    - Central crystals (found in 50% of patients) in a ring, disc, or comma shape form annulus during first to second decade of life
    - Dense arcus ring forms during third to fourth decade of life
  - ii. Exceptions to standard rules for dystrophy
    - Associated with systemic hypercholesterolemia
    - Only dystrophy associated with systemic disease

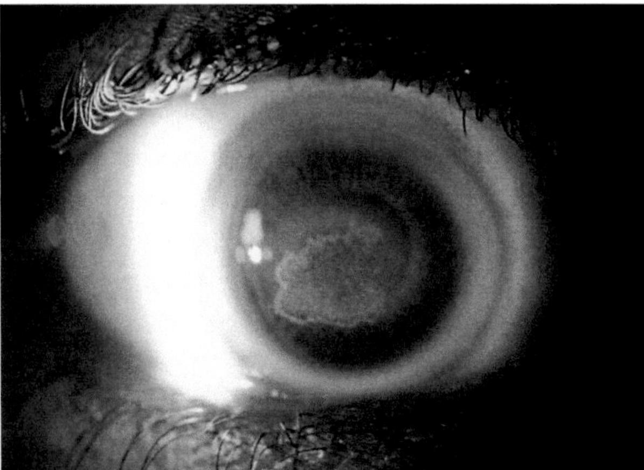

FIGURE 5.49 Central crystalline dystrophy (of Schnyder), an anterior stromal dystrophy associated with systemic hypercholesterolemia (only dystrophy associated with systemic disorder) producing an annulus of central corneal crystal and a dense arcus ring.

  - iii. Potential complications
    - Over 50 years old significant reduction in photopic vision
    - Cardiovascular risks of hyper-cholesterol
  - iv. Management
    - Refer to general medicine
    - Monitor ocular changes annually
  - v. Prognosis
    - Good systemically with proper controls
    - Ocular signs not reversible, even with systemic control
- e. Thiel–Behnke corneal dystrophy (TBCD)
  - i. Clinical features
    - Childhood onset
    - Flecks or irregularly scattered sub-epithelial opacities and progressing to honeycomb pattern
    - Centrally located
    - Epithelial erosions through 20 years of life and then decrease
  - ii. Exceptions to standard rules for dystrophy: none
  - iii. Potential complications: vision loss later in life due to scarring
  - iv. Management: superficial keratectomy or PTK
  - v. Prognosis: recurrence possible after treatment

4. *Deep (Posterior) Stromal Dystrophies*

- a. Central cloudy dystrophy (of Francois)
  - i. Clinical features
    - Fuzzy gray areas in deep central stroma called crocodile shagreen
    - Slight polygonal pattern
    - Most patients asymptomatic
  - ii. Exceptions to standard rules for dystrophy: none
  - iii. Complications: none
  - iv. Management: none
  - v. Prognosis: excellent
- b. Posterior amorphous corneal dystrophy (PACD)
  - i. Clinical features
    - Gray sheets develop across stroma
    - First decade
    - Occasional endothelial mosaic disruption
    - Associated with iris abnormalities (e.g., iris corneal adhesions, corectopia)
    - Slowly or non-progressive
  - ii. Exceptions to standard rules for dystrophy: extends to periphery
  - iii. Complications: may reduce VA to about 20/40
  - iv. Management: none
  - v. Prognosis: good
- c. Pre-Descemet's corneal dystrophy (PDCD)
  - i. Clinical features
    - Deep punctate or filamentous gray opacities
    - Indentations in Descemet's membrane
    - Fine "flour-like" dusting of gray specks of varying size and shapes
      - Dendriform
      - Boomerang
      - Circular
      - Comma
      - Linear
    - All shapes may be in same cornea
    - May be annular or diffuse pattern
  - ii. Exceptions to standard rules for dystrophy

- May present in older age initially (probably degeneration called corneal farinata)
- May extend to periphery
- Questionable hereditary pattern
- Found with other dystrophies

iii. Complications: none

iv. Management
- Rule out degeneration versus dystrophy
- Diagnosis other combined dystrophies

v. Prognosis: excellent

5. *Full-Thickness Stromal Dystrophies*

a. Macular (Groenouw's II) corneal dystrophy (MCD) (Figure 5.50)

i. Clinical features
- Diffuse ground-glass haze
- Focal gray or white opacities
- Increases to full thickness by teens
- Eventually spreads to Descemet's membrane and endothelium

ii. Exceptions to standard rules for dystrophy
- Autosomal-recessive type (more severe)
- Extends to periphery

iii. Complications
- VA reduces substantially before 50 years old
- Corneal guttata with secondary erosions (a late occurrence in course)

iv. Management
- Treat erosions
- Keratoplasty for VA

v. Prognosis: guarded

b. Fleck corneal dystrophy (FCD) (François–Neetens)

i. Clinical features
- Congenital or by 2 years of age
- Asymmetry between eyes
- Gray to white ring, oval, "wreath" or comma-shaped spots
- Lesions remain stable from early years
- Usually, asymptomatic

ii. Exceptions to standard rules for dystrophy: extends to periphery but less opacities compared to central cornea

iii. Complications
- Occasional congenital lens opacity
- Occasional dermoids

iv. Management: none

v. Prognosis: excellent

6. *Posterior Corneal Dystrophies*

a. Fuchs' (late) endothelial dystrophy (Figure 5.51)

i. Clinical features
- Slowly progressive disorder of aging
- Three levels of guttata (depressions in endothelium, best seen by retroillumination)
  - Few scattered guttata (20 to 30 years of age)
  - Early endothelial dystrophy: increasing guttata (30 to 40 years of age)
  - Late (Fuchs') endothelial dystrophy: guttata plus other signs (age greater than 40 years)
- Pigment dusting on endothelium
- Stromal edema and thickening (variable) first appears as blue-gray stromal haze with striae (vertical lines) and progresses to ground glass appearance
- Epithelial edema (variable)
  - Microcystic (diffuse)
  - Wet, ground-glass effect (bedewing)
  - Bullae (bullous keratopathy; see Figure 5.43)
- Pain, photophobia, and epiphora from ruptured epithelial bullae
- Advanced edema produces subepithelial connective tissue opacities (permanent)

ii. Exceptions to standard rules for dystrophy
- Much higher prevalence in females (postmenopausal)
- Late-age onset
- Some forms extend to periphery with age
- Appears as multilayer involvement
- May be far more common (in milder forms) than traditionally reported

iii. Complications
- Generally reduces VA in advancing stages
- Increased stromal edema (thickening) in AM (secondary to closed lid edematous effect)

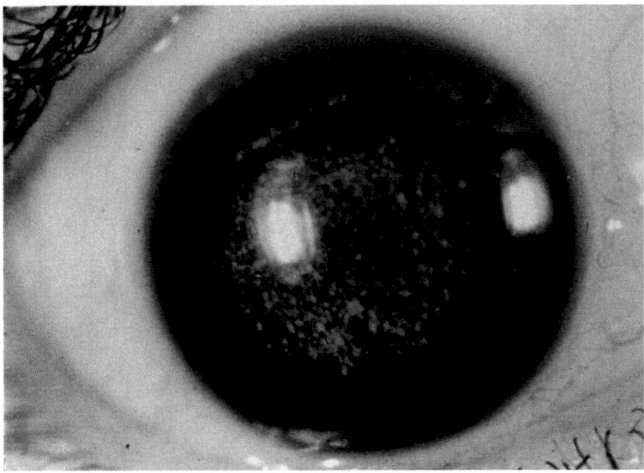

FIGURE 5.50 Macular dystrophy (Groenouw's II), a full-thickness stromal dystrophy demonstrating focal gray and white and central opacities, usually causing a substantial visual reduction.

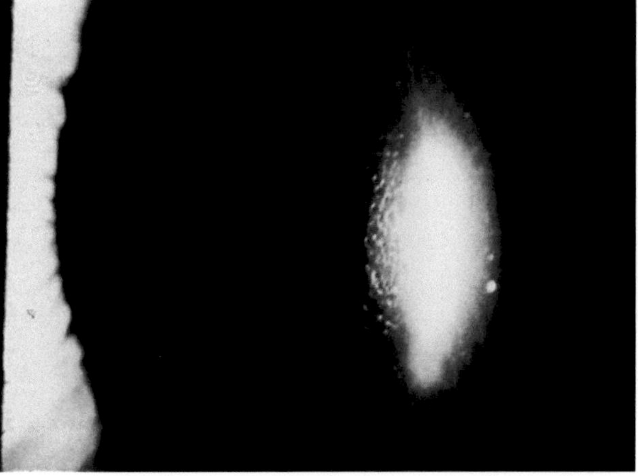

FIGURE 5.51 Fuchs' endothelial dystrophy (corneal guttata) presented under slit-lamp biomicroscopic specular reflection (and retroillumination). Also referred to as early endothelial dystrophy in younger patients (under 30 to 40 years of age).

produces VA fluctuation with transient increases in myopic errors
- Advanced edema (and bullous keratopathy) produce AM erosions (morning syndrome). The four morning syndromes are
  - Marginal keratitis (toxic staphylococcal)
  - EBMD
  - RCE
  - Fuchs' endothelial dystrophy
- Prolonged untreated edema produces connective tissue clouding of cornea
- Familial keratoconus has been associated

iv. Management (with symptoms or advancing signs)
- Warm packs for edema
- Hypertonic saline (drops and hs ointment)
- Hot air (hair) blow dryer in AM
  - 5 to 10 minutes at arms-length
  - Keep moving dryer back and forth
- Increased minus prescription for AM use if indicated
- Pupil dilation to increase light pathway around central clouding may help
  - Sometimes increased luminance is interpreted as increased VA
  - Use a sympathomimetic dilator (2.5% phenylephrine) to avoid cycloplegia
  - Tropicamide will require higher add due to cycloplegic effect
- Bandage soft lenses
  - With chronic discomfort and erosions
  - Definitely with bullous keratopathy
- Surgical options
  - Repair endothelium/Descemet's membrane via Descemet stripping endothelial keratoplasty (DSEK) or Descemet stripping automated endothelial keratoplasty (DSAEK)
    - Less invasive than PK
  - Penetrating Keratoplasty (PK)
    - If VA in better eye non-functional
    - If dystrophic changes spreading to periphery with increased density
    - Follow patient every 3 to 6 months
- Genetic counseling in severe cases

vi. Prognosis
- Most cases remain stable and respond to simple antiedema therapies
- Endothelial keratoplasty works well

b. Posterior polymorphous corneal dystrophy (of Schlicting)

i. Clinical features
- Grouped vesicles of varying shape and distribution
  - Peripheral ring distribution
  - Focal wedge
  - Diffuse "Swiss cheese" pattern
- Gray thickenings of Descemet's between vesicles
  - Often produce linear patterns
  - Lines tend to present as parallel pairs (resembling railroad tracks)
- Congenital or very early onset
- Very slow changes if any
- Usually asymptomatic

ii. Exceptions to standard rules for dystrophy
- Occasional ring pattern
- Occasional congenital presentation
- Suggested association with mesodermal dysgenesis syndromes

iii. Complications
- Mild stromal or epithelial edema
- Rare reduction in VA to 20/30
- Increased risk of glaucoma due to iris and posterior corneal adhesions

iv. Management
- Hypertonics for edema if indicated
- PK if edema is severe
- Annual IOP checks throughout life

v. Prognosis: good

c. Congenital hereditary endothelial corneal dystrophy

i. Clinical features
- Recessive form (congenital) with nystagmus
- Dominant form (onset during first to second decade of life) with no nystagmus
- Diffuse haze to ground-glass edema (stromal and epithelial)
- Increased corneal thickness (2 to 3×)
- "Peau d'orange" (orange peel) effect of Descemet's

ii. Exceptions to standard rules for dystrophy
- Congenital recessive form
- Extends to periphery
- Appears as multilayer involvement
  - Occasionally mistaken for interstitial keratitis
  - Interstitial keratitis defined as full-thickness infiltration, stromal thinning, and neovascularization
  - Dystrophy (all types) shows no true infiltrates, thinning, or neovascularization

iii. Complications
- Secondary epithelial reactions cause pain and photophobia
- Frequently progressive to blindness by early age

iv. Management
- Refer early for keratoplasty to reduce risk of amblyopia
- Strongly recommend genetic counseling

v. Prognosis
- Poor for recessive forms
- Guarded for the dominant forms (see Table 5.7)

d. X-linked endothelial corneal dystrophy

i. Clinical features
- Congenital ground glass corneal clouding
- Males more affected than females and severe opacification associated with nystagmus
- Slowly progressive and band keratopathy develops peripherally in adulthood

ii. Exceptions to standard rules for dystrophy
- Advanced cases have sub-epithelial band keratopathy

iii. Complications
- Band keratopathy

iv. Management
- PK if vision significantly reduced

v. Prognosis: good

D. Epithelial Basement Membrane Disorders (EBMD)

1. *Historical Background*

a. Funny-looking changes in the epithelium (intraepithelial) were first noted by Vogt during the 1920s

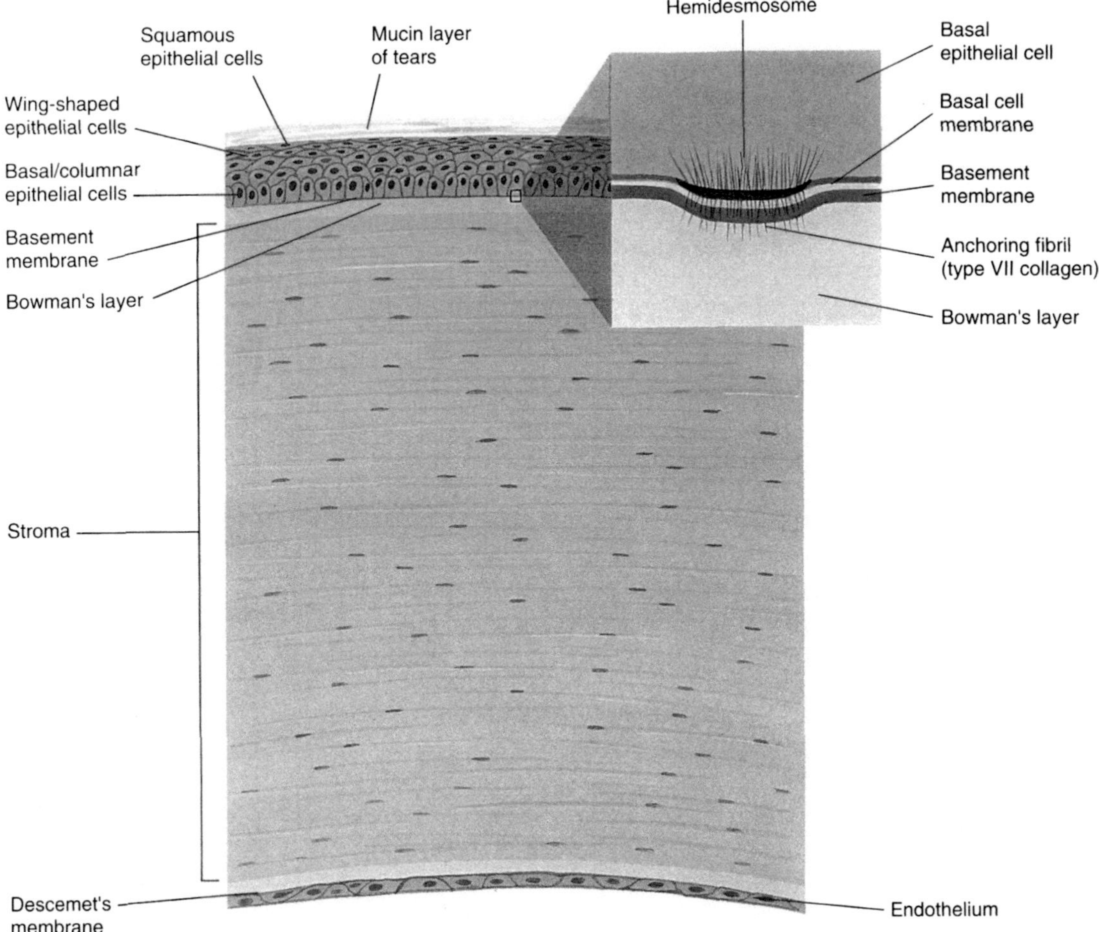

FIGURE 5.52 Diagrammatic corneal anatomy. Epithelial layer consists of mucin layer of tears, squamous epithelial cells, wing-shaped epithelial cells, basal (columnar-shaped) epithelial cells, and epithelial basement membrane. Stromal layer consists of Bowman's layer (condensed collagen fibers), stroma (loose collagen fibers), Descemet's membrane, and endothelium.

b. Again reported by Guerry during the 1950s as rare (1/4000) findings
c. Cogan et al. documented microcysts (dots) as part of an "epithelial dystrophy" during the 1960s
   i. Called it Cogan's microcystic dystrophy
   ii. More generic term for findings became map-dot-fingerprint dystrophy
d. Finally, during the 1970s, many investigators began to describe these findings as EBMD
   i. Since majority of cases have no documented inheritance, the changes are considered degenerative or secondary to trauma
   ii. Prevalence reported at approximately 2% to 6%
e. Increased prevalence (from Guerry, in the 1930s, to Laibson, in the 1970s) probably a result of improved slit-lamp instrumentation and capabilities
f. Better understanding of etiology was a product of advanced electron microscopic techniques during the 1970s

2. *Anatomy of the Epithelial Basement Membrane*

a. Also called the basal lamina
b. Separates the epithelial cells from Bowman's layer
c. Thin mucoproteinous membrane secreted by basal epithelial cells
   i. Takes 8 to 12 weeks to form or re-secrete membrane
   ii. Thus, loss or damage to membrane requires extended period (much greater than expected hours for squamous epithelium and days for deeper epithelial cells to regenerate)
d. Function of basement membrane is to attach epithelial cells firmly to stroma (Bowman's layer)
   i. Does so on epithelial side by fibrils called hemidesmosomes which extend into epithelium
   ii. On stromal side, fine fibrils (anchoring fibrils of type VII collagen) bind membrane and epithelium down to Bowman's layer
f. Thus, the contemporary concept of corneal anatomy differs slightly from traditional
   i. Epithelial layer
      - Mucin layer
      - Squamous epithelial cells
      - Wing-shaped epithelial cells
      - Basal (columnar shaped) epithelial cells
      - Epithelial basement membrane
   ii. Stromal layer
      - Bowman's layer (condensed collagen fibers)
      - Stroma (loosening collagen fibers increasing from anterior to posterior)
   iii. Descemet's membrane
   iv. Endothelium

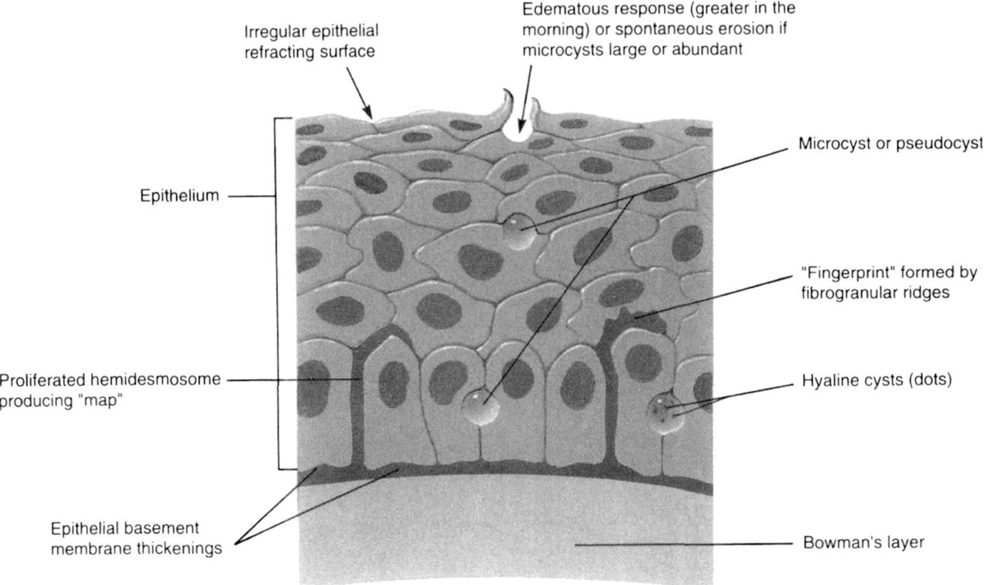

FIGURE 5.53 Diagram of intraepithelial histopathology of EBMD.

3. *Histopathology*

a. Basal epithelial cells produce abnormal finger like projections off basement membrane
   i. Generate off hemidesmosome thickenings
   ii. Thickenings and projections produce intraepithelial "map" configurations by slit-lamp examination (most common finding)
   iii. Projections with fibroglandular ridges produce "fingerprint" patterns (least common finding)
b. Loosening of surrounding deep epithelial cells from thickenings and fingerlike projections with their intraepithelial bendings, trap epithelial cells and debris to form microcysts (actually non-walled "pseudocysts")
   i. Microcysts appear clinically, under slit lamp as "dots" (common with maps)
   ii. Migration of microcysts to surface produce subjective and objective corneal signs and symptoms ("morning syndrome") and epithelial erosions
c. All these intraepithelial changes create an irregular epithelial surface
   i. Clinical result is negative NaFl staining
   ii. When extensive, results are irregular astigmatism and reduced best correctable VA
d. Changes exaggerated in diabetes

4. *Clinical Considerations*

Subjective

- Onset of symptoms may be insidious, subacute, or acute
- Often Objective signs will be noted without symptoms (especially in general examination patients)
  1. More frequently, symptoms will be reported (in varying degree) with no objective signs
  2. Probably subclinical findings
- Appears to be slightly more common in females
- Wide range of symptoms depending on degree of condition (Table 5.8)
  1. Mild degree
     a. Usually asymptomatic
     b. Mild, short-lived corneal irritation on waking ("morning syndrome")
  2. Moderate degree
     a. Morning syndrome or chronic corneal irritation
     b. May be awakened during sleep by reaction
     c. Transient or constant visual fluctuation
     d. Mild to moderate photophobia and glare
  3. Severe degree
     a. Reduced best correctable visual acuity
     b. History of spontaneous (non-traumatic) nonpainful epithelial erosions
     c. Slow epithelial healing time with re-erosions during treatment
     d. RCE syndrome (morning syndrome; Section II. C. 6.)

Objective

- Usually bilateral presentation
  1. One eye may be more advanced than the other
  2. One eye may show no signs at all
- Findings seen best under high magnification, indirect, or retroillumination
  1. Even easier and more vivid with dilated pupil
  2. Observable without dilation, *but*
     a. Must have good slit-lamp illumination and optics in dark room
     b. Must know what to look for and be looking
- Occasionally signs are subtle, difficult to find
  1. If subjective symptoms present and you have ruled out other causes, follow cornea closely (especially after trauma), and they will probably show up in time
  2. Sometimes symptoms (e.g., morning syndrome) show up before physical signs
- Negative staining frequently presents early (alone or before other signs)
  1. Instant tear breakup over same area(s) after each blink frequently in horizontal, linear cascades
  2. Different from TBUT (tear-breakup time) in dry eye syndrome, which is not an instantaneous process
  3. Valuable differential diagnostic tool for EBMD versus dry eye (TBUT; Table 5.9)
- Maps (usually central but could reach periphery; Figure 5.54)

TABLE 5.8 Clinical Summary of Epithelial Basement Membrane Disorders (EBMDs)

	Mild	Moderate	Severe
Subjective	AM Irritation	AM Irritation Chronic irritation Reduced (±) BVA Photophobia	AM Irritation Chronic irritation Reduced (±) BVA Photophobia Irregular astigmatism Spontaneous erosion RCE after injury Slow corneal healing
Objective	No observable signs Bilateral (occasionally unilateral) Maps or dots Fingerprints (rare) Negative staining	Bilateral (occasionally unilateral) Maps or dots Fingerprints (rare) Negative staining Tramlines "Mare's tail" Positive staining Diffuse epithelial edema	Bilateral (occasionally unilateral) Maps or dots Fingerprints (rare) Negative staining Tramlines "Mare's tail" Positive staining Diffuse epithelial edema Dendrites or filaments Spontaneous erosion Brawny edema
Assessment	Keratitis sicca Dry eye syndrome Fuchs' endothelial dystrophy Other epithelial or endothelial dystrophy	Keratitis sicca Dry eye syndrome Fuchs' endothelial dystrophy Other epithelial or endothelial dystrophy Cogan's degeneration Traumatic aggravant	Keratitis sicca Dry eye syndrome Fuchs' endothelial dystrophy Other epithelial or endothelial dystrophy Cogan's degeneration Traumatic aggravant Infection or inflammation Other degenerations
Plan	Advise and educate patient Hypertonic drops	Advise and educate patient Evaluate family Hypertonic drops and ointments, Soft lens wear	Advise and educate patient Evaluate family Hypertonic drops and ointments, Bandage soft lens wear (disposable) RCE therapy Phototherapeutic keratectomy (PTK) Anterior stromal puncture
Follow-up	PRN Annual check	PRN Annual check Every 3 months with SL Every 6 months with SL	PRN Annual check Every 3 months with SL Every 6 months without SL Every 4 to 6 weeks with bandage

Abbreviations: BVA, best visual acuity; RCE, recurrent corneal erosion; SL, soft lens.

TABLE 5.9 Comparison of NaFL Tear Breakup Time (TBUT) and Other Common Findings in Dry Eye or Keratoconjunctivitis Sicca (KCS) Syndrome versus Findings in Epithelial Basement Membrane Disorders (EBMD)

Finding to Compare	Dry Eye/KCS Syndrome	EBMD
Subjective presentation	Mid to late day and increasing irritation	Irritation on waking ("morning syndrome")
Objective signs	Associated with tear film dysfunction Band region superficial punctate keratitis Tear meniscus variations Mucoid debris	Intraepithelial signs (when observable) Maps Dots/microcysts Fingerprints
Schirmer testing	Positive or negative	Always negative
NaFl pattern		
Appearance	Positive staining	Negative staining
Timing	<10 sec/>1 sec (TBUT)	Instantaneous
Configuration	Round or oval and enlarging with time	Linear and cascading
Location	Random position after each blink	Stationary position after each blink

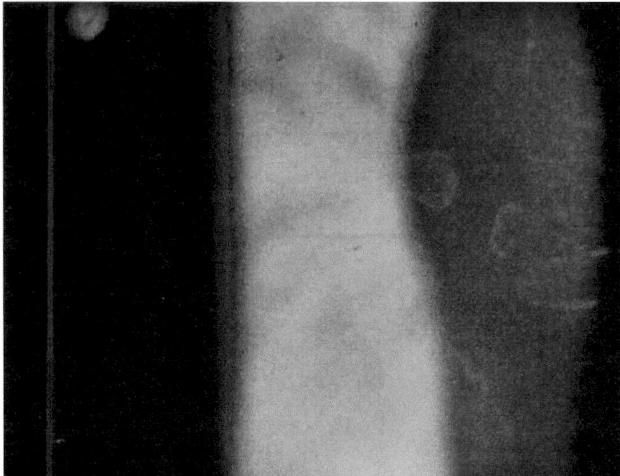

FIGURE 5.54 Map configuration (in EBMD) viewed by slit-lamp biomicroscopy under direct retroillumination.

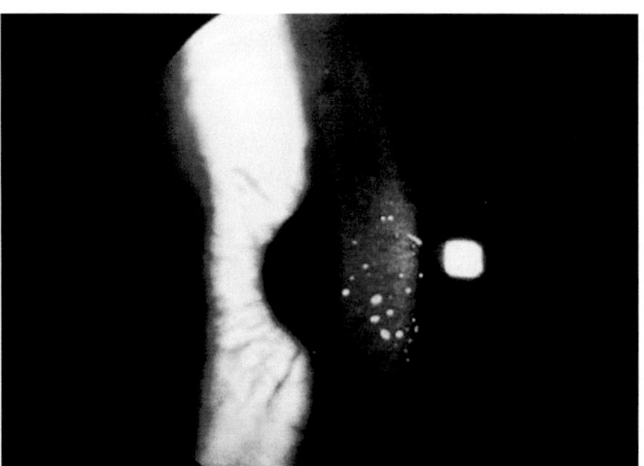

FIGURE 5.55 Dots (in EBMD) presenting in the inferior pupillary zone in a grouping ("archipelago") with a subtle, surrounding, amorphous haze.

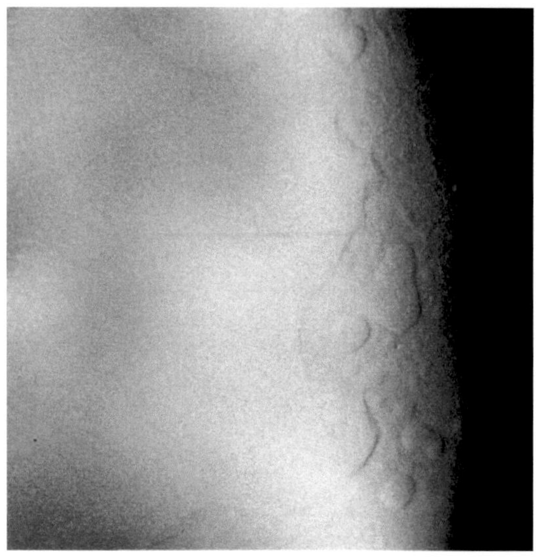

FIGURE 5.56 Microcysts (in EBMD) are vividly revealed with slit-lamp biomicroscopy under indirect specular reflection. These microcysts ("pseudocysts") represent spaces between deep epithelial cells created by irregularities in the basement membrane.

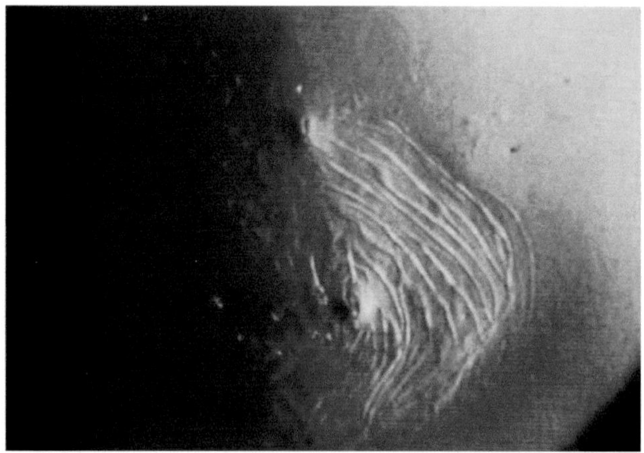

FIGURE 5.57 Fingerprint configurations (in EBMD) are the least common of EBMD signs and are found most commonly in older patients. They represent fibrogranular ridges on the surface of the basement membrane.

1. Grayish patches or sheets of clear zones, geographic lines, and amorphous patterns
2. May be distinct lines or have fading edges
3. Thicken and become denser with aging or recurrent corneal erosions
4. Size and shapes of patterns vary from short (<1 mm) to long (>3 mm), round, oval, sinuous, irregular
5. Frequently present with associated dots

- Dots (usually inferior central or just below pupil border) (Figures 5.55 and 5.56)
  1. Grayish (hyaline-filled) microcysts or clear fluid-filled cysts
  2. Round ameboid, or comma shaped
  3. Often found in multiple clusters
  4. May be pinpoint but never much larger than 0.5 mm to 1 mm
  5. Sometimes form polygonal type rows, or "nets"
  6. Negative staining when intraepithelial
     a. Will stain positive if they erupt
     b. Will also be symptomatic at that point
  7. Seen frequently with maps
- Fingerprints (larger patterns and usually central; Figure 5.57).
  1. Swirled refractile lines resembling a thumb print on corneal epithelium
  2. Look like "shift lines," "slipped rug," or "tramlines" seen in other corneal conditions (e.g., bullous keratopathy, ulcers)
  3. Clear to gray with indirect or retroillumination
  4. Least common presenting sign in EBMD
  5. May appear alone or with maps or dots
  6. Occasionally lines come off central point (dot), giving appearance of a "mare's tail"
- As condition advances, complications can occur on epithelial surface and anterior stroma
  1. Positive NaFl staining
  2. Edematous clouding and bullae
  3. Dendriform (infiltrative) keratitis
  4. Filamentary keratitis

5. "Brawny" (brownish) edema
   a. Especially after trauma and RCE
   b. Persists for months to years with RCE
6. Spontaneous (non-traumatic) epithelial erosions
   a. Usually "biggies" (25% to 50% corneal surface involvement)
   b. Usually followed by RCE
   c. Typically situated at inferior cornea
   d. May be loosely associated with Hudson–Stahli's line (e.g., frequency, risk?)
7. Once epithelium compromised in advanced conditions, increased risk of infection
8. Advanced EBMD with RCE can also produce an anterior stromal haze and potential scarring

- RCE complications can be predicted quite well with relative accuracy by checking Bell's phenomenon
  1. Positive EBMD clinical findings with a negative Bell's phenomenon (eyes do not roll up ward on forced lid closure) indicates significant risk (>75%) for spontaneous corneal erosion
  2. Simple test: hold upper lids firmly with thumbs and ask patient to shut lids forcefully while you observe eye movements
  3. Negative Bell's with EBMD findings indicates need for preventive therapy with or without symptoms

Assessment

(See also Appendix 3)

- Rule out dry eye or keratitis sicca–type syndromes (Figure 5.58)
  1. Sicca symptoms usually increase in later day versus EBMD morning syndrome
  2. Sicca stains positively with NaFl and rose bengal/lissamine green vs negative NaFl staining and negative rose bengal in EBMD
  3. TBUT less than 10 seconds (but greater than instantaneous) vs instantaneous breakup of tears (cascading) in EBMD (see Table 5.9)

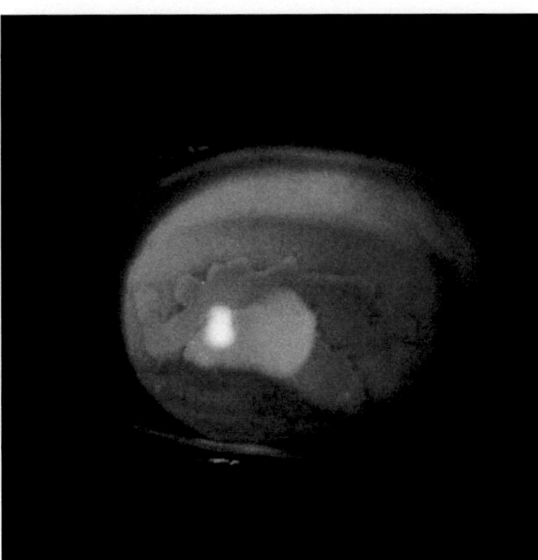

FIGURE 5.58 Cascade sodium fluorescein staining of a linear nature (versus rounder, amorphous patterns) represents the negative staining effect usually produced by visible or submicroscopic epithelial basement membrane changes.

  4. Presence of band SPK and other keratoconjunctivitis sicca signs vs. map-dot-fingerprint changes in EBMD
- Rule out epithelial (and endothelial) dystrophies
- Rule out Cogan's microcystic degeneration
- Rule out corneal infection or inflammation
  1. Diagnose "by the company they keep"
  2. Good history is critical
- Rule out corneal degenerations

Plan: Epithelial Basement Membrane Disorders

(See also Appendix 4)

- In advanced presentations or positive findings in patients under 20 years of age, consider dystrophy etiology
  1. Examine other family members
  2. Advise, educate, and counsel family
- In asymptomatic presentations (with positive clinical findings and normal Bell's phenomenon)
  1. Advise and educate patient as to findings
  2. Instruct on possible symptoms and care
- In asymptomatic presentations (with positive clinical findings and absent Bell's phenomenon)
  1. Advise and educate patient as to findings and as to increased risk of spontaneous erosion
  2. Instruct on possible symptoms and care
  3. Discuss prophylactic (mild) therapies as optional and available (patient's decision)
- Mild symptoms (morning syndrome) with or without objective signs
  1. Treatment optional
  2. Hypertonic ointment at bedtime
  3. Warm packs ad lib
  4. Hypertonic solution (2% or 5%) ad lib
- Moderate symptoms with or without objective signs
  1. Hypertonic saline drops q3–4h daily
  2. Hypertonic saline ointments at bedtime
  3. Antiedema therapies (heat) in AM
  4. Consider contact lens wear, if BVA reduced
- Severe symptoms or complications (e.g., RCE, reference Chapter 5, Section F)
  1. Treat uncomplicated symptoms with same regimen as moderate, at more frequent dose rates
  2. For spontaneous erosions and RCE
     a. Use standard abrasion protocol
     b. Avoid prolonged patching (more than 2 to 3 days); it causes edema complications
     c. Run minimum 1-week post-abrasion course of hypertonic ointment q2–3h and hs
     d. Consider bandage soft lens for RCE
  3. Use prophylactic tobramycin drops qid during any complication with epithelial compromise
  4. Treat any secondary infection or inflammation appropriately, avoiding steroids if possible
  5. PTK (see Chapter 7)
     a. A study of 58 eyes who failed with conventional medical therapy underwent PTK
        i. Patients with visual symptoms after treatment was 13% and increased to 20% after 3 years post-treatment
        ii. Pain from recurrence was 21% after treatment and 10% on average 10 months post-treatment
        iii. 90% of patients re-epithelialize within 7 days (100% by 14 days) with no infections

6. Anterior stromal puncture (with needle or laser)
    a. Generally good results
    b. Procedure produces minimal (puncture) scarring which seems to serve as alternative anchoring mechanism for overlying cellular epithelium

Follow-Up

- Asymptomatic and mild cases followed routinely
- Moderate cases, PRN *or*
    1. Every 3 months with contact lens wear
    2. Every 6 months without contact lens wear
- Manage severe cases closely during acute complications or bandage lens therapies
- After complications phase, carefully advise and educate patient on early signs and symptoms and monitor corneal integrity every 3 months
- Remember to explain chronic nature of condition
    1. No cures
    2. Long-term prognosis guarded, but prognosis for individual episodes of complications and pain are generally favorable for complete resolution (average time approximately 6 to 12 weeks, but could take up to 1 year)
    3. Substantial risk of exacerbation

5. Concepts and Controversies[38,39]

a. In 1981, Werblin et al. documented significantly greater frequencies than in previously reported map-dot-fingerprint changes in corneas
    i. 43% of the general population
    ii. 76% (or greater) in patients over 50 years of age
b. In late 1983, Alvarado was able to prove that the human epithelial basement membrane thickens substantially through membrane reduplication in focal areas from 20 years of age and older (almost 100% thickening from 20 to 60 years of age)
    i. The thickening occurs in all individuals
    ii. The process is aggravated or accelerated by trauma or chronic irritation (cell injury and death)
        - Abrasion
        - Ulceration
        - Infection or inflammation
        - Contact lenses (as chronic irritant)
        - Corneal surgery (e.g., radial keratotomy)
    iii. Changes below 20 years of age (infrequent) are probably primary (dystrophic) changes, unless an aggravant is present
    iv. Membrane thickening weakens attachments and even "buries anchoring fibrils" over time, producing "significant disruption in terms of adhesion and stability of the corneal epithelium"
    v. Thus, EBM changes are age related, very prevalent, perhaps universal, and varying in degree of clinical appearance and significance (i.e., signs and symptoms)
c. Suggestion
    i. Retain EBMD as the mnemonic device
    ii. But instead of Epithelial Basement Membrane Dystrophy, broaden the mnemonic to Epithelial Basement Membrane Disorders
        - Dystrophic (<2% to 6% from 20 years of age and up)
        - Acquired (variable frequency at all ages)
        - Degenerative (frequency as high as 50% from 20 years of age and older and greater than 50% from 60 years of age and up)

E. Keratoconus[40–43]

Subjective

- Sometimes referred to as corneal ectasia or ectatic cornea (connotes thinning and bulging)
- Patient begins to demonstrate slow, insidious, refractive changes, and reduced BVA over months to years
    1. First signs usually about 15 to 25 years of age
    2. The younger the age of onset, the higher the risk for progression and severe disease
    3. Progressive refractive changes
    4. With increasing age most patients' progression will eventually slow and stabilizes in their fourth decade
- Frequent history of asthma, allergies, atopias, with reports of chronic eye rubbing
    1. Supports mechanical (environmental) etiology
    2. Hereditary etiology also possible
- Most cases remain painless unless secondarily complicated (e.g., epithelial breakdown, hydrops)
- Increasing irregular astigmatism and higher order optical aberrations cause:
    1. Serious problems with glare and visual discomfort
    2. Monocular diplopia
- Mild to moderate photophobia
- May have familial tendencies

Objective

- Noninflammatory bulging and thinning of cornea
- Early clinical signs (other than frequent, irregular refractive changes and reducing BVA) are usually subtle and difficult to discern
- Bilateral condition with one eye usually less involved or completely arrested (forme fruste)
- Earliest signs are refractive and visual
    1. Retinoscopy produces scissor-type reflex
    2. Irregular, asymmetric astigmatic changes occur with each subsequent refraction
    3. Keratometry readings begin to steepen (most common course) and mires begin to distort
    4. Corneal topography will begin to show conic shape, irregular astigmatism, and higher order aberrations
    5. BVA will be reduced with spectacle correction and improved by pinhole, stenopaic slit, and rigid contact lenses
- Progression can be monitored by corneal topography (e.g., changes in maximum simulated central keratometry and irregularity indexes)
- With advancing changes, the central to inferior (most frequent) cornea will begin to present a bulging, protruding profile (Munson's sign; Figure 5.59)
- Mild to moderate stromal thinning can be observed early at or proximal to the bulging "cone" area
- Eventually, a brownish-orange ferrous ring will be observable at the base (or 360°) of the cone (Fleischer's ring)
- Fine, fibrillary lines will begin to be noticed at the subepithelial and anterior stromal levels
- The posterior cornea will reveal slightly thicker, vertically oriented stress lines or Vogt lines (striae, disappear

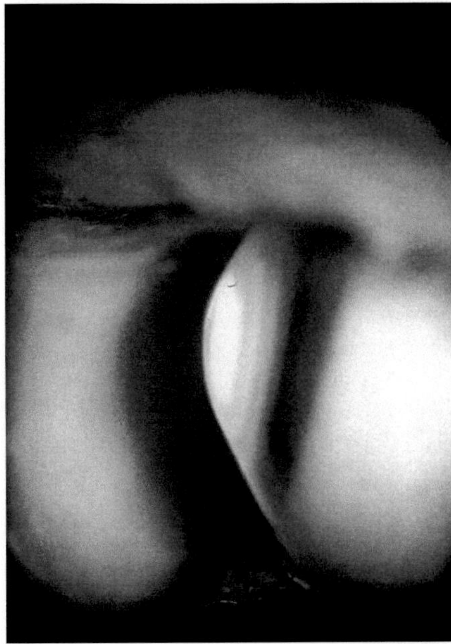

FIGURE 5.59 Keratoconus (Munson's sign) is obvious in this patient on profile view of the cornea. Note the slight inferior displacement of the apex of the cone.

with external pressure applied to globe), usually centrally and frequently aligned with the minus axis of the refractive cylinder

- Stromal nerve fibers (in irregular orientation) will appear more prominent (central and peripheral)
- In advanced cases, scarred corneal lamellae may appear at Bowman's and anterior stromal levels
- Rarely, in advanced cases, corneal hydrops occurs
  1. Breaks in posterior cornea cause dense edema
  2. Onset can be acute and painful
  3. Full-thickness stromal edema can dramatically reduce vision
  4. Resolution occurs (with no specific therapy) over 2 to 3 months with guaranteed scarring
- Risk of perforation is almost nil

Assessment

- Rule out other thinning disorders
  1. Marginal furrow (peripheral in older patient)
  2. Pellucid (inferior limbal)
  3. Terrien's (superior and usually acute onset)
- Rule out keratoglobus (thinning and bulging to periphery)
- Differentiate posterior keratoconus findings
  1. Usually congenital
  2. Thinning occurs from posterior surface toward anterior with early disruption of endothelium and resultant stromal edema
  3. Probably a form of ICE syndrome (mesodermal)
- Rule out herpes simplex disciform keratitis by history and clinical findings
- Rule out associated systemic syndromes

Plan: Keratoconus

- There is no known specific treatment, cure, or prevention for this unknown etiologic ectatic condition
- Visual treatment with spectacle lenses or soft contact lenses may help in early stages or mild cases
- Advanced changes require visual correction through custom contact lenses
  1. Custom soft lenses for astigmatism and custom thickness (e.g., Hydrocone, KeraSoft, and SpecialEyes)
  2. Standard rigid gas permeable (RGP) contact lenses (mild)
  3. Specially designed RGPs are required as corneal curvature and irregular astigmatism increases
     a. Piggy backing: RGP on top of a soft lens
     b. Special design RGP (e.g., Rose K) (mild to moderate)
     c. Hybrid (RGP center with soft lens skirt, e.g., SynergEyes) (mild to moderate)
     d. Scleral gas permeable lens (moderate to severe)
- Corneal cross linking (CXL) is used to reduce risk of progression
  1. An important consideration for younger (<18 years old) patients since progression is more likely and severe than adults
  2. To be eligible must have clear central cornea and thinnest corneal reading >400 microns
  3. Epithelium is removed (Dresden method) (other method is performed with epi on) and cornea is bathed in riboflavin for 30 minutes followed by 30 minutes of UV-A irradiation
     a. With epithelial removal (Dresden method) patient may experience pain, stromal haze, temporary vision loss, and infections
     b. The "epi on" procedure has fewer side effects but is not as effective since riboflavin does not penetrate the stroma as well compared to "epi off"
  4. Prevents progression by increasing corneal rigidity
  5. Studies have shown improved best corrected VA and reduced maximum corneal curvature following CXL
  6. Studies have shown keratoconus stabilization in pediatric population over time (up to 3–5 years post-CXL)
  7. Does not stop all progression on all patients
  8. May still need rigid lenses for best corrected vision
- Intrastromal corneal ring segments (e.g., Intacs)
  1. Plastic rings (1 or 2) are inserted into corneal stroma
  2. Require clear 6 mm central cornea with corneal thickness >450 microns
  3. Can reduce corneal steepness and decrease irregular astigmatism
  4. Contraindicated in young patients due to higher probability of progression
  5. May still need rigid lenses for best corrected vision
- Care for acute or painful hydrops is usually conservative with limited use of medication
  1. Extensive antiedema therapies
  2. Prophylactic antibiotics if epithelial surface is severely compromised
  3. Rarely, a short-course topical steroid may be of value to reduce scarring
     a. However, risk of retarded healing with steroid may contraindicate its use
     b. Should be avoided
- Primary indication for deep anterior lamellar keratoplasty (DALK) should be functional need or severe cosmetic distress

1. Indicated when better functioning eye is below acceptable (patient) standards with best visual correction system (contact lens)
2. Indicated when scarred cornea is emotionally or psychologically unacceptable to patient
3. Prognosis for corneal graft is generally good to excellent in adults but is contraindicated in young patients due to poor prognosis

Follow-Up

- Monitor active refractive changes every 6 months
- Monitor contact lens patients closely
- Post-keratoplasty patients usually require contact lens correction and close monitoring

F. Pellucid Marginal Degeneration[44]

Subjective

- Rare condition of unknown etiology
- A progressive, bilateral, noninflammatory corneal ectasia
- Age onset ranges from 20–50 years old, predominately male
- Symptomatic when vision decreases due to increasing irregular astigmatism/higher order aberrations
- Maybe a peripheral form of keratoconus

Objective

- Inferior corneal thinning (noninflammatory) is most common location from 4 to 8 o'clock, 1–2 mm from the limbus in a crescent shape
- The cornea separating the limbus and thin area is normal
- The ectasia is above the thinnest section of cornea
- Corneal topography shows inferior peripheral steepening extending into the mid-periphery and image resembles "kissing-doves" or "crab claws"
- May be a peripheral form of keratoconus

Assessment

- Rule out other marginal degenerations
- No risk of perforation or significant scarring

Plan and Follow-Up: Pellucid Marginal Degeneration

- As condition progresses best corrected vision will be reduced due to increased irregular, against-the-rule astigmatism
  1. Large diameter rigid gas permeable (RGP) lenses
  2. RGP-soft hybrid lens for RGP intolerant patients
  3. Scleral lenses for RGP intolerant patients
- Corneal surgeries
  1. Penetrating keratoplasty (PK)
     a. Large diameter must be used due to peripheral thinning and increases risk of graft rejection and high post-op astigmatism
  2. Deep anterior lamellar keratoplasty (DALK)
     a. Better post-op visual acuity compared to PK
  3. Other options include intrastromal rings and corneal crosslinking
  4. No consensus on best surgical option for CL intolerant patients

G. Pigmentations

1. Arlt's triangle (brownish coloration)
   a. Triangular-shaped pigment deposition at 6-o'clock position on posterior cornea
   b. Pathognomonic of old uveitis
2. Brawny edema (brownish coloration)
   a. Brownish edematous haze in epithelium
   b. Pathognomonic of EBMDs or recurrent corneal erosions
3. Ferry's line (orangish-brown coloration)
   a. Ferric ions around a surgical filtering bleb
   b. No pathognomonic indications
4. Fleischer's ring (orangish-brown coloration)
   a. Ferric ions around or at base of cone in keratoconus
   b. No additional pathognomonic indications regarding keratoconus or other conditions
5. Goar's line
   a. Pigment granules forming horizontal line on inferior cornea
   b. Pathognomonic for pigmentary glaucoma
6. Hemosiderosis
   a. Intracorneal or posterior corneal surface blood staining
   b. Pathognomonic for
      i. Intracorneal bleed (neovascularization)
      ii. Hyphema (posterior surface staining)
7. Hudson–Stahli's line (orangish-brown coloration (Figure 5.60)
   a. Level of Bowman's layer in band region of cornea where margins of lids meet on blink; may be produced by migration of tear film ions over time into line from blinking action
   b. More frequent in males
   c. Frequency parallels age (e.g., age 20 = 20%, 30 = 30%)
   d. Three typical presentations
      i. Faint segmented line
      ii. Continuous distinct line
      iii. Line with surrounding (whitish-yellow) opacities
   e. Frequent site of spontaneous or recurrent corneal epithelial erosions

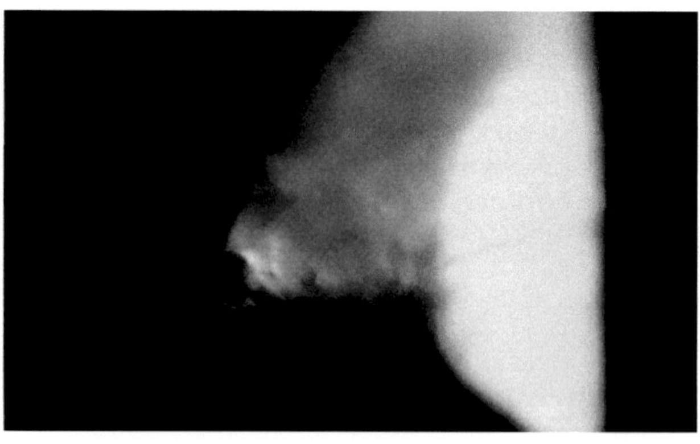

FIGURE 5.60 Hudson–Stahli line in the inferior third of the cornea (at approximate site of the closed lid margin juncture) with associated whitish-yellow deposits. These common brownish-orange lines increase in frequency with age and may appear as continuous from limbus to limbus, segmented, or with deposits.

8. Kayser–Fleischer ring (orangish coloration)
   a. Posterior corneal (and anterior angle) ring
      i. Best observed by gonioscopy
      ii. Advanced presentations may be grossly visible or observed by slit lamp alone
   b. Copper deposition specifically pathognomonic of Wilson's hepatolenticular disease
9. Keratitic (keratic) precipitates (white or pigmented)
   a. Endothelial surface pigment cells
   b. Almost universal with age
   c. May be pathognomonic (check history and associated findings) for
      i. Uveitis
      ii. Trauma
      iii. Aging
10. Keratomelanocystosis (striate melanokeratosis)
   a. Pigmented spokes radiating into cornea from limbal juncture
   b. Seen mostly in dark-skinned patients
   c. Usually greater inferiorly, especially at 4- and 8-o'clock positions
   d. Pathognomonic for
      i. Trauma
      ii. Infection
      iii. Focal, toxic inflammation (e.g., Staphylococcus at 4- and 8-o'clock positions)
11. Krukenberg's spindle (brownish coloration)
   a. A vertical spindle-shaped pigment deposition on inferior one third to one half posterior cornea
   b. Pathognomonic for
      i. Old uveitis
      ii. Pigment dispersion syndrome
12. Salmon patch (orangish coloration)
   a. Discoloration of mid-stroma in interstitial keratitis (usually 3 to 6 weeks after onset)
   b. Pathognomonic of syphilitic keratitis
13. Sampaolesi's line
   a. Pigment granules are deposited at Schwalbe's line
   b. Pathognomonic for pigmentary glaucoma
14. Stocker's line (orangish-brown coloration)
   a. Ferric ions at leading edge of pterygium
   b. No pathognomonic indications to pterygium or other conditions
15. "Tattooing" (variable colorations)
   a. Staining of mucocutaneous membranes by heavy metallic substances or certain drugs
   b. Usually diagnosed through history

III. Inflammatory Conditions

A. Sterile (Superficial) Keratitis[45]

(See also Chapter 2)

Background Information

Subjective

- Presentation of corneal symptoms with no associated history of corneal injury, irritation, or foreign body
- Corneal symptoms usually reported in one of three classic descriptions
  1. Report of a "sandy, gritty" feeling in eye(s)
  2. Description of a foreign-body sensation
  3. Report of "something under upper lid"
     a. Effect of upper lid pressure during blink
     b. Worth everting upper lid to rule out any possibility of tarsal foreign body
- Symptoms are generally acute or subacute
- Always conduct careful, comprehensive history to help establish non-traumatic etiology (toxic, physiological, or contact lens wear related)
- Associated symptoms may also help establish etiology
  1. Inflammatory pain and congested feeling
  2. Allergic (hypersensitivity) itching
  3. Viral burning sensation

Objective

- Designation superficial keratitis assumes primary disease process limited to the superficial squamous epithelial layer of cornea
  1. Secondary effects, such as edema and infiltration, may be limited to deeper cellular epithelial layers and anterior stroma
  2. Full-thickness stromal involvement should be considered deep keratitis with different diagnostic, therapeutic, and prognostic implications
- Classic physical finding usually termed superficial punctate keratitis (SPK)
  1. Epithelial surface irregularities cause by multiple etiologic factors and mechanics
     a. Superficial epithelial erosions (SEE) or superficial punctate staining (SPS)
        i. Usually well-defined punctate dots
        ii. May be confluent, grayish accumulations of necrotic cellular debris on epithelial surface (e.g., keratitis sicca or erosion under a contact lens)
        iii. Frequently stains with rose bengal/lissamine green/NaFl
     b. Microcystic (physiological) edema as distinct cysts or diffusely distributed pinpoint staining dots (SME)
        i. Cysts (intercellular pseudocysts, usually 1 mm or less) may or may not stain with NaFl
        ii. Diffuse intracellular edema may stain as discrete superficial punctate dots and/or diffuse hyperfluorescence
     c. Infiltrative (inflammatory) punctate staining usually presents as larger, surface dots with ill-defined borders (due to surrounding edema)
        i. Includes inflammatory/infiltrative white blood cells, inflammatory debris (proteins, cells, etc.), and edema
        ii. Generally will present with some degree of limbal, conjunctival vasodilation (redness)
  2. All types cause squamous cell juncture breaks that stain with NaFl as small punctate dots (from pinpoint in size to 1 to 2 mm for some infiltrates)
  3. Often small punctate dots can concentrate into a focal confluent patch of stain and appear as a single larger lesion (focal epithelial defect)
- Infiltrates (white blood cells) can remain as superficial (punctate infiltrates) or may penetrate deeper (intraepithelial)
  1. Intraepithelial infiltrate (partial or full cellular epithelial thickness including cuboidal and columnar cells)

a. Usually focal, sterile, toxic, or immune response (e.g., sterile staphylococcal toxic marginal infiltrate)
   i. Considered focal epithelial defect
   ii. Compromise of cellular epithelial protective barrier
b. May be diffuse (e.g., toxic, medicamentosus, SPK of Thygeson) in variable sizes
   i. Small, well-defined, non-staining infiltrates that do not break surface, but may raise focal epithelium to produce negative NaFl pattern (break in surface fluorescence) with a surrounding "halo" appearance (see Table 5.12)
   ii. Larger infiltrates will break surface integrity and stain positively
c. Infiltrative material may produce a linear (or branching) dendritiform pattern (Table 5.12)
   i. May be flat or raised with positive staining
   ii. Non-ulcerative infiltrative dendrite (vs herpes simplex epithelial ulcerative dendrite)

2. Subepithelial infiltrate (between epithelium and anterior surface of Bowman's layer of anterior stroma)
   a. Usually associated with virus (lymphocytes)
   b. Proximity to anterior stroma may result in mild stromal scar secondary to antigen–antibody reaction over prolonged exposure
      i. Scar(s) often mistaken for infiltrates
      ii. Process can occur with any infiltrate
   c. Contact lens peripheral ulcer (see Table 5.15)
      i. Usually associated with extended soft lens wear
      ii. Patients report irritation, foreign-body sensation, and sometimes mild photophobia
      iii. A single, focal subepithelial/anterior stromal infiltrate, 1–2 mm round with overlying NaFl staining in peripheral cornea; sectorial hyperemia; anterior chamber is clear; usually leaves a scar
3. Stromal infiltration can also occur, usually secondary to superficial corneal infiltrative process
   a. Superficial stimulus (sterile or infectious toxic antigen) can penetrate into stroma (even through intact epithelium) for numerous reasons
      i. Highly virulent (especially certain bacteria in high concentration and/or prolonged exposure)
         - Streptococcus
         - Gonococcus
         - *Haemophilus influenzae*
      ii. High concentrations, prolonged exposure, or chronic replenishment of the toxin (e.g., staphylococcal exotoxins)
      iii. Toxins of small molecular size (proteins, chemical, and viruses)
      iv. Migratory toxin (e.g., the trophozoite stage of acanthamoeba)
   b. Also, toxins from systemic causes may enter the stroma through superficial diffusion into the tear film, with subsequent penetration through the epithelium, or simply through deep limbal blood vessel diffusion directly into the stroma
   c. Stromal infiltrative presentations include multiple routes (above), multiple levels, and variable patterns
      i. Anterior stromal (e.g., staphylococcal toxins)
      ii. Deep stromal (e.g., herpetic, systemic causes)
      iii. Full thickness (e.g., variable)
      iv. Wessely or immune ring (from antigen–antibody response to penetrating toxin)
      v. Interstitial keratitis (90% syphilitic), producing a triad (syndrome) of stromal infiltration, stromal neovascularization, and stromal thinning

- Chronic superficial toxic or hypersensitive irritation will tend to stimulate translimbal immunological vascular responses
  1. Increased prominence of limbal arcades
  2. Pannus (superficial neovascular process with formation of a fibrous bed)
  3. Neovascularization (deeper, fine, weak, terminal arborizing vessels)

Assessment

- Diagnose superficial keratitis "by the company it keeps," both subjectively and objectively
  1. Bacterial
  2. Viral
  3. Toxic or hypersensitive (immunological)
  4. Contact lens wear associated
  5. Mechanical
  6. Irritative
  7. Systemic manifestations
  8. Other associated clinical findings
- Geographic (topographic) pattern of SPK usually of significant differential diagnostic value in superficial keratitis (localization of predominance of SPK)
  1. Diffuse SPK (in approximate order of frequency) (Figure 5.61)

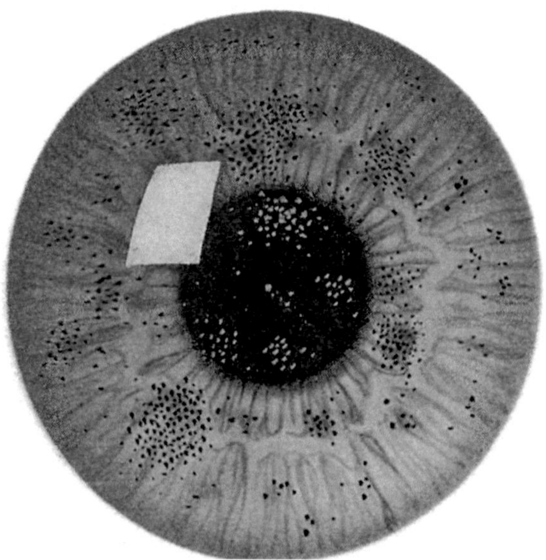

FIGURE 5.61 Diffuse SPK pattern of punctate infiltrative sites staining with NaFl on superficial squamous epithelial layer.

   a. Adenovirus
   b. Toxic staphylococcal reaction
   c. Medicamentosa (reaction to diagnostic or therapeutic eyedrops)
   d. Herpes simplex
   e. Herpes zoster
   f. SPK of Thygeson
   g. Verrucae
   h. Molluscum contagiosum
2. Inferior SPK (in approximate order of frequency) (Figure 5.62)
   a. Toxic staphylococcal reaction
   b. Trichiasis (usually vertical or irregular FBT)
   c. Medicamentosa (gravitational effect)
   d. Entropion (same pattern as trichiasis)
3. Band-region SPK (usually epithelial erosions) (Figure 5.63)
   a. Dry eye syndrome
   b. Keratoconjunctivitis sicca
   c. Exposure
      i. Lagophthalmos
      ii. Radiation burns
      iii. Chemical burns
      iv. Neurotropic
4. Superior SPK (in approximate order of frequency) (Figure 5.64)
   a. Atopic keratoconjunctivitis
   b. Superior limbic keratoconjunctivitis (SLK)
   c. Inclusion (chlamydial) keratoconjunctivitis
   d. Vernal keratoconjunctivitis
   e. Trachoma (old scarring or active stage)
5. Ulcerative keratitis deeper (stromal) and usually infectious (e.g., bacterial, fungal)

- Combine topographic, geographic differential diagnostic considerations with the "level" of infiltration for safest and most effective diagnostic and management approaches (Tables 5.10–5.12)
  1. Superficial, squamous epithelial level
  2. Intraepithelial, cuboidal, and columnar epithelial level

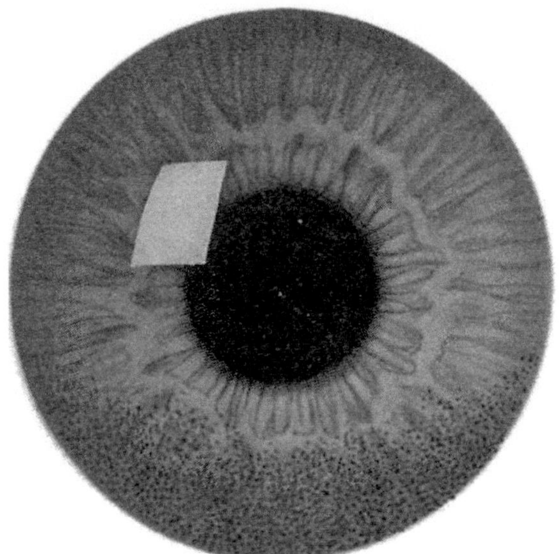

FIGURE 5.62 Inferior SPK pattern most often associated with staphylococcal toxins (sterile) from the lid margins.

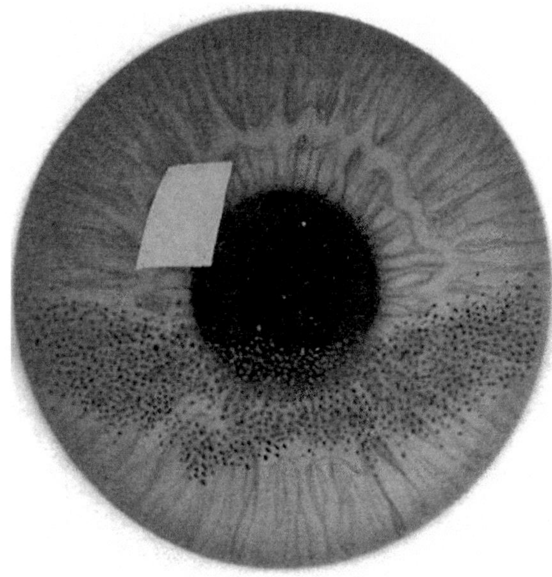

FIGURE 5.63 Band region SPK pattern or more accurately (and more commonly) superficial epithelial erosion (SEE) from drying or exposure of the band region of the cornea.

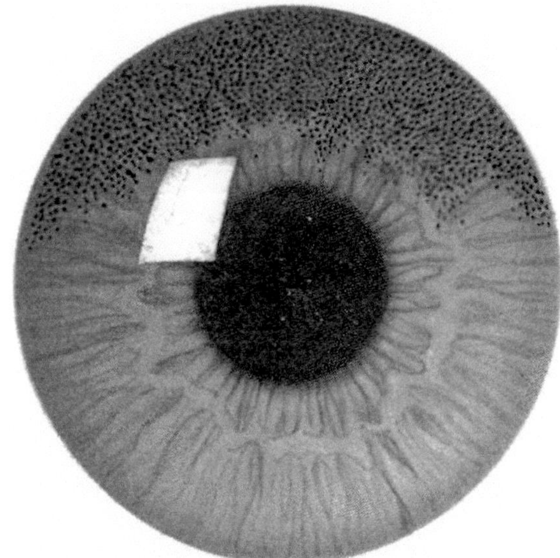

FIGURE 5.64 Superior SPK pattern associated with immune or autoimmune disorders, often of an idiopathic nature.

  3. Subepithelial (at Bowman's layer) level
  4. Stromal level (anterior, mid, deep, or full thickness)
- Most important differential consideration in assessing superficial keratitis is differentiating infiltration (process) from ulceration (process)
  1. Infiltrative keratitis usually superficial (epithelial) and non-infectious (sterile on culture)

Plan and Follow-Up: Sterile (Superficial) Keratitis

- Aminoglycoside(s) (e.g., gentamicin, tobramycin) and fluoroquinolones as therapeutic or prophylactic agent

TABLE 5.10 Superficial Corneal Findings and Prescription Options in Common Anterior Segment Diagnoses

Etiology	Differential Diagnosis	Sx		Tears			Squamous Epithelium								
		Contributing History	Corneal Irritation	Breakup Time/Neg. Staining	Rose Bengal Stain	Filaments	Superior SPK	Band SPK	Inferior SPK	Diffuse SPK	Peripheral SPK	Focal SPK	Band Keratopathy	Limbal Follicles	Pannus
Irritation/Injury	Corneal abrasions	X	X			X						X			
	Blunt injury	X										X			
	Burns	X	X		X	X		X		X		X			X
	Dry eye/KCS syndrome		X	X	X	X		X		X		X	X		
	Recurrent corneal erosion (RCE)	X	X	X								X			
Noninflammatory Conditions	Degenerations			X	X	X						X	X		
	Dellen	X		X											
	Dystrophies									X		X			
	EBMDs		X	X		X			X	X		X			
	Keratoconus			X											
	Systemic complications	X											1	X	X
Inflammatory Conditions, Sterile	Acne rosacea						X		X	X	X				X
	Atopic keratoconjunctivitis	X	X				X	X			X			X	X
	Contact lens complications	X				X			X	X	X	X			X
	Giant papillary conjunctivitis (GPC)		X			X	X								
	Medicamentosa	X	X	X					X						
	SLK of Theodore or SL		X	X			X			X	X	X			
	Staphylococcal exotoxic keratitis		X	X		X		X	X	X	X	X			X
	SPK of Thygeson			X		X				X					
	Terrien's marginal degeneration		X				X								X
	Toxic keratitis		X	X				X	X	X	X	X			X
	Vernal keratoconjunctivitis	X	X			X	X			X		X		X	X
Inflammatory Conditions, Infectious	Acanthamoeba keratitis	X	X							X		X			
	Adenoviral keratitis		X	X						X					
	Bacterial keratitis (corneal ulcer)		X									X			X
	Chlamydial keratoconjunctivitis	X	X				X		X	X	X				
	Fungal keratitis	X	X		X							X			
	Herpes simplex (HSV)keratitis				X					X		X			
	Herpes zoster ophthalmicus		X		X					X		X			

Abbreviations: Sx, Symptoms; BUT, breakup time: SPK, superficial punctate keratitis; KCS, keratoconjunctivitis sicca: EBMDs, epithelial basement membrane disorders; SLK, superior limbic keratoconjunctivitis; SL, soft lens; NSAID, nonsteroidal anti-inflammatory drug.

1. Minimum standard for acute or subacute keratitis
2. Minimum therapeutic dosage, qid for 5 to 7 days depending on diagnosis and degree of presentation
3. Minimum prophylactic dosage, bid for 2 to 3 days
4. Limit fluoroquinolones to more advanced or gram-negative and pseudomonal risk cases

- Topical steroids are indicated in superficial corneal involvements, including cellular or tissue damage, destruction, infiltration, or scarring being produced by non-infectious-induced immune response
  1. Contraindicated in infectious (ulcerative) keratitis or any superficial keratitis of suspicious origin
  2. With suspicion (of infection or ulceration) or risk factors for ulcer, do not introduce steroids for minimum of 24 to 48 hours or until clinical picture or cultures reveal non-infectious etiology
  3. Research suggests that in culture positive, gram-positive staphylococcal corneal ulceration, infiltrative white blood cells (polymorphonuclear WBCs) may have an equal or even more pronounced collagenolytic effect on the stroma than the proliferating staphylococcal bacterial itself
     a. If such is the case, immediate introduction of a combination (antistaphylococcal/corticosteroid) topical agent (e.g., 0.03% Tobramycin/0.1% Dexamethasone) is appropriate in staphylococcal corneal ulceration to fight the infection and the infiltrative destruction simultaneously
     b. Similar studies done on gram-positive streptococcus, gram-negative bacteria including Pseudomonas, and fungal infection continue to show a *contraindication* of early steroid usage in such infections

TABLE 5.10 (CONTINUED)

Cuboidal and Columnar Epithelium												Basement Membrane							Prescription Options									Follow-Up		
Edema	Dots	Microcysts	Bullae	Dendrites	Ulceration	Thinning	Hypoesthesia	Sub-Epithelial Infiltrates	Intra-Epithelial Infiltrates	Phlyctenule	Epithelial Splitting	Maps	Fingerprints	Epithelial Erosion	Indolent Ulcer	Melanocytosis	Hemosiderosis	Ferric Lines	Pressure Patch	Soft Lens Bandage	Topical Anti-Infective	Topical Steroid	Antihist./Mast Cell Stabilizer	Topical NSAIDs	Lubricant	Hypertonic	Oral Agents	24 Hours	3–5 Days	Variable
X	X	X		X		X			X			X	X	X			X		X	X	X					X	13	X	X	
X			X														X									X		X		
X		X			X	X									X			X			X	10		14	X	X	13	X	X	
X					X										X					X		X			X	X				X
X	X	X										X	X	X	X			X	X	X						X	13	X	X	X
X	X	X	X			X						X	X					X							X	X				X
						X													X	X					X				X	X
x	X	x	X									X	X	X						X										X
X	X	X		X								X	X	X				x	x	X						x				x
						x												X							X					X
X		X				4	5	X	X	7							X													X
X						X		X			X			X								X		X			14			X
X					3				X		X				X					X		X	X	X	X	X	15		X	
X		X		X	X			X	X		X									X			X	X	X	X			x	x
X		X							X																					X
						X												x				X			X				X	
									X											X	X	X			X				X	X
X				x				X	X	X	X										X	X				X	X			X
							X		X											X		X		X	X					X
						X																X							X	X
X		X						X	X		X											X	X		X	X			X	X
X					X										X							X	X	X	X		15		X	X
X				X		X		X													X							17		
X								X													x				X				X	
x					X	X									X					X	9						13	17		
								X																			14	18		X
X					X	X									X						X						13	17		
X				2		X	X								X						X	11			X		16	X	X	
X				X	X	X	X	X	X						X						X	X		X			16		X	X

Notes: 1 = hyperparathyroidism; 2 = ulcerative; 3 = shield ulcer; 4 = interstitial keratitis (syphilis); 5 = neurotropic; 6 = Epstein-Barr (mononucleosis); 7 = tuberculosis; 8 = Drug reservoir; 9 = fortified or fluoroquinolone; 10 = first 5 days; 11 = stromal HSV; 12 = after 5 days; 13 = analgesic NSAID; 14 = tetracycline/doxycycline/azithromycin; 15= antihistamine/decongestant; 16 = oral antiviral; 17 - consider hospitalization; 18= refer for medical consultation.

- Contact lens wear associated (including contact lens peripheral ulcer)
  1. If mild, consider daily lens wear only (no overnight wear), more frequent lens replacement (e.g., daily disposable), switch to hydrogen peroxide disinfecting solution (multipurpose solutions may be toxic) for reusable lenses, and lenses with greater lubricity (e.g., Acuvue Oasys, 2 weeks; Acuvue Oasys, 1 Day; and Dailies Total 1)
  2. If moderate to severe, temporarily discontinue lens wear and treat appropriately with antibiotics and/or steroids as stated above; upon resolution consider other contact lens wearing options described above in 1.
- Lubricants are valuable adjunctive agents with or without other therapy
  1. Can be used to monitor a suspicious keratitis
  2. Tend to reduce subjective corneal symptoms
  3. Should not be used exclusively (e.g., without prophylactic antibiotic) in acute or subacute keratitis (SPK with inflammation)
- Hypertonic saline (drops or ointments) can be used to reduce secondary epithelial edema
  1. Not effective in deeper stromal edemas
  2. Not effective in larger (than SPK) epithelial defects
- Standard cycloplegic-dilation therapy may be indicated in moderate to severe SPKs to reduce risk of (or actual) secondary anterior uveitis
  1. Prostaglandins (inflammogenic agents) released in aqueous with any degree of corneal insult
  2. High probability of secondary anterior uveitis in moderate to severe superficial keratitis
  3. Minimum dosage, tid (e.g., 1% tropicamide, 2% or 5% homatropine) based on degree of corneal and anterior chamber sign and symptoms

TABLE 5.11 **Management of Infiltrative Keratitis by Level and Degree**

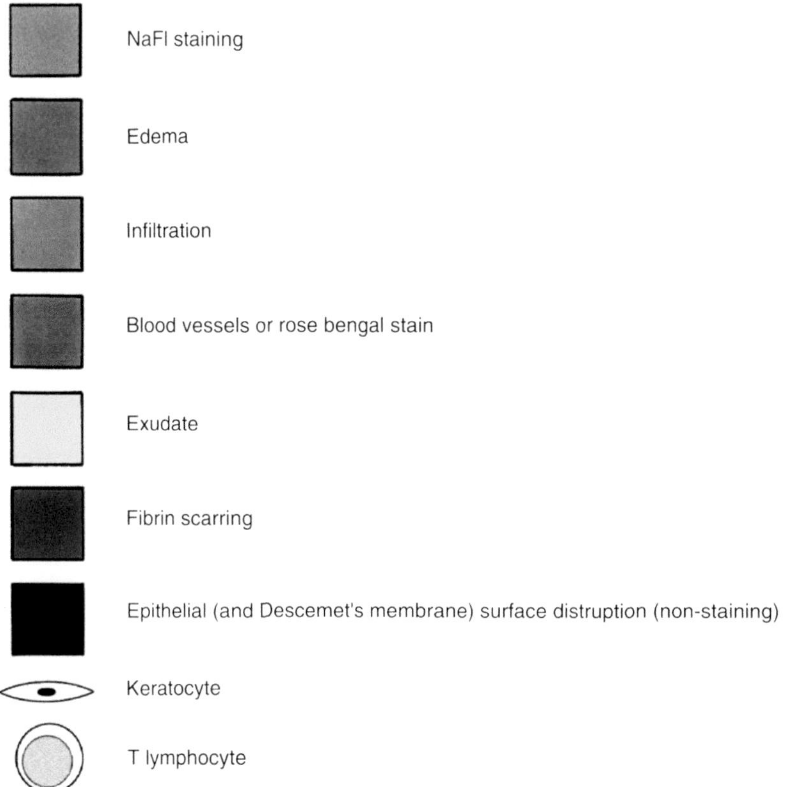

SUPERFICIAL EPITHELIAL KERATITIS (SPK)

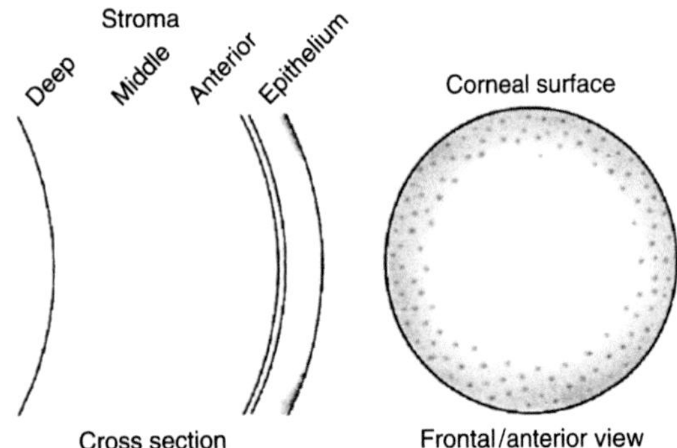

(See also Figure 5.70)

Management Considerations	Mild	Moderate	Severe
Antigen (?)	Staphylococcal (infection)	Tears/protein	Mechanica/toxic
Contact lens care	Modify lens wear	Temporary discontinue	Temporary discontinue
Irrigate/lubricate	bid to tid	tid to qid	qid to q2h
Cold pack	tid to qid	qid to q4h	q2–4h
Antibiotic	—	Tobramycin?	Tobramycin qid
Steroid/combination	—	Consider if noninfectious	If suspicious lesion, wait 24–48 hours
Other	Antistaphylococcal	Antistaphylococcal 5% NaCl qid	Antistaphylococcal 5% NaCl qid
RTC	2–4 wk	1–2 wk	5–7 days

(Continued)

TABLE 5.11 (CONTINUED) **Management of Infiltrative Keratitis by Level and Degree**

Diffuse

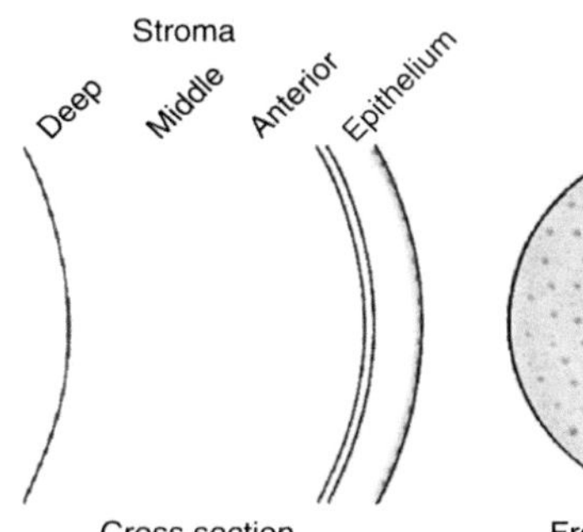

Corneal surface

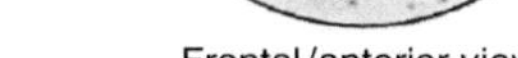

Cross section

Frontal/anterior view

(See also Figure 5.72)

Management Considerations	Mild	Moderate	Severe
Antigen (?)	Staphylococcal/solution	Virus/edema	Mechanical/toxic/virus
Contact lens care	Temporarily discontinue	Temporarily discontinue	Surface quality?
Irrigate/lubricate	Lubricate qid	Lubricate q2–4h	Lubricate qh
Cold pack	qid to q4h	q2–4h	qh
Antibiotic	—	Tobramycin?	Topical tobramycin qid
Steroid/combination	—	Consider if noninfectious	If suspicious lesion, wait for 24–48 hours
Other	Antistaphylococcal	Antistaphylococcal 5% NaCl qid	Antistaphylococcal 5% NaCl qid Ibuprofen 400 mg/qid
RTC	1–2 wk	5–7 days	3–5 days

Confluent

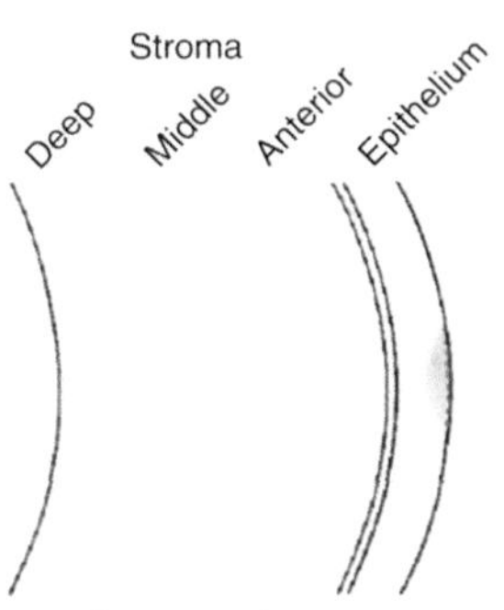

Corneal surface

Cross section

Frontal/anterior view

(See also Figure 5.73)

Management Considerations	Mild	Moderate	Severe
Antigen (?)	Mechanical/toxic	Toxic/virus	Bacteria?
Contact lens care	Change lens material/increase replacement frequency?	Temporarily discontinue	Temporarily discontinue
Irrigate/lubricate	Lubricate qid	Lubricate q2–4h	Lubricate qh
Cold pack	qid to q4h	q2–4h	
Antibiotic	Topical tobramycin?	Topical tobramycin?	Topical tobramycin qid
Steroid/combination	—	—	If suspicious lesion, wait 24–48 hours
Other	Antistaphylococcal (infection) 5% NaCl tid	Antistaphylococcal (infection) 5% NaCl qid	Antistaphylococcal (infection) 5% NaCl q2–4h Ibuprofen 400 mg/qid
RTC	7–10 days	5–7 days	3–5 days

(*Continued*)

TABLE 5.11 (CONTINUED) **Management of Infiltrative Keratitis by Level and Degree**

Focal

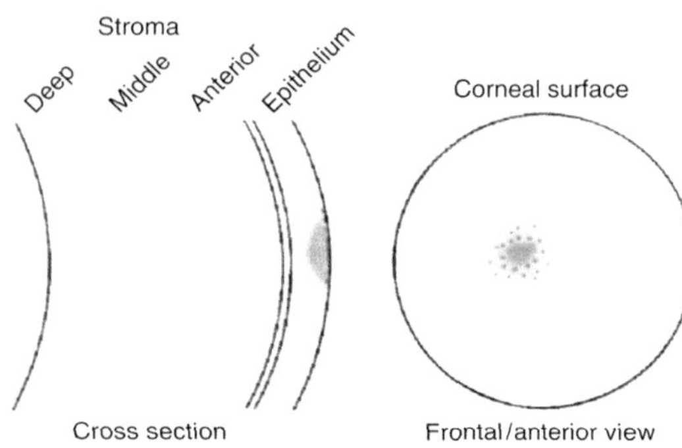

(See also Figure 5.74)

Management Considerations	Mild	Moderate	Severe
Antigen (?)	Mechanical/toxic	Toxic/bacteria?	Assume bacteria
Contact lens care	Temporarily discontinue	Temporarily discontinue	Temporarily discontinue
Irrigate/lubricate	Lubricate qid	—	—
Cold pack	qid to q4h	q2–4h	qh
Antibiotic	Ak-Bac-Poly ointment hs	Tobramycin qid?	Gentamicin or tobramycin or Ciloxan q2–4h
Steroid/combination	—	If suspicious lesion, wait 24–48 hours	If suspicious lesion, wait 24–48 hours
Other	Antistaphylococcal (infection)	Antistaphylococcal (infection)	Antistaphylococcal (infection)
			Topical NSAID?
		Oral ibuprofen?	Ibuprofen 400 mg/qid
			Cycloplege/dilate tid to q2–4h
RTC	5–7 days	3–5 days	24–48 hr

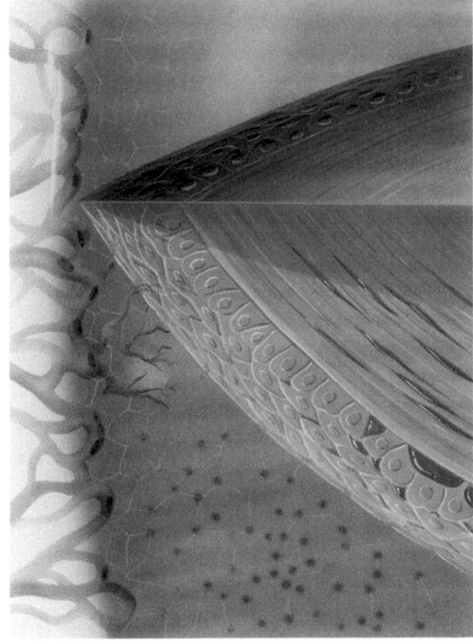

Superficial Epithelial Keratitis (SPK)

(Continued)

TABLE 5.11 (CONTINUED) **Management of Infiltrative Keratitis by Level and Degree**

INTRAEPITHELIAL KERATITIS

Marginal

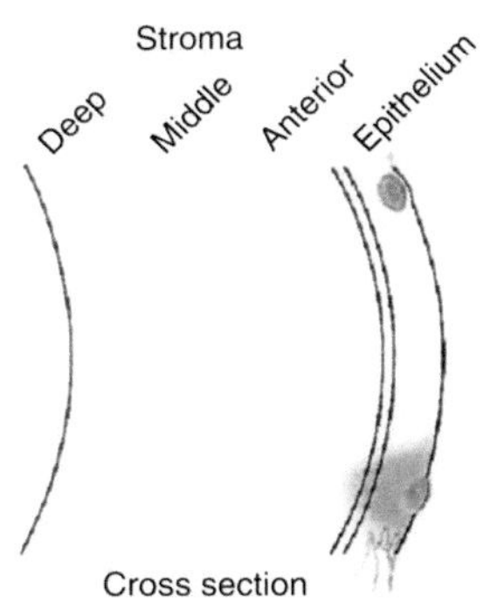

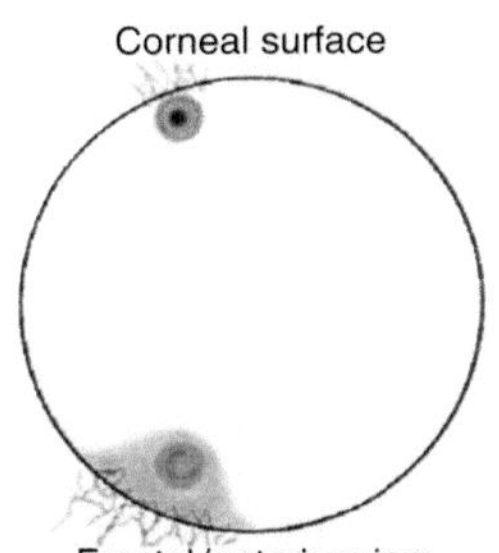

(See also Figure 5.66)

Management Considerations	Mild	Moderate	Severe
Antigen (?)	Staphylococcal/edema	Staphylococcal/toxic	Staphlococcal (infection for sure)
Contact lens care	Temporarily discontinue	Temporarily discontinue	Temporarily discontinue
Irrigate/lubricate	Irrigate tid	Irrigate qid	Irrigate qid
Cold pack	qid to q4h	q2–4h	qh
Antibiotic	Tobramycin qid?	Tobramycin qid	Tobramycin q2–4h
Steroid/combination	Rarely after 7 days	If presumed noninfectious Tobradex q4h	After 2–5 days if needed
Other	Antistaphylococcal (infection)	Antistaphylococcal (infection) Oral ibuprofen? Cycloplege/dilate qid?	Antistaphylococcal (infection) Ibuprofen 400 mg/qid Cycloplege/dilate qid? Culture/sensitivity if resistant
RTC	5–7 days	3–5 days	24–48 hr

Multiple and Diffuse

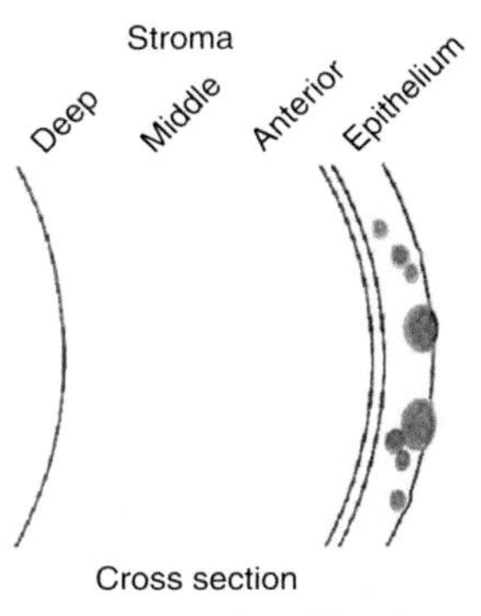

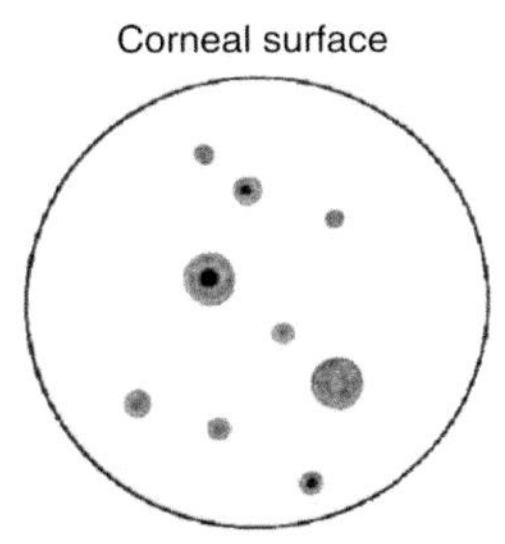

(See also Figure 5.71)

Management Considerations	Mild	Moderate	Severe
Antigen (?)	Solutions	Toxic/edema	Thygeson's superficial punctate keratitis?
Contact lens care	Rx daily disposable	Temporarily discontinue	As bandage?
Irrigate/lubricate	Lubricate qid	Irrigate and lubricate qid	Lubricate q2–4h
Cold pack	tid to qid	qid to q4h	q2–4h
Antibiotic	—	Tobramycin qid with positive NaFl	Tobramycin q4h with positive NaFl
Steroid/combination	Rarely	If presumed noninfectious TobraDex q4h	If presumed noninfectious TobraDex q4h
Other		5% NaCl q2–4h Cycloplege/dilate qid?	Cycloplege/dilate qid?
RTC	7–10 days	5–7 days	3–5 days

(Continued)

TABLE 5.11 (CONTINUED) **Management of Infiltrative Keratitis by Level and Degree**

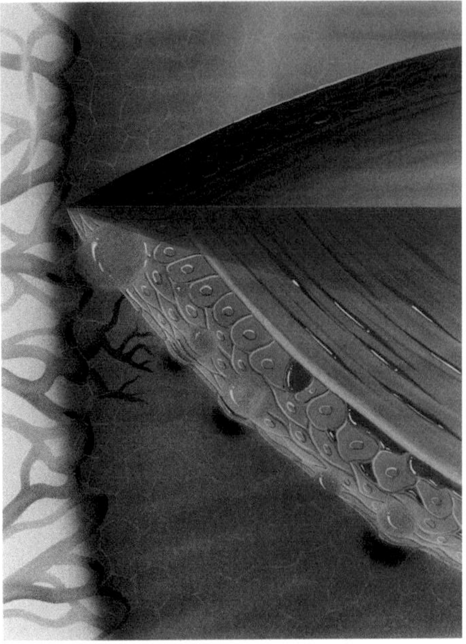

Intraepithelial Keratitis

Dendritic (Infiltrative)

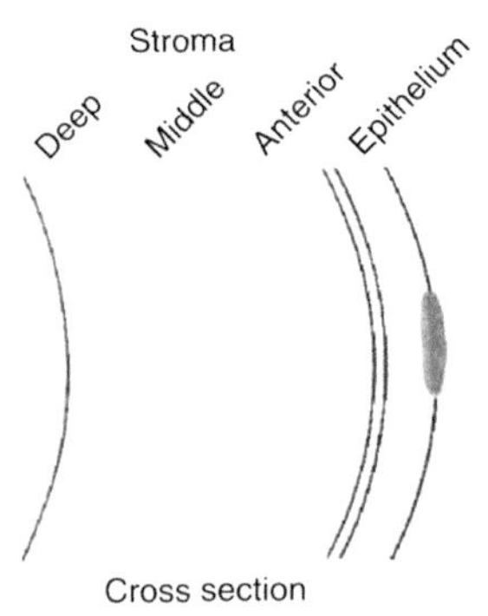

(See also Figure 5.90)

Management Considerations	Mild	Moderate	Severe
Antigen (?)	Edema/HSV?	Rule out HSV ulcer	Rule out Acanthamoeba
Contact lens care	Temporarily discontinue	Temporarily discontinue	Temporarily discontinue
Irrigate/lubricate Cold pack	Lubricate with positive NaFl tid to qid	Lubricate with positive NaFl qid to q4h	Lubricate with positive NaFl q2–4h
Antibiotic	—	Topical tobramycin qid with positive NaFl	Topical tobramycin q4h with positive NaFl
Steroid/combination	—	After 7–10 days	After 7–10 days?
Other	5% NaCl qid	5% NaCl q2–4h Cycloplege/dilate qid? Viroptic q2h? Culture/sensitivity?	5% NaCl qh Cycloplege/dilate qid? Viroptic q2h? Culture/sensitivity? Corneal consultation?
RTC	7 days	3–5 days	24–48 hr

(*Continued*)

TABLE 5.11 (CONTINUED) **Management of Infiltrative Keratitis by Level and Degree**

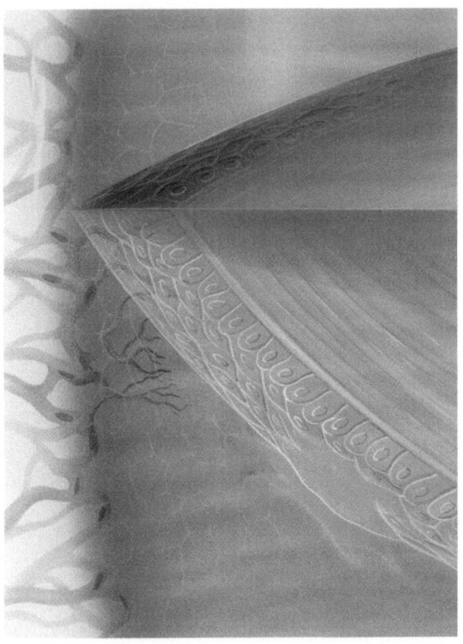

Dendritic (Infiltrative) Intraepithelial Keratitis

Dendritic (Ulcerative)

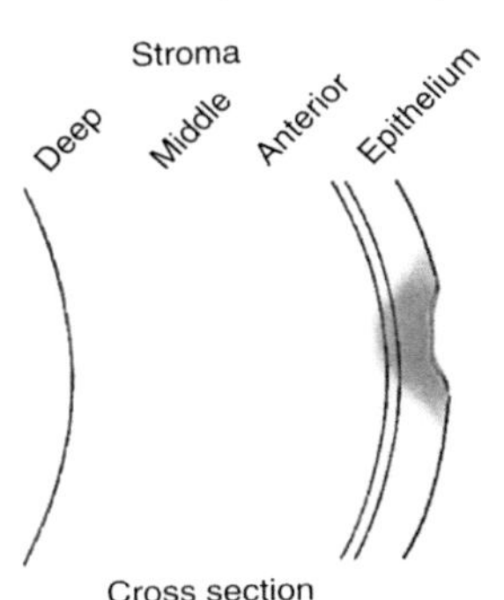

(See also Figure 5.87)

Management Considerations	Mild	Moderate	Severe
Antigen (?)	Edema/HSV?	Rule out HSV ulcer	Rule out Acanthamoeba
Contact lens care	Temporarily discontinue	Temporarily discontinue	Temporarily discontinue
Irrigate/lubricate Cold pack	Lubricate with positive NaFl tid to qid	Lubricate with positive NaFl qid to q4h	Lubricate with positive NaFl q2–4h
Antibiotic	—	Topical tobramycin qid with positive NaFl	Topical tobramycin q4h? with positive NaFl
Steroid/combination	—	After 7–10 days	After 7–10 days?
Other	5% NaCl qid	5% NaCl q2–4h Cycloplege/dilate qid? Viroptic q2h? Oral antiviral? Culture/sensitivity?	5% NaCl qh Cycloplege/dilate qid? Viroptic q2h? Oral antiviral? Culture/sensitivity? Corneal consultation?
RTC	7–10 days	3–5 days	24–48 hr

(*Continued*)

TABLE 5.11 (CONTINUED) **Management of Infiltrative Keratitis by Level and Degree**

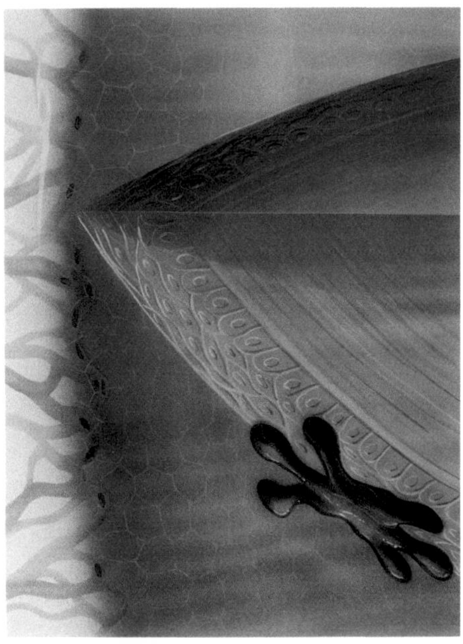

Dendritic (Ulcerative) Intraepithelial Keratitis

SUBEPITHELIAL KERATITIS

Without Stromal Involvement

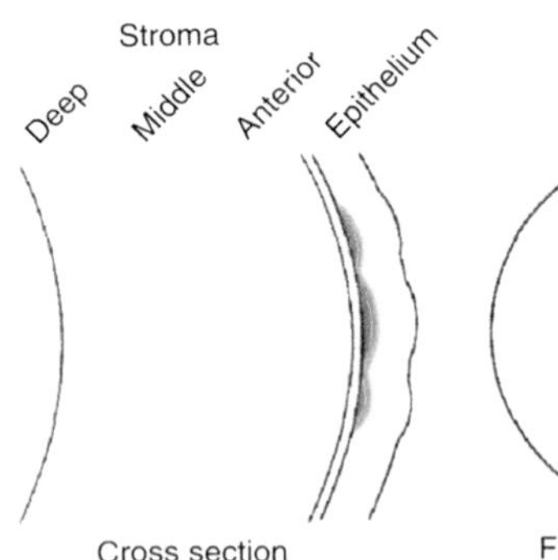

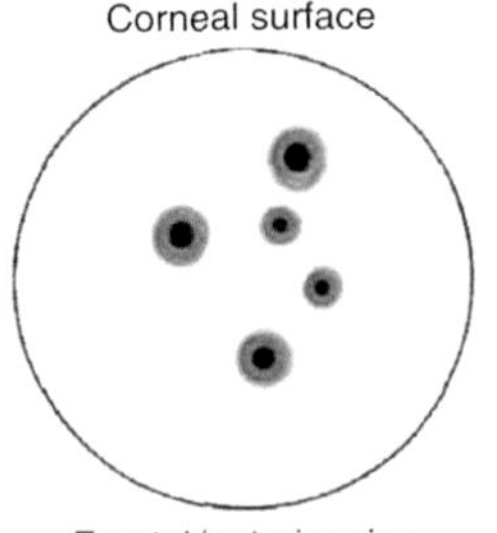

(See also Figure 5.84)

Management Considerations	Mild	Moderate	Severe
Antigen (?)	Edema/toxic	Edema/virus	Virus/Chlamydia?
Contact lens care	Temporarily discontinue	Temporarily discontinue	Temporarily discontinue
Irrigate/lubricate	Irrigate and lubricate tid with negative stain	Irrigate and lubricate qid with negative stain	Irrigate and lubricate q4h with negative stain
Cold pack	tid to qid	qid to qh4	q2–4h
Antibiotic	—	Topical tobramycin qid	Topical tobraymycin q2–4h
Steroid/combination	Rarely	After 1 wk qid	If visual acuity < 20/60 q2–4h
Other	5% NaCl tid	5% NaCl qid	5% NaCl q2–4h
		Oral ibuprofen?	Ibuprofen 400 mg/qid
		Cycloplege/dilate qid?	Cycloplege/dilate qid
RTC	1–2 wk	5–7 days	3–5 days

(Continued)

TABLE 5.11 (CONTINUED) **Management of Infiltrative Keratitis by Level and Degree**

With Stromal Involvement

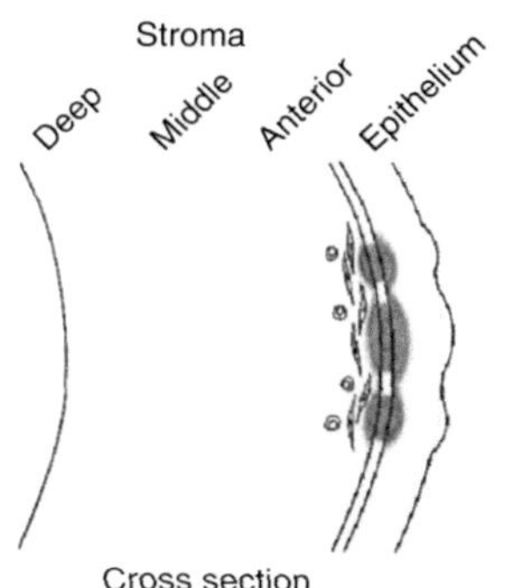

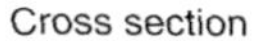

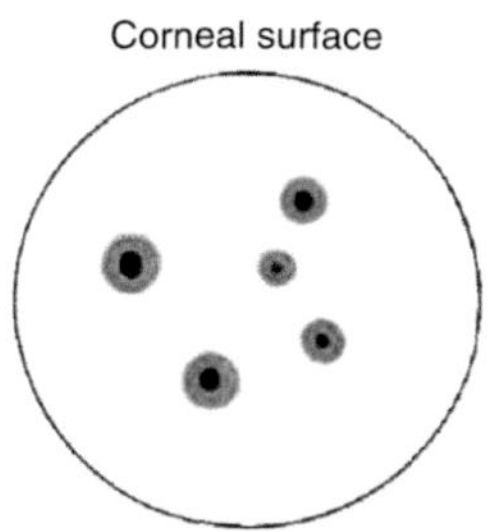

(See also Figure 5.85)

Management Considerations	Mild	Moderate	Severe
Antigen (?)	Edema/toxic	Edema/virus	Virus/Chlamydia?
Contact lens care	Temporarily discontinue	Temporarily discontinue	Temporarily discontinue
Irrigate/lubricate	Irrigate and lubricate tid with negative stain	Irrigate and lubricate qid with negative stain	Irrigate and lubricate q4h with negative stain
Cold pack	tid to qid	qid to q4h	q2–4h
Antibiotic	—	Topical tobramycin qid	Topical tobramycin q2–4h
Steroid/combination	qid for 7–10 days	qid for 7–10 days	q2–4h for 1–2 wk
Other	5% NaCl tid	5% NaCl qid Oral ibuprofen? Cycloplege/dilate qid?	5% NaCl q2–4h Ibuprofen 400 mg/qid Cycloplege/dilate qid
RTC	7–10 days	5–7 days	3–5 days

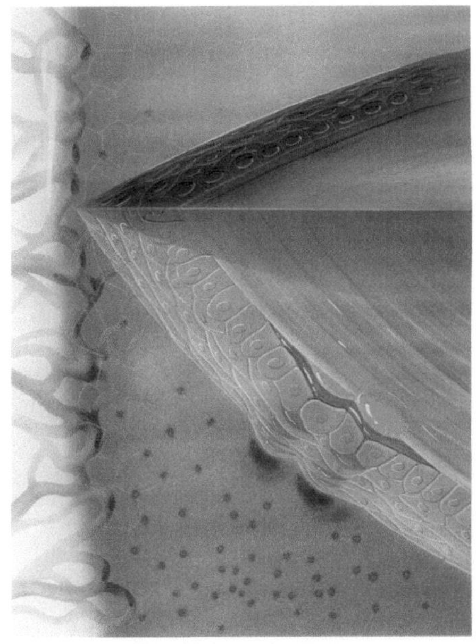

Subepithelial Keratitis

(Continued)

TABLE 5.11 (CONTINUED) **Management of Infiltrative Keratitis by Level and Degree**

STROMAL KERATITIS

Anterior

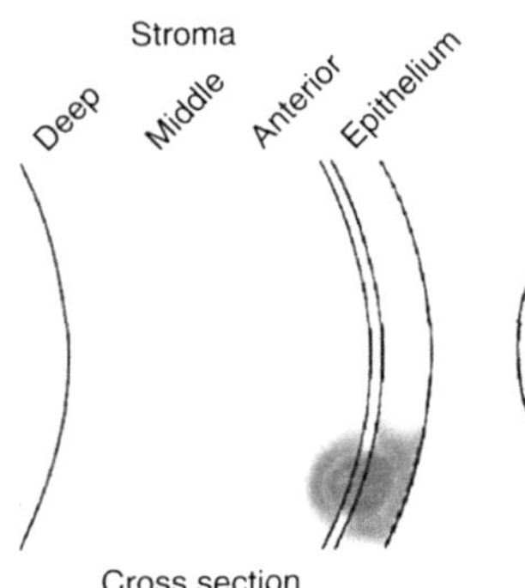

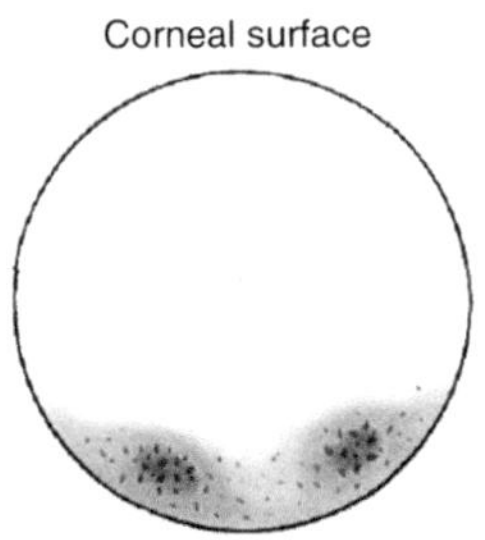

(See also Figure 5.75)

Management Considerations	Mild	Moderate	Severe
Antigen (?)	Mechanical/edema	Toxic/virus Other infection	Gram-positive/negative bacteria Acanthamoeba/other
Contact lens care	Temporarily discontinue	Temporarily discontinue	Prolonged discontinue
Irrigate/lubricate	—	Irrigate qid	Irrigate q2–4h
Cold pack	tid to qid	qid to q2–4h	qh
Antibiotic	Tobramycin qid with positive NaFl	Tobramycin q4h with positive NaFl	Tobramycin q2–4h with positive NaFl
Steroid/combination	With clear epithelia qid 7–10 days	With clear epithelia qid for 1–2 wk	With clear epithelia q2–4h for 1–2 wk
Other		Culture/sensitivity	Culture/sensitivity Corneal consultation?
RTC	5–7 days	3–5 days	24–48 hr

Wessely or Immune Ring

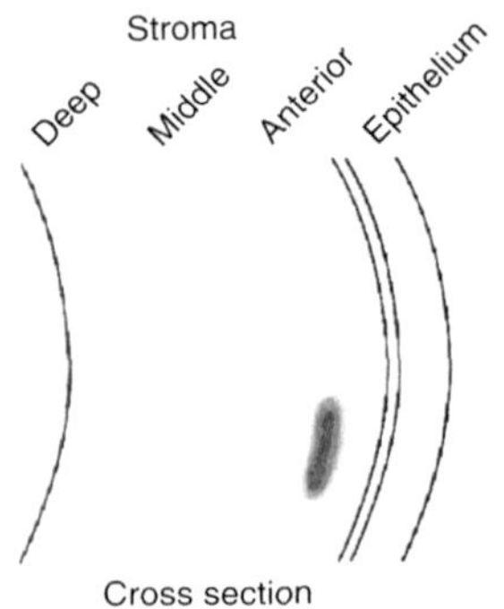

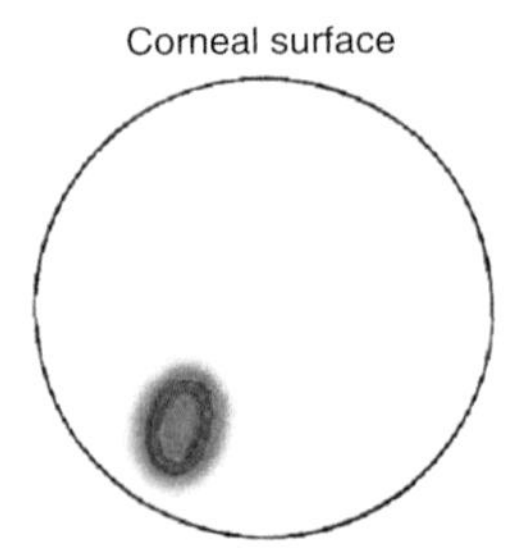

(See also Figure 5.94)

Management Considerations	Mild	Moderate	Severe
Antigen (?)	Staphylococcal/toxic	Staphylococcal/parasites	Fungi/Acanthamoeba
Contact lens care	Temporarily discontinue	Temporarily discontinue	Prolonged discontinue
Irrigate/lubricate	Irrigate tid	Irrigate qid	Irrigate q2–4h
Cold pack	tid to qid	qid to q2–4h	qh
Antibiotic	AK-Poly-Bac ointment hs	Topical tobramycin qid	Topical tobramycin q4h
Steroid/combination	—	qid for 1–2 wk?	q2–4h for 1–2 wk
Other	Antistaphylococcal (infection)	Antistaphylococcal (infection) Corneal consultation? Antiparasitics? Antifungals?	Antistaphylococcal Corneal consultation? Antiparasitics? Antifungals? Corneal biopsy?
RTC	5–7 days	5–7 days	3–5 days

(*Continued*)

TABLE 5.11 (CONTINUED) **Management of Infiltrative Keratitis by Level and Degree**

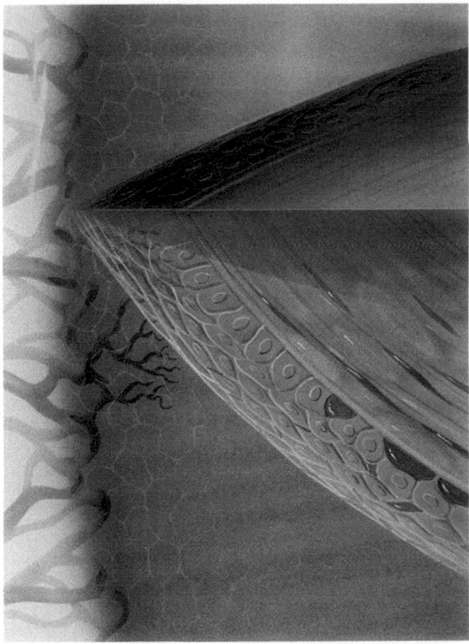

Stromal Keratitis

Deep

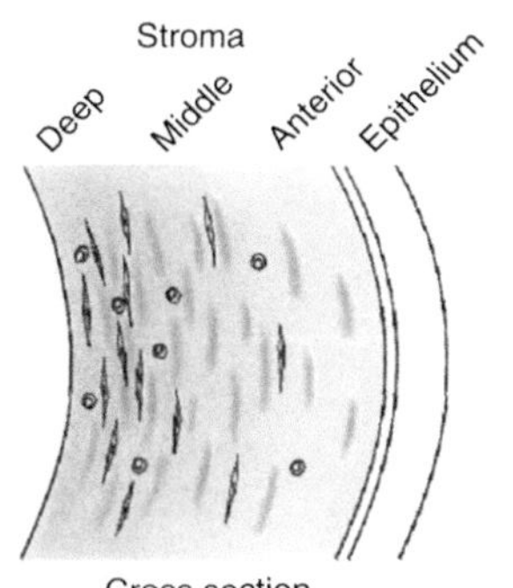

Corneal surface

Frontal/anterior view

(See also Figure 5.73)

Management Considerations	Mild	Moderate	Severe
Antigen (?)	Edema/systemic	Dyst/deg/HSV	Any infection
Contact lens care	Temporarily discontinue	Prolonged discontinue	Prolonged discontinue
Irrigate/lubricate	—	—	—
Cold pack	—	—	—
Antibiotic	Gentamicin qid with positive NaFl	Tobramycin q2–4h with positive NaFl	Ciprofloxacin q2h with positive NaFl
Steroid/combination	With clear epithelia qid for 7–10 days	With clear epithelia qid for 1–2 wk	With clear epithelia q2–4h for 1–2 wk
Other	Culture/sensitivity?	Culture/sensitivity? Corneal consultation?	Culture/sensitivity? Corneal consultation?
RTC	5–7 days	3–5 days	24–48 hr

(*Continued*)

TABLE 5.11 (CONTINUED) **Management of Infiltrative Keratitis by Level and Degree**

Interstitial

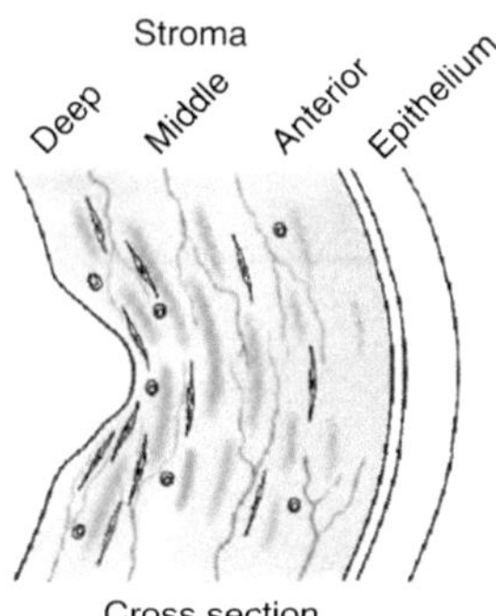

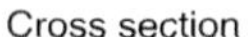
Cross section

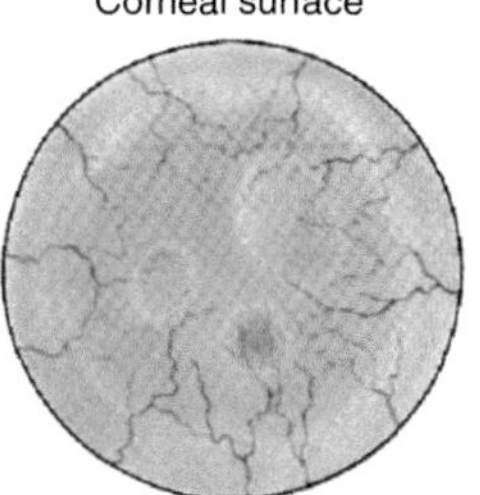

Frontal/anterior view

(See also Figure 5.96)

Management Considerations	**Mild**	**Moderate**	**Severe**
Antigen (?)	Syphilis/HSV	Syphilis/HSV	Syphilis/HSV
Contact lens care	Discontinue with inflammation	Temporarily discontinue	Prolonged discontinue
Irrigate/lubricate	—	—	—
Cold pack	—	—	—
Antibiotic	—	—	—
Steroid/combination	qid for 2–4 wk	q4h for 30 days	q2–4h for 30–90 days
Other	Antivirals? Medical referral	Antivirals? Medical referral Systemic penicillin	Antivirals? Medical referral Systemic penicillin
RTC	2–4 wk	Per consultant	Per consultant

Ulceration

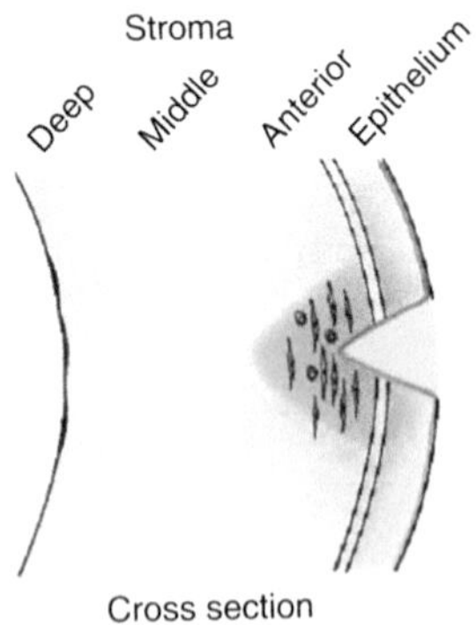

Cross section

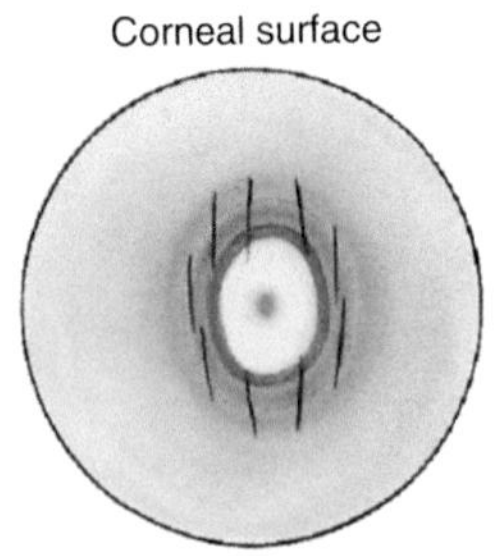

Frontal/anterior view

Management Considerations	**Mild**	**Moderate**	**Severe**
Antigen (?)	Steroid/infection	Gram-positive bacteria	Gram-negative bacteria
Contact lens care	Temporarily discontinue	Prolonged discontinue	Prolonged discontinue
Irrigate/lubricate	—	—	—
Cold pack	—	—	—
Antibiotic	Besifloxicin qh plus loading dose	Fortified gentamicin, tobramycin, and besifloxacin q30 min	Fortified vancomycin, tobramycin, and besifloxacin q30 min
Steroid/combination	With clear epithelia qid for 7–10 days	On negative culture qid for 1–2 wk	On negative culture q2–4h for 1–2 wk
Other	Cycloplege/dilate q4h Culture/sensitivity?	Cycloplege/dilate q2h Culture/sensitivity? Corneal consultation	Cycloplege/dilate q2h Culture/sensitivity? Corneal consultation Hospitalization
RTC	24 hr	Per consultant	Per consultant

(Continued)

TABLE 5.11 (CONTINUED) **Management of Infiltrative Keratitis by Level and Degree**

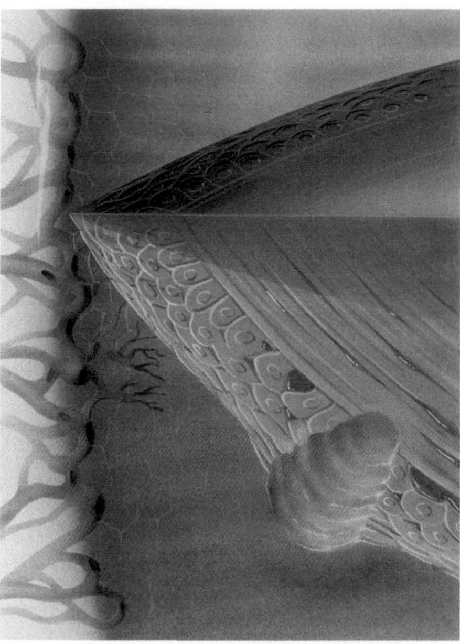

Corneal Ulcer

TABLE 5.12 **Contact Lens-Related Keratitis**

	Superficial	Intraepithelial	Subepithelial
In White Eyes			
Prominent diagnostic features	SPK Microcystic edema	NaFl "halos" Small, well-defined sites	Negative NaFl Larger, ill-defined sites
Probable cause	Lens care solutions, Sterile toxins Mechanical/dry	Sterile toxins, SPK of Thygeson	Adenoviral Anterior stromal scarring?
Lens wear and management or drug options	Daily wear including disposable, Increase lens replacement frequency Hydrogen peroxide disinfection, Lid and ocular surface hygiene, Lubrication	Daily wear including disposable, Increase lens replacement frequency, Hydrogen peroxide disinfection	Temporarily D/C
Lens re-wear options	Change lens material	Change lens material	Re-wear schedule 1 week after full resolution
In Red Eyes			
Prominent diag-nostic features	Prominent limbal vasculature, SPK Microcystic edema	Deeper limbal flush, Bulbar hyperemia, Small, well-defined sites	Diffuse conjunctival hyperemia, Follicles Increased lacrimation Positive lymph node enlargement Larger, ill-defined sites
Probable cause	Toxic/immune sterile Staphylococcal infection Mechanical/dry	Sterile toxic immune response Medicamentosa solutions Preservatives	Adenoviral, Chlamydial
Lens wear and management or drug options	Temporarily D/C Lid and ocular surface hygiene Lubrication Cold packs	Temporarily D/C, Hydrogen peroxide disinfection Lubrication Cold packs, Topical anti-inflammatory	Temporarily D/C Possible topical or oral (chlamydia) anti-inflammatory Lubrication Cold packs
Lens re-wear options	Full-time in 1–2 weeks; consider options above	Full-time in 1–2 weeks; consider options above	Monitor q 3–5 days, Re-wear schedule 1 week after resolution; consider options above

Abbreviations: SPK, superficial punctate keratitis; D/C, discontinue.

- Heat is useful adjunctive therapy to reduce ciliary muscle spasms and to promote epithelial healing
- Oral medications are rarely indicated in superficial keratitis because of the avascular nature of the cornea and subclinical tear level concentrations
- Complications from superficial keratitis are usually non-epithelial, but rather a product of compromised surface epithelial defense mechanisms, tissue damage from immune responses, and secondary anterior stromal infiltration and scarring
  1. Secondary infectious or ulcerative complications
  2. Risk of toxic or hypersensitive, antigen–antibody immune responses causing anterior stromal damage

Clinical Conditions

(See Tables 5.10–5.12)

1. Atopic Keratoconjunctivitis[46,47]

Subjective

- Greater in men, age range approximately 20 to 50
- Frequently an active or inactive (history of) atopic dermatitis in patient and family
- Always report itching (moderate to severe) with "insatiable" need to rub the eyes vigorously
  1. Often results in excoriated tissue leading to further discomfort
  2. May also be associated with increased risk of keratoconus
- Symptoms persist year-round (as opposed to vernal or seasonal conditions)
- Additional burning sensation, pain, photophobia, foreign-body sensation, and non-specific irritation are frequently reported

Objective

- Always a bilateral condition
- Discharge includes tearing and often thicker, white, stringy mucoid accumulations in ocular surface
- Lids are usually moderately edematous and mild to moderately erythematous
  1. Also secondary excoriation
  2. Occasionally, chronic edema produces hardening of soft tissues (induration) and leathery textures
- Inferior palpebral conjunctiva produces moderate to dramatic papillary changes
- Bulbar conjunctiva varies from no hyperemia to mild or moderate degrees, but no chemosis
- Corneal findings are concentrated superiorly
  1. Limbal infiltrates (usually circumlimbal)
  2. Trantas' dots
     a. Usually about 1 to 2 mm round, slightly raised whitish dots (eosinophilic accumulations)
     b. Rarely more than two to five present on limbus
  3. Moderate to severe SPK
  4. Chronic forms may show prominent limbal arcades, pannus, and neovascularization
- Long-term complications generally produce an anterior stromal haze and scarring
  1. Superior arcus-like band may develop (called pseudogeronotoxon)
  2. Sterile ulceration ("shield ulcer") can occur (usually shallow, oval, and horizontally oriented)
- Superior tarsus generally spared of advanced changes
- Reports of increased frequency of premature cataracts

Assessment

- Rule out vernal keratoconjunctivitis (seasonal)
- Rule out SLK (no dermatitis or atopic history)
- Rule out giant papillary conjunctivitis (dramatic superior tarsal involvement)

Plan: Atopic Keratoconjunctivitis

- Cold packs as frequent as possible
- Oral antihistamines or decongestants (non-prescription)
- Topical 1% prednisolone (dramatically effective) or 0.5% loteprednol
  1. Dosage q2–4h for short course (maximum 7 to 10 days)
  2. Taper to antihistamine/mast cell stabilizer combination agents
  3. Loteprednol has fewer side effects than prednisolone and should be considered due to chronic nature of disease
- Oral steroids maybe needed for severe cases
- Lubricants may provide increased comfort initially

Follow-Up

- Counsel and advise patient on chronic nature
- Condition does self-limit over time, but may take many years
- Minimize topical steroids by using only during acute phases and running short courses, replaced as soon as possible with antihistamine/mast cell stabilizer combination agent
  1. Run minimum 6- to 8-week courses at qid
  2. Taper and monitor for exacerbations every 6 months
  3. Advise patient to reinstitute steroid therapy at first sign of symptoms or PRN appointments

2. Bacterial Keratitis

a. Synonyms
   i. Bacterial ulcer
   ii. Central corneal ulcer
   iii. Corneal ulcer
   iv. Infectious keratitis
   v. Microbial keratitis

3. Contact Lens-Related Keratitis

a. Secondary to mechanical, physiological, and immune responses to contact lens wear
b. Inclusive considerations
   i. See Tables 5.10–5.12
   ii. Infiltrative keratitis
   iii. Infectious keratitis

4. Filamentary Keratitis

Subjective

- A secondary non-specific diagnosis resulting from a primary precipitating clinical condition that disrupts corneal epithelial integrity
- Onset may be acute, subacute, or insidious
- Symptoms range from annoying (in chronic, low grade forms) to severe in acute presentations
- Corneal foreign-body sensation (as lid tugs on filaments with each successive blink)
- Symptoms of primary causative disease process may also be present

Objective

- Dead epithelial cells combine with mucin debris to form chains (helices) in the form of small round buds and elongated threads (or filaments) from 1 to 3 mm or greater (Figure 5.65)
    1. One end of filament becomes adherent to dry spot on cornea
    2. Unattached portion of filament hangs loosely over corneal surface and moves slightly with the blink
- Filaments tend to accumulate on corneal region most aggravated by underlying, primary disease process (often superior, under upper lid)
- Filaments (or buds) stain with both NaFl and rose bengal/lissamine green
- Signs of primary disease usually associated with filamentary findings

Assessment

(See also Appendix 2)

- Determine primary, underlying, causative disease
- Most common possibilities (see Table 5.10)
    1. Atopic keratoconjunctivitis
    2. Burns to cornea (radiation, thermal, chemical)
    3. Dry eye or keratitis sicca syndromes
    4. Epidemic keratoconjunctivitis
    5. EBMDs
    6. Herpes simplex keratitis
    7. Herpes zoster ophthalmicus
    8. Mechanical (chronic) corneal irritation (e.g., poor contact lens surfaces or edges, tarsal FB)
    9. Postoperative response
    10. Prolonged pressure patching
    11. RCE
    12. SLK
    13. SPK of Thygeson
    14. Vernal keratoconjunctivitis

Plan: Filamentary Keratitis

- Treat primary, underlying disease
- Reduce or remove in situ filaments

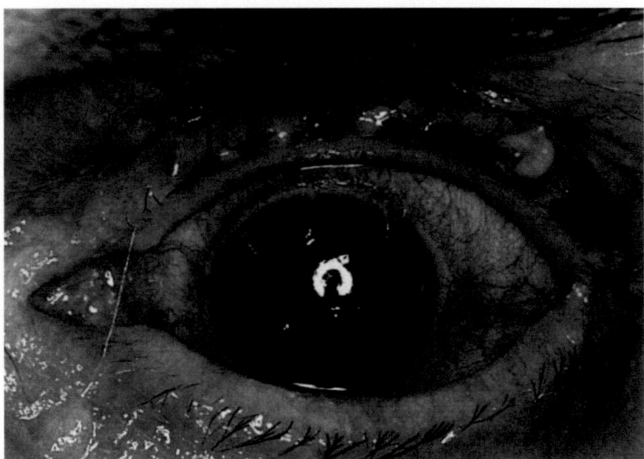

FIGURE 5.65 Filamentary keratitis in the superior portion of a cornea demonstrating multiple filamentary strands made up of dead epithelial cells in a mucoid helix attached to a dry or raised spot on the epithelium.

1. Heavy lubrication will reduce filaments over a 3- to 5-day period
2. Short-term pressure patch (in non-prolonged patch cases) usually melt existing filaments
3. Mechanically remove filaments
    a. Grasp at base with jeweler's forceps and lift off cornea with upward twist
    b. Gently swab or roll filament onto a wetted cotton-tipped applicator in upward sweep
4. Acetylcysteine (Mucomyst) 1× or qid for 24 to 48 hours
5. Bandage soft lens for 24 to 48 hours

Follow-Up

- Manage primary condition appropriately
- Advise patient on risk of recurrence and PRN recheck

5. Infiltrative Keratitis

a. Synonyms
    i. Marginal infiltrative keratitis
    ii. Marginal keratitis
    iii. Marginal ulcer (misnomer)
    iv. Staphylococcal infiltrative keratitis
    v. Sterile infiltrative keratitis
    vi. Sterile keratitis
    vii. Toxic keratitis
b. Management (see Table 5.12)

6. Keratoconjunctivitis Sicca Syndromes

Refer to Section I. D. for a complete discussion.

7. Marginal Keratitis

Background Information

a. Synonyms
    i. Marginal infiltrative keratitis
    ii. Marginal staphylococcal keratitis
    iii. Marginal ulcer (misnomer)
    iv. Staphylococcal infiltrative keratitis
    v. Sterile infiltrative keratitis
b. Usually caused by infiltrative immune response to staphylococcal exotoxins (usually from inferior lid margin glands)
    i. Most vulnerable sites at 4- and 8-o'clock positions of peripheral cornea (approximately), where the lid margin crosses corneolimbal juncture (4/8 syndrome)
    ii. Exotoxins are enzymes that produce superficial sterile toxic (infiltrative/immune) responses
    iii. Result in intraepithelial infiltrates on mid-peripheral cornea (usually inferior) (see Table 5.12)
        - Raised lesions due to accumulated excess of infiltrative cells and debris
        - Lesions are always "islands" on peripheral cornea with clear interval (called interval of Vogt) between limbus and distal border of lesion (antigen–antibody, immune complex response)
c. Corneal lesion (infiltrate) is sterile response to bacterial (staphylococcal) toxins on corneal surface
    i. Keratitis is sterile keratitis, as opposed to infectious keratitis, which has live bacteria on, or in, the cornea (producing ulceration)
    ii. Cultures of sterile infiltrative keratitis will be negative, even though primary cause is Staphylococcus

iii. Clinical diagnosis (of symptoms, risk factors, and physical signs) usually more useful than laboratory work (versus necessity for cultures in ulcers)

d. Appropriate therapy for infiltrative or immune process is to reverse the infiltration and "melt" the excess accumulated infiltrative cells and debris by immunosuppressing the tissue with corticosteroids (see Chapter 2)
   i. Simultaneous antistaphylococcal therapy helps reduce primary cause of toxins with resultant immune response and its adverse corneal tissue effects and potential risk of scarring
   ii. Ulcerative process requires deep stromal immune response to reduce penetration and thus contraindicates immunosuppressive corticosteroid use

Subjective

- Acute or subacute presentation (on waking)
- Usually unilateral
- Frequent history of previous occurrences (usually subacute and self-limiting)
- Classic corneal symptoms
  1. "Sandy, gritty" sensation
  2. FB sensation
  3. "Something under upper lid"
- History of staphylococcal lid disease (subclinical, chronic, subacute, or acute)
- Visual acuity rarely affected
- Generally a painful, watery eye with or without photophobia
- Consider infectious keratitis risk factors in history

Objective

- Staphylococcal toxic (sterile) infiltrative response at the peripheral corneal margin (Figure 5.66)
- Lesions are most often found inferiorly
  1. Most common at 4- and 8-o'clock positions, where inferior lid margin intersects limbus (4/8 syndrome)
  2. May also be superior or circumlimbal
- Lesions may be single or multiple, usually ranging in size from approximately 0.5 to 1.5 mm (maximum; Figure 5.67)
  1. Multiple lesions may combine into an elongated circumlimbal single appearing lesion
  2. Any combination of single, elongated, and even 360° infiltrative lesions possible
- Infiltrative lesions are *always* island(s) on the corneal periphery with clear corneal tissue between distal border of lesion and limbus (interval of Vogt)
  1. Surrounding edema (when dense) may cloud interval
  2. But NaFl staining pattern will reveal lesion as a distinctly (brighter) staining "island"
  3. If "island" appears large and depressed (vs flat or raised), consider ulceration possibilities (Figure 5.68)

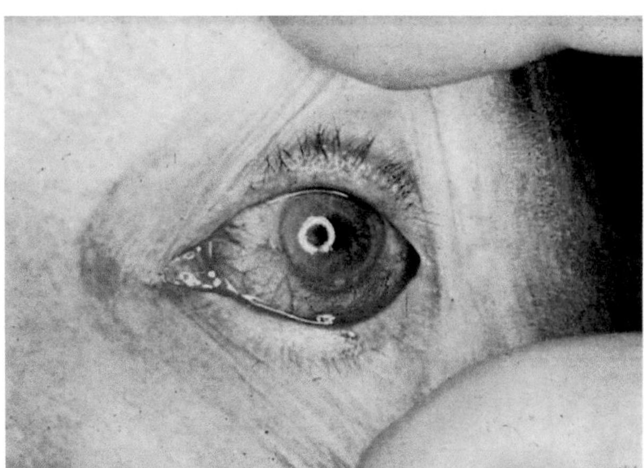

FIGURE 5.66 Intraepithelial marginal infiltrate presenting as a midperipheral island with an associated leash of conjunctival vessels at the 4-o'clock position of the left eye.

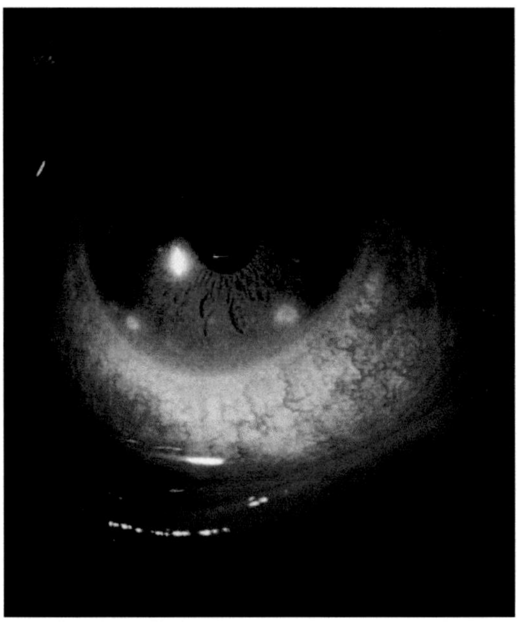

FIGURE 5.67 "4/8 syndrome," or the common staphylococcal toxic effects at the 4- and 8-o'clock positions on the bulbar conjunctiva and the face of the cornea where the lid margins cross the limbal junctures. Here marginal infiltrates appear on the cornea in a classic "4/8 syndrome" (and one at 9:30).

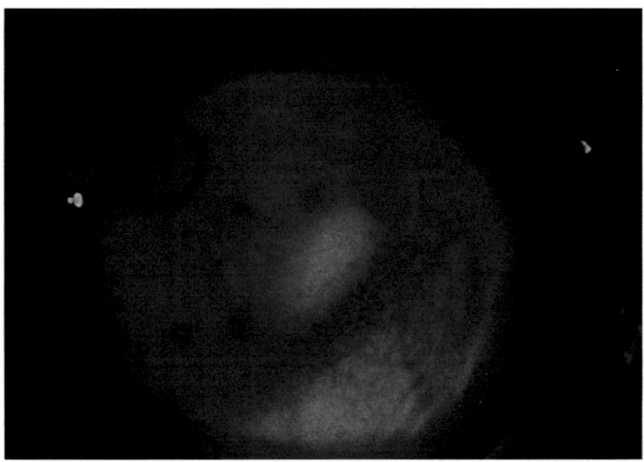

FIGURE 5.68 Marginal infiltrate with diffuse NaFl staining surrounding brightly staining central infiltrate. Such edema could suggest ulceration unless central core is recognized as infiltrative accumulation without stromal invasion.

   a. Staphylococcus
   b. Streptococcus
   c. Gram-negative infection
- May present only as a superficial punctate keratitis
  1. Variable quantity and quality (fine to coarse) SPK (punctate NaFl staining of squamous epithelium)
  2. Most frequent presentation concentrated on inferior corneal surface (toward lower limbus; Figure 5.69)
  3. May also present as diffuse SPK (entire cornea surface)
  4. Frequently localized areas of SPK (greater inferiorly, especially at 4 or 8 o'clock) may become dense and confluence into "patches" of NaFl staining (prodromal sign of toxic marginal infiltrative keratitic response)
- Bulbar conjunctiva produces moderate to severe superficial hyperemic, injected vessel patterns
  1. Usually greatest inferiorly
  2. Most common to have "leashes" (radiating pattern) of vessels ranging from 15 to 90° pointing directly toward infiltrated marginal corneal area
- Superficial injected conjunctival vessels often cross corneolimbal juncture (inflammatory or immune response)
  1. Produce prominent limbal arcades and ultimately superficial corneal vascularization (pannus)
  2. Chronic (inflammatory or immune) vascular response can begin to produce deeper, fine vessel tufts with terminal branching into anterior (and deep) corneal stroma (neovascularization)
- Surrounding corneal edema usually mild to moderate
  1. Produces a haze around infiltrate (especially in subacute and chronic cases)
  2. Usually 0.5 to 1 mm diameter
  3. Mostly epithelial edema, but could also involve anterior stroma (up to half-stromal thickness)
- Occasionally radiating pigmented spokes (keratomelanocytosis) may be associated
- Proximal or adjacent subepithelial infiltrates may develop secondarily
- Chronic, subacute, delayed, or undertreated lesions may produce anterior stromal (antigen–antibody) infiltration
  1. Usually result in anterior stromal focal hazes and nebula (faint opacification)

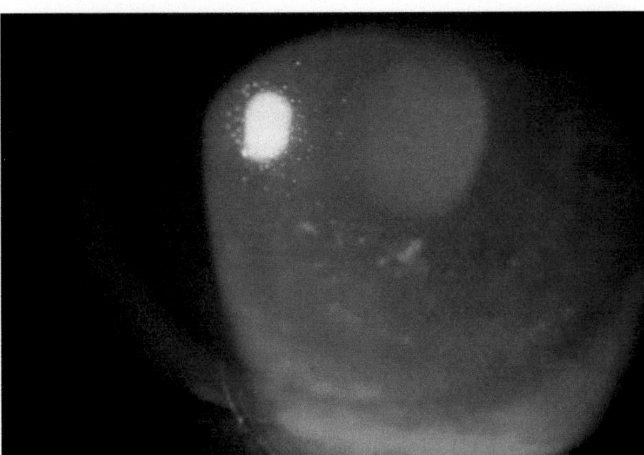

FIGURE 5.69 Inferior (peripheral) superficial punctate keratitis (SPK) most frequently associated with sterile staphylococcal toxins from the eyelids.

  2. May also produce leukomatous anterior stromal scar(s) (often noted in subclinical presentation)
- Rarely, staphylococcal toxins or other toxic agents may progress (by resisting immune defense mechanisms) to produce anterior stromal necrosis (tissue destruction and loss)
  1. This must be considered a "sterile ulcer," as opposed to the more common sterile infiltrate
  2. Sterile ulcer (as with infectious ulcers) is a more advanced, depressed, pale gray lesion, usually 1 to 2 mm in diameter
  3. Sterile ulcers should be treated and managed under infectious keratitis guidelines

Assessment

- Differentiate from infectious keratitis
- Rule out other peripheral corneal lesions
- Rule out sterile ulceration
  1. More advanced and intense response
  2. Loss of anterior stromal substance
  3. Infiltrate is raised lesion (on slit-lamp examination) vs depressed (ulcerative) appearance
  4. Infiltrate stains superficially (from breaks in squamous epithelial cell junctures) and clears within minutes
  5. Ulcers stain deeply (into stroma) and tend to produce an amorphous spreading pattern to stain over following minutes

Plan: Marginal Keratitis

(See also Appendix 4)

- Clinical presentations *without* significant infectious risk factors
  1. For mild presentations (mild to moderate symptoms and one or few small (≤0.5 mm) superficial lesions
     a. Warm packs qid for 7 to 10 days
     b. Tobramycin (or gentamicin) or antibiotic-steroid combination (e.g., tobramycin 0.3%/dexamethasone 0.01%) drops tid to qid for 5 to 7 days
     c. Bacitracin ointment on lid margins or hypochlorous acid 0.1% tid to qid
     d. Return check in 3 to 5 days or PRN
  2. For moderate presentations, moderate to severe symptoms with 0.5 to 1 mm lesion(s)
     a. Cycloplege/dilate with 1% tropicamide qid
     b. Tobramycin (or gentamicin) drops q2–4h
     c. One percent prednisolone drops qid or antibiotic-steroid combination (e.g., 0.3% tobramycin and 0.1% dexamethasone) q2–4h
     d. Warm packs and bacitracin ointment or hypochlorous acid 0.1% (as with mild)
     e. Return check 2 to 3 days or PRN
  3. For severe presentations (severe symptoms and larger, suspicious-looking lesions)
     a. Cycloplege and dilate with 5% homatropine or cyclopentolate 1% tid
     b. Loading dose
        i. Delivered in office during first visit
        ii. 1 gtt tobramycin or fourth generation fluroquinolone (e.g., moxifloxacin, gatifloxacin, besifloxacin) every minute ×5 (5 dosages)
     c. Extended dose

i. Delivered by patient (or advocate) at home
ii. 3 gtt tobramycin or fourth generation fluroquinolone (at 1-minute intervals) every 1–2 hours for 24 hours (asking patient to wake q1–2h throughout the night)
d. Return check within 24 hours of initial visit
e. Do not introduce steroids in severe presentations for the first 24 to 48 hours
i. Risk of infectious ulcerative process, especially with any risk factors, indicates withholding early steroid use
ii. Secondary risk of anterior stromal infiltration, causing mild peripheral scarring attributable to delayed immunosuppression preferable to risk of aggravating possible early ulcer

- Clinical presentations *with* multiple or significant infectious risk factors
  1. For mild presentations
     a. Warm packs qid
     b. Gentamicin or tobramycin drops q4h
     c. Bacitracin ointment or hypochlorous acid 0.01% on lid margins tid to qid
     d. Return check within 24 to 48 hours or PRN
  2. For moderate and severe presentations
     a. Same as for severe presentation without infectious risk factors
     b. Seriously consider culturing cornea before administering antibiotic therapy
     c. If degree of clinical suspicion is high, based on multiple, suggestive ulcerative signs, follow guidelines for infectious keratitis immediately

Follow-Up

- *Without* infectious risk factors
  1. Mild conditions on return check (3 to 5 days)
     a. Stable or improving: reduce and discontinue plan within 7 to 10 days
     b. If worse, increase plan to moderate level
     c. After control and discontinued therapy, advise "staph risk-reduction program" (see Figure 3.1)
     d. Prognosis: usually complete resolution with no scarring and minimal risk of recurrence
     e. Recheck in 6 to 12 months or PRN
  2. Moderate conditions on return check (2 to 3 days)
     a. Stable or improving: reduce and discontinue plan within 10 to 14 days
     b. If worse, increase plan to severe level
     c. After control and discontinued therapy, advise "staph risk-reduction program"
     d. Prognosis: usually complete resolution, with slight risk of recurrent staphylococcal problems
     e. Recheck in 6 months or PRN
  3. Severe conditions on return check (within 24 hours)
     a. Stable: continue for additional 24 hours
     b. Improving: introduce moderate level plan (with steroid) and reduce slowly and discontinue over 2- to 3-week period, depending on response
     c. If worse, culture (if not done initially) and introduce bacterial keratitis treatment plan
     d. After control and discontinued therapy, advise on continued risk of reinfection and need for "staph risk-reduction program"
     e. Prognosis: probable anterior stromal peripheral leucomatous scar (usually minimally apparent)
     f. Recheck in 3 months or PRN
- *With* infectious risk factors
  1. Mild conditions on return check (within 24 to 48 hours)
     a. Stable or improving: reduce and discontinue plan within 7 to 10 days
     b. If worse, increase to severe level plan
     c. Advise and educate patient regarding specific infectious risk factors and introduce appropriate care when indicated
     d. Prognosis: no risk of scarring and with proper care and control of risk factors, minimal risk of recurrence
     e. Return check in 3 to 6 months or PRN
  2. Moderate to severe conditions on return (within 24 hours)
     a. Stable: continue for additional 24 hours
     b. Improving: introduce moderate level plan (with steroid) and reduce slowly and discontinue over 2- to 3-week period, depending on response
     c. If worse, culture (if not done initially) and introduce bacterial keratitis treatment plan
     d. Advise and educate patient regarding specific infectious risk factors and introduce appropriate care when indicated
     e. Prognosis: probable anterior stromal peripheral leucomatous scar (usually minimally apparent) and with proper care and control of risk factors, mild to moderate risk of recurrence
     f. Return check within 3 months after complete discontinuation of all medical therapies, or PRN

8. *Neurotrophic Keratitis*[48–50]

Background

- Rare corneal degenerative disease caused by damage to CN V (trigeminal)
- Caused by herpes simplex/zoster keratitis, diabetes, multiple sclerosis, chemical burns, corneal surgical (e.g., LASIK) damage, and neurosurgical procedures
- Loss of corneal sensitivity, impaired epithelial wound healing, and impaired lacrimation reflex
- Difficult and challenging to treat

Subjective

- Usually unilateral
- Patient is asymptomatic due to loss of corneal sensitivity
- If epithelial defect/edema centrally located, patient will report blurred vision
- Need detailed ocular and medical history

Objective

- Presents in 3 stages
- *Stage 1*
  1. Decrease tear breakup time
  2. Punctate epithelial erosions, superficial neovascularization, and stromal scarring
  3. Decreased corneal sensitivity
     a. Take a cotton swab and tease out strand of cotton
     b. Touch uninvolved eye and tell patient that represents a 10 on a 1–10 scale of sensation

   c. Touch involved eye (same corneal location) and ask patient to rate on same 1–10 scale
- *Stage 2*
  1. Persistent epithelial defect; rolled, loose edges of epithelium
  2. Stromal edema and Descemet's folds
  3. Cell and flare: sterile hypopyon
  4. Patient needs to be followed carefully due to lack of pain and possible ulcer progression
- *Stage 3*
  1. Stromal ulceration, corneal melting, and perforation

Assessment

Rule out other causes
  1. Lagophthalmos and exposure keratitis
  2. Blepharitis
  3. Topical drug toxicity
  4. Large, persisting epithelial lesions must be evaluated for microbial etiology

Plan: Neurotrophic Keratitis

- *Stage 1*
  1. Preservative artificial tears and ointment at night
  2. Punctal occlusion
- *Stage 2* (promote healing)
  1. Autologous serum
  2. Amniotic membrane (patch for smaller defects, graft for larger defects)
     a. Provides mechanical protection and contains growth factors
  3. Bandage soft lens
  4. Scleral gas permeable contact lens
     a. Provides mechanical protection and fluid-filled chamber
  5. Oxervate
     a. Recombinant growth factor solution (FDA approved)
     b. 6 drops (every 2 hours)/day for 8 weeks
  5. Topical antibiotic for prophylaxis
- *Stage 3*
  1. Corneal specialist referral
  2. Cyanoacrylate glue/graft amniotic membrane for small perforations
  3. Penetrating keratoplasty for large perforation

Follow-Up

- Goal is to prevent progression and promote ocular surface healing
- *Stage 1*
  1. Follow-up 5–7 days
- *Stage 2*
  1. Follow-up 24–48 hours
  2. With significant improvement, follow-up every 3–5 days until resolved
- *Stage 3*
  1. Daily or hospitalization may be required

9. Phlyctenular Keratoconjunctivitis[51]

Subjective

- Usually unilateral presentation
- Delayed-type hypersensitivity reaction to various antigens
- Acute or subacute onset of symptoms
- Classic corneal symptoms
  1. Sandy, gritty feeling
  2. FB sensation
  3. "Something under upper lid"
- Frequently associated with staphylococcal signs and symptoms
- Visual acuity minimally affected
- Variable degrees of lacrimation and photophobia

Objective

- Phlyctenule (or phlycten) is localized, superficial, infiltrative reaction (Figure 5.70)
  1. A raised, circumscribed, focal accumulation of infiltrative cells and debris, leading to fibrin formation
  2. Caused by superficial epithelial toxins
  3. Lesion associated with variable degrees of surrounding edema and hyperemia
- Lesions may form at any site on ocular surface
  1. On bulbar conjunctiva away from limbus, phlycten produces phlyctenular conjunctivitis
  2. When proximal to limbus, phlycten may extend onto peripheral cornea, producing phlyctenular keratoconjunctivitis
- Most common sites for limbal phlyctenules are the inferior circumlimbal areas, especially the 4- and 8-o'clock positions (4/8 syndrome)
- Usually, injected bulbar conjunctival vessels create "leash" of hyperemia pointing toward lesion
  1. Vessels may overlie corneal portion of phlycten
  2. May produce a superficial pannus onto cornea
- Occasionally (not common), multiple phlyctenules may develop simultaneously
- Size of phlyctenules vary considerably
  1. Width may range from 1 to 4 mm
  2. Extension onto cornea may range from 1 to 3 mm
- Rarely, mucopurulent discharge will be associated
- Generally, corneal surface surrounding phlyctenule will demonstrate variable degrees of toxic SPK

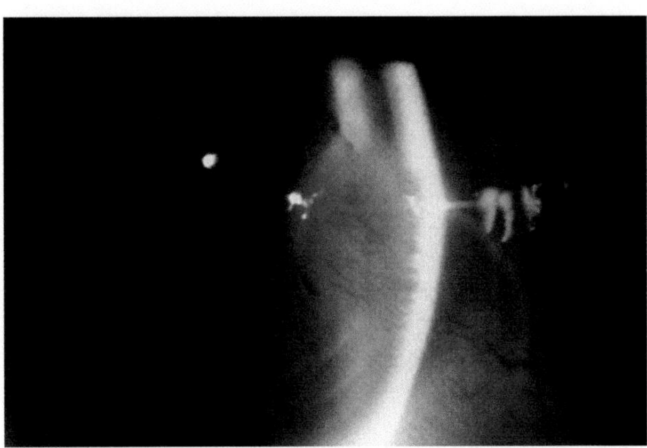

FIGURE 5.70 Phlyctenular keratoconjunctivitis producing an elevated, fingerlike projection of fibrous tissue across the limbal juncture, onto the peripheral cornea, with overlying pannus (proliferating superficial vessels). Most common etiologies include tuberculosis in developing worldwide endemic areas and Staphylococcus in more industrialized countries.

Assessment

- Older sources generally associate phlyctenular keratoconjunctivitis with tuberculosis
  1. Probably correct regarding worldwide distribution
  2. In industrialized, developed countries (e.g., United States), 75% of cases are toxic staphylococcal reactions
  3. Nonetheless, rule out history of tuberculosis (TB), especially in areas of increasing prevalence (including United States)
  4. Other possible antigens such as parasites, worms, fungus, and viruses
- Rule out other peripheral inflammatory corneal reactions
  1. Marginal keratitis: midperiphery (island) lesion without raised conjunctival portion
  2. Limbal infiltrates (e.g., vernal, atopic): limited to corneolimbal tissue, with no conjunctival (raised) portion
  3. Others: usually keratitis rather than keratoconjunctivitis (associated conjunctival lesion)
- Rule out non-inflamed, raised corneolimbal lesions
  1. Such as pterygium, degenerations
  2. Usually insidious versus acute and not inflamed

Plan: Phlyctenular Keratoconjunctivitis

- Topical steroids (e.g., prednisolone) in relatively high dosages (q3–4h) to "melt" phlyctenule quickly and minimize risk of anterior stromal scarring
- Prophylactic gentamicin drops qid for 5 to 7 days
- Antibiotic-steroid combo drops (e.g., 0.3% tobramycin/0.5% loteprednol) q2–3h as an alternative treatment
- For moderate to severe presentations (extensive corneal involvement), cycloplege and dilate with 1% tropicamide, 5% homatropine, or cyclpentolate 1% during acute phase
- If Staphylococcus likely cause, add bacitracin ointment or hypochlorous acid 0.01% (e.g., Avenova) on lids bid to qid
- Recheck within 3 to 5 days depending on steroid dosage

Follow-Up

- Phlyctenule should show quick response and reversal
  1. If not, increase steroid dosage
  2. On improvement, continue steroid until complete reduction of raised fibrin lesion and (it is hoped) total resolution of corneal (anterior stromal) haze
- Often, permanent anterior stromal leucomatous hazy scar will persist with or without overlying pannus (and rarely, neovascularization)
- Full course of therapy may run up to 2 to 4 weeks
  1. Monitor closely during treatment for steroid complications
  2. Taper therapy once phlycten or scarring maximally reduced
- If staphylococcal toxins determined (or assumed) cause, advise and prescribe "staph risk-reduction program" (see Figure 3.1)
- Recheck within 6 months or PRN

10. Sterile Keratitis

a. Synonyms
   i. Hypersensitivity (immune) keratitis
   ii. Infiltrative keratitis
   iii. Marginal infiltrative keratitis
   iv. Marginal keratitis
   v. Marginal ulcer (misnomer)
   vi. Staphylococcal infiltrative keratitis
   vii. Sterile infiltrative keratitis
   viii. Sterile ulcer
   ix. Toxic keratitis
b. See appropriate diagnosis (per synonym)

11. Thygeson's Superficial Punctate Keratitis (SPK)[52,53]

Subjective

- Etiology unknown (associated with virus and antigen–antibody response)
- Greatest frequency in young adult females (15 to 40 years of age)
- Usually mild symptomatic reports (if at all) of transient sandy, gritty sensation
- Occasional mild to moderate photophobic reaction
- Any reports of symptoms usually remit and exacerbate over short periods of 4- to 6-week duration
- Patients begin to remain relatively asymptomatic in later years of disease process, with remission periods becoming longer and exacerbations shorter and milder
- Disease tends to self-limit over a 4- to 7-year period
- Often diagnosed during routine examination because of its asymptomatic nature

Objective

- Generally bilateral, but greater in one eye
- Diffuse SPK with slightly greater concentration in central corneal regions
  1. SPK may be fine or coarse, sparse, or dense
  2. When dense, visual acuity is reduced
  3. When coarse or dense, confluence of NaFl staining may produce large patches and spots on corneal surface
- Slightly raised, whitish-gray, granular intraepithelial opacities frequently develop with subsequent exacerbations of disease
  1. Produce negative staining patterns (i.e., break up NaFl pattern directly over epithelial surface above opacity with distinctive "halos" around negative staining lesions (Figure 5.71)
  2. Recurrences of opacities often change with reactivation of keratitis

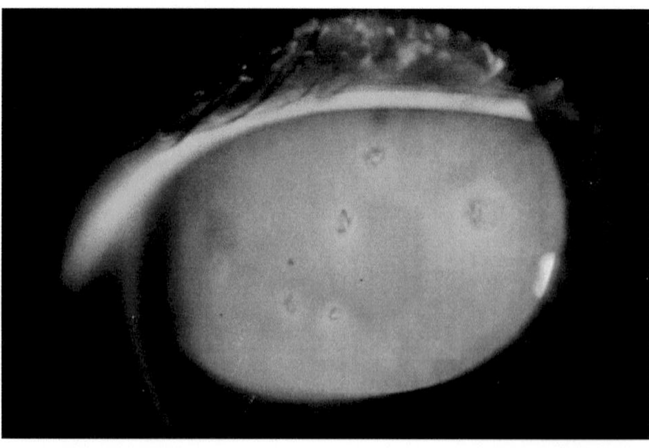

FIGURE 5.71 Multiple intraepithelial infiltrates demonstrating a sodium fluorescein pattern with hyperfluorescent "halos" around negative staining points associated with each raised epithelial site overlying diffuse, intraepithelial infiltrates.

a. Position of lesions may change
b. Size of lesions may change
c. Shapes of lesions may change

- Eyes tend to remain white and clear in the presence of distinct keratitis, which would normally produce a secondary conjunctival inflammatory response
- Beyond the primary SPK, eyes show no associated signs of any infectious or inflammatory disease process
  1. SPK of Thygeson "keeps no company"
  2. One of the only forms of keratitis that "keep no company"

Assessment

- Rule out other causes of SPKs (Figure 5.72)
  1. Bacterial
  2. Viral
  3. Sterile
- If patient wears contact lenses, rule out lens-associated causes of SPK
  1. Material-related causes
  2. Solution-related causes
  3. Mechanical, physiological, toxic causes (Figures 5.73 and 5.74)

Plan: Thygeson's Superficial Punctate Keratitis

(See also Appendix 4)

- Mild to moderate SPKs may require lubrication therapy only, with close monitoring for complications
- For moderate to severe degrees of SPKs (with or without symptoms)
  1. Heavy lubrication (6 to 10 times per day)
  2. Topical steroids (q2–4h for 10–14 days or more)
     a. Occasionally condition may not respond to steroids
     b. Discontinue use if no response in 3–4 weeks
  3. Topical tacrolimus 0.03% twice daily for 2 weeks or cyclosporine 2% have been used as alternative to steroids
  4. Bandage soft lens useful in medically non-responsive cases or symptomatic patients

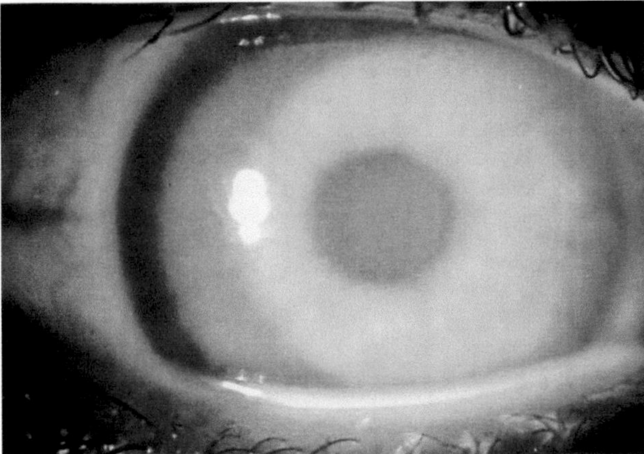

FIGURE 5.72 Diffuse superficial punctate keratitis (SPK) associated with numerous etiologies including viral, staphylococcal, and toxic (e.g., medicamentosa) causes.

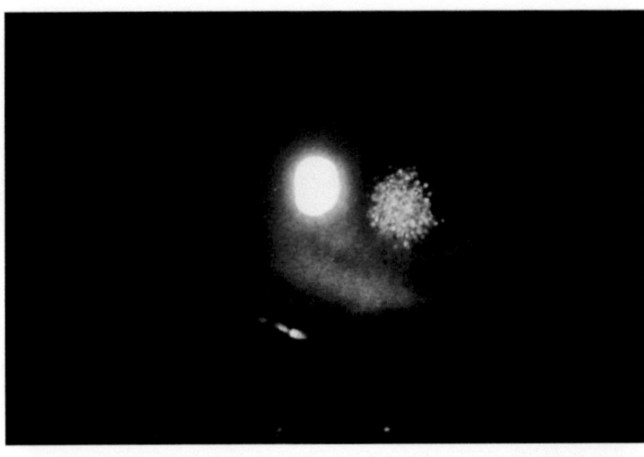

FIGURE 5.73 Confluent superficial punctate keratitis (SPK) representing a concentrated area of SPK associated with a localized toxic stimulus (e.g., toxin on a contact lens surface).

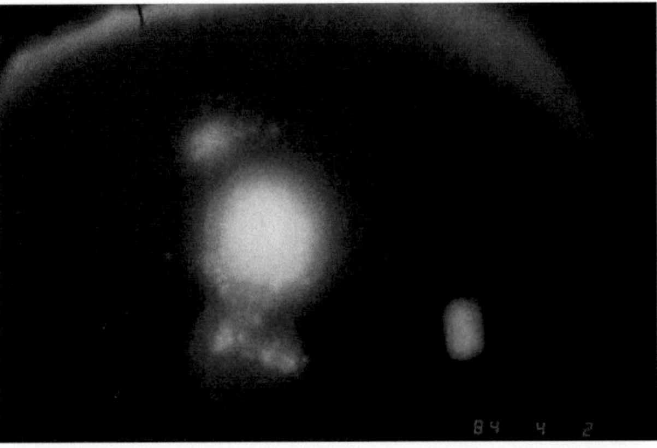

FIGURE 5.74 Focal epithelial defect is a densely, concentrated area of SPK associated with prolonged and/or more virulent, localized toxic stimuli causing full-thickness epithelial compromise from combined infiltration and inflammatory edema.

     a. Soft contact lens wearers who present with SPK of Thygeson may be kept on lens wear (as bandage) with close monitoring (every 4 to 6 weeks or PRN)
     b. With any therapy of moderate to severe degree SPK, add prophylactic gentamicin or tobramycin drops bid to qid (also in conjunction with bandage lens wear)

Follow-Up

- Advise and educate patient as to unknown etiology, clinical course, chronicity, risks, and prognosis of condition
- Treat moderate to severe degrees only during periods of exacerbations with patient instructed to report initial symptoms (if present) or signs (e.g., vision) of each episode
- Without contact lens wear, recheck every 4 to 6 months or PRN
- With contact lens wear (cosmetic or therapeutic), recheck every 4 to 6 weeks or PRN

12. *Viral Keratoconjunctivitis*

A complete discussion of viral keratoconjunctivitis begins in Section III. C.

B. Infectious Keratitis (Corneal Ulcers)

Background Information

1. Synonyms
   a. Bacterial corneal ulcer
   b. Bacterial keratitis
   c. Central corneal ulcer
   d. Corneal ulcer
   e. Microbial keratitis
   f. Ulcerative keratitis

Subjective

- Symptoms are usually acute to hyperacute including corneal irritation and uveitic (deeper) pain
- Whereas traumatic histories (injury and irritation) help differentiate etiology of superficial corneal epithelial disease (e.g., inflammatory, or immune response from irritation or injury), epithelial injury is a major risk factor in the diagnosis of infectious keratitis
- Risk-factor analysis is the most important means of early assessment of infectious keratitis
  1. Helps differentiate between early physical signs of sterile versus infectious keratitis
  2. Helps differentiate between possible causes of infectious keratitis (e.g., bacterial versus fungal)
  3. Helps determine the significance of symptoms (e.g., FB sensation in a non-compliant, extended wear contact lens patient with old, months or years, lenses versus a non-lens-wearing patient)
- Risk-factor analysis for infectious keratitis (Table 5.13)
  1. Symptom-related risk factors (in approximate order of increasing risk)
     a. Mild, non-specific irritation
     b. Burning sensation (toxins from microbe?)
     c. Lacrimation
     d. Photophobia
     e. Reduced visual acuity
     f. History of corneal injury
     g. FB sensation
     h. Continuing foreign-body sensation in contact lens patient after lens removal
     i. Pain
  2. Contact lens-related risk factors (in approximate order of increasing risk)
     a. Non-compliance (e.g., regarding wear, care)
     b. Poor hygiene
     c. Extended wear
     d. Lenses not frequently replaced
     e. Dirty lens surfaces
     f. Contaminated solutions
     g. Dirty cases
  3. Health-related risk factors (in approximate order of increasing risk)
     a. Diabetes
     b. Warm climates
     c. Staphylococcal toxins
     d. Dry eye syndromes
     e. Immune-compromised patients, such as acquired immune deficiency syndrome (AIDS)
     f. Post-surgical corneas
     g. Topical steroids
     h. Mechanical irritation (corneal trauma)
     i. Focal epithelial defects

Objective

- Infectious keratitis indicates the presence of a viable infectious organism (microbe) living and proliferating both on and in the cornea (Figure 5.75)
  1. Bacteria
  2. Virus
  3. Fungi
  4. Protozoa (e.g., Acanthamoeba)
- Critical indication for laboratory analysis along with clinical assessment
  1. Cytology (histopathology)
  2. Cultures and sensitivities
  3. Specimens (ideally) should be taken before any treatment is rendered
     a. Often not the case because of initial non-infectious diagnosis or secondary infection
     b. Laboratory workup still useful after commencement of therapy for differential diagnostic purposes and for resistant organisms
- Active proliferating microbes usually render pathological effect on corneal stroma, with resultant deep keratitis reactions versus superficial epithelial keratitis, which is

TABLE 5.13 Risk Factors in Infectious Keratitis: Subjective[a]

Risk	Symptom-Related Risk Factors	Contact Lens-Related Risk Factors	Health-Related Risk Factors
Increasing risk[b]	Mild irritation Burning Lacrimation	Noncompliance Poor hygiene procedures	Diabetes Warmer climates Staphylococcal toxins Dry eye syndromes Immune-compromised
	---------------	---------------	---------------
↓	Photophobia Reduced visual acuity Foreign-body sensation Foreign-body sensation continues (or increases) after contact lens removal Pain	Extended wear Lenses not replaced frequently Dirty lenses Contaminated solutions Dirty cases	Postsurgical corneas Topical steroids Mechanical irritation Focal epithelial defects

[a] History, symptoms, and risk factor analysis.

[b] Dotted lines in risk factor categories indicate author's levels of significant concern. Risk factors below --------------- lines, in combination with corneal lesion(s), should be considered as no less than moderate (to severe) presentations.

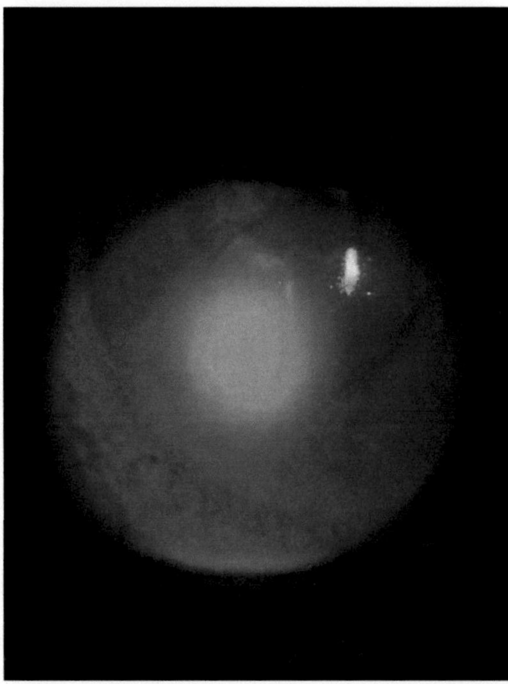

FIGURE 5.75 Infectious corneal ulcer in a midperipheral cornea with numerous suspicious diagnostic signs of corneal ulceration including size of the lesion (greater than 2 mm diameter), inner border of lesion greater than 2 mm in from the limbus, and dense stromal edema and infiltration.

usually sterile (toxins rather than live organisms on cornea, except for some viruses)

- Toxic by-products (e.g., enzymes) of polymorphonuclear WBCs and/or the active, proliferating microbial organisms (e.g., endotoxins of gram-negative bacteria: Pseudomonas) produce ulcer or necrotizing effect to stromal substance versus epithelial infiltrative reaction in superficial keratitis (see Table 5.12)
- Deep stromal reaction associated with infectious ulcerative keratitis produces deep (usually 50% to full stromal thickness) infiltrative or immune response to proliferating toxic (proteolytic) enzymes of offending organism
    1. Immune defense system is attempting to neutralize toxins and protect stromal tissue
    2. Because of virulence of organism and depth of reaction, immune system produces more dramatic and diffuse response than to the focal, localized, superficial toxins (usually staphylococcal exotoxins) associated with superficial keratitis (the "innocent bystander effect," described below)
- Most corneal ulcers tend to develop centrally, farther away from the immediate influence of the immune system (probably avoiding such influence) from the vascular supply at the limbus; thus, the immune system is further obligated to produce a more disseminated, pronounced, deep infiltrative response to effect neutralization of the offending organism and protection of the stromal tissue (from further ulceration)
    1. Not to say that some highly virulent organisms can also seed peripherally on the cornea and succeed in overcoming at least the initial effects of the peripheral corneal immune system response (proximal, immune complex, and Langerhans cells)
        a. Highly virulent organisms can overcome these defense mechanisms
        b. Immune-compromised eyes can also be vulnerable
            i. Compromised from systemic causes
            ii. Eyes treated with topical steroids
    2. In either case, such a pronounced, deep infiltrative or immune response produces a significantly more dramatic and disseminated clinical inflammatory reaction than that of a localized superficial epithelial infiltrative response
- Because of this intense inflammatory reaction, occurring in response to the ulcerative process, considerable adverse associated findings to the cornea and adjacent anatomy ("innocent bystanders") are produced (despite the attempted benefits being administered by the immune defense mechanism)
    1. Lid edema and erythema
    2. Conjunctival hyperemia and chemosis
    3. Corneal
        a. Edema (epithelial and stromal)
        b. Infiltration (deep stromal)
        c. Neovascularization (as chronic response)
        d. Posterior corneal keratic precipitates
        e. Folds in Descemet's membrane (striae)
    4. Anterior chamber
        a. Uveitic response (cells and flare)
        b. Endophthalmitis (sterile hypopyon, accumulated white blood cells in chamber)
        c. Increased IOP (secondary to angle congestion)

Assessment

- The primary diagnostic consideration is the accurate differentiation between infectious ulcerative keratitis and sterile infiltrative keratitis
    1. Definition of *ulcer(ation)*: a local defect, or excavation, of the surface of an organ or tissue, which is produced by sloughing of inflammatory necrotic tissue (Figure 5.76)
    2. Definition of *infiltration*: the diffusion or accumulation in a tissue or cells of substances not normal to it or in amounts more than the normal (Figure 5.77)
- Differential diagnosis is established by three steps
    1. Careful history and risk-factor analysis (see Table 5.13)
    2. Detailed physical examination
    3. Categorizing patient based on combined assessment of history, symptoms, and risk factors (subjective) relative to physical examination (objective)
- Risk categories for infectious keratitis
    1. Low risk: few subjective or objective findings
    2. Medium risk: risk factors in the presence of suspicious physical findings
    3. High risk: significant risk factors combined with ulcerative finding(s)
- Comparison of sterile infiltrate to corneal ulcer (see Table 5.15)
- After establishing a definitive diagnosis of infectious keratitis, next step is to attempt to differentiate type of infectious keratitis (Table 5.14)
    1. Clinical differential sometimes difficult
    2. Laboratory workup essential (e.g., cytology, cultures, and sensitivities)

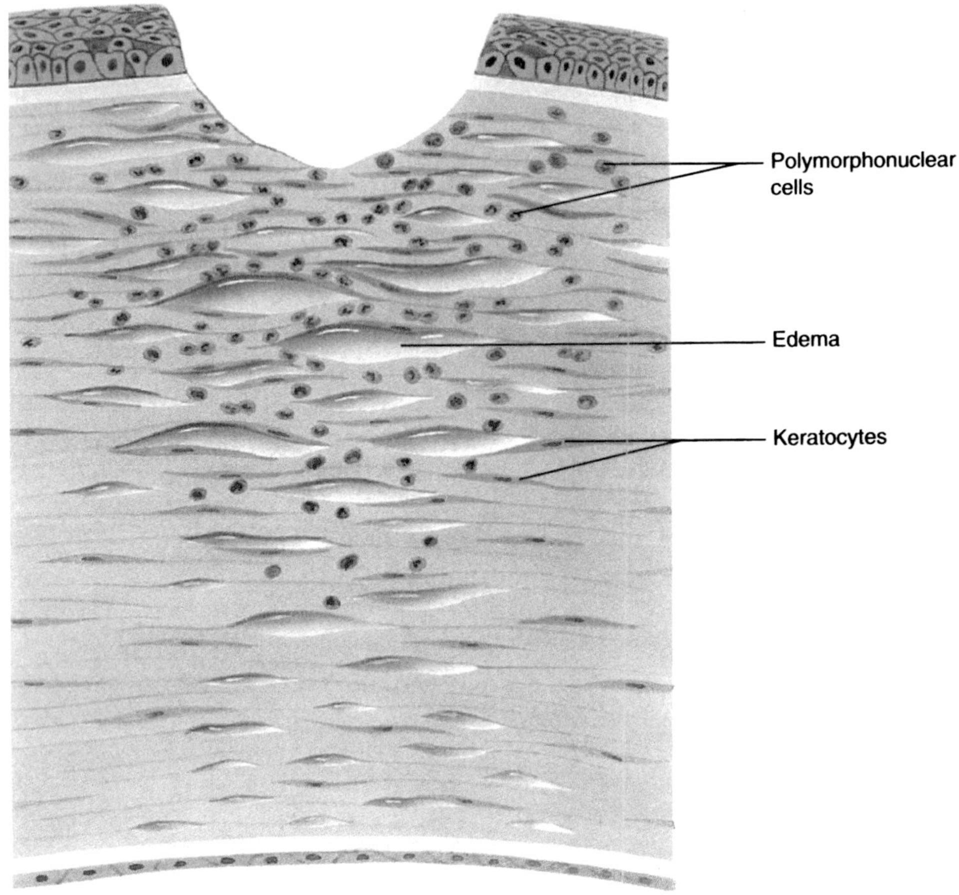

FIGURE 5.76 Histopathology of corneal ulceration demonstrates the compromised epithelial surface with deep stromal PMN infiltration and ultimate destruction of stromal matrix.

- After establishing specific type of infectious keratitis, next step is to attempt to differentiate specific category, family, genus, species, depending on infectious etiology (see specific types of infectious keratites)

Plan and Follow-Up: Infectious Keratitis

- Hospitalization or diligent home care is necessary for all forms of infectious keratitis
    1. Primary concerns are for patient compliance and cooperation with frequency, complexity, intensity, and toxic risks of indicated therapies
    2. Skilled nursing care may be needed for proper administration of most treatment plans associated with infectious keratitis
- The most effective method of delivering drugs in infectious keratitis is topical administration
    1. Speed of infectious or ulcerative process on the avascular cornea necessitates topical drug use in high concentration
    2. Oral and intravenous medications do not deliver effect rapidly enough or in high enough concentration (through tears, aqueous, or translimbal effects) as compared with topical agents
        a. May be used if there is significant risk of corneal perforation
        b. Theory is to bathe the posterior corneal tissue with high concentrations in aqueous
    3. Depot injections (subconjunctival or subtenons) may also be used in severe clinical presentations
- Oral tetracyclines may have some value in corneal ulceration as an anticollagenolytic agent
- Immunosuppressive agents (corticosteroids) are *contraindicated* in active infectious ulceration
    1. Immune system is serving a positive function during active ulcerative process by helping to neutralize toxins and reduce further stromal penetration
    2. Immunosuppression would reduce effect and permit increased penetration and possible perforation
    3. Notwithstanding positive functions of immune system response, deep stromal infiltrative activity potentiates permanent (full-thickness) stromal scarring
        a. This is considered an unavoidable sequalae of corneal ulceration
        b. However, until all infectious organisms and their associated toxins are neutralized and destroyed by appropriate anti-infective agents, the immune system is the singular defense mechanism working to protect the cornea
    4. Once infectious agents are neutralized (as determined by negative culturing) or reepithelization,

steroids then become *indicated* to reduce any further stromal damage and scarring

- Unfortunately (for patient and practitioner), the most appropriate and effective therapy for most forms of infectious keratitis (in fact, any stromal infiltrative, ulcerative, or traumatic insult) usually results in permanent corneal scarring
  1. Such scarring (especially in central ulceration) virtually guarantees the risk of cosmetic awareness and permanent functional (vision) loss
  2. Negative sequelae of permanent cosmetic scar and functional loss (although unavoidable) are often cause for patient dissatisfaction and distress
  3. Substantial potential for such negative outcomes should be considered by the primary eye care provider on diagnosis and before treatment
     a. Explain diagnosis in clear and simple terms
     b. Firmly advise patient of need for care
     c. Discuss nature and goals of treatment
     d. Carefully and clearly define the associated risks and prognosis of the condition (with and without proper care)
     e. Recommend and coordinate the most appropriate (e.g., corneal specialist) and accessible professional care for treatment and management of the patient
     f. Contemporaneously (at that very moment) document all clinical information, care, instructions, advice, and recommendations at initial visit and all subsequent visits

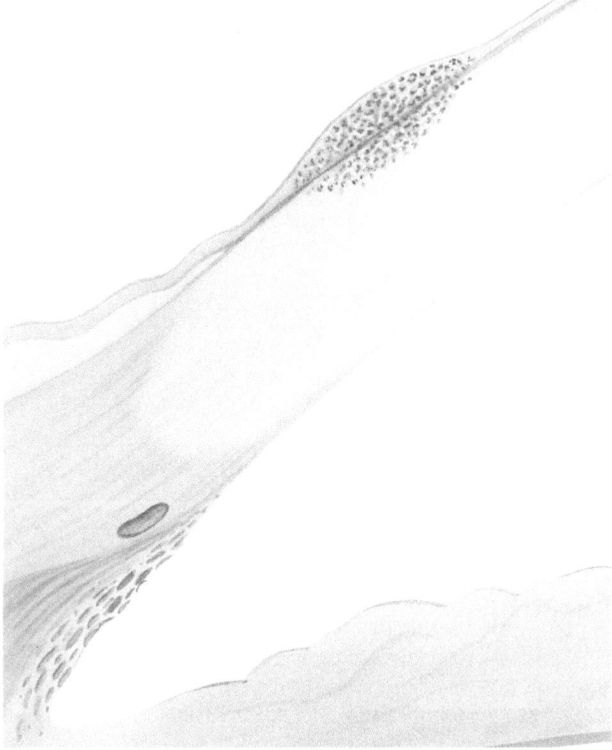

FIGURE 5.77 Histopathology of corneal infiltration demonstrates accumulation of PMNs (intraepithelial) with risk of secondary ulceration to stromal surface.

1. Acanthamoeba Keratitis[54]

Subjective

- A ubiquitous protozoan capable of infecting injured corneas or corneas of contact lens patients
- History usually includes some form of corneal trauma

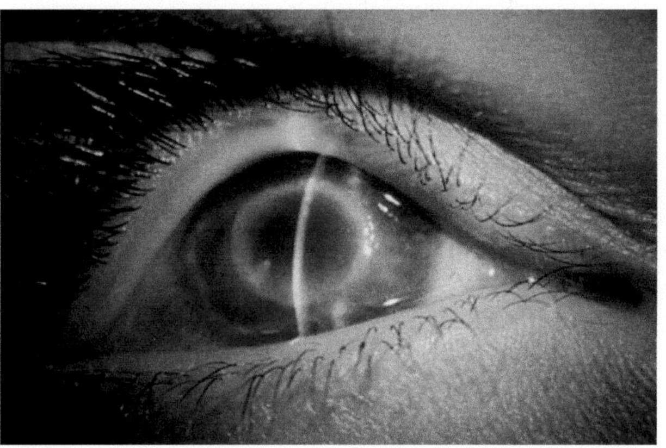

FIGURE 5.78 Acanthamoeba keratitis producing a dense, stromal ring infiltrate in a soft contact lens wearer. Early stages included a severely painful epithelial dendrifom keratitis (see Figure 5.90), followed by stromal infiltration (ring keratitis) and stromal "melting" (polymorphonuclear proteolysis).

TABLE 5.14 Differential Diagnosis of Nonbacterial Infectious Keratitis: Assessment

Differential Diagnosis	Subjective	Objective	Assessment	Plan	Prognosis
Herpes simplex (HSV) stromal keratitis	Burning irritation Recurrent history(?)	Dendrite possible Stromal infiltration	Disciform Immune (Wessely) ring	Antiviral agents Steroids	Bad!
Fungal keratitis	History of vegetative injury	Spores and hypha Serpiginous	Mooren's ulcer Marginal infiltrate	Natamycin Other antifungal agents	Worse!
Acanthamoeba	History of trauma	Localized infiltrate progressing to stromal ring ulcer	Usually mistaken for HSV stromal keratitis	Biguanides	Even worse!
	Poor contact lens hygiene Solution contaminates		Nonresponsive	Penetrating keratoplasty	

[a] Differential diagnosis (ruling out).

- Exposure to stagnant water sources (e.g., lake), swimming pools, hot tubs, and so forth, have been reported as risk factors
- Contaminated contact lens solutions have become somewhat notorious risk factors
- Pain is acute and often far more dramatic than early physical signs might suggest
- History often includes non-responsiveness to steroid therapy or anti-infective medications

Objective

- Early signs may be limited to epithelial disruption non-responsive to standard anti-infective regimens
- Associated inflammatory reactions include anterior uveitis and scleritis
  1. Advancing conditions produce hypopyon, hyphema, and potential scleral "melt"
  2. Steroids may mitigate inflammation but may not resolve condition
- Corneal involvement involves five levels over days to weeks with little response to standard medical regimens
  1. Epithelialitis with radial neuritis
  2. Circumscribed stromal infiltrative or inflammatory responses
  3. Anterior stromal disease (stromal infiltrates or radial infiltrates)
  4. Deep stromal disease
  5. Ring infiltrate (only 50% of patients will develop and in advanced stage)
- Stromal "melt" can occur, and descemetocele can lead to perforation
- Other associated findings vary with intensity of progressing infectious corneal involvement
  1. Conjunctival chemosis
  2. Pseudomembranes
  3. Preauricular lymphadenopathy
  4. Psuedodentrites (infiltrative)
- Degree of clinical signs, although chronic, may wax and wane despite treatment modalities

Assessment

- Differentiate sterile versus infectious keratitis (see Table 5.14)
- Standard bacterial cultures prove negative
  1. However, acanthamoeba is a bacterial parasite
  2. *Escherichia coli* culture will grow organism
  3. Quick, easy test for clinical use
- In vivo confocal microscopy can identify cysts easily
- Polymerase chain reaction (PCR) techniques are available
- Corneal smears under immunofluorescent microscopy with a "calcuflour" agent considered an accurate diagnostic test
- Early differential diagnosis usually difficult
  1. Often made *ex juvantia* (from lack of response to other forms of therapy)
  2. Risk factor analysis critical in early corneal infections not responding to other therapies
- Rule out all other conditions that might mimic infectious keratitis
- Most common misdiagnosis
  1. Herpes simplex for epithelial disease
  2. Stromal herpes simplex for stromal disease

Plan and Follow-Up: Acanthamoeba Keratitis

- Consider and coordinate the most appropriate professional resource(s) for care and management
- Provide patient with proper advice and instructions
- Acanthamoeba cysts (dormant form) difficult to treat due to being encased in a proteoglycan coat
- Medical therapies generally ineffective
- No single drug exists that treats cysts and trophozoites
- Multiple therapies suggested in literature
  1. Biquanides are the first line of treatment
     a. PHMB and chlorhexidine are used in combination (reported to be effective against both cysts and trophozoites)
  2. Hexamidine 0.1% (Desomedine)
  3. Dibromopropamidine 0.15%
  4. Propamadine isethionate (Brolene)
  5. Ketoconazole (Nizoral)
  6. Neomycin (Neosporin)
- Adjunctive therapies include
  1. Topical steroid use is controversial
  2. Pain relievers
- Surgical intervention (corneal grafting) is usually the long-term prognosis in all cases
  1. For pending corneal perforation
  2. Therapeutic with medically uncontrolled central infection
  3. Resultant scarring

2. *Bacterial Keratitis*[55–58]

Background Information

a. Synonyms
   i. Bacterial ulcer
   ii. Central corneal ulcer
   iii. Corneal ulcer
b. Bacteria generally categorized as gram-positive and gram-negative
   i. Most common gram-positive corneal infectors
      - Staphylococcus (multiple species)
      - *Streptococcus pneumoniae* or *pyogenes*
   ii. Most common gram-negative corneal infectors (in approximate decreasing order of frequency)
      - *Pseudomonas aeruginosa*
      - Moraxella
      - *Neisseria gonorrhoeae* (with venereal disease)
      - *Haemophilus influenzae* (common in children)
      - Morax–Axenfeld (higher risk in alcoholics)
      - Others
        - *Serratia marcescens*
        - Enterobacteriaceae
        - *Proteus vulgaris*
        - Klebsiella
        - *Escherichia coli*
        - Corynebacterium
c. Most common cause of all bacterial keratitis is Pseudomonas
   i. Greater in warmer (southern) climates
   ii. Clinical "rule of thumb" is to assume Pseudomonas until proven (by culture) otherwise
d. Highest-risk ulcer patients are contact lens wearers (hydrogel and silicone hydrogel)
   i. Annual incidence in daily wear soft approximately 0.04%
   ii. Annual incidence in extended wear soft about 0.2%

   iii. Parents with children in diapers are at greater risk of infection by some gram-negative, gastrointestinal bacteria
   iv. Children
e. Other risk categories
   i. Nutritionally deprived patients
   ii. Immune-compromised patients
f. Generally, Staphylococcus (gram-positive) tends to produce less intense and slower developing ulcers because of its exotoxic (versus endotoxic) nature
   i. Streptococcus and the gram-negative bacteria that produce endotoxins are more virulent corneal infectors, developing more rapidly, with hyperacute signs and symptoms and greater risk of corneal damage
   ii. Pseudomonas is the notorious gram-negative corneal infector because of its virulent endotoxins, rapid proliferation, ubiquitous, opportunistic nature (especially in warm, moist environments), and its ability to destroy corneal stroma within minutes to hours after entering the cornea
      - The only (minimal) "good news" about Pseudomonas is that it cannot penetrate an intact corneal epithelial surface
      - It requires a "focal epithelial defect" to enter and begin to infect and ulcerate corneal stroma

Subjective

- Unilateral, acute presentation
- History usually includes at least one (but usually multiple) risk factors (see Table 5.13)
   1. Most common risk factor tends to be history of recent trauma causative of a focal epithelial defect
   2. Recent contact lens manipulations (procedures) can be considered traumatic event
- Other corneal disease states may be considered predisposing factors for ulceration
   1. Superficial keratites
   2. Marginal infiltrate (as focal epithelial defect)
   3. Dry eye or keratitis sicca syndromes
- Rate of progression of ulcer varies with bacteria (in increasing order of speed of progression)
   1. Staphylococcus (usually over days)
   2. Streptococcus (usually within 1 to 2 days)
   3. Most gram-negatives (usually within 24 hours)
   4. *Neisseria gonorrhoeae* (usually within 12 to 24 hours)
   5. Pseudomonas (within hours)
- Pain usually develops subacutely (within days) to acutely (within minutes to hours)
- Symptoms usually follow typical sequence, especially in contact lens wearers
   1. Non-specific irritation
   2. Burning sensation (toxins of bacteria)
   3. Lacrimation
   4. Photophobia (secondary to corneal edema)
   5. Reduced vision (from edema and infiltration)
   6. FB sensation
      a. May develop early without contact lens wear
      b. With contacts (especially soft), bandaging effect can artificially reduce FB sensation late into ulcerative process
   7. Continued (or increasing) FB sensation on contact lens removal or over extended time period (hours to days)
   8. Dull, aching (inflammatory or uveitic) pain
- Evaluate carefully for all risk factors

Objective

(See Table 5.15)

- Eyelids
   1. Staphylococcus usually produces mild to moderate edema and erythema with frequent associated staphylococcal lid signs (marginal crustation, tylosis)
   2. Streptococcal and gram-negative bacteria usually produce severe lid reactions
      a. Pronounced inflammatory response
      b. Pseudoptosis
      c. Preseptal cellulitis
   3. *Haemophilus influenzae* often produces a bluish, purplish preseptal flush in acute phase
   4. Gonorrhoeae (and other hyperacute purulent bacteria) may accumulate discharge under a "stuck-shut" lid during sleep and present a "ballooning" lid on waking (and examination)
      a. Separate lids slowly and carefully
      b. Purulence has tendency to projectile outward on release of lid margins
- Conjunctiva
   1. Bulbar conjunctival reaction is usually a severe crimson-violet, red (violaceous) hyperemia involving greater than 180°, usually 360°
   2. Chemosis ranges from mild elevation of portions or all the bulbar conjunctiva (<1 mm) to dramatic "watchglass" (bulbar conjunctiva grossly elevated and overlapping peripheral cornea) effects
   3. Streptococcus, and some gram-negatives will occasionally produce hemorrhages on the bulbar conjunctiva
   4. Palpebral conjunctiva usually produces mild to moderate papillary (velvety type) changes
   5. Amount of mucopurulent discharge varies considerably according to bacteria, intensity of infection, and duration of infection
      a. Staphylococcal discharge ranges from nothing at all to moderate amounts
      b. Streptococcus and gram-negative bacteria tend to produce moderate to copious amounts of discharge
      c. Often, a mucous plug congests and overlies the ulcer site on the corneal surface
      d. Gonorrhea is most notorious for its hyperacute mucopurulent nature
- Corneal epithelium during active ulceration (Figure 5.79)
   1. Ulceration usually destroys epithelial surface (and anterior stromal substance) early in the process, producing a depressed, "excavated" lesion
      a. Staphylococcus tends to produce well-defined borders, creating a clearly circumscribed lesion
      b. Streptococcus and gram-negative bacteria produce indistinct "fuzzy" edges to the ulcer
      c. Edges of ulcers frequently show an overhang effect of necrotic epithelial tissue
      d. NaFl stain will pool at the site initially and spread amorphously into a geographic stromal pattern within minutes
   2. Ulcer is usually about 2-mm diameter or greater
   3. Position on the corneal surface varies

TABLE 5.15 Sterile versus Infectious Keratitis: Objective

Findings	Sterile Infiltrate		Infectious Ulcer
Eyelids			
Edema	Minimal		Ptosis
Erythema	Faint		Crimson red
Conjunctiva			
Injection	15–90°		>180°
Intensity	Pink to red		Crimson to violet
Exudate	Lacrimation		Mucopurulence
Cornea (day 1)			
Epithelial defect			
Size	≤1 mm		>2 mm
Position	≤2 mm off limbus		>3 mm in from limbus
Depth	Epithelial		>50% thickness
Height	Raised		Depressed
Edges	Well defined		Fuzzy
NaFl	Superficial (as "island")		Deep
Lucency	Nebula (haze)	**THE GRAY ZONE**	Macula to opaque
Edema			
Size	>2 mm (surrounding "island")		>50% of surface
Intensity	Epithelial		>50% stromal thickness
Folds in Descemet's membrane	None		>2
Infiltration	Superficial		Full stromal thickness
Neo vascularization/Pannus			
Area	0–30°		0–360° (late)
Length	0–2 mm		0–4 mm (late)
Anterior chamber			
Cells and flare	None to trace		Countable to dense
Hypopyon	None		>1 mm
Other			
Pupil size	PERRLA		Miotic
Intraocular pressure	Normal range		Usually raised
Best visual acuity	Unaffected		≤20/50

[a] Clinical signs and physical examinations.

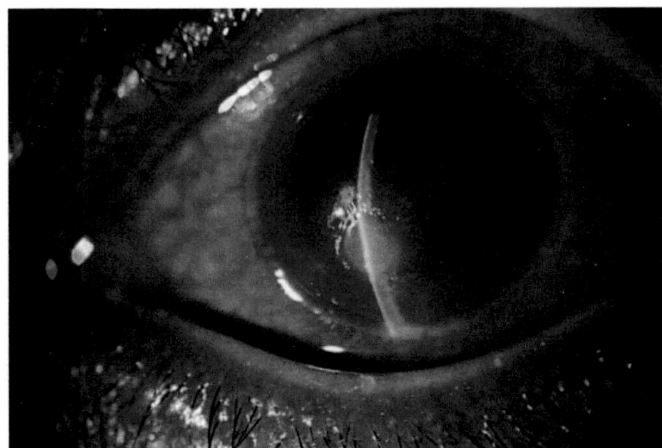

FIGURE 5.79 Bacterial corneal ulcer presenting a densely infiltrated stromal lesion in the inferior portion of an acutely inflamed cornea and anterior segment with 4+ bulbar conjunctival hyperemia, corneal edema, posterior corneal congestion, and a 3+ (cells and flare) anterior chamber reaction.

   a. Most common location is centralward, away from the vascular or immune effects of the limbus (synonym: central ulcer)
   b. Virulent organisms may be able to overcome such effects and seed themselves at the corneal periphery (perhaps, using a sterile infiltrate as their focal epithelial defect for entry; Figure 5.80)
4. Rarely, additional ulcers (satellite lesions) may develop on cornea during disease process

- Corneal stroma during active ulceration
  1. Corneal edema (epithelial and stromal) usually covers more than 50% of the cornea and affects at least 50% of the stromal thickness
     a. Produces a whitish-gray corneal haze
     b. Advancing edema creates secondary fold in Descemet's membrane (striate keratitis)
  2. Infiltration occurs under and around the entire ulcer in a classic deep and dense pattern
     a. Depth is usually 50% to full-thickness stroma
     b. Density ranges from hazy to opaque

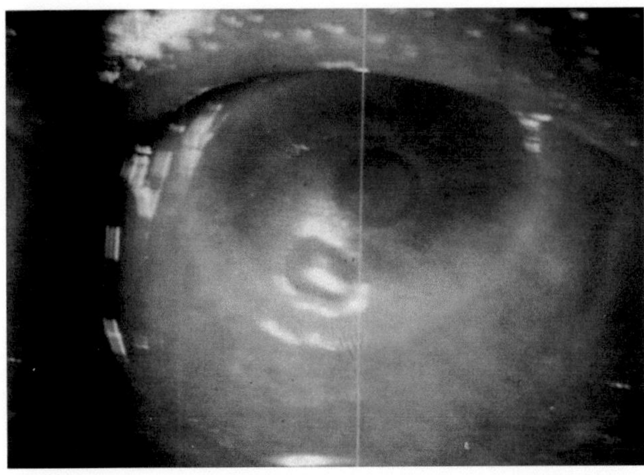

FIGURE 5.80 Gonococcal corneal ulcer in a rapidly deteriorating, untreated (for 48 hours), hyperacute red eye with copious mucopurulent discharge. Laboratory cultures confirmed *Neisseria gonorrhoeae* and corneal perforation resulted in spite of aggressive, fortified antibiotic therapy.

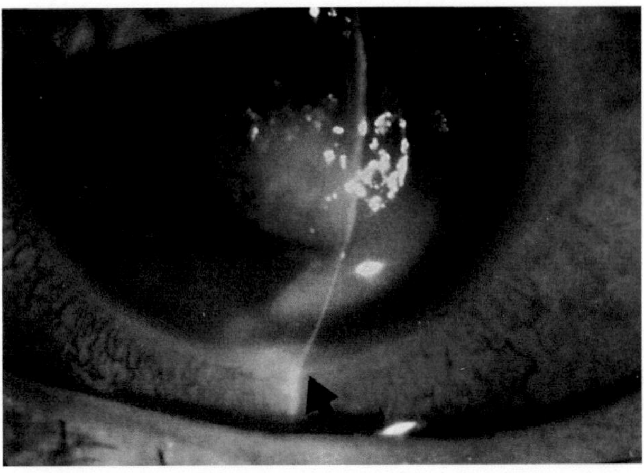

FIGURE 5.81 Endophthalmitis with overlying, exudative mucoid plug filling a depressed ulcerative lesion in the central corneal stroma. The associated hypopyon arrow is the defining clinical sign in endophthalmitis and frequently denotes gram-negative infection (serratia marcesans in this case).

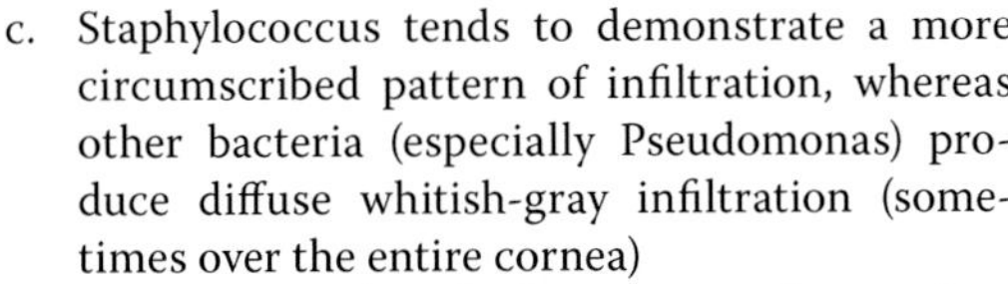

    c. Staphylococcus tends to demonstrate a more circumscribed pattern of infiltration, whereas other bacteria (especially Pseudomonas) produce diffuse whitish-gray infiltration (sometimes over the entire cornea)
    d. Pseudomonas has also been reported as producing ring infiltration or ulceration
  3. Highly virulent organisms, resistant bacteria (to selected antibiotics), and delayed treatment can lead to additional stromal complications
    a. Stromal abscess
    b. Descemetoceles
    c. Stromal melting
    d. Corneal perforation
- Posterior cornea during active ulceration
  1. Striate keratitis (folds in Descemet's membrane)
  2. Keratic precipitates (white blood cells on endothelium)
  3. Fibrin plaques (infiltrative or inflammatory debris)
  4. Pseudoguttata-like formations
- Anterior chamber during active ulceration
  1. Anterior uveitic reaction (cells and flare) always present, ranging from trace reaction to dense (fibrinous) anterior chamber reaction
  2. Staphylococcus tends to produce mildest uveitic response, rarely presenting a measurable hypopyon (Figure 5.81)
  3. Sterile hypopyon (endophthalmitis), accumulation of white blood cells producing an opaque fluid level in the inferior aqueous, varying in height, presents in most advanced bacterial keratitis
- Other associated findings during active ulceration
  1. Neovascularization may develop in varying degrees in delayed or untreated corneal ulcers
  2. IOP frequently begins to rise during active ulceration secondary to anterior angle congestion
  3. Miotic pupils are often noted during acute phase
  4. VA is almost always reduced significantly, usually below 20/40

Assessment

- Follow step-by-step approach
  1. Analyze risk factors (see Table 5.13)
  2. Careful physical examination
  3. Categorize patient risk
- Differentiate sterile infiltrate (e.g., contact lens peripheral ulcer) from corneal ulcer (see Table 5.15)
- Differentiate bacterial keratitis from other forms of infectious keratitis
- (see Table 5.15)
- Cultures and sensitivities
  1. Positive laboratory workup is always reassuring
  2. Negative laboratory workup is inconclusive
  3. With negative cultures, best to rely on clinical data and presumptive diagnosis
- "Assume the worst" (Pseudomonas) until proven otherwise or correct
- Beware of the three bacteria that can penetrate intact corneal epithelium (no focal epithelial defect necessary for corneal invasion and ulceration)
  1. Streptococcus (especially in children)
  2. *Haemophilus influenzae* (especially in children)
  3. *Neisseria gonorrhoeae* (venereal disease in adults and transmissible to newborns)
- Do not forget to assess less obvious risk factors
  1. Alcoholism (increased risk for moraxella)
  2. Parents of kids in diapers (increased risk of gastrointestinal gram-negative bacteria)
  3. Venereal disease (increased risk of gonococcus, chlamydia, herpes)
  4. Systemic risks (e.g., diabetes, immunosuppressive oral medications)
  5. Dirty hands in kids (or adults)

Plan: Bacterial Keratitis

(See also Appendices 4 and 6)

- Consider and coordinate the most appropriate professional resource(s) for care and management

- Provide patient with proper advice and instructions
- Hospitalization should be considered based on the best interest and needs of the patient determined through reasonable and prudent professional judgment
  1. Considerations should include risk of patient noncompliance, need for supervised care, access to hospital care, and cost
  2. Medicolegal considerations are based on minimum standard of care for the given conditions in that community
- Cultures and sensitivities (before any treatment)
  1. Cultures (and smears for cytology, if available) should be collected from lids, conjunctiva, cul-de-sac, corneal scrapings, and (if applicable) contact lenses, solutions, and accessories
  2. On return of a positive culture, treatment can be adjusted or maintained, depending on results
  3. But initial treatment should be intensive, broad-spectrum antibiosis with specific emphasis on antipseudomonal therapy
- Cycloplege and dilate with 1% atropine q2–4h or 5% homatropine ql–2h
- Minimum of two fortified aminoglycosides commonly used
  1. Must include gentamicin and tobramycin
  2. Commercial (proprietary) concentrations usually 3 mg/mL
  3. Fortified concentrations equal 10 to 15 mg/mL
     a. Add 1 mL of injectable gentamicin or tobramycin to 5-mL bottle of commercial strength of the same drug to yield a fortified concentration
     b. Procedure can also be done with 1 mL of injectable cephalosporin in 4 mL of balanced, sterile saline (for 50 mg/mL fortification)
     c. Fortified solutions are unstable beyond 3 to 5 days
     d. Fortified strengths usually produce secondary toxic medicamentosa
     e. Another option is fortified Vancomycin (optimal gram + coverage) and fortified tobramycin (optimal gram–coverage)
  4. Can be compounded by pharmacist or, if circumstances dictate, prepared in office (for short course, 24-hour maximum use per preparation) by using dilute sterile injectable products as eyedrops such as tobramycin (Nebcin) and gentamicin (Garamycin)
  5. Standard dosage every 15 to 30 minutes around the clock
- Alternative dosage regimen of aminoglycosides reported as equally effective as every 30 minutes (and useful if outpatient care indicated or necessary)
  1. Loading dose
     a. Delivered in office during initial visit
     b. One drop fortified tobramycin every minute ×5 (5 dosages)
  2. Extended dose
     a. Delivered by patient (or advocate) at home
     b. 3 gtt fortified tobramycin (at 1-minute intervals) ql–2h for 24 hours (asking patient to wake q2h throughout the night)
  3. Beware of toxicities with frequent or fortified dose levels necessary in ulcer care
- Fluoroquinolones, particularly besofloxacin for bacterial keratitis, should be considered for use as the first drug of choice in any keratitis that has cultures positive for gram-negative bacteria (particularly Pseudomonas), or has significant risk factors and/or clinical indications of gram-negative infection
  1. Has been shown to be safe and highly effective
  2. Apply same alternative loading and extended dosage regime as described above for aminoglycosides for the first 2 days, and then reduce to 2 gtts qh for 2 days, and then q4h for 10 to 14 days or until complete reepithelialization (no staining)
  3. One study reported similar efficacy with besofloxacin qid versus fortified aminoglycosides (Vancomycin and tobramycin) q1h
- Subconjunctival and subtenons injections of aminoglycosides often provided in advancing cases of bacterial keratitis
- Oral doxycycline (as an anticollagenolytic agent) may be prescribed at 100 mg bid
- Oral and IV antibiotics are usually indicated in ulcers with significant threat of corneal perforation
- Additional oral penicillins, cephalosporins, tetracycline, and so forth, are indicated in venereal organisms (e.g., gonorrhea)
  1. Patient should also be referred to primary physician
  2. Sexual partners must be identified and treated
- If pain is severe, OTC NSAIDs or oral narcotic analgesics are indicated

Follow-Up

- Re-culturing should be conducted within 48 hours after commencement of therapy and every 24 hours thereafter until negative cultures are established
  1. On negative culture, topical steroids should be introduced at q3–4h
  2. If bacterial keratitis diagnosis was presumptive (i.e., without positive cultures), steroids should be withheld for minimum of 2 to 3 days
  3. SCUT (steroids for corneal ulcers trial) compared topical prednisone to placebo after 48 hours of topical antibiotic treatment
     a. At 3 months sub-group analyses showed some patients had a better visual outcome and smaller scar size (except Nocardia infections) than placebo
- Active ulcerative process could persist (even with full medical therapy) for weeks to months
  1. Usually a result of resistant strains to aminoglycosides/fluroquinolones used or available
  2. Resultant full-thickness stromal scarring almost ensured
  3. Corneal (stromal) melt and perforation always major risk
- Penetrating keratoplasty often required after resolution of active infectious process
- Continued patient education, advice, and counseling essential for proper patient management

3. *Fungal Keratitis*[59]

Background Information

a. Synonyms
   i. Fungal ulcer
   ii. Mycotic keratitis
b. Tends to mimic other forms of infectious keratitis

c. More difficult to treat than bacterial infection
d. Generally rare, but more prevalent in certain "risk areas"
    i. Southern and southwestern states
    ii. Temperate climates
    iii. Farming communities
e. Most common infectors
    i. Fusarium
    ii. Candida
    iii. Aspergillus
f. Frequently found in compromised hosts
    i. Steroid (oral or topical) users
    ii. Anticancer therapy
    iii. AIDS patients
g. Notorious as a lacrimal apparatus infector

Subjective

- Most common presentation includes a history of vegetative injury to the cornea (e.g., plants)
- Careful medical history useful to assess risk
    1. Use of steroids
    2. Immunosuppressive diseases
    3. Diagnosis of (or major risk factors for) AIDS
- Insidious to rapid onset of corneal symptoms

Objective

- Usually a dirty grayish infiltrate (raised)
    1. More frequently on peripheral cornea
    2. Serpiginous ("creeping") ulcerative process on corneal surface usually moving along the periphery, but may move centralward as well
- Ulcerated area has rough textured surface
- Feathered edge to ulcerated area, with branching hyphae and spores at the leading edge
- Satellite lesions are common (high magnification)
- Degree (width and depth) of surrounding infiltration varies with virulence of organism
- Other associated findings are relative to degree
    1. Conjunctival hyperemia
    2. Posterior corneal infiltration
        a. Folds and fibrin
        b. Endothelial plaques
        c. Immune rings (Wessely)
    3. Anterior chamber reaction
        a. Cells and flare
        b. Fibrin
        c. Hypopyon (common)

Assessment

- Laboratory diagnosis essential
- Rule out sterile infiltrative keratitis
- Rule out other forms of infectious keratitis (see Table 5.15)
- Valuable differential test for serpiginous type ulceration (fungal and Mooren's ulcers) is a combined fluorescein–rose bengal staining technique
    1. Serpiginous ulcer has active (live-vital cells) leading edge and necrotic (dead-devitalized) rear edge
    2. Leading edge will stain with fluorescein only, while rear edge will stain with rose bengal

Plan and Follow-Up: Fungal Keratitis

- All antifungal therapies (topical and systemic) include extremely toxic medications
- Consider management by corneal specialist skilled in use of antifungal drugs
- Some antifungal drugs used include
    1. Topical natamycin 5% (Natacyn) only FDA-approved antifungal medication
    2. Nystatin (non-ophthalmic preparation)
    3. Voriconazole
        i. Topical has shown to be effective against fungal infections but mycotic ulcer treatment trial (MUTT I) demonstrated natamycin better outcome visual acuity and lower rate of corneal perforation
        ii. In MUTT II the addition of oral Voriconazole medication did not improve treatment over topical medication only
    4. Amphotericin B (non-ophthalmic preparation)
        i. Extremely toxic
        ii. Medicamentosa usually within 7 days
    5. Owing to vast number of potential fungal infective organisms, resistant strains are common, and therapy and response is highly unpredictable

4. Herpetic Keratitis

A complete discussion of herpetic keratitis follows in the next section.

C. Viral Keratoconjunctivitis

Background Information

Refer to Chapter 4, "Viral (and Other Follicular) Conjunctivitis, Adenoviral Types," under "Background Information," for a complete discussion (see also Table 5.10).

1. Epidemic Keratoconjunctivitis[60–66] *(EKC)*

Background Information

a. Epidemic keratoconjunctivitis (EKC) is arguably the most common contagious clinical condition managed in primary eye care practice
    i. Highly contagious nature in its early (milder) phases causes "epidemic" spreading potential
    ii. Most patients do not realize, or underestimate, communicable nature because of mild symptoms and clinical signs during early contagious phase
b. Virus transmitted by direct or indirect contact (e.g., from a contaminated towel, hand, in-office instruments, cell phones, computer keyboards) with the infected tissues or tears
c. Patient will shed active virus for 10–14 days after onset of symptoms
d. Virus can survive for up to 1 month outside of the body
e. EKC is traditionally associated with adenovirus 8
    i. Each year new strains are presenting increasing frequency and virulence of EKC-type syndromes
    ii. Other EKC adenoviruses: 37, 53, 54, 56, 64
f. Originally, EKC syndrome was a fairly definitive set of clinical parameters and findings
    i. Called EKC rule of 8's
        - Adenovirus 8 most common
        - First 8 days (conjunctivitis stage) most contagious
        - Eighth day, corneal SPK presentation
        - Eight days later (sixteenth day), SEIs
    ii. Time sequences are rough approximations
    iii. With increasing numbers and virulence of EKC type adenoviruses, exceptions to the rule of 8's are becoming quite frequent

- Conjunctivitis stage may be shorter than 8 days or completely absent with contagious period being prodromal or during the keratitic phase
- Keratitic phase (SPK and SEI) may be immediate or within days (rather than weeks)

Subjective

- Most common viral presentation (in practice) because of intensity and duration (resulting in patient concern)
- Frequently seen as an "epidemic" (outbreak and spread within a given period of time)
- Usually a common denominator is (ultimately) recognized as potential contaminating source of environment
  1. Family
  2. Neighborhood
  3. Workplace
  4. School
  5. Hospital
  6. Eye doctor's office!
- Age range is usually 15 to 18 years or older
  1. Classic differential for PCF (usually in children)
  2. However, more virulent strains are transmissible to children under age 15 (in increasing numbers)
- Never any significant systemic signs or symptoms associated (as with the PCF syndrome)
  1. Strictly an ocular reaction
  2. Any systemic associations are probably coincidental in that adenoviruses producing EKC are not known for any substantial systemic reactions
- Classic viral-type symptoms in milder presentations
  1. Non-specific irritation
  2. Burning sensation
- Day of presentation (for care) varies with intensity
  1. Milder, more common forms, within 5 to 10 days
  2. Virulent forms (e.g., 37) within 3 to 5 days
- Degree of symptoms varies with intensity and duration
  1. Incubation time varies between 5–12 days
  2. Milder presentations vary from phase to phase
     a. First 8 days: mild to moderate symptoms of non-specific irritation, burning, and photophobia
     b. Second 8 days: moderate to severe burning, photophobia, corneal irritation, and blurring
     c. After 14 to 18 days: blurring may persist or increase slightly while irritation, burning, and photophobia begin to diminish
  3. Virulent forms are highly symptomatic within days
     a. Corneal irritation, photophobia, and epiphora may be severe in 3 to 5 days
     b. Symptoms will increase without therapy

Objective

- Vision varies with time and intensity
  1. Milder forms produce slight fluctuations during the first week from 20/20 to 20/30
  2. Second week (SPK stage) shows moderate reductions to approximately 20/40
  3. After about 16 days, reduction (secondary to SEI stage) can vary from 20/30 to 20/60 or less
  4. In virulent conditions, acuity can fall dramatically at any stage (usually within days rather than weeks) to 20/100 or less
- Most common presentation is unilateral with second eye (70% of patients) usually infected (to lesser degree than primary) by autoinoculation during the first week
- Eyelid(s) usually mild to moderately edematous, depending on virulence of ocular viral reaction
- Early (and persisting) signs typical of viral conjunctivitis
  1. Purplish-pinkish bulbar hyperemia
  2. Starts at inner canthus (in milder forms)
  3. Tearing, serous discharge
  4. Reduced TBUT (with risk of secondary exposure SPK)
  5. Follicular palpebral (inferior) conjunctivitis
  6. Preauricular lymph enlargement or adenopathy
- Bulbar conjunctival reaction varies significantly with virulence of virus
  1. Purplish-pink in mild to moderate forms
  2. Hemorrhagic changes in severe forms (11, 19, 37)
- Pseudomembranes (infiltrative cells combined with mucin and fibrin) form in more virulent presentations (Figures 5.82 and 5.83)

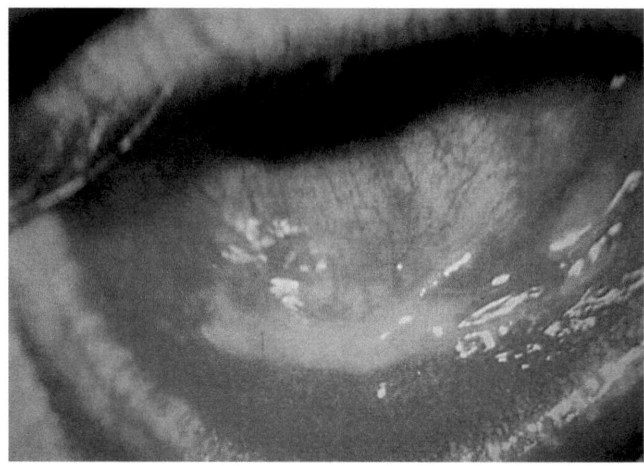

FIGURE 5.82 Pseudomembrane is an accumulation of fibrinous/mucoid material loosely connected by fibrin strands to the underlying true membrane. This moderate accumulation in the inferior cul-de-sac of a viral conjunctivitis was successfully removed by gentle manipulation with a wetted cotton-tip applicator.

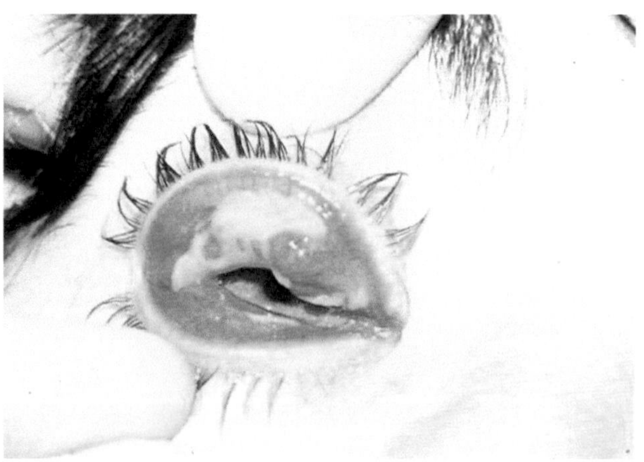

FIGURE 5.83 Severe pseudomembrane formations are found in advanced ocular surface inflammations such as a virulent epidemic keratoconjunctivitis. Removal is usually painful (even with topical anesthetic) and best accomplished by gently peeling off small sections with a jeweler's forceps.

1. Mild forms show film over palpebral conjunctiva
2. Moderate forms produce coagulates (usually inferior cul-de-sac)
3. Severe involvement covers parts or all of the palpebral conjunctiva with dense, opaque, whitish sheets of exudative-like material
4. All forms are adherent by fibrinous adhesions to "true" underlying mucous membranes
5. Can lead to symblepharon formations

- Keratitis usually begins to develop after about 6 to 8 days (1 week) from initial conjunctival hyperemia
  1. Usually diffuse SPK
  2. May vary from fine to coarse punctate spots
  3. Virulent viruses will present a much faster keratitis (sometimes simultaneous with conjunctivitis)
- SEIs usually begin to develop within 14 to 16 days or about 2 weeks
  1. Again, virulent forms will produce keratitic complications much faster than typical syndrome
  2. SEIs are flat accumulations of infiltrative white blood cells (especially lymphocytes) some surrounding edema and inflammatory debris (Figure 5.84)
     a. No proliferating viral cells present in SEIs
     b. This suggests that SEI keratitis may be the postinfectious inflammatory clinical phase of the EKC syndrome
  3. Number from few to "countless" (with increasing virulence; Figure 5.85)
  4. Central localization is most common but may also present peripherally as well
     a. May be central and peripheral
     b. Not usually peripheral only
  5. SEIs do not stain with NaFl
     a. Secondary stain may occur in large, dense spots that disrupt overlying cells
     b. Secondary disruption of epithelial surface may result in a negative (breaking up of) staining pattern or positive staining
  6. Edges of EKC SEIs are usually indistinct
  7. Vary from pale, hazy subepithelial level spots to dense, opaque anterior stromal level leucomas

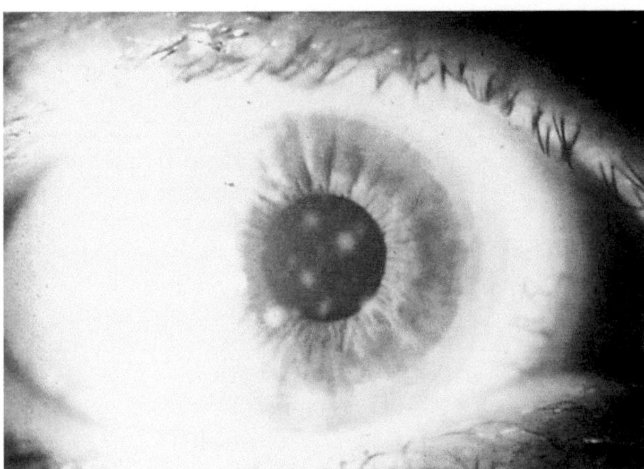

FIGURE 5.84 Subepithelial infiltrates in the central cornea (pupillary zone) appearing large, with ill-defined (edematous) borders.

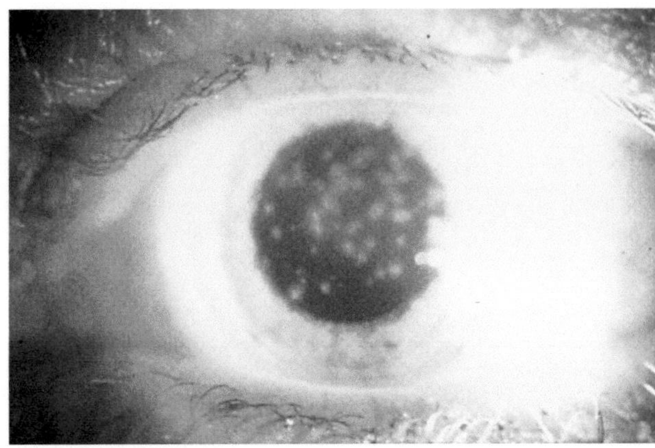

FIGURE 5.85 Dense subepithelial infiltration is the hallmark corneal finding in epidemic keratoconjunctivitis. Amount of infiltration varies considerably (see Figure 5.84) with virulence of the infecting virus and degree of infection.

     a. Subepithelial level SEIs will blanch with or without therapy in weeks to months
     b. Anterior stromal level spots may or may not blanch over weeks to years (if ever), some resulting in translucent to opaque scars from anterior stromal fibrogenic, antigen–antibody reaction to overlying infiltrative subepithelial response
- Depending on virulence of virus and corneal involvement, secondary anterior uveitis will vary from no response to florid reactions

Assessment

(See also Appendix 3)

- EKC can present difficult and misleading diagnostic assessments
  1. Mild forms (or stages) that can be banal in appearance but that are nonetheless highly contagious may be underestimated or neglected
  2. Severe forms that are easily misdiagnosed and often overtreated out of concern for potential damage and progression, are usually self-limiting and in a noncommunicable stage
- Rule out bacterial, atopic, toxic keratites by the subjective and objective "company they keep"
  1. EKC is so common that it may appear in combination with other keratites
  2. As parasitic infection, it may be exacerbated with any form of ocular surface stress (e.g., disease)
- Differentiate EKC from PCF
  1. By age (PCF in 5 to 15 versus EKC in over 15)
  2. EKC has no systemic involvement versus PCF
  3. Rule of 8's usually helpful (despite exceptions)
- Compare course of events by time to other viral conditions (see Table 5.16)
- Rule out SPK of Thygeson
  1. SPK of Thygeson "keeps no viral company"
  2. Usually asymptomatic with white eye
  3. Remits and exacerbates for years
- Rule out herpes simplex (HSV) keratitis
  1. History of recurrences (in adults)
  2. Dendritic ulcer (75% to 80% of time)

TABLE 5.16 Comparison of Forms of Viral Keratoconjunctivitis (by Time)

Time Interval (days)	Non-Specific	PCF	EKC	Herpes Simplex
1–3	Mild	Mild	Moderate	Moderate to severe
4–6	Mild	Moderate	Moderate to severe	Severe (75% dendrite)
7–10[a]	Improving	Moderate (occasional superficial punctate keratitis)	Moderate to severe (with superficial punctate keratitis)	Moderate (with therapeusis)
11–14	Resolved	Improving	Moderate (with supportive therapy)	Improving (with therapeusis)
14–21	Resolved	Resolved	Subepithelial infiltrates	Improving (with therapeusis)
22–28	Resolved	Resolved	Improving	Resolved (with therapeusis)

[a] Return visit during this interval usually confirms diagnosis.

3. Corneal hyposensitivity test
   a. Pronounced corneal hypoesthesia in recurrent HSV epithelial keratitis
   b. Could also be present in severe forms of EKC
- Rule out Epstein–Barr (mononucleosis) virus, which has been reported to mimic EKC
- AdenoPlus (RPS ADP; Rapid Pathogen Screening Inc) an in-office diagnostic tool
  1. Tear sample taken in the office and results provided in 10 minutes
  2. Company sponsored clinical trial data showed very accurate for EKC
  3. However, subsequent independent trials have questioned its accuracy
- Laboratory workup (e.g., serotypes) not usually done due to well-defined clinical picture over a time period usually shorter than that necessary to establish viral titer in the laboratory

Plan: Epidemic Keratoconjunctivitis

(See also Appendix 4)

- All first presentation viral conjunctivitis or keratoconjunctivitis should be treated as suspect EKC
  1. Presume a contagious, communicable infection
  2. Advise patient of contagious nature and instruct
     a. Do not touch or rub eyes
     b. Use separate towels, sheets, pillowcases
     c. If in unavoidable contact situation (e.g., work, school), discontinue activities until confirmed diagnosis or follow-up visit
  3. Advise carefully of possibility of eye and vision "getting worse before it gets better"
     a. Increased likelihood of EKC if initial presentation is "hot"
     b. Increased likelihood if "pink eye" in family or school or workplace (i.e., "it's going around")
- There is no FDA-approved treatment for EKC
- Theoretically, no treatment at all required for EKC
  1. All presentation will be self-limiting (through autoimmune defense mechanism)
  2. However, most EKC produces enough discomfort, inflammation (secondary to immune response), and patient concern that supportive or palliative care is indicated
  3. Moderate to severe forms require therapy for support as well as some protection against secondary tissue changes and potential scarring of SEIs areas from immune response
  4. Certainly all secondary associated reactions (e.g., anterior uveitis) require appropriate therapy
- Pseudomembranes should be removed for patient comfort and more rapid recovery
  1. Mild forms can be brushed off with wetted cotton swabs
  2. Moderate to severe forms can be "peeled off"
     a. Anesthetize area with topical anesthetic (1 gtt every 15 seconds) 4× over pseudomembrane
     b. Peel (from edges) slowly with jeweler's forceps
     c. Petechial hemorrhages (small conjunctival bleeds) may result from fibrin adhesions during removal (don't worry)
     d. Patient will report discomfort during procedure
  3. Irrigate tissues copiously with ophthalmic irrigator after removal
- Supportive or palliative measures
  1. Cold packs (q3–4h)
  2. Topical decongestants or astringents (q3–4h)
  3. Ocular lubricants (mucomimetic agents) q3–4h
  4. Irrigation with ophthalmic irrigator or cold water (q3–4h)
  5. Aspirin or ibuprofen (in lieu of contraindication)
- Use of topical antibiotics is optional but recommended
  1. No proven "prophylactic" value
  2. However, some research supports antibiotic as a "therapeutic" measure against viral spread, penetration, duration, and recurrence
  3. In either case, antibacterial coverage on a compromised corneal surface is always clinically reassuring (better to be safe than sorry!)
- Early antiviral agents (e.g., idoxuridine, vidarabine, trifluridine) are of no value against adenoviruses
  1. However, treatment of early viral conjunctivitis or keratoconjunctivitis (3 to 5 days old) with a relatively toxic antimetabolite is questionable
  2. Topical ganciclovir is a newer antiviral (e.g., herpes simplex, varicella virus, cytomegalovirus, Epstein–Barr)
     a. FDA approved for herpes simplex keratitis
     b. Invitro studies have shown it to be effective against variety of adenovirus
     c. In a small study topical ganciclovir 0.15% (Zirgan) trended better than placebo for EKC signs and symptoms but not statistically significant
- Povidone-iodine irrigation
  1. "Off-label" treatment for EKC
  2. Povidone-iodine 5% (Betadine) is a broad spectrum antibiocide used in ophthalmic surgery

3. The goal is to reduce viral load and reduce shedding
4. In-office process
   a. Use nitrile gloves during this process since patient is highly contagious
   b. Anesthetize ocular surface with 1–2 drops topical anesthetic
   c. Instill 1 drop NSAID
   d. Instill 4–5 drops of Povidone-iodine 5%
   e. Have patient keep eye shut for 1 minutes and roll eyes around to spread solution over ocular surface including lid swabbing
   f. Irrigate eye thoroughly with sterile saline
   g. Instill 1 drop NSAID post-irrigation
5. Advise patients that may have some discomfort (e.g., burning, stinging, irritation) 12–24 hours post-procedure

- The use of topical steroids in EKC is a "delicate" decision
  1. Not indicated in mild forms
  2. Loteprednol as effective as dexamethasone for SEI treatment with less adverse effects
  3. In severe forms there may be no alternative
     a. Reduces inflammation and potential scarring
     b. Makes patient more comfortable
     c. Blanches SEIs and improves vision
     d. Reduces pseudomembranous response
     e. However, as immunosuppressive on a virus
        i. Reduces immune response to virus
        ii. Steroids have been reported to enhance virus with resultant increased risk for rebound and recurrent patterns of SEIs and reinfection
        iii. If HSV dormant in tissue, steroid could aggravate that condition as well
  4. In moderate degree EKC, consider pros and cons of steroid use and base decision on following criteria and judgments (individually or any combination)
     a. If VA falls below 20/40 to 20/60
     b. If SEIs appear dense (anterior stromal) with risk of fibrinogenic scarring
     c. If inflammatory response is severe enough to threaten tissue damage
     d. If significant secondary anterior uveitis develops
     e. If patient discomfort is uncontrollable by other means
- NSAIDs not likely to have antiviral effects
- Cyclosporin A 0.5–2% "off label" results have been inconsistent
  1. May be used as a steroid sparing agent in mild recurring disease or as a method to taper steroid use
- Tacrolimus 0.3% drops or 0.2% ointment "off label" has been shown to be effective against SEIs in small sample size studies
- Finally, always take careful personal (and office) precautions against contagious or infectious patients
  1. Wash hands thoroughly after care with water and alcohol
  2. Clean instruments
     a. Consider postponing tonometry on infectious conditions during acute stages (unless necessary)
     b. All other instruments and equipment can also be contaminated directly or indirectly
     c. Sodium hypochlorite (1:10 bleach dilution) soak (maximum 5 minutes to reduce prism damage) recommended for tonometer tip disinfection if disposable tips are not used
  3. Advise office personnel of necessary precautions

Follow-Up

- Recheck in 7 to 10 days after initial presentation (unless severe or corneal presentation)
- Subsequent recheck should be based on progress or advancement of clinical course
  1. Monitor cornea at least weekly until resolution of SPK phase
  2. Monitor SEIs at least monthly until resolved or stable (anterior stromal scars)
- Release to PRN after thorough education, advice, and instruction of exacerbation
- If patient is a contact lens wearer
  1. Discontinue lens wear during acute phase
  2. Restart lens wear (new lens and new case if reusable lens) (if gas permeable lenses, clean thoroughly and soak in hydrogen peroxide for 1 hour and then rinse thoroughly with sterile saline solution) after negative corneal staining for 5 to 7 days
  3. If condition exacerbates within 1 to 2 weeks after restarting lens wear, discontinue wear, wait for 5 to 7 days, and replace lenses if hydrophilic material
  4. During exacerbation periods (secondary to aggravants or stress factors), discontinue contact lens wear during acute phase and 3 to 5 days post
     a. Re-wear after exacerbations
     b. Always recheck cornea before restarting lens wear

2. Herpes Simplex Virus (HSV)

Background Information

a. Most common virus in humans (only natural host)
b. There is a global incidence of 1.5 million cases and 40,000 of these causing severe vision loss in the United States per year (leading infectious cause of blindness)
c. Two forms of virus: herpes simplex virus type 1 (HSV-1) (oral) and herpes simplex virus type 2 (HSV-2) (genital)
   i. Original theory was 90% of HSV infections "above the waist" were HSV-1 and 90% "below the waist" were HSV-2
   ii. Current statistic uncertain, since dramatic increases in occurrence of HSV-2 (genital herpes)
   iii. Thus, ocular infections can possibly have an HSV-2 (genital) association (check history)
d. Higher incidence with females compared to males
e. Sources of HSV infections
   i. Primary infection
   ii. Recurrent infection (after primary attack)
   iii. Transmission from symptomatic or asymptomatic carrier
f. Transmission is through direct contact
   i. Mostly saliva and mouth contact
   ii. Also contact with active skin lesions (vesicles)
   iii. Incubation period approximately 1 week
g. Most common site of infection is mucocutaneous border of lips
   i. Classic fever blister or cold sore
   ii. Route to trigeminal ganglion and ultimately eye (although far less frequent than mouth)
   iii. Corneal epithelium is frequent site through this route
h. Primary HSV attacks uncommon but dramatic

  i. Mostly in children and young adults
  ii. Usually conjunctivitis with eyelid vesicles
  iii. Older age ranges protected by immunity
- i. Greatest risk for primary infection from 6 months of age to 5 to 10 years of age (as immunity begins to develop)
  i. 70% of children infected by 5 years of age
  ii. 90% of these infections remain subclinical
  iii. 70% immune to HSV by 15 to 25 years of age
  iv. 90% immune to HSV by 60 years of age
- j. Recurrence will occur in 25% of HSV infections
  i. One-third will recur once or more per year
  ii. Two-thirds will recur once or more every 2 years
  iii. Males recur 50% more than females
  iv. Sources of infection, age, race, and so forth, are not considered factors in recurrent potential
  v. Climate may be a factor in that recurrences are more frequent in fall and winter
  vi. Recurrent infection can present ocularly despite non-ocular primary infection
- k. Increasing data suggest that recurrent potential is related to the strain of infecting HSV
  i. Thus, statistics work against recurrent patients
    - Primary HSV attack: 25% risk of recurrence
    - First recurrence: 50% risk of recurrence
    - Second recurrence: 75% risk of recurrence
    - Third recurrence: 100% risk of recurrence
- l. Aggravating or inciting factors for recurrence
  i. Sunlight (UV)
  ii. Trauma (especially localized to ocular area)
  iii. Extreme heat or cold
  iv. Fever
  v. Steroids
  vi. Infectious disease (systemic or ocular)
  vii. Surgery
  viii. Epilation
- m. HSV replicates in corneal epithelium only
  i. However, substantial tissue destruction and inflammatory reaction in the stroma can be produced by the immune response to the virus
  ii. Factors influencing the intensity of the host immune response (stromal infiltration) are unpredictable
    - Genetic factors
    - HLAs
    - Atopias (familial tendencies) such as hay fever, eczema, and asthma
    - Other unknown factors
  iii. To what degree the host response is necessary and beneficial to viral control (in epithelium cells) versus stromal inflammation, infiltration, ulceration, and scarring is unknown
    - Such information is key to steroid considerations in treatment
    - Too little steroid would permit excessive stromal destruction and scarring
    - Too much steroid would permit the epithelial infection to proliferate and trigger a cycle of increasing adverse clinical responses
- n. Fortunately, most HSV ocular disease presents as epithelial keratitis, which is relatively controllable with antiviral or antimetabolite drugs
  i. Usually no deep stromal immune reactions
  ii. Occasionally, anterior stromal reaction (metaherpetica) controllable with adjunctive steroid therapy
  iii. Rarely, virus may show primary clinical response to the stroma (e.g., disciform keratitis) with significant and relatively uncontrollable tissue destruction
- o. In summary, HSV is poorly understood with a highly varied and unpredictable clinical course
  i. May actually be considered a spectrum of five distinct clinical disease entities
    - Primary epithelial (infectious) disease
    - Recurrent epithelial (infectious) disease
    - Metaherpetic (postinfectious inflammatory) disease
    - Stromal (sterile immune) disease
    - Disciform (sterile disease of questionable etiology)
  ii. Primary HSV infection is usually limited to epithelial disease (due to an immature immune system or lack of preexisting circulating antibodies)
  iii. Recurrent HSV infection may occur in any form
  iv. The diagnosis and management of HSV keratitis must include the identification of the form(s) of disease and appropriate management for each form

a. *Primary HSV/Epithelial Keratitis*[67–70]

Subjective

- Usually infants and young children (5 to 15 years of age)
  1. Rare in adults but may be increasing with increasing HSV-2 (genital) infections
  2. Autoinoculation from open genital lesion to eye
- Occasional history of 2-day to 2-week contact with infected host (with or without active lesion)
- Mild to moderate fever or malaise (versus recurrent form with no systemic response)
- Usually, "red eye" is secondary issue (rarely severe) and treated prophylactically with antibiotic drops) by attending pediatrician or primary physician
  1. Mild foreign-body sensation
  2. Mild photophobia
  3. Unilateral
  4. Burning irritation

Objective

- Skin lesions (vesicles or pustules) most prominent clinical feature
  1. Greatest in and around mouth (mucocutaneous border of lips)
  2. Often adjacent to lid margins (single or grouped)
  3. Often buried between lashes
- Lid usually mildly to moderately swollen
- Moderate to severe lymphadenopathy
  1. Preauricular node (ipsilateral)
  2. Frequently dramatic face and neck adenopathy
- Usually moderate follicular conjunctivitis
- In more severe eye involvements
  1. Bulbar conjunctival hemorrhages
  2. Pseudomembranes
  3. Phlyctenules
- Keratitis *always* epithelial (never stromal)
  1. Immature immune system precludes host immune response to stroma
  2. Conversely, immature (absent) immune response produces relative increase in viral infectious activity in epithelial cells

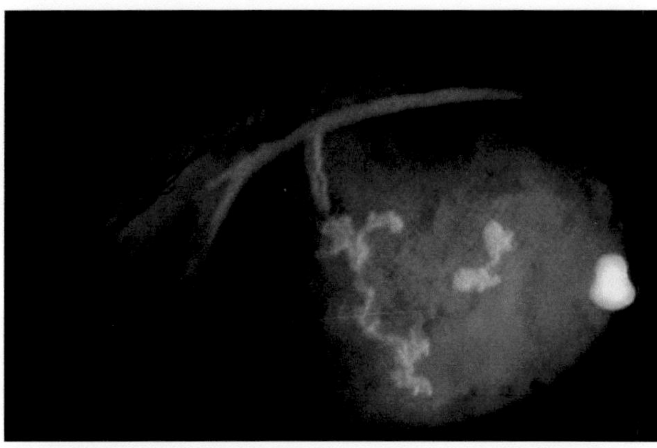

FIGURE 5.86 Herpes simplex epithelial keratitis with prominent ulcerative dendrites and diffuse epitheliopathy with positive and negative sodium fluorescein staining.

- Corneal findings are fairly predictable
  1. Fine to coarse diffuse SPK
     a. Occasionally regional patches
     b. Sometimes greater inferiorly
  2. Dendrites (when present) may be quite large and multiple (Figure 5.86)
     a. Attributable to poor immune protection
     b. Stain with rose bengal
  3. Often multiple subepithelial infiltrates
     a. Central or peripheral
     b. Appear within 1 to 2 weeks, depending on severity of keratitis

Assessment

(See also Appendix 3)

- Rule out bacterial infections
  1. Staphylococcal (papillae versus follicles)
  2. Impetigo (adenopathy too pronounced)
- Rule out pharyngoconjunctival fever (PCF)
  1. Corneal involvement too severe
  2. Skin lesions (to eye or remote)
- Rule out chlamydia (no mucopurulence)
- Rule out epidemic keratoconjunctivitis (EKC)
  1. Wrong age range
  2. No rule of 8's
  3. Systemic involvement (malaise and fever)
- Rule out herpes zoster
  1. Pain not so severe
  2. Vesicles to pustules versus ulcerations
  3. Midline not respected

Plan: Primary HSV/Epithelial Keratitis

(See also Appendix 4)

- Co-manage with pediatrician or patient's primary physician
- Skin lesions should be mildly abraded (washcloth) and treated with Acyclovir ointment
  1. Dosage q4h for 21 days
  2. Alternate therapy: alcohol scrubs tid for 14 to 21 days
- Supportive systemic therapy (e.g., Acyclovir, aspirin, ibuprofen)
- Cycloplegia and dilation if indicated
- Treatment (only with keratitis)
  1. Antiviral drops
     a. Viroptic
        i. 9×/day while ulcer is active
        ii. 5×/day for prophylactic use
        iii. 21-day maximum usage due to epithelial toxicity
     b. Ganciclovir 0.15% (Zirgan)
        i. 5×/day while ulcer is active
        ii. 3×/day for prophylactic use
        iii. Less toxic than Viroptic
     c. "Off label" oral acyclovir (400 mg 5×/day for 7–10 days) or Valacyclovir (500 mg tid for 7–10 days) has been as effective as topical treatment with less toxicity
     d. No additional benefit prescribing both oral and topical drugs, therefore prescribe only one

Follow-Up

- Recheck every 3 days, until cornea is clear
- Recheck every 5 days, until skin lesions resolve
- Be watchful for complications
  1. Bacterial or fungal (rare) superinfection
  2. Secondary preseptal cellulitis
  3. Stromal involvement
     a. Best to get corneal specialist consultation
     b. Avoid steroids
- Advise patient (or parents) on recurrence risks
- Routine rechecks or PRN

b. *Recurrent HSV Keratitis*[71–73]

i. Epithelial Disease

Subjective

- History of previous attacks is most useful diagnostic tool in recurrent HSV infections
- Careful history may reveal primary HSV infection in first recurrent episodes
  1. Previous ocular involvement (mild or severe)
  2. Fever blister or cold sore
  3. Mouth ulcerations
  4. Previous (or active) vesicular skin lesions
     a. Periocular
     b. Mouth or skin
     c. Genital region
- Consider other aggravating stress factors
- Corneal pain and irritation ranges from absent to severe
  1. Usually more severe in initial recurrences
  2. Diminishes with subsequent attacks owing to increasing corneal hypoesthesia
- Variable photophobic response
- Burning irritation
- Vision reduction varies with intensity of keratitis

Objective

- General findings in all epithelial forms
  1. Always unilateral (bilateral very rare)
  2. Follicular conjunctivitis
  3. Moderate to severe bulbar hyperemia
  4. Occasional bulbar conjunctival hemorrhages
  5. Occasional pseudomembranes
  6. Ipsilateral preauricular lymphadenopathy

7. Tearing (serous) discharge
8. Quick TBUT
9. Keratitis
10. Secondary anterior uveitis (relative to intensity of keratitis)

- Dendriform keratitis (75% to 80% frequency; Figure 5.87)
  1. Starts as dense coalescing of focal SPK (Figure 5.88)
  2. Usually fine, linear branching pattern forms with overhanging, pale, flat margins
     a. Usually about 0.1 to 1.0 mm wide
     b. Varies from 1 to 2 mm, up to 10 mm long
  3. Demonstrates classic rounded endings to each linear branch (called "terminal end bulbs")
  4. May be single or multiple lesions
  5. Associated with surrounding SPK
  6. Located centrally or peripherally
     a. Peripheral dendrites are more resistant to treatment
     b. Thicker corneal nerve involved
  7. Stains with rose bengal (variable)
  8. Frequently a mild to moderate stromal edema surrounds dendrite
  9. Reaction usually remains superficial and localized
  10. Corneal hypoesthesia develops and increases with each recurrent attack
  11. True dendritic "ulceration" of epithelium versus infiltrative forms of dendriform keratitis (Table 5.17; Figures 5.89 and 5.90)

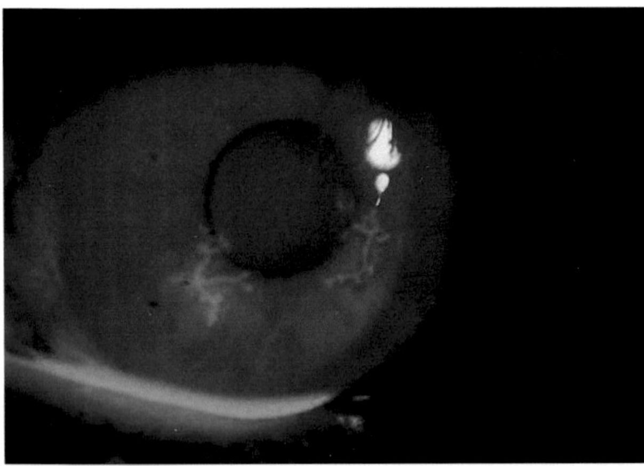

FIGURE 5.87 Herpes simplex ulcerative dendrites (2) stained with sodium fluorescein. Note the obvious terminal end bulbs" on most of the branches of each lesion.

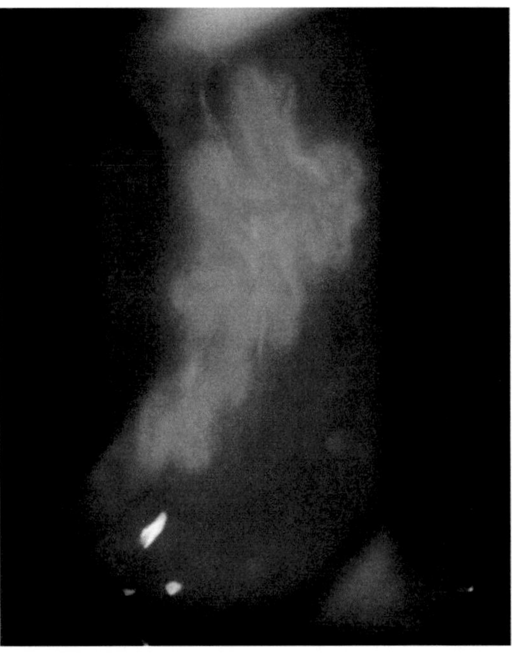

FIGURE 5.89 Sodium fluorescein ulceration test in a herpes simplex dendrite demonstrating geographic or amorphous spreading of the stain into the deeper surrounding epithelium and underlying stroma. Infiltrative dendrites (see Figure 5.90) shed fluorescein stain within minutes resulting in superficial, threadlike, epithelial patterns.

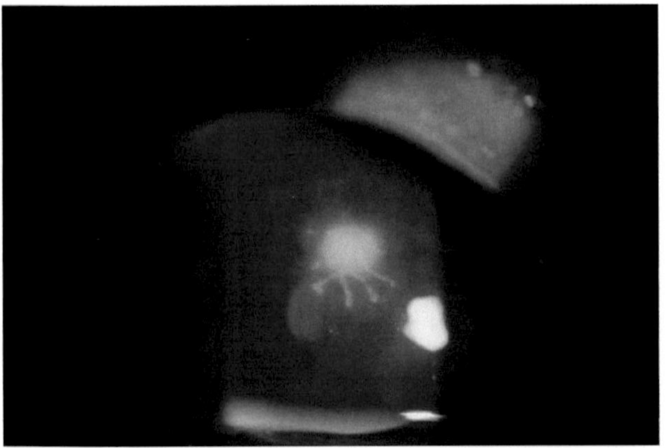

FIGURE 5.88 Proliferating dendrites emanating over 48 hours from a dense, focal patch of sodium fluorescein stain on a cornea. About 15% to 20% of herpes simplex dendrites may present initially as diffuse or focal superficial punctate keratitis (SPK). Corneal sensitivity testing in diagnostic evaluations of SPK can reduce inappropriate steroid use in HSV keratitis.

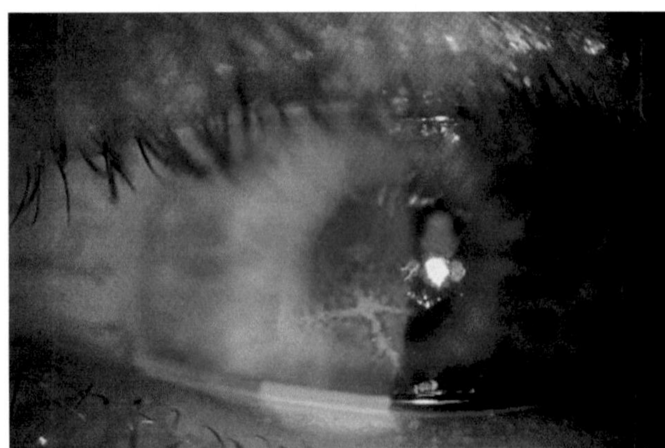

FIGURE 5.90 Infiltrative dendritic keratitis produced during the migratory, trophozoite, epithelial stage of acanthamoeba keratitis. Numerous etiologies are associated with infiltrative dendrites (sometimes referred to as "pseudodendrites"), whereas only herpes simplex virus produces ulcerative dendrites (linear, branching lesions).

Assessment

(See also Appendix 3)

- Differentiate primary versus recurrent HSV by history, age, systemic involvement (in primary HSV)
- Check for corneal sensitivity (decreases with each recurrent attack)
- Rule out bacterial and other possible infectious keratites (cultures, if necessary)
- Rule out other viral keratites
- The presence of a dendrite should always raise suspicion of epithelial HSV keratitis
- However, HSV is the only condition that will produce a true ulcerative dendritic keratitis
- All other forms of dendriform keratitis are infiltrative keratites (see Table 5.17)
  1. Recurrent corneal erosion
  2. Keratitis sicca
  3. SLK of Theodore
  4. SPK of Thygeson
  5. Atopic keratoconjunctivitis
  6. Vernal keratoconjunctivitis
  7. Herpes zoster ophthalmicus
  8. Others
- Under slit-lamp examination
  1. Ulcerative dendrite will be depressed versus infiltrative dendrite being raised
  2. Within 2 to 4 minutes after instillation, NaFl stain undermines ulcerative dendrite versus shedding effect over infiltrative dendrite

Plan: Epithelial HSV Keratitis

(See also Appendix 4)

Primary Care (Table 5.18)

- Some practitioners debride all dendrites
  1. Studies indicated medical therapy equally effective with or without debridement
  2. Occasional risk of spreading virus with debridement procedure
- Treat aggressively with antiviral agents (to reduce risk of metaherpetic phase)
  1. IDU (e.g., Stoxil) and vidarabine ointment (e.g., Vira-A) no longer available
  2. Trifluridine drops (e.g., Viroptic), acyclovir ointment (US "off label"), and ganciclovir gel (e.g., Zirgan) are probably equally effective and are the preferred topical drugs.
     a. Viroptic arrests dendrites in 3 to 5 days
     b. Acyclovir ointment can cause stinging upon instillation and extended blurred vision
     c. Viroptic more toxic than Zirgan and irritates more upon instillation and therefore use should be limited
- Dosages
  1. Viroptic drops
     a. q2h for 48 to 72 hours and patient waking as frequently as possible during night to reinstill drops
     b. Reduce to q3–4h after 3 to 5 days or on dendrite regression
  2. Zirgan gel
     a. Q3h for 48 to 72 hours
     b. Reduce to tid after 3 to 5 days or on dendrite regression
  3. "Off label" oral acyclovir (400 mg 5×/day for 7–10 days) or Valacyclovir (500 mg tid for 7–10 days) has been as effective as topical treatment with less toxicity and are less expensive
  4. Dendrites usually begin to regress to "islands"
  5. Live virus supposedly present if rose bengal staining persists (?)
  6. Continue topical treatment for 14 to 21 days or until rose bengal and NaFl negative, tapering during last week of treatment
- Beware of antiviral toxicity with Viroptic (usually at 5 to 8 days)
  1. Follicles
  2. Chemosis
  3. Fine to coarse SPK
  4. Retarded epithelial (dendritic) healing
- Cycloplege or dilate (standard dosages), if indicated
- Cold packs and ad lib
- Ocular lubricants qid
- Topical antibiotic drops as prophylactic (optional)

Follow-Up

- Secondary care requires close management and ongoing monitoring by the specialty provider
- Primary care should be followed closely
  1. Every 24 to 48 hours during first week
  2. Every 3 to 5 days during second week (resolving)
  3. Weekly for 2 to 3 weeks after resolution
- Contact lens re-wear should be like approach with EKC
- Long-term management includes careful instruction to patient on recurrent nature of condition
  1. Use "red eye" criteria, not corneal pain, as patient's guideline for assessing recurrence

TABLE 5.17 Differential Diagnosis of Herpes Simplex (HSV) Epithelial Dendritic Ulceration from Epithelial Infiltrative Dendrites

HSV Ulcerative Dendrites	Infiltrative Dendrites
Terminal end bulbs	Blunt or tapered endings
Absorbs stain into deep epithelium and anterior stroma	Sheds stain superficially on blinking
Slightly depressed	Slightly raised
Corneal hypoesthesia	Normal corneal sensitivity
Edges stain with rose bengal	Usually NaFl staining only
Generally an appearance of epithelial erosion appearance	Usually minimal epithelial damage or erosion
	Variable per diagnosis
Keeps viral "company"	

TABLE 5.18 Day-by-Day Flowchart for Primary Care Management of Epithelial Herpes Simplex Keratitis

Time Interval	Corneal Findings	Standard Treatment	Possible Complications	Treatment Additions and Adjustments
Day 1–2	1. Hypoesthesia 2. Coarse diffuse SPK 3. Coalescing dendrite(s)	1. Antiviral drops q1–2h (24 hour continuous) or Oral antiviral 2. Antibiotic/cycloplege and dilate qid 3. Ocular lubricant qid 4. Warm packs ad lib 5. Aspirin ad lib	1. Secondary bacterial or fungal infection	1. Culture eye 2. Add antibiotic or antifungal
Day 3–4	1, 2 *plus* 4. Ulcerative dendrite(s)	Continue all steps 1–5	1 *plus* 2. Anterior stromal edema 3. Anterior uveitis	1, 2 *plus* 3. Cycloplege and dilate (increase) No steroids! 4. Increase hot packs
Day 5–6	1, 2, 4 *plus* 5. SPK decreasing 6. Dendrite(s) stable	Continue 2–5 *plus* 6. Oral antiviral or Antiviral drops q3–4h with ointment at hs	1–3 *plus* 4. SPK increasing[a] 5. Dendrite worsening[a]	1–4 *plus* 5. Change antiviral agent
Day 7–10	1, 5 *plus* 7. Dendrite resolving	Continue 2–6	1–5 *plus* 6. Deep stromal edema	1–4 *plus* 6. Recheck every 24 hours
Day 11–14	1 *plus* 8. Negative rose bengal	Continue 3 and 4 *plus* 7. antibiotic bid 8. Antiviral qid 9. Patient counseling re: HSV	1–6 *plus* 7. Stromal infiltration 8. Metaherpetic ulceration	7. Add topical steroid (lid) 8. Consider ophthalmological consult
Day 15–21	1 *plus* 9. Cornea negative	10. D/C antibiotic 11. Antiviral tid	1, 3–8 *plus* 9. Neovascularization	9. Consult with ophthalmologist or corneal specialist
Day 22–28	1 *plus* 10. Cornea remains negative	12. D/C antivirals 13. Schedule weekly for weeks 5 and 6	1, 3–9 *plus* 10. Stromal keratitis	10. Refer to corneal specialist
Week 5–6	1 and 10	14. Recheck PRN or 6 months	Recurrence(s)	11. Dig in!

[a] Probable drug toxicity.
Abbreviations: SPK, superfical punctate keratitis: HSV, herpes simplex virus; D/C, discontinue.

2. Corneal pain will decrease (sometimes to zero) with subsequent recurrent attacks and possibly be neglected by patient
3. Acyclovir (400 mg bid) and valacyclovir (500 mg qd) have been shown to reduce the rate of recurrent disease

- Recheck every 6 months for 1 year and then annually or PRN

ii. *Metaherpetic Disease*

Subjective

- Always a history of epithelial HSV disease
- May be active dendritiform epithelial involvement or inactive recurrent disease

Objective

Metapherpetic (trophic) keratopathy (less common; Figure 5.91)

1. Chronic "sterile" indolent ulceration secondary to epithelial (dendriform) keratitis
   a. Probably caused by damage to basement membrane and possibly live virus or viral toxins "embedding" in membrane
   b. Antigen–antibody (immune) response to live virus (or toxins) produces sterile, indolent ulcerative process and anterior stromal damage

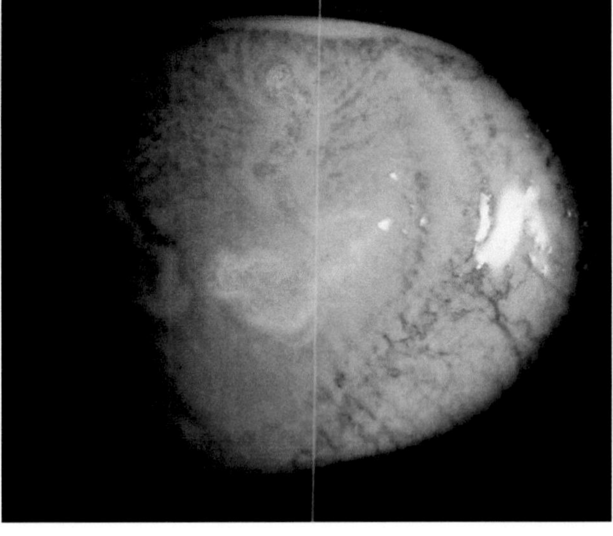

FIGURE 5.91 Metaherpetic disease stems from untreated epithelial herpes simplex keratitis, which can lead to toxic (or herpetic viral?) invasion of the epithelial basement membrane as quickly as 14 to 21 days. Disease results in trophic or indolent epithelial ulceration (poor adhesion of cells to basement membrane) and potential immune response and scarring of the anterior stroma.

   c. Resultant clinical condition is considered a postinfectious inflammatory response (noninfectious)
2. Epithelial ulcer shape is usually oval, ameboid, or geographic (amorphous shape)
3. Edges are distinctly raised, thickened, gray borders appearing rolled or heaped
4. Size of ulcer varies from 2 to 8 mm
5. Frequently vertically oriented in longer axis
6. Stains brilliantly with rose bengal
7. Produce moderate to dramatic anterior stromal response (infiltration and edema)
   a. Usually beneath and more diffuse than overlying dendrites(s)
   b. If persistent (i.e., viral toxins "embedded" for 6- to 8-week life of basement membrane), could produce collagenolytic scarring and corneal melting (postinfectious inflammation)
8. Chronic nature may produce neovascularization

Assessment

- Differentiated from dendritic form by
  1. Shape and edges
  2. Diffuse and deeper stromal response
  3. Persistence in lieu of antiviral therapy
- Differentiated from stromal forms by
  1. Persistent NaFl and rose bengal staining (Figure 5.92)
  2. Chronic epithelial involvement

Plan: Metaherpetic HSV Keratitis

- Consider care by most appropriate practitioner
- Treatment should include (but not necessarily be limited to) any or all of the following

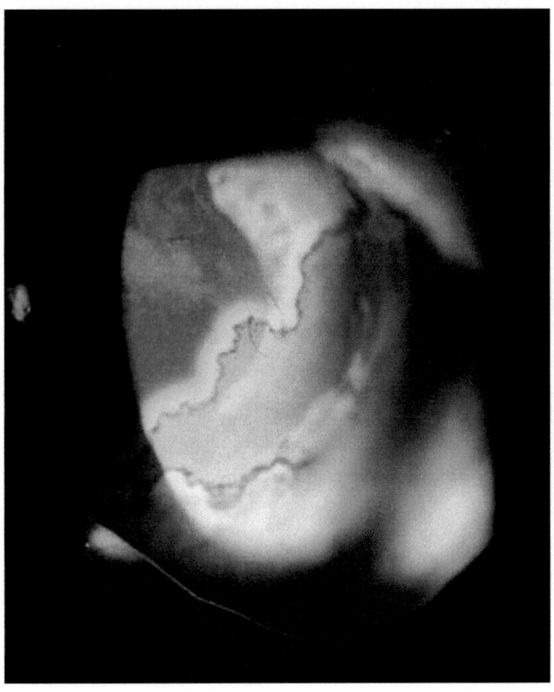

FIGURE 5.92 Rose bengal stain in metaherpes presents a vivid diagnostic picture as it stains the exposed, toxic/infected (?) epithelial basement membrane.

  1. Debridement (repeated as indicated)
  2. All primary care steps described for epithelial HSV disease
  3. Different class(es) of antiviral drugs (topical and oral) at full strength for full cycles and recycles
  4. Topical steroids (along with antivirals)
  5. Bandage soft contact lenses
  6. Intermittent pressure patching
  7. Heavy lubrication therapy
  8. Acetylcysteine (Mucomyst) for corneal melting
  9. Cyanoacrylate glues
  10. Surgery (as a last resort)
      a. Conjunctival flap
      b. Keratoplasty (guarded-to-poor prognosis)

Follow-Up

- Secondary care requires close management and ongoing monitoring
- Primary care should be followed closely
  1. Every 24 to 48 hours during first week
  2. Every 3 to 5 days during second week (resolving)
  3. Weekly for 2 to 3 weeks after resolution
- Contact lens re-wear should be similar to approach with EKC
- Long-term management includes careful instruction to patient on recurrent nature of condition
  1. Use "red eye" criteria, not corneal pain, as patient's guideline for assessing recurrence
  2. Corneal pain will decrease (sometimes to zero) with subsequent recurrent attacks and possibly be neglected by patient
- Recheck every 6 months for 1 year and then annually or PRN

iii. *Stromal HSV Keratitis*

Subjective

- History is usually quite apparent regarding recurrent epithelial or stromal keratitis
  1. Recurrent epithelial HSV keratitis almost always associated with stromal (interstitial) form
  2. Disciform usually has no epithelial history
- Pain may vary from epithelial types
  1. Frequently corneal pain may be absent or minimal (owing to corneal hypoesthesia from multiple recurrences)
  2. Usually deep, throbbing (headache) pain caused by secondary keratouveitis
- Vision is almost always substantially reduced
  1. Loss is insidious in stromal forms
  2. Subacute loss in disciform type
- Clinical presentation usually insidious versus acute onset in epithelial responses
  1. Acute or subacute epithelial response may occur after stromal presentation
  2. In disciform, epithelial response rarely follows stromal involvement

Objective

- Intensity varies widely (Figure 5.93)
- Stromal infiltration with mild to moderate edema
  1. Deep to full-thickness infiltrates
  2. Infiltration substantially exceeds edema
- Neovascularization (usually deep stromal)

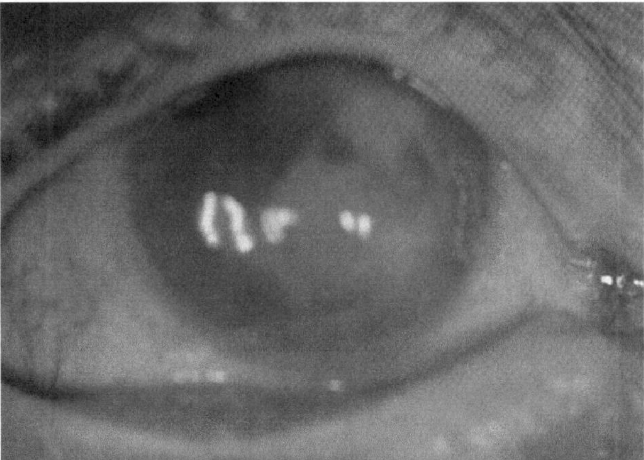

FIGURE 5.93 Stromal herpes simplex disease is a destructive, sterile immune response to herpes simplex virus, active in the corneal epithelium or even dormant in the ciliary ganglion or nerves. As a sterile infiltrative keratitis (no active virus in the stroma), steroids are valuable in reducing an often irreversible proteolysis (stromal melting) and corneal neovascularization.

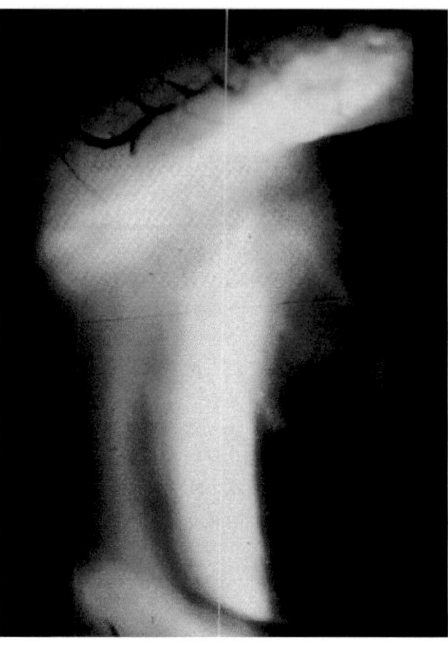

FIGURE 5.94 Immune (Wessely) ring in the superior temporal anterior corneal stroma. This ring suggests a toxic etiology produced by an antigen–antibody reaction to a toxin penetrating into the stromal matrix.

   1. Vessels may reveal active (whole blood) flow
   2. Vessels may be empty and gray in appearance ("ghost vessels")
- Patchy infiltrative response resulting in permanent scarring
- Ulcerative necrosis can develop as creamy homogeneous stromal breakdown (to abscess)
   1. Produces localized (or diffuse) areas of stromal thinning
   2. Could lead to corneal "melting"
- Wessely rings (antigen–antibody reactions) in anterior stroma are frequently seen (partial or complete infiltrative annular rings; Figure 5.94)
- Edema usually causes ground-glass appearance and corneal thickening
- Corneal endothelium is usually involved
   1. Keratic precipitates (infiltrative and pigment debris)
   2. Guttata
   3. Fibrin plaques
- Epithelial edema (diffuse and bullous) is probably a product of endothelial disruption
- Keratouveitis is always present (secondary response)
   1. Associated trabeculitis (with IOP increase) in severe cases
   2. Red blood cells (microhyphema) may be seen among cells and flare in chamber
- Descemetocele formations occur in advanced cases

Assessment

(See also Appendix 3)

- Most deep (interstitial) keratitis in non-syphilitic patients is presumed HSV stromal keratitis
   1. Thus, fluorescent treponemal antibody absorption test (FTA-ABS) in inactive cases
      a. Indicates active versus inactive syphilitic infection
      b. Also, positive for congenital or acquired forms
   2. FTA-ABS plus venereal disease research laboratory (VDRL) test in active cases
      a. VDRL indicates only active process
      b. This would confirm syphilitic involvement versus possible false-positive FTA-ABS taken alone
- Differentials beyond syphilis for stromal HSV keratitis are limited and quickly ruled out by epithelial involvement or history
   1. Rule out herpes zoster
   2. Systemic disease associations
   3. Bacterial causes
- Rule out stromal corneal dystrophies
   1. Classic triad of interstitial keratitis (infiltration, neovascularization, and thinning) is not present in dystrophy

Plan and Follow-Up: Stromal HSV Keratitis

(See also Appendices 4 and 6)

- Recurrent nature, guaranteed scarring (with resultant cosmetic effect and functional loss), and need for extensive, ongoing steroid therapy, with attendant epithelial risks, indicates need for appropriate corneal (specialist) care (Table 5.19)
   1. Secondary ophthalmological care
   2. Tertiary corneal specialist care
- Specialty care will probably include (but not be limited to) any or all the following steps
   1. Topical steroids during active infiltrative periods without ulceration with concomitant oral antiviral agents to reduce or control epithelial infection
      a. May need 10+ weeks of treatment including steroid taper based on patient progress
   2. Cycloplegia-dilation when indicated

TABLE 5.19 **Clinical Signs and Levels of Care in Herpes Simplex Keratitis**

Degree	Primary HSV Infection	Recurrent HSV Ocular Infections				
		Epithelial	Metaherpetic	Stromal	Disciform	Complications
Mild	Fever Dermatoses Lid swelling Viral conjunctivitis SPK SEI	Dermatoses Viral conjunctivitis Lymphadenopathy SPK	Dermatoses SPK	Dermatoses Dendrites SPK	Dermatoses Dendrites SPK	Drug toxicity Secondary cataract Secondary dermatoses, infections Bacterial Fungal
Moderate	Malaise Lymphadenopathy Phlyctenules Conjunctival hemorrhages Pseudomembranes Dendrites	Conjunctival hemorrhages Pseudomembranes Dendrites Anterior stromal edema Anterior uveitis	Nonresponsive dendrite(s) Stromal edema Stromal scarring	Epithelial edema Endothelial guttata Keratic precipitates Immune (Wessely) ring	Granular infiltrates Keratic precipitates Immune (Wessely) ring Central edematous stromal disk Descemet's folds	Keratouveitis Trabeculitis Vasculitis Secondary glaucoma
Severe	Systemic reactions	Stromal infiltration Neovascularization	Indolent ulcer Stromal infiltration Neovascularization Stromal melting	Deep infiltration Endothelial plaques Neovascularization Necrosis or abscess Corneal melting	Dense edematous stromal disc Neovascularization Corneal melting	Super infection Bacterial Fungal Hypopyon Descemetocele Corneal melting Perforation

Note: No shading indicates primary care, light shading indicates opthalmological care, and dark shading indicates corneal specialist.
Abbreviations: HSV, herpes simplex virus; SPK, superficial punctate keratitis; SEI, subepithelial infiltrates.

3. Prophylactic antibiotics
4. Oral acyclovir or valacyclovir may be of value in reducing recurrences
5. Penetrating keratoplasty when indicated
   a. Should be withheld for case of corneal melting and perforation risks
   b. Should not be considered strictly for cosmetic or functional reasons
   c. Guarded to poor prognosis with interstitial forms, especially with neovascularization moving centralward
   d. Oral antiviral agents used post-op have reduced corneal graft failure

- Ongoing management should be co-managed with specialist due to likelihood of recurrences
- Prognosis
  1. Generally poor
  2. Highly unpredictable, often unremitting, and invariably destructive

iv. *HSV Endothelial (Disciform) Keratitis*

Subjective

- Usually no history of epithelial HSV, but may manifest epithelial findings (e.g., SPK, dendrite)
- Stromal (interstitial) disease occasionally associated (active or inactive)
- Usually no pain with patient presenting for visual reasons or possible red eye concerns

Objective

- Frequently presents with no history or presence of epithelial keratitis (Figure 5.95)
- Usually centrally located, dense edematous (not infiltrative as in interstitial type) stromal disc
  1. Etiology of edema (versus infiltrates) is uncertain
  2. Reaction is known to be a type IV (delayed hypersensitivity) response
- Presents with a uniformly rounded disc-shaped stromal involvement with well defined borders (versus diffuse stromal, interstitial type)
- Disc may have a Wessely ring around it (see Figure 5.94)
- Fine granular infiltrates are occasionally scattered elsewhere in stroma
- Folds in Descemet's membrane are usually apparent
- Moderate keratouveitis and keratic precipitates usually present

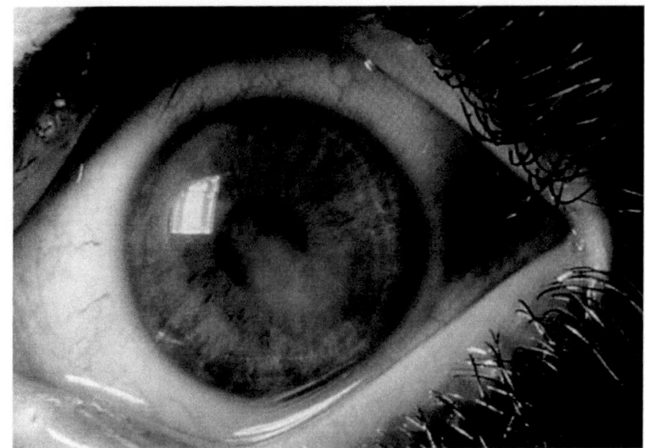

FIGURE 5.95 Disciform herpes simplex keratitis is caused by the development of a sterile, edematous, mid to deep stromal lesion of a disciform (disc-shaped) nature. Etiology is poorly understood, and treatment varies from monitoring to antiedema therapies, from conservative (hot packs and hypertonics) to aggressive (steroids and immunosuppressives) approaches.

- No necrosis or neovascularization (as in interstitial, stromal form)
- Secondary epithelial response may occur in cases with advanced endothelial changes

Assessment

HSV endothelial (disciform) keratitis is almost exclusively considered herpetic (with or without epithelial involvement)
1. Rule out herpes zoster
2. Systemic causes
3. Bacterial causes (ulcer)

Plan and Follow-Up: HSV Endothelial (Disciform) Keratitis

- Recurrent nature, guaranteed scarring (with resultant cosmetic effect and functional loss) and need for extensive, ongoing steroid therapy, with attendant epithelial risks, indicates need for appropriate corneal (specialist) care (see Table 5.19)
  1. Secondary ophthalmological care
  2. Tertiary corneal specialist care
- Specialty care will probably include (but not be limited to) any or all the following steps
  1. Topical steroids during active periods with concomitant oral antiviral agents
  2. Cycloplegia-dilation when indicated
  3. Heat to reduce edematous disc
  4. Penetrating keratoplasty when indicated
     a. Should be withheld for case of corneal melting and perforation risks
     b. Should not be considered strictly for cosmetic or functional reasons
     c. Oral antiviral agents used post-op have reduced corneal graft failure
- Ongoing management should be co-managed with specialist due to likelihood of recurrences
- Prognosis
  1. Guarded to poor
  2. Highly unpredictable, often unremitting, and invariably destructive

3. *Herpes Zoster Ophthalmicus (HZO)*[74–78]

Background Information

a. Varicella-type virus infecting dorsal root ganglion
   i. Virus called chickenpox in children
   ii. Virus called shingles in adults
b. Estimated 1 in 3 adults in United States will develop shingles (herpes zoster) in their lifetime
c. 8–20% of shingle patients will develop HZO
d. Shingle's incidence is increasing probably due to aging population with inherent immune senescence and immunosuppression by medications or diseases (e.g., AIDS)
e. Two possible means of contagious spread
   i. Reactivation of latent virus (in ganglion)
   ii. Contact with (externally) infected host
f. Usually effects first division of trigeminal (fifth) cranial nerve
   i. Most often attacks frontal branch of ophthalmic nerve
   ii. Can attack nasal branch of ophthalmic nerve or (less commonly) maxillary or mandibular branch of trigeminal
   iii. Nasal branch gives off nasociliar branch to eye and tip of nose
   iv. Vesicle on tip of nose (Hutchinson's sign) indicates nasociliary involvement and thus, higher risk of ocular involvement (HZV ophthalmicus)
g. Ocular involvement is highly variable and can mimic almost any anterior segment disease
   i. Must differentiate by history, subjective pain, and accompanying lid signs
   ii. Must be especially careful in differentiating HSV

Subjective

- Usually a 2-week incubation period after contact with an infected source
- Distinctive history of severe pain associated with classic lid signs
- Patient may report history of associated systemic signs
  1. Headache
  2. Malaise
  3. Fever
  4. Chills
- Pain usually severe because of associated neuralgia, which is usually dramatic in the primary attack and remits and exacerbates chronically with or without recurrent objective signs
- Some systemic diseases may leave patient vulnerable to (opportunistic) secondary herpes zoster infection
  1. Occasionally such secondary clinical manifestations may give altered subjective and/or objective presentations from classic primary signs and symptoms
     a. Mild to no pain
     b. No objective signs with severe pain
  2. Notorious disease categories for such variable presentations of zoster include cancers (particularly lymphomas) and AIDS

Objective

- Lid signs are usually prodrome to ocular involvement
  1. With vesicle at tip of nose (Hutchinson's sign), about a 75% risk of ocular involvement
  2. Without vesicle, risk approximately 25%
- All ocular signs are non-specific and mimic many other external ocular diseases
- Usually follicular conjunctivitis presents earliest
  1. Lymphadenopathy varies from mild to severe
  2. Pseudomembranes (and true membranes) common in severe involvements
- Scleritis can develop and advance to "melting" stage
- Keratitis highly variable
  1. Diffuse SPK usually occurs early and may persist for months to years
  2. Chronic epithelial (trophic type) ulcerations are common and create substantial risk of secondary infection
  3. Dendriform keratitis mimics HSV epithelial keratitis
     a. Dendrite is infiltrative versus ulcerative
     b. Dendrite has tapered endings versus "terminal end bulbs"
     c. Only HSV dendrites are ulcerative with terminal end bulbs
  4. Corneal hypoesthesia may occur (mimicking HSV) producing reduced subjective corneal irritation
  5. Interstitial stromal keratitis

   a. Infiltration (anterior to full thickness)
   b. Neovascularization
   c. Thinning (with risk of stromal "melting")
- Anterior uveitis almost certain with keratitis
- Hyphema occasionally associated with uveitis
- Sympathetic ophthalmia possible
- Posterior segment involvement (e.g., chorioretinitis) occasionally associated with progressive, unremitting forms
- Congestive glaucoma (trabeculitis) frequently part of advanced anterior segment involvements

Assessment

(See also Appendix 3)

- Because of the highly variable presentations of HZO and its tendency to mimic almost any anterior segment disease, technically every anterior segment disorder must be ruled out
  1. A formidable task, except for classic HZO presentation
  2. HZV produces a definitive pattern of severe pain associated with distinctly unilateral (dramatic midline "respect") lid involvement
- Carefully rule out HSV keratitis, which is mimicked more than any other corneal involvement
  1. Pain, lid signs, and infiltrative dendrite usually most helpful differentials
  2. Beware of a secondary (overlying) HSV infection
- HZV involvement is often associated with systemic immunosuppressive diseases and cancers
  1. Evaluate history and risk factors carefully
  2. Medical workup may be useful with risk factors
  3. Subjective and/or objective presentations may vary from classic patterns

Plan: Herpes Zoster Ophthalmicus

(See also Appendix 6)

- Medical, dermatological, and ophthalmic specialists (depending on severity) are indicated with HZV
- Treatment ranges from supportive therapies to tertiary procedures based on severity of condition
- Supportive therapies
  1. Warm or cold packs
  2. Domeboro packs
  3. Alcohol therapy (on skin for mild involvements to "oral" for pain relief to retrobulbar injection for severe cases)
- Topical prophylactic (and therapeutic) antibiotics
- Topical Zirgan has been used off-label for dendritic infiltrative keratitis
- Topical steroids (with advancing corneal involvement)
  1. Do not use too early, but don't consider steroids contraindicated for epithelial varicella infection (versus HSV epithelial infection)
  2. If steroid used, continually reevaluate HSV risk
- Cycloplegia-dilation based on uveitic reactions
- Oral antiviral agents have a dramatic positive effect on HZV course both objectively and for pain relief when used in first 3 to 5 days for immunocompetent patients
  1. Acyclovir (Zovirax) 800 mg 5×/day for 7–10 days or
  2. Valacyclovir (Valtrex) 1000 mg tid for 7–10 days or
  3. Famciclovir (Famvir) 500 mg tid for 7–10 days
  4. Can be used with other oral medications as well
     a. Oral steroids
     b. NSAIDs
     c. Narcotic analgesics
- Nonsteroidal anti-inflammatories useful for pain relief (aspirin or ibuprofen)
- Oral steroids (from 30 to 60 mg with taper) useful in more advanced cases (should be administered with physician's co-management)
- Narcotic pain control often indicated
- Oral immunosuppressive (anticancer) medications used both experimentally and clinically in severe cases
- Corneal melting and perforation risks treated nonsurgically whenever possible
  1. Bandage soft contact lenses
  2. Cyanoacrylate adhesives

Follow-Up

- HZV is notorious for its persistence and recurrence
  1. Destructive nature accentuated with each attack
  2. Pain is often unrelenting with and without clinical activity (post-herpetic neuralgia)
  3. Postherpetic neuralgia (PHN) (persistent pain lasting more than 90 days after onset) can be reduced or eliminated with early (within 3 days of onset) oral antiviral intervention at first presentations and even recurrent attacks in some cases
     a. PHN is worse when acute pain is severe, patient is older, and ophthalmic involvement
- Long-term complications
  1. Corneal scarring
  2. Glaucoma
  3. Cataracts
  4. PHN
- Risk of permanent corneal damage (i.e., scarring) is directly proportional to severity of condition, overall ocular signs, and stromal involvement
- HZV presents a poor postoperative (keratoplasty) surgical risk (e.g., chronic inflammation, graft rejection)
  1. Preferable to postoperative complications, often a neovascular and pannus overgrowth is allowed to develop
  2. Alternative would be conjunctival flap
- Advise patient carefully on all aspects of disease
  1. Recurrent, chronic nature
  2. Postherpetic neuralgia
  3. Permanent scarring risks
  4. Highly variable, ongoing ocular complications
- Recheck eye every 6 months or PRN
- In 2018 FDA approved an inactivated (non-live) recombinant vaccine (Shingrix) intramuscular injection in 2-shot series 2–6 months apart
  1. Recommended for immunocompetent patients >50 years old
  2. 97% effective to prevent shingles for 50–70 year olds and 90% effective for >70 years
  3. 91% effective to prevent postherpetic neuralgia for 50–70 year olds and 89% effective for >70 years
  4. Can be done even with prior shingle outbreaks

4. Non-Specific Adenoviral Keratoconjunctivitis

Subjective

- Extremely common in children and adults
- Mostly unilateral, but may show contralateral autoinoculation

- Patient rarely presents for care because of mild, usually subclinical, symptoms (e.g., mild burning or non-specific irritation at inner canthal region)
- Duration of mild acute phase is short (3 to 5 days)

Objective

- Mild, diffuse, or regional (may be greater nasalward) superficial, bulbar pinkish injection
- Mild to moderate follicular response on inferior palpebral conjunctiva
- Eye(s) may show mild to moderate amount of hyperlacrimation
- Vision is not affected
- Corneal epithelium usually remains negative
  1. Occasionally, a fine diffuse SPK
  2. Most often only a few scattered punctata
- No preauricular lymph node enlargement or adenopathy

Assessment

(See also Appendix 3)

- Rule out other forms of conjunctivitis and keratoconjunctivitis
  1. Bacterial (meaty red and mucopurulent)
  2. Allergic (itching and edema)
  3. Toxic or hypersensitive (chronic versus acute)
  4. Others (by "the company they keep")
- Compare course of events (by time) to other more specific forms of viral keratoconjunctivitis (see Table 5.16)

Plan: Non-Specific Adenoviral Keratoconjunctivitis

(See also Appendix 4)

- Usually not treated because patient never presents
- Reassure and treat supportively
  1. Cold packs bid or tid (optional)
  2. Cold water irrigation (ad lib)
  3. Lubricating drops qid

Follow-Up

- For children, instruct parent or caretaker on dormant viral nature
  1. Recurrences should be monitored
  2. Non-specific adenoviral infection can be early reservoir for subsequent EKC virus
- Return checks not indicated, unless patient requests

5. *Pharyngoconjunctival Fever (PCF)*[79,80]

Subjective

- Pharyngoconjunctival fever (PCF) is a viral syndrome associated with adenovirus 3
  1. Also associated (to lesser degree) with other adenoviral strains
  2. Occasionally adenovirus 4 and 7
- Only ocular surface involvement with a distinct, relatively predictable systemic association
  1. Almost always a recent history of an upper respiratory condition (pharyngitis)
     a. Sore throat
     b. Congestion (throat or chest)
     c. Cough
  2. Low- to moderate-grade fever (usually 99 to 101 °F)
- Most common in children 5 to 15 years of age (±3 years)
- Occasionally referred to as Beal's conjunctivitis
- Frequently called "pink eye" by patients and nurses
- May present with a recent exposure to swimming pool (or hot tubs)
  1. Called "swimming pool" conjunctivitis
  2. Adenovirus transmitted through fecal material in poorly chlorinated water
- Although most common in children, if syndrome fits (e.g., pharyngitis, fever, history of hot tub), adults should also be considered candidates

Objective

- Similar to viral conjunctivitis forms
- Usually mild to moderate viral signs
  1. Purplish-pinkish bulbar hyperemia
  2. Starts at inner canthus and spreads
  3. Tearing (serous) discharge
  4. Quick TBUT (which can lead to secondary staining)
  5. Follicular palpebral changes
  6. Preauricular lymph enlargement or lymphadenopathy
- Corneal involvement is usually mild (sometimes absent)
  1. Fine, diffuse SPK or scattered punctata
  2. Rarely, a few, small subepithelial infiltrates

Assessment

(See also Appendix 3)

- Rule out other forms of conjunctivitis and keratoconjunctivitis
  1. Bacterial (meaty red and mucopurulent)
  2. Allergic (itching and edema)
  3. Toxic or hypersensitive (chronic versus acute)
  4. Others (by "the company they keep")
- Compare course of events (by time) with other more specific viral keratoconjunctivites (see Table 5.16)
- Three helpful considerations in differentiating PCF from other viral keratoconjunctivites
  1. Ages 5 to 15
  2. It is a systemic syndrome (i.e., pharyngitis, fever)
  3. A swimming pool or a hot tub history (also in EKC)
- Do corneal hyposensitivity ("cotton wisp") test to differentiate from recurrent herpes simplex keratitis
  1. Make cotton wisp from cotton ball or swab
  2. Firmly brush wisp over unaffected cornea and define response to patient as a 10 on a 1–10 scale
  3. Then brush affected cornea (using same pressure and region), and ask patient to quantify sensation on a 1–10 scale
  4. Response of 5 or less indicates corneal hypoesthesia (i.e., reduced corneal sensitivity), which is suggestive of recurrent herpes simplex keratitis
- Laboratory workup (e.g., serotyping) is not usually done in primary clinical setting due to relative obvious clinical presentation and delay (up to 2 weeks for final viral titers) in results

Plan: Pharyngoconjunctival Fever

(See also Appendix 4)

- Advise patient of viral diagnosis
- Explain non-curable nature of virus
  1. Benign course with no permanent damage
  2. Self-timing course (usually about 10 to 14 days)

3. No curative therapy, only supportive and palliative measures
4. Possibility of contagious nature (EKC)
   a. Always assume the worst (EKC) until time and physical findings prove otherwise
   b. Instruct carefully not to rub or touch, to use of personal towels and sheets, and so forth

- Advise patient that "this may get worse before it gets better!" (i.e., possibility of EKC)
- Supportive, palliative measures
  1. Cold (for symptom relief) packs
  2. Ocular lubricants
  3. Irrigation (ophthalmic solutions or cold water)
  4. Decongestants or astringents (optional)
  5. If systemic signs and symptoms still present, therapy for pharyngitis and fever (per physician)

Follow-Up

- Recheck in 7 to 10 days after report of first symptoms
  1. Reducing signs and symptoms indicates no EKC
  2. Increasing clinical course suggests EKC
- If cornea involved, recheck 10 to 14 days after confirmation (at first recheck visit) of non-EKC conditions
- Advise patient of dormant, obligate, parasitic nature of adenovirus (lies dormant in tissue) and recurrent potential with various stress factors
- Routine follow-up or PRN

D. Miscellaneous Keratitis

1. Acne (Ocular) Rosacea[81–84]

Background Information

a. Syndrome of unknown etiology involving the skin and eyes (ocular rosacea)
b. Approximately 60–70% of rosacea patients will have ocular signs and symptoms
c. Very common anterior segment disease, frequently misdiagnosed or undiagnosed
   i. Misdiagnosed because findings treated as separate entities rather than as part of a syndrome (defined as a predictable collection of clinical entities)
      - 57% of patients with excised chalazia were found to have acne rosacea
      - 20% of patients develop ocular signs first
      - 53% develop skin lesions first
      - 27% develop eye and skin signs simultaneously
   ii. Eye signs need not be proportional to skin manifestations and vice versa (either may predominate)
d. Often mimics (and is misdiagnosed as) staphylococcal blepharitis and blepharoconjunctivitis
   i. Frequently associated with overlying staphylococcal involvement
   ii. Additional signs (i.e., syndrome) become diagnostic
e. Etiology unknown, but many theories
   i. Bacterial (especially Staphylococcus)
   ii. Climatic exposure (e.g., sun, wind, heat, cold)
   iii. Psychosomatic (anxiety, depression, neurosis)
   iv. Gastrointestinal disorder (dietary)
   v. Disorder of vasodilation (vasomotor disturbance)
   vi. Sebaceous gland abnormalities (hypertrophy, stagnation)
   vii. *Demodex folliculorum*

Subjective

- Usually no previous family or personal history of full syndrome (combined eye and skin involvement)
- Greatest frequency in 30- to 60-year age range, but may also be found in children
  1. Early skin signs most common in females
  2. Overall syndrome slightly greater in females
- Most common in patients with fair complexions
- Appears to be more frequent in Scot–Irish descendants and in those of northern European origin
  1. But can be found in all patients
  2. Being reported with increased frequency in Black patients (previously believed rare)
- Histories of recurrent lid manifestations ("styes" or recurrent chalazia and hordeoli, chronic marginal blepharitis, especially resistant to standard therapy)
- Symptoms are usually synonymous with level of involvement and associated complications
  1. Blepharitis stage may produce only cosmetic concerns
  2. Conjunctival stage usually produces burning and non-specific irritation (typical of conjunctivitis)
  3. Keratitis produces classic corneal symptomatology
- Suspicion and ultimate diagnosis are possible only with careful history and uncovering of active or inactive combination of classic eye and skin signs

Objective

- Mild to moderate ocular (or skin) manifestations are far more common than severe involvements
  1. Chronic blepharitis: mild and most common ocular manifestation
  2. Blepharoconjunctivitis: moderate manifestation
  3. Blepharokeratoconjunctivitis: moderate to severe
  4. Lids are always involved, either alone, with conjunctiva, or with conjunctiva and cornea
- Specific ocular manifestations (in approximate increasing order of occurrence)
  1. Chronic marginal blepharitis (mimicking Staphylococcus)
  2. Telangiectatic vessels (on lid margins, mimicking seborrheic blepharitis)
  3. Chalazia and hordeoli (usually recurrent)
  4. Plugged meibomian gland orifices (meibomian gland dysfunction) without inflammation
  5. Meibomitis (inflammation of meibomian glands)
  6. Conjunctival hyperemia
     a. Tends to produce a 360° superficial (non-uveitic) circumcorneal flush
     b. Occasionally associated with tearing/serous discharge
  7. Prominent limbal arcades (also 360° pattern)
  8. Peripheral SPK (usually fine to moderately dense)
  9. Tear film disorders (frothing, quick TBUT)
  10. Pannus (360° pattern, usually 1 to 2 mm onto cornea)
  11. Neovascularization (360° anterior stromal)
  12. Epithelial edema (peripheral and diffuse)
  13. Microcysts (peripheral and diffuse)
  14. Peripheral epithelial basement membrane changes
      a. Maps-dots-fingerprints
      b. Differ from other typical EBM changes in their peripheral (versus classic central) location
      c. Tend to produce recurrent corneal erosions

15. Ill-defined subepithelial infiltrates (peripheral)
16. Peripheral (to diffuse) anterior stromal infiltration and hazing
17. Anterior uveitis (acute or chronic)
18. Episcleritis and scleritis
19. Peripheral corneal thinning but perforation is rare

- Specific dermatological (skin) manifestations (in approximate increasing order of occurrence)
  1. Erythematous "flushing" of skin
     a. Confined to limited "flush areas" only
        i. Cheeks
        ii. Forehead
        iii. Nose
        iv. Chin
        v. Neck
     b. Aggravated by certain substances, elements
        i. Alcohol and certain ingested foods (e.g., spicy) and drink (variable among patients)
        ii. Wind, heat, cold, sunlight, airborne elements
        iii. Anxiety, stress, excitement, depression
        iv. Menopause
        v. Physical exercise
  2. Telangiectasia
     a. Prominent, dilated superficial capillary vessels on skin surface
     b. Limited to "flush areas"
  3. Papules
     a. Small (approximately 1 to 3 mm) raised, red skin nodules
     b. Limited to "flush areas"
  4. Pustules (usually small and non-inflamed)
  5. Sebaceous gland hypertrophy
     a. Thickened, irregular, erythematous skin texture
     b. Limited to "flush areas"
  6. Rhinophyma
     a. Concentration of all skin findings with thickened, swollen tissue encompassing an area ranging from the tip of the nose to the entire nose
     b. Sometimes called the "W.C. Fields look"

Assessment

(See also Appendix 3)

- Mimics many lid and anterior segment disorders
- Key to definitive diagnosis is "syndrome" findings
  1. Eye and skin findings
  2. Manifested simultaneously or one part of syndrome present (eye or skin) with positive history of other components
  3. If other components not (yet) manifested, diagnosis may be difficult, if not impossible (initially)
- If any of classic clinical signs of rosacea are treated as individual entities and do not respond to standard therapies, consider rosacea diagnosis
  1. Especially in 30- to 60-year-old patients
  2. Especially with increased risk factors
     a. Fair complexion
     b. Northern European heritage
- If clinical signs are too vague and confusing, ultimate definitive diagnosis should be considered by a dermatologist

Plan: Acne (Ocular) Rosacea

(See also Appendix 6)

- Warm compresses, lubricating drops and gels, lid hygiene (e.g., lid wipes)
- Oral treatment for rosacea syndrome with ocular manifestations is
  1. Oral tetracycline; dosage 250 mg bid to qid for 3 to 4 weeks
  2. Oral doxycycline at 50 to 100 mg qd to bid for 6 to 12 weeks
     a. For long term maintenance and less GI upset, use ORACEA (FDA approved) qd (30 mg immediate release plus 10 mg delayed release doxycycline) or doxycycline "off label" 20 mg or 50 mg qd to bid
  3. Azithromycin is an alternative oral drug (if tetracycline or doxycycline contraindicated)
- "Off label" topical cyclosporin 0.05% has shown improvement in symptoms, eyelid signs, and tear function and is an alternative treatment for this chronic condition to avoid complications of long-term tetracycline treatment
- Topical metronidazole 0.75% applied to lid margin bid has been used "off label"
- Omega-3 fatty acids improve meibomian gland secretion
- Specific ocular complications should be treated according to standard, appropriate therapies
  1. Topical tetracyclines may or may not have any substantial value if used without oral counterpart (especially in moderate to severe involvements)
  2. Topical steroids are indicated (and usually do provide significant benefits) in ocular surface inflammation (e.g., keratitis, episcleritis) and other inflammatory complications (e.g., uveitis)
- In severe conditions (with significant skin involvement), patient should be urged to seek dermatological consultation and care
- Corneal perforations managed with sutures, adhesive glue, conjunctival flaps, and keratoplasty
- Advise and educate patient carefully on unknown etiology of disease and chronicity of complications

Follow-Up

- Most patients will respond initially to oral (and, if indicated, topical) medications over approximately a 4-week dosage period
  1. If non-responsive, additional 2 to 4 weeks indicated
  2. Unfortunately, some patients may not respond
  3. Non-responsive patients should receive close ocular and dermatological management by specialist
- Responsive patients often (more than 50% of the time) reactivate within approximately a 6-month to 2-year period and require retreatment
  1. About 50% of remaining patients will continue to reactivate intermittently for extended periods
  2. Some patients will require low-dose maintenance regimens for indefinite periods to control frequent recurrences
  3. Most patients will eventually self-limit (usually by 50 to 60 years of age)
- Patients with chronic mild to moderate lid involvement should be maintained on standard antistaphylococcal lid care procedures (see Figure 3.1)

- Severe cases (with extensive ocular and eye involvement) and non-responsive cases should be comanaged with dermatologist or patient's primary physician

2. *Chlamydial (Adult Inclusion and Inclusion Blennorrhea) Keratitis*[85,86]

Background Information

a. Trachoma family organism (TRIC)
b. Called inclusion conjunctivitis in adults and inclusion blennorrhea in newborns
c. Incubation period of approximately 4 to 12 days
d. Produces combined viral and bacterial signs
e. Similar to viruses, organism is an obligate intracellular parasite (with dormant recurrent potential)
f. More benign clinical course than trachoma
g. An oculogenital disease
    i. Transmitted eye to eye or hand to eye
    ii. From infected mother to baby (2% to 5% of newborns)
    iii. Non-chlorinated swimming pools (reported in Europe)
    iv. Associated with hot tub use
h. Frequency increasing dramatically

Clinical Presentation

Subjective

For Adult Inclusion Conjunctivitis

- Sexually active adults (especially from 15 to 25 years of age) are prime candidates
- History of prolonged (2- to 4-week) bacterial conjunctivitis signs and symptoms
- Non-responsive or remitting and exacerbating with use of standard topical antibiotic therapies
- Mild to moderate foreign-body sensation, tearing, photophobia, mucopurulent discharge, crusting of lashes
- Unilateral presentations more common than bilateral
- No significant visual loss or disturbance (in mild to moderate forms)
- History of non-gonococcal genitourinary (or urethral or urinary) tract infection
    1. Discharge with negative culture for *Neisseria gonorrhoeae*
    2. Patient often denies active infection but may admit to recent history of discharge

For Neonatal Inclusion Blennorrhea

- Most frequent cause of conjunctivitis in infants
    1. Usually within 15 days of birth
    2. Incubation period produces delay in clinical manifestation
    3. Discharge, redness, and swollen eyelids
- Usually positive history of maternal infection
- Risk of birth canal transmission from infected mother is greater than 20%
- Baby frequently presents an associated pneumonia-like upper respiratory infectious (URI) syndrome

Objective

For Adult Inclusion Conjunctivitis

- Incubation (dormancy) period of 1 to 3 weeks
- Bacterial-like signs
    1. Papillary changes on palpebral conjunctiva
    2. Mild to moderate mucopurulent discharge (less on waking)
    3. Meaty red bulbar hyperemia (usually without hemorrhagic changes)
    4. Diffuse SPK (usually greater superiorward)
    5. Corneal signs may linger and ultimately self-limit within 6 to 12 months (without scarring)
- Viral-like signs
    1. Dramatic follicular conjunctivitis (greatest in inferior cul-de-sac)
    2. Occasional conjunctival chemosis
    3. Preauricular lymph enlargement (usually non-tender)
    4. Occasionally pseudomembrane formations in more severe presentations
    5. Diffuse SPK (greater superiorward) of variable density and degree
    6. Superior micropannus
    7. EKC-like subepithelial infiltrates (greater superiorward and peripherally)
- Secondary anterior uveitis usually develops in the cases with more advanced corneal involvement
- Occasionally patient may report an associated ipsilateral otitis media (earache on same side)

For Neonatal Inclusion Blennorrhea

- Similar signs to adult form
- Follicles and corneal infiltrates take longer to develop (6 to 8 weeks) owing to immature immune system
- Laboratory workup (done more frequently in infants than in adults) will reveal cytoplasmic inclusion bodies from conjunctival scrapings
- May show systemic involvements in prolonged disease (usually URI-type responses)
- Prolonged, untreated corneal involvement could lead to pannus and permanent scarring

Assessment

(See also Appendix 3)

Laboratory assessment (of conjunctival scrapings) should be considered in infants or severe cases
1. Attempt to isolate cytoplasmic inclusion bodies
2. Difficult laboratory procedure (especially for non-ophthalmic labs) with frequent false negatives

For Adult Inclusion Conjunctivitis

- Rule out bacterial keratoconjunctivitis
    1. Usually history most significant differential (i.e., sexually active adult with active or history of recent urinary tract involvement)
    2. Non-responsive to standard topical antibiosis and chronicity usually suggestive in risk categories
- Rule out viral keratoconjunctivitis
    1. Again, history significant
    2. Chronicity of acute or subacute phases of chlamydial infection substantially longer than viral (EKC) syndromes

For Neonatal Inclusion Blennorrhea

- Rule out gonococcal infection
    1. Best done through culturing (patient and mother)
    2. Gonorrhea tends to produce immediate (day 1 or 2) clinical response versus delayed (5 days or greater) chlamydial reaction
- Rule out viral etiologies (uncommon in newborns)

Plan: Chlamydial Keratitis

(See also Appendix 6)

For Adult Inclusion Conjunctivitis

- Oral azithromycin 1 g 1× dose
- Oral doxycycline 100 mg bid × 15 to 30 days
- Avoid doxycycline in pregnant females and even in women of childbearing age (who may be uncertain or unaware of early pregnancy)
    1. Documented risk of discoloration of developing calcium (e.g., teeth) tissue
    2. Azithromycin (1 g) alternative

For Neonatal Inclusion Blennorrhea

- Co-manage patient with pediatrician or primary physician
- Azithromycin 20 mg/kg orally qd × 3 days
- Definitely no use of tetracycline (same reasons as stated above)

Follow-Up

- Patients, mothers of patients, and sexual partners must be advised and counseled as to venereal disease
- All patients and associated parties should be advised of the need for medical care
- Clinical signs of conjunctivitis may take 2 to 3 months to resolve completely (with treatment)
- Corneal findings (SPK and subepithelial infiltrates) may persist for 6 to 12 months
- Monitor clinical findings every 2 to 4 weeks until complete resolution
    1. Withhold contact lens re-wear for 2 to 4 weeks after resolution of acute clinical presentation
    2. If reinfection occurs with lenses, discontinue temporarily, and replace lenses on re-wear
    3. Monitor re-wear closely if subepithelial infiltrates persist
- Advise patient on dormant obligate parasitic nature of organism and risk of recurrences

3. Interstitial Keratitis[87,88]

Subjective

- Acute or chronic presentation
    1. Acute form, usually in childhood or early adulthood, includes painful red eye with sudden decrease in vision
    2. Chronic conditions usually reveal long-standing history of disease (ocular and systemic)
- Careful medical and ocular history required
    1. Any form of serious systemic disease (acute or chronic)?
    2. History of any venereal diseases (clinical or laboratory diagnoses)?
    3. History of previous red eye episodes or reduced vision?

Objective

- Usually unilateral presentation
- Preponderance of findings frequently superiorward
- Acute conditions present as red, inflamed eye ranging from circumcorneal flush to sclerouveitic intensity
- Cornea always presents with triad of findings (Figure 5.96)
    1. Corneal infiltration (and edema in acute forms)
        a. Usually from limbus toward central cornea

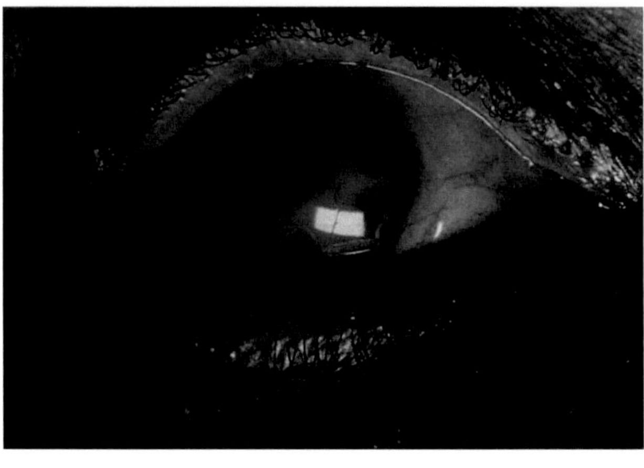

FIGURE 5.96 Interstitial keratitis is a syndrome of three corneal findings—stromal infiltration, thinning, and neovascularization—most often associated with systemic syphilis.

        b. Feathered borders (intrastromal)
        c. Effects visual acuity when central
    2. Corneal thinning
        a. Most apparent in the chronic forms
        b. From the posterior surface forward
        c. Small (1 mm) to large, diffuse involved areas
    3. Deep stromal (full-thickness) neovascularization
        a. Range from peripheral to central encroachment
        b. Usually entering from superior 180° of limbus
        c. May appear with active blood flow or no blood ("ghost vessels") in chronic, inactive forms
- Corneal stromal nerves may be segmentally thickened (beaded appearance)
- Anterior angle and/or iris may reveal fleshy nodules

Assessment

- 90% of all interstitial keratitis is caused by syphilis
    1. Can present as acute ocular infection from 5 to 15 years after systemic infection
        a. Can also present insidiously after infection
        b. In congenital forms usually presents by 15 years of age
    2. Check for external leutic signs
        a. Saddle nose bridge
        b. Hutchinson's triad
            i. Notched incisor teeth
            ii. Deafness (Cogan's syndrome)
            iii. Interstitial keratitis
    3. FTA-ABS, VDRL, and other lab work required
- Rule out dystrophies and degenerations
    1. Usually bilateral
    2. Corneal triad not present

Plan and Follow-Up: Interstitial Keratitis

- Refer to medical specialist for systemic treatment
- Consider referral to corneal specialist for care
    1. Guaranteed scarring and vision loss
    2. Generally poorly responsive to therapies
    3. Non-specific topical therapy includes cycloplegia/dilation, steroids (up to qh for acute presentations), and topical tacrolimus "off label"
- Corneal transplant frequently required with good prognosis

4. *Mooren's Ulcer*[89,90]

Subjective

- Acute or subacute painful presentation
- Photophobia and blurred vision due to astigmatism
- Two forms
  1. Older patients present with a unilateral, less severe inflammation
  2. Younger patients (rare) present a bilateral, severe type
- May have a higher frequency among Black patients

Objective

- Inflammatory (presumed autoimmune etiology) peripheral, serpiginous (creeping) type ulceration of unknown etiology (refer to "Fungal Keratitis," under "Assessment" for serpiginous ulceration test)
- Usually starts inferior and then spreads
- A progressing ulcer will have anterior yellowish-white infiltrates at ulcer edge
- Usually a lateral to medial limbal presentation
- No discharge associated with stromal ulceration
- Often neovascularization develops early
- Chronic cases have stromal scarring and irregular astigmatism reducing vision

Assessment

(See also Appendix 3)

- Major risk of scarring and possible perforation
- Rule out other marginal degenerations
  1. Marginal furrow (painless)
  2. Pellucid (inferior)
  3. Terrien's (superior)
- Rule out marginal staphylococcal keratitis (no thinning)
- Rule out fungal keratitis (traumatic history)

Plan and Follow-Up: Mooren's Ulcer

- Responds poorly to therapies including steroids
- Frequently unrelenting course for 6 to 12 months
- Refer to corneal specialist

5. *Photoablation Keratitis*[91–94]

Background Information

a. Excimer lasers have been used for over 25 years to perform a variety of refractive surgery procedures (e.g., photorefractive keratectomy [PRK], laser-assisted in situ keratomileusis [LASIK], etc.; refer to Chapter 7), which attempts to neutralize refractive error through corneal molding and sculpting by photoablation laser techniques
b. Photoablation is also being used to correct corneal surface defects through a procedure termed phototherapeutic keratectomy (PTK)
c. While excimer ablations have as their endpoint correction of refractive error (PRK), or correction of corneal surface defects (PTK), the corneal immune response to the procedure (inflammatory response) produces a keratitis
   i. The inflammatory response incorporates the traditional "corneal remodeling" effects
   ii. Additionally, some poorly understood immunologic effects also result in clinical variations in the keratitis
d. Improved instrumentation and surgical techniques have significantly reduced complications and improved endpoint predictability and stability
e. Problems do, however, persist as immediate, intermediate, and long-term/chronic problem

Clinical Course

(After the photoablation procedure)

a. *Remodeling effect 1:* epithelial hyperplasia
   i. Postprocedural epithelial thickening recontours corneal shape
   ii. Clinical result: undeterminable degree of photorefractive neutralization effect
b. *Remodeling effect 2:* keratocytic activation
   i. Keratocytes activated by circulating inflammatory white blood cells synthesize new collagen fibrils and fibroblasts
   ii. Clinical result: anterior stromal haze (diffuse lamellar keratitis) and risk of fibrin scarring
c. *Remodeling effect 3:* copolymerization effect
   i. Fibronectin and type III collagen copolymerize with type I collagen to form small reticular fibrils versus normal type I replacement fibrils
   ii. Clinical result: changes in interfibrillary (distances) relationships in the stromal matrix produce optical interferences and irregularities (more stromal haze)
d. *Remodeling effect 4:* GAG concentration alteration
   i. Relative concentrations of stromal glycosaminoglycans (GAGs) increase
   ii. Clinical result: alteration in interfibrillary uniformity and spacing in the matrix (more stromal haze)
e. *Remodeling effect 5:* recontouring of anterior stromal lamellar matrix
   i. Newly formed stromal fibrils (type III replacing type I from remodeling effect 3) may weaken anterior stromal lamellar matrix and produce recontouring by forces of the increased concentrations of GAGs (from remodeling effect 4)
   ii. Clinical result: reduction in photoablation refractive effects (and more anterior stromal hazing)
f. *Remodeling effect 6:* collagenase enzyme synthesis
   i. Keratocytes also synthesize a collagenase enzyme that can degrade small reticular fibrils (types III and VII)
   ii. Clinical results
      - Potentially positive effect of reducing the replacement of type I collagen fibrils by type III (remodeling effect 3)
      - Potentially negative effect of reducing type VII (epithelial basement membrane anchoring fibrils), and producing epithelial instability
g. Corneal wound healing and immune response is greater with PRK compared to LASIK
h. Corneal wound healing and immune response is greater with femtosecond laser compared to microkeratome but has been reduced with newer lasers and reduced energy used for flap creation
i. Diffuse lamellar keratitis
   i. A sterile inflammatory response with granular white infiltrates at the flap interface of varying densities
   ii. Few patients are treated for DLK after 1-week post-op

j. Management approaches to potentially negate remodeling effects include the use of postprocedural topical steroids for 3 to 6 months or longer
   i. To reduce stromal haze (diffuse lamellar keratitis)
   ii. To reduce the risk of fibrin scarring
   iii. To stabilize the refractive endpoint

Clinical Considerations

Subjective

- Diurnal variations
- Reduced vision
- Night vision problems
- Halos and glare (light scatter throughout cornea)
- Insidious hyperopic shifts

Objective

- Immediate complications
  1. Risk of infectious keratitis
  2. Keratitis due to endothelial compromise
  3. Recurrent corneal erosion (RCE) syndrome (for procedures that remove the epithelium prior to ablation)
- Intermediate complications
  1. Wound contraction and scarring
  2. Under- or over-correction and refractive regression
  3. Reduced resistance to blunt injury and corneal rupture (not a risk in laser photoablation procedures without a flap created)
  4. Induced astigmatism
  5. Corneal hazing (diffuse lamellar keratitis)
  6. Transient light sensitivity syndrome (TLSS)
     a. Only with femtosecond laser created flaps
     b. Photophobia with minimal or no inflammation
  7. Neovascularization at incision sites
  8. Subepithelial fibrosis
- Long-term problems and risks
  1. Increased ongoing risk of fungal and gram-negative keratitis
  2. Risk (about 19%) of chronic RCE syndrome
  3. Chronic endothelial/physiological edematous problems
  4. Secondary infiltrative keratitis from chronic neovascularization

Assessment

Other refractive therapies
  a. Surgical
     i. Astigmatic (or arcuate) keratotomy (AK): *aka* limbal relaxing incisions (LRI)
     ii. Laser thermal procedures
     - Laser thermal keratoplasty (LTK)
     - Conductive keratoplasty (CK)
     iii. Other intracorneal procedures
     - Small incision lenticule extraction (*SMILE*)
     - Intrastromal corneal ring segments (ICRS) (*aka* Intacs)
  b. Non-surgical
     i. Orthokeratology
     ii. Contact lenses
     iii. Spectacle lenses

Plan and Follow-Up: Photoablation Keratitis

- Long-term steroid management
  1. Deep lamellar keratitis (DLK)
     a. 1 to 2+: Steroid drops q4 h
     b. 2 to 3+: Steroid drops q2 h
     c. 3 to 4+: Lift flap, irrigate, steroid drops q2h
- Contact lens or spectacle assistance

6. Superior Limbic Keratoconjunctivitis (SLK)[5]

Background Information

a. Disease originally described by Theodore in 1963 (frequently called SLK of Theodore)
b. Etiology unknown
c. Frequently (up to 50%) associated with hyperthyroidism

Subjective

- Generalized ocular irritation, burning, foreign-body sensation, and discomfort
- Symptoms and frequency of SLK of Theodore slightly more prevalent in women
- Most common age range is 20 to 50 years of age
- SLK of Theodore tends to remit and exacerbate over 5- to 10-year period

Objective

- Mostly bilateral presentations, with one eye usually more advanced than the other
- Lid spasms frequently associated
- Prominent superior bulbar hyperemia (Figure 5.97)
  1. Usually follows "corridor" pattern from insertion of superior rectus muscle to corneolimbal juncture
  2. Occasionally, chemosis develops over injected area and along limbal border
- Superior tarsal palpebral papillary changes
  1. Dense
  2. Not large "giant" papillae as in vernal or giant papillary conjunctivitis
- Fine superior SPK pattern
  1. When abundant, will coalesce to patches
  2. Positive NaFl and rose bengal stain
  3. Often associated with prominent limbal arcades and developing pannus
- Occasional dendriform infiltrates (pseudodendrites)

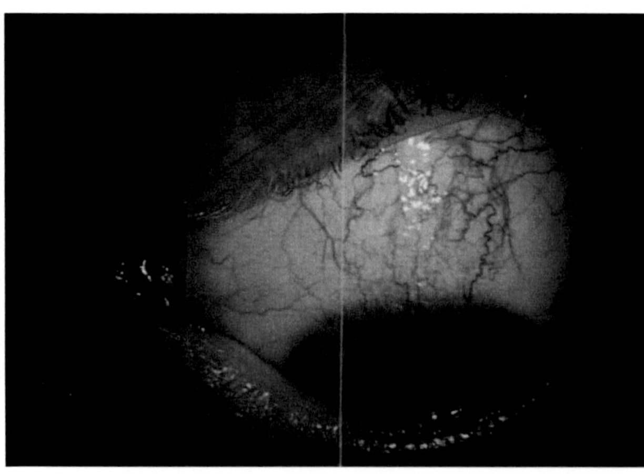

FIGURE 5.97 Superior limbic keratoconjunctivitis (SLK) presents with bilateral, superior bulbar hyperemia often following a "corridor" along the insertion of the superior rectus muscle. The disease is poorly understood with questionable etiologies (e.g., hyperthyroidism) with non-specific therapies.

- Superior subepithelial infiltrates may form in chronic or severe presentations
- Filament formations may occur on superior cornea

Assessment

(See also Appendix 3)

- Rule out GPC
  1. More dramatic, larger "giant" papillae
  2. Usually less bulbar conjunctival involvement
  3. Usually less (if any) corneal involvement
- Rule out vernal keratoconjunctivitis
  1. More frequent in younger males
  2. Tranta's dots on superior limbus

	SLK of Theodore
1. Age	Middle age
2. Sex	Women greater
3. Systemic	Hyperthyroidism
4. Symptoms	Irritation
5. Bulbar	Superior conjunctivitis hyperemia
6. Tarsal conjunctivitis	Dense papillae
7. Limbus	Chemosis
8. Cornea	Superior SPK
	Pseudodendrites
	SEIs
	Filaments

Plan: Superior Limbic Keratoconjunctivitis

(See also Appendix 4)

- Disease is usually self-limiting over 5- to 10-year period
- For mild cases artificial tears and gels and punctal occlusion for increased lubrication
- In mild to moderate cases, topical antihistamine/mast cell stabilizers or NSAIDs qid 3 to 4 weeks
- Autologous serum tears can be effective but must be used long term and cost is an issue
- In moderate to severe presentations, topical steroids qid for 10 to 14 days often effective for subjective and objective signs
  1. Sometimes steroids have little or no effect
  2. Do not overuse (i.e., beyond 2 to 3 weeks)
- Severe cases may require advanced therapies
  1. 0.5% silver nitrate painted onto superior conjunctiva and tarsus often effective (reasons uncertain)
     a. Relief usually for about 4 to 6 weeks, then recurrence likely
     b. Careful with application (do not touch cornea)
     c. Irrigate copiously after about 3 to 5 minutes
  2. Cryotherapy used in very severe cases
- Moderate to severe levels of the disease may also be treated with large-diameter bandage soft contact lenses

SLK (Adjunctive Therapies)

- Cold packs
- Oral NSAIDs (as prostaglandin inhibitors) in lieu of contraindications
  1. Aspirin (3 g/day)
  2. Ibuprofen (400 mg qid)
- Oral antihistamine-decongestants

Follow-Up

- Patients with SLK of Theodore should be advised of 5- to 10-year chronicity with remitting and exacerbating clinical episodes

7. Terrien's Marginal Degeneration[95]

Subjective

- Occurs in males, usually over 40 years of age
- Patients usually asymptomatic unless inflammatory or irregular astigmatism blurs vision

Objective

- Slowly progressive, bilateral (usually asymmetric) condition
- Begins superior nasal as fine anterior stromal opacities (similar appearance as arcus senillus) and mild superficial neovascularization
- Proceeds circumferentially with corneal thinning that produces a gutter
- Usually just superior but can spread to inferior quadrant
- In later stages a yellowish-white lipid can be seen at edge of advancing gutter formation
- There is a clear area of corneal between thinning and limbus
- Thinning is usually extensive, leading to corneal distortions and permanent visual loss due to irregular against-the-rule astigmatism
- Acute presentations produce secondary inflammation and subsequent neovascularization of affected area

Assessment

- Rule out other marginal degenerations
- Rule out inflammatory causes
  1. Mooren's ulcer
  2. Fungal ulcer (history of trauma)
  3. Rheumatoid disease

Plan and Follow-Up: Terrien's Marginal Degeneration

- Heavy topical steroids may or may not help
- If thinning progresses to precarious stage or vision correction is no longer adequate with CL, consider penetrating keratoplasty (PK) or lamellar keratoplasty (LK) for protection
- Condition usually stabilizes (with permanent scarring) after initial attack

8. Trachoma

Complete discussion in Chapter 4, Section III.

9. Vernal Keratoconjunctivitis[96–98]

Subjective

- Seasonal disease presenting mostly in warmer weather
- Young males peak incidence age 4–7 (age range 12 to 30, slightly greater in Black patients) in hot, dry climates at highest risk
- Usually a family or personal history of allergies
- Disease has a remitting and exacerbating history with a self-limiting nature usually within 5 to 10 years after initial attack
- Primary, overriding presenting symptom is itching with secondary corneal FB sensation
- Patient usually reports burning, mucous discharge, and photophobia

Objective

- Mostly bilateral presentations
- A palpebral, limbal, and mixed presentation
- Frequently associated with secondary lid congestion and a pseudoptosis
- Discharge is characteristically thick, ropy, whitish-yellow strands of dense mucus
  1. Covers superior tarsus and conjunctiva
  2. Spreads over cornea
  3. Accumulates at inner canthus
- Generalized bulbar hyperemia
- Giant papillary ("cobblestone") conjunctivitis on the superior tarsal plate
- Most common corneal involvement is superior SPK
  1. Usually fine and scattered in upper third corneal region
  2. Increases in density at limbal area (from about 10- to 2-o'clock position)
  3. Rarely can worsen to erosions and shield ulcers
  4. Associated with keratoconus
- Occasional filamentary formations (superiorly)
- Disease presents numerous limbal forms with mild to severe subjective and objective presentations
  1. Mild forms will demonstrate small to moderately sized limbal follicles or infiltrates of a circumlimbal nature ranging from 1 to 3 mm in length with little corneal involvement
     a. Called limbal vernal infiltrate or follicle
     b. Conjunctival injection usually limited to leash of vessels associated directly with limbal infiltrate
     c. Usually no severe conjunctival or corneal involvement
  2. More advanced, generalized forms of vernal keratoconjunctivitis frequently present a limbal form of disease called Horner–Trantas dots
     a. Found most on superior limbus
     b. Puffy, white, round dots about 1 to 2 mm in size
     c. May be flat or slightly raised (in more advanced disease)
     d. Accumulations of eosinophils from type I immune response

Assessment

(See also Appendix 3)

- Rule out atopic keratoconjunctivitis (year-round versus seasonal vernal presentations)
- Rule out SLK (usually a milder, less symptomatic presentation)
- Rule out GPC
  1. Less symptomatic
  2. More related to cause (e.g., soft lenses) versus seasonal allergic response
  3. Clinically less severe
- Rule out infectious causes (by seasonal nature and itching)

Plan: Vernal Keratoconjunctivitis

(See also Appendices 4 and 6)

- Mild forms can be managed with allergen avoidance, lubricants, and antihistamine/mast cell stabilizers (work best if started prior to symptoms in anticipation of seasonal recurrence)
- Moderate to severe forms respond dramatically well to topical steroids
  1. Ester-based steroids (e.g., 0.5% loteprednol) q2–4 h for 7 days preferable over 1% prednisolone due to the better safety profile and recurrent nature of disease to minimize steroid ocular side effects
  2. Duration may be prolonged in severe cases
  3. Taper steroids to lowest maintenance dose and continue low (maintenance) dose for 4 to 6 weeks
     a. Maintenance dose can be as low as 1 gtt 3×/week
     b. Less than maintenance dose will result in exacerbation of disease
     c. After 4 to 6 weeks, attempt to further taper to 0
  4. In long-term chronic disease pharmacy compounded cyclosporine 0.5 to 2% and tacrolimus 0.03% ointment are used "off-labeled" to minimize steroid side effects
     a. 0.1% cyclosporin (Verkazia) qid FDA approved for VK July 2021
- Blinding disease (active corneal shield ulcers, severe limbal inflammation, and limbal stem cell deficiency) difficult to treat
- Other adjunctive therapies (with steroids)
  1. Cold packs
  2. Topical antihistamine/mast cell stabilizers
  3. Oral antihistamines-decongestants
  4. Oral NSAIDs may have some value during acute and subacute phases
  5. Oral steroids for non-responsive patients

Follow-Up

- Milder generalized (and vernal) forms usually respond very quickly and completely to steroids within 1 week
  1. Mild generalized forms may or may not require maintenance regimens (with steroids or antihistamine/mast cell stabilizers)
  2. Limbal vernal forms do not require maintenance regimens beyond initial steroid for 5 to 7 days (then complete taper)
- Patients with more severe forms should be carefully advised of the chronic nature of their disease with remissions and exacerbations over extended period of years (5 to 10?)
  1. Severe disease may not remit completely, even with maintenance steroids
  2. Rarely, patient may require additional immunotherapy (e.g., desensitizations, immunosuppressive agents)
- Advise patients in remission to report symptoms on exacerbation or recheck annually
- Best never to allow open-ended use or self-prescribing (restarting) steroid therapy without recheck visit

IV. Common Corneal Surgical Procedures

(See also Chapter 7, "Pre- and Postoperative Management of Refractive Procedures")

A. History

Indication

1. Therapeutic: treat disease process
2. Stabilize cornea: threat of perforation
3. Optical: to improve vision due to scarring, irregular astigmatism/higher order aberrations, and surface irregularities (refractive only procedures will be discussed in Chapter 7)

B. Superficial Keratectomy[99–102]

- Used to treat anterior corneal disease such as recurrent corneal erosions, superficial cornea opacities and corneal dystrophies and degenerations
- Manual keratectomy
  1. Topical anesthesia usually used
  2. Epithelial debridement and basement membrane removal with Weck cell sponge or blade
  3. Carefully polish Bowman's membrane with Weck cell sponge or a diamond burr polishing drill
     a. Do not damage Bowman's membrane as this can cause scarring
  4. Bandage soft contact lens is used to promote re-epithelialization
  5. Antibiotic-steroid drops used qid for 1–3 weeks
- Phototherapeutic keratectomy (PTK) (specific post-op care discussed in Chapter 7)
  1. Topical anesthesia usually used
  2. Used to treat recurrent corneal erosions, superficial corneal opacities (depth up to 100 microns), and corneal dystrophies and degenerations
  3. More expensive than manual kerectomy since involves excimer laser compared to simple surgical instruments
  4. The excimer laser emits high energy UV light to photo ablate corneal tissue with minimal thermal damage to adjacent tissue
     a. Each laser pulse ablates 0.25 microns of tissue depth
     b. Very precise surgical tool
  5. Procedure
     a. If epithelium is not smooth, debridement is performed (blade or 20% alcohol) and a masking agent (e.g., dextran 0.1% or HPMC 0.7%) is applied prior to PTK
     b. If epithelium is smooth but underlying stroma is rough, epithelium left in place
     c. Focal smoothing can be performed for defects (e.g., nodules) that rise above the epithelium
     d. Can be combined with an amniotic membrane graft
  6. Complications
     a. Disease recurrence
     b. Refractive shift
        i. Central flattening will induce hyperopic shift and will be larger with deeper and wider ablations
        ii. Peripheral flattening can induce myopia or irregular astigmatism
        iii. Deep ablations can cause hazing and scarring

C. Intrastromal Corneal Ring Segments (ICRS)[103,104]

(Specific post-op care discussed in Chapter 7.)

- Used to treat keratoconus and post-LASIK ectasia
- Intacs, Keraring, and Ferrara rings are common ICRS
- ICRS are inserted through a channel created with mechanical dissection or femtosecond laser
- Vary in radii, thickness, and arc length
- Flatten corneal curvature and reduce asymmetry (e.g., high order aberrations)
- A reversible procedure: the rings can be removed if necessary
- Has been combined with other procedures such as CXL and PRK
- Usually does not eliminate need for refractive correction (e.g., gas permeable lens for irregular astigmatism)

D. Corneal Cross Linking (CXL)

(Refer to Chapter 5, Section II, E)

E. Lamellar Keratoplasty (LK)[105–107]

- Specific procedure depends on diseased corneal layer
- Reduces healing time and complications compared to PKP
- Automated lamellar therapeutic keratoplasty (ALTK)
  1. For anterior and mid stromal opacities with healthy endothelium
  2. Microkeratome dissects graft and host cornea
  3. Host posterior cornea and endothelium remains
- Deep anterior lamellar keratoplasty (DALK)
  1. For deep stromal opacities with healthy endothelium
  2. Post-op complications
     a. Descemet's rupture
     b. Graft rejection low (5–8%)
- Posterior lamellar keratoplasty (PLK)
  1. Healthy cornea except endothelium
  2. Peripheral self-sealing wound induced by microtome for graft insertion
  3. Descemet stripping endothelial keratoplasty (DSEK)
     a. Host Descemet/endothelial complex is stripped and replaced with Descemet/endothelial and thin layer of posterior stroma donor tissue
     b. Host tissue is folded and inserted into anterior chamber
     c. Graft is centered, and an air bubble is introduced to tamponade donor tissue to host tissue
     d. Descemet's automated stripping endothelial keratoplasty (DSAEK)
        i. Technique modified to use microkeratome to remove host tissue
  4. Descemet membrane endothelial keratoplasty (DMEK)
     a. Only diseased endothelium and Descemet's membrane is removed and replaced with host endothelium tissue
     b. Faster recovery, better visual outcome, and lower rejection rate compared to DSAEK
     c. Higher surgical skill required since donor tissue difficult to uncurl, greater endothelial cell loss, greater re-bubbling rate
  5. Post-op complications
     a. Graft dislocation most common post-op complication (20–30%) that needs to be managed with re-air bubbling
     b. Pupillary block glaucoma (caused by residual air bubble)
     c. No suture complications because none are used
     d. Better visual outcome (no induced post-op astigmatism) than PKP
     e. Hyperopic shift approximately 1–1.5 D
     f. Epithelial ingrowth at host/donor interface
     g. Graft rejection 7–9% and less clinically evident as compared to PKP
     h. Long-term graft failure not well documented due to these techniques being only approximately 15 years in existence
- 21st century has shown a decrease in PKP and an increase in LK due to less invasive surgery with better outcomes and reduced complications

- Newest techniques
  1. Pre-Descemet's endothelial keratoplasty (PDEK)
     a. Composed of 5–8 layers of compact collagen plus Descemet's/endothelial complex
     b. Easier to handle
     c. Tissue unfolds easier in eye
     d. Tissue can be collected from any age category
  2. Bowman layer transplant (BLT)
     a. After epithelial debridement donor Bowman membrane is onlayed to patient's Bowman's membrane
     b. Used to treat PRK post-op corneal haze
     c. Used to treat keratoconus to add mechanical strength to cornea and reduce ectasia
  3. Intraoperative optical coherence tomography (iOCT)
     a. Guides every step of surgery from tissue trephination to host/donor interface
  4. Femtosecond laser-assisted lamellar keratoplasty (FALK)
     a. Sharp and accurate cuts of donor and host cornea
     b. Better epithelial healing and less post-op astigmatism
  5. Bioengineered corneas
     a. Keratoprosthetics
        i. A PMMA front (optics) and back plate is sandwiched between a donor cornea (e.g., Boston keratoprosthetics)
        ii. Option for patients who are not PKP candidates (e.g., history of multiple graft failures)
     b. Tissue engineered hydrogels
     c. Bioengineered corneal lenticule for implantation
     d. Artificial cornea in clinical trials

F. Penetrating Full-Thickness Keratoplasty (PKP or PK)[108,109]

- Earliest corneal surgery performed
- For full-thickness opacities and dystrophies with endothelial involvement
- Entire corneal thickness is transplanted
- Topical steroids and antibiotics are used in post-op recovery
  1. Steroids will be slowly tapered over months and may be continued qd indefinitely especially if IOP does not increase
- Complications
  1. Graft failure (three most frequent reasons)
     a. Rejection
     b. Infection
     c. Glaucoma
  2. Suture complications
  3. Graft/Host junction weakness
  4. High post-op astigmatism
  5. Long healing time
  6. Catastrophic complications due to open globe surgery

References

1. Wipperman JL, Dorsch JN. Evaluation and management of corneal abrasions. *Am Fam Physician*. 2013;87(2):114–120
2. Sánchez-González JM, López-Izquierdo I, Gargallo-Martínez B, De-Hita-Cantalejo C, Bautista-Llamas MJ. Bandage contact lens use after photorefractive keratectomy. *J Cataract Refract Surg*. 2019;45(8):1183–1190. doi:10.1016/j.jcrs.2019.02.045
3. Mukherjee A, Ioannides A, Aslanides I. Comparative evaluation of Comfilcon A and Senofilcon A bandage contact lenses after transepithelial photorefractive keratectomy. *J Optom*. 2015;8(1):27–32. doi:10.1016/j.optom.2014.02.002
4. Bizrah M, Yusuf A, Ahmad S. An update on chemical eye burns. *Eye*. 2019;33(9):1362–1377. doi:10.1038/s41433-019-0456-5
5. Burrow MK, Patel BC. Keratoconjunctivitis. In: *StatPearls*. Treasure Island: StatPearls Publishing; February 25, 2021
6. Matossian C, McDonald M, Donaldson KE, Nichols KK, MacIver S, Gupta PK. Dry eye disease: consideration for women's health. *J Womens Health*. 2019;28(4):502–514. doi:10.1089/jwh.2018.7041
7. Willcox MDP, Argüeso P, Georgiev GA, et al. TFOS DEWS II tear film report. *Ocul Surf*. 2017;15(3):366–403. doi:10.1016/j.jtos.2017.03.006
8. Bang SP, Son MJ, Kim H, Lee YH, Jun JH. In vitro validation of the tear matrix metalloproteinase 9 in-situ immunoassay. *Sci Rep*. 2020;10(1):15126. Published 2020 Sep 15. doi:10.1038/s41598-020-71977-w
9. Tashbayev B, Utheim TP, Utheim ØA, et al. Utility of tear osmolarity measurement in diagnosis of dry eye disease. *Sci Rep*. 2020;10(1):5542. Published 2020 Mar 26. doi:10.1038/s41598-020-62583-x
10. Hessen M, Akpek EK. Dry eye: an inflammatory ocular disease. *J Ophthalmic Vis Res*. 2014;9(2):240–250
11. Ervin AM, Law A, Pucker AD. Punctal occlusion for dry eye syndrome. *Cochrane Database Syst Rev*. 2017;6(6):CD006775. Published 2017 Jun 26. doi:10.1002/14651858.CD006775.pub3
12. Ji MH, Moshfeghi DM, Periman L, et al. Novel extranasal tear stimulation: pivotal study results. *Transl Vis Sci Technol*. 2020;9(12):23. Published 2020 Nov 17. doi:10.1167/tvst.9.12.23
13. Wander AH, Koffler BH. Extending the duration of tear film protection in dry eye syndrome: review and retrospective case series study of the hydroxypropyl cellulose ophthalmic insert. *Ocul Surf*. 2009;7(3):154–162. doi:10.1016/s1542-0124(12)70310-5
14. Messmer EM. The pathophysiology, diagnosis, and treatment of dry eye disease. *Dtsch Arztebl Int*. 2015;112(5):71–82. doi:10.3238/arztebl.2015.0071
15. Messmer EM. The pathophysiology, diagnosis, and treatment of dry eye disease. *Dtsch Arztebl Int*. 2015;112(5):71–82. doi:10.3238/arztebl.2015.0071
16. Chalmers RL, Begley CG, Caffery B. Validation of the 5-item dry eye questionnaire (DEQ-5): Discrimination across self-assessed severity and aqueous tear deficient dry eye diagnoses. *Cont Lens Anterior Eye*. 2010 Apr;33(2):55–60. doi: 10.1016/j.clae.2009.12.010. Epub 2010 Jan 25. PMID: 20093066
17. Fraunfelder FT, Sciubba JJ, Mathers WD. The role of medications in causing dry eye [published correction appears in J Ophthalmol. 2019 Mar 4;2019:2989680]. *J Ophthalmol*. 2012;2012:285851. doi:10.1155/2012/285851
18. Pan Q, Angelina A, Marrone M, Stark WJ, Akpek EK. Autologous serum eye drops for dry eye. *Cochrane Database Syst Rev*. 2017 Feb 28;2(2):CD009327. doi: 10.1002/14651858.CD009327.pub3. PMID: 28245347; PMCID: PMC5510593
19. Murri MS, Moshirfar M, Birdsong OC, Ronquillo YC, Ding Y, Hoopes PC. Amniotic membrane extract and eye drops: a review of literature and clinical application. *Clin Ophthalmol*. 2018 Jun 18;12:1105–1112. doi: 10.2147/OPTH.S165553. PMID: 29950805; PMCID: PMC6012548
20. Pflugfelder SC, de Paiva CS. The pathophysiology of dry eye disease: what we know and future directions for research. *Ophthalmology*. 2017;124(11S):S4–S13. doi:10.1016/j.ophtha.2017.07.010
21. Craig JP, Nelson JD, Azar DT, Belmonte C, Bron AJ, Chauhan SK, de Paiva CS et al. The TFOS dry eye workshop II: executive summary. *Ocul Surf*. 2017;15(4):802–812. doi:10.1016/j.jtos.2017.08.003
22. Camodeca AJ, Anderson EP. Corneal foreign body. 2021 Apr 26. In: *StatPearls* [Internet]. Treasure Island: StatPearls Publishing; 2021 Jan–. PMID: 30725662

23. Miller DD, Hasan SA, Simmons NL, Stewart MW. Recurrent corneal erosion: a comprehensive review. *Clin Ophthalmol.* 2019;13:325–335. Published 2019 Feb 11. doi:10.2147/OPTH.S157430
24. Moshirfar M, Hastings J, Ronquillo Y. Megalocornea. 2021 Apr 14. In: *StatPearls* [Internet]. Treasure Island: StatPearls Publishing; 2021 Jan. PMID: 32119261
25. Bhat YR, Sanoj KM. Sclerocornea. *Indian Pediatr.* 2005 Mar;42(3):277. PMID: 15817979
26. Munjal A, Kaufman EJ. Arcus Senilis. 2020 Dec 28. In: *StatPearls* [Internet]. Treasure Island: StatPearls Publishing; 2021 Jan–. PMID: 32119257
27. Al-Hity A, Ramaesh K, Lockington D. EDTA chelation for symptomatic band keratopathy: results and recurrence. *Eye.* 2018;32(1):26–31. doi:10.1038/eye.2017.264
28. Pricopie S, Istrate S, Voinea L, Leasu C, Paun V, Radu C. Pseudophakic bullous keratopathy. *Rom J Ophthalmol.* 2017;61(2):90–94. doi:10.22336/rjo.2017.17
29. He Z, Campolmi N, Gain P, Ha Thi BM, Dumollard JM, Duband S, Peoc'h M, Piselli S, Garraud O, Thuret G. Revisited microanatomy of the corneal endothelial periphery: new evidence for continuous centripetal migration of endothelial cells in humans. *Stem Cells.* 2012 Nov;30(11):2523–34. doi: 10.1002/stem.1212. PMID: 22949402
30. Moshirfar M, Villarreal A, Ronquillo Y. Furrow degeneration. 2021 Jan 21. In: *StatPearls* [Internet]. Treasure Island: StatPearls Publishing; 2021 Jan–. PMID: 32491464
31. Chu WK, Choi HL, Bhat AK, Jhanji V. Pterygium: new insights. *Eye.* 2020;34(6):1047–1050. doi:10.1038/s41433-020-0786-3
32. Fonseca EC, Rocha EM, Arruda GV. Comparison among adjuvant treatments for primary pterygium: a network meta-analysis. *Br J Ophthalmol.* 2018 Jun;102(6):748–756. doi: 10.1136/bjophthalmol-2017-310288. Epub 2017 Nov 16. PMID: 29146761
33. Aljindan MY, Bamashmoos MA, AlShamlan RA, AlOdaini AA, Alabdullatif HA. Atypical presentation of salzmann nodule: a case report and literature review. *Cureus.* 2021;13(6):e15397. Published 2021 Jun 2. doi:10.7759/cureus.15397
34. Paranjpe V, Galor A, Monsalve P, Dubovy SR, Karp CL. Salzmann nodular degeneration: prevalence, impact, and management strategies. *Clin Ophthalmol.* 2019;13:1305–1314. Published 2019 Jul 25. doi:10.2147/OPTH.S166280
35. Klintworth GK. Corneal dystrophies. *Orphanet J Rare Dis.* 2009;4:7. Published 2009 Feb 23. doi:10.1186/1750-1172-4-7
36. Weiss JS, Møller HU, Aldave AJ, et al. IC3D classification of corneal dystrophies--edition 2 [published correction appears in Cornea. 2015 Oct;34(10):e32]. *Cornea.* 2015;34(2):117–159. doi:10.1097/ICO.0000000000000307
37. Moshirfar M, Bennett P, Ronquillo Y. Corneal dystrophy. In: *StatPearls.* Treasure Island: StatPearls Publishing; August 11, 2021
38. Werblin TP, Hirst LW, Stark WJ, Maumenee IH. Prevalence of map-dot-fingerprint changes in the cornea. *British J Ophthalmol.* 1981;65(6):401–409.
39. Alvarado J, Murphy C, Juster R. Age-related changes in the basement membrane of the human corneal epithelium. *Invest Ophthalmol Vis Sci.* 1983;24(8):1015–1028.
40. Shetty R, Kaweri L, Pahuja N, et al. Current review and a simplified "five-point management algorithm" for keratoconus. *Indian J Ophthalmol.* 2015;63(1):46–53. doi:10.4103/0301-4738.151468
41. Rathi VM, Mandathara PS, Dumpati S. Contact lens in keratoconus. *Indian J Ophthalmol.* 2013;61(8):410–415. doi:10.4103/0301-4738
42. Choi JA, Kim MS. Progression of keratoconus by longitudinal assessment with corneal topography. *Invest Ophthalmol Vis Sci.* 2012;53(2):927–935. Published 2012 Feb 23. doi:10.1167/iovs.11-8118
43. Mukhtar S, Ambati BK. Pediatric keratoconus: a review of the literature. *Int Ophthalmol.* 2018;38(5):2257–2266. doi:10.1007/s10792-017-0699-8
44. Sahu J, Raizada K. Pellucid marginal corneal degeneration. In: *StatPearls.* Treasure Island: StatPearls Publishing; July 19, 2021
45. Efron N, Morgan PB. Rethinking contact lens associated keratitis. *Clin Exp Optom.* 2006;89(5):280–298.
46. Baab S, Le PH, Kinzer EE. Allergic conjunctivitis. In: *StatPearls.* Treasure Island: StatPearls Publishing; March 23, 2021
47. La Rosa M, Lionetti E, Reibaldi M, et al. Allergic conjunctivitis: a comprehensive review of the literature. *Ital J Pediatr.* 2013;39:18. Published 2013 Mar 14. doi:10.1186/1824-7288-39-18
48. Versura P, Giannaccare G, Pellegrini M, Sebastiani S, Campos EC. Neurotrophic keratitis: current challenges and future prospects. *Eye Brain.* 2018;10:37–45. Published 2018 Jun 28. doi:10.2147/EB.S117261
49. Sheha H, Tighe S, Hashem O, Hayashida Y. Update on cenegermin eye drops in the treatment of neurotrophic keratitis. *Clin Ophthalmol.* 2019;13:1973–1980. Published 2019 Oct 7. doi:10.2147/OPTH.S185184
50. Semeraro F, Forbice E, Romano V, Angi M, Romano MR, Filippelli ME, Costagliola, C. Neurotrophic keratitis. *Ophthalmologica.* 2014;231(4):191–197.
51. Wiriyachai T, Boonsathorn S, Apiwattanakul N, Assawawiroonhakarn S. A rare case of primary sinonasal tuberculosis presented with phlyctenular keratoconjunctivitis in a pediatric patient: A case report and literature review. *Medicine.* 2021;100(7):e24787. doi:10.1097/MD.0000000000024787
52. Tang XJ, Liu Q, Pi LH, Chen XK, Chen L. Thygeson's superficial punctate keratitis (TSPK): a paediatric case report and review of the literature. *BMC Ophthalmol.* 2021;21(1):64. Published 2021 Jan 29. doi:10.1186/s12886-020-01790-6
53. Priyadarshini SR, Roy A, Das S. Thygeson's superficial punctate keratopathy: A review and case series. *Indian J Ophthalmol.* 2021;69(4):806–811. doi:10.4103/ijo.IJO_1624_20
54. Lorenzo-Morales J, Khan NA, Walochnik J. An update on Acanthamoeba keratitis: diagnosis, pathogenesis and treatment. *Parasite.* 2015;22:10. doi:10.1051/parasite/2015010
55. Austin A, Lietman T, Rose-Nussbaumer J. Update on the management of infectious keratitis. *Ophthalmology.* 2017;124(11):1678–1689. doi:10.1016/j.ophtha.2017.05.0
56. Tena D, Rodríguez N, Toribio L, González-Praetorius A. Infectious keratitis: microbiological review of 297 cases. *Jpn J Infect Dis.* 2019;72(2):121–123. doi:10.7883/yoken.JJID.2018.269
57. Stapleton F, Keay L, Edwards K, et al. The incidence of contact lens-related microbial keratitis in Australia. *Ophthalmology* 2008;115:1655–1662
58. Zaguia F, Ross M, Darvish M, Deschenes J. Besifloxacin ophthalmic suspension in patients with bacterial keratitis: a prospective, randomized clinical study. *Invest Ophthalmol Vis Scie.* 2018;59(9):3659–3659.
59. Prajna NV, Mascarenhas J, Krishnan T, et al. Comparison of natamycin and voriconazole for the treatment of fungal keratitis. *Arch Ophthalmol.* 2010;128(6):672–678. doi:10.1001/archophthalmol.2010.102
60. Yabiku ST, Yabiku MM, Bottós KM, Araújo AL, Freitas Dd, Belfort R Jr. Uso de ganciclovir 0,15% gel para tratamento de ceratoconjuntivite adenoviral [Ganciclovir 0.15% ophthalmic gel in the treatment of adenovirus keratoconjunctivitis]. *Arq Bras Oftalmol.* 2011;74(6):417–421. doi:10.1590/s0004-27492011000600007
61. Huang J, Kadonosono K, Uchio E. Antiadenoviral effects of ganciclovir in types inducing keratoconjunctivitis by quantitative polymerase chain reaction methods. *Clin Ophthalmol.* 2014;8:315–320. Published 2014 Jan 30. doi:10.2147/OPTH.S55284
62. Labib BA, Minhas BK, Chigbu DI. Management of adenoviral keratoconjunctivitis: challenges and solutions. *Clin Ophthalmol.* 2020;14:837–852. Published 2020 Mar 17. doi:10.2147/OPTH.S207976
63. Jonas RA, Ung L, Rajaiya J, Chodosh J. Mystery eye: Human adenovirus and the enigma of epidemic keratoconjunctivitis. *Prog Retin Eye Res.* 2020;76:100826. doi:10.1016/j.preteyeres.2019.100826
64. Okumus S, Coskun E, Tatar MG, et al. Cyclosporine a 0.05% eye drops for the treatment of subepithelial infiltrates after epidemic keratoconjunctivitis. *BMC Ophthalmol.* 2012;12:42. Published 2012 Aug 18. doi:10.1186/1471-2415-12-42

65. Berisa Prado S, Riestra Ayora AC, Lisa Fernández C, Chacón Rodríguez M, Merayo-Lloves J, Alfonso Sánchez JF. Topical tacrolimus for corneal subepithelial infiltrates secondary to adenoviral keratoconjunctivitis. *Cornea*. 2017;36(9):1102–1105. doi:10.1097/ICO.0000000000001279
66. Junk AK, Chen PP, Lin SC, Nouri-Mahdavi K, Radhakrishnan S, Singh K, Chen TC. Disinfection of tonometers: a report by the American academy of ophthalmology. *Ophthalmology*. 2017;124(12):1867–1875.
67. Herpetic Eye Disease Study Group. Acyclovir for the prevention of recurrent herpes simplex virus eye disease. *N Engl J Med*. 1998;339(5):300–306. doi:10.1056/NEJM199807303390503
68. Rowe AM, St Leger AJ, Jeon S, Dhaliwal DK, Knickelbein JE, Hendricks RL. Herpes keratitis. *Prog Retin Eye Res*. 2013;32:88–101. doi:10.1016/j.preteyeres.2012.08.002
69. Lobo AM, Agelidis AM, Shukla D. Pathogenesis of herpes simplex keratitis: The host cell response and ocular surface sequelae to infection and inflammation. *Ocul Surf*. 2019;17(1):40–49. doi:10.1016/j.jtos.2018.10.002
70. Tabbara KF, Al Balushi N. Topical ganciclovir in the treatment of acute herpetic keratitis. *Clin Ophthalmol*. 2010;4:905–912. Published 2010 Aug 19. doi:10.2147/opth.s8666
71. White ML, Chodosh J. Herpes simplex virus keratitis: a treatment guideline. In: *The American Academy of Ophthalmology Clinical Guidelines*. June 2014.
72. Chou TY, Hong BY. Ganciclovir ophthalmic gel 0.15% for the treatment of acute herpetic keratitis: background, effectiveness, tolerability, safety, and future applications. *Ther Clin Risk Manag*. 2014;10:665–681. Published 2014 Aug 20. doi:10.2147/TCRM.S58242
73. Colin J, Hoh HB, Easty DL, et al. Ganciclovir ophthalmic gel (Virgan; 0.15%) in the treatment of herpes simplex keratitis. *Cornea*. 1997;16(4):393–399
74. Minor M, Payne E. Herpes zoster ophthalmicus. In: *StatPearls*. Treasure Island: StatPearls Publishing; August 11, 2021
75. Kong CL, Thompson RR, Porco TC, Kim E, Acharya NR. Incidence rate of herpes zoster ophthalmicus: a retrospective cohort study from 1994 through 2018. *Ophthalmology*. 2020;127(3):324–330. doi:10.1016/j.ophtha.2019.10.001
76. Policy statement: recommendations for herpes zoster vaccine for patients 50 years of age and older. *Ophthalmology*. 2018;125(11):1813–1816
77. Tran KD, Falcone MM, Choi DS, et al. Epidemiology of herpes zoster ophthalmicus: recurrence and chronicity. *Ophthalmology*. 2016;123(7):1469–1475. doi:10.1016/j.ophtha.2016.03.005
78. Peng L, Du B, Sun L, Zhao Y, Zhang X. Short-term efficacy and safety of prednisone in herpes zoster and the effects on IL-6 and IL-10. *Exp Ther Med*. 2019;18(4):2893–2900. doi:10.3892/etm.2019.7898
79. Ghebremedhin B. Human adenovirus: Viral pathogen with increasing importance. *Eur J Microbiol Immunol (Bp)*. 2014;4(1):26–33. doi:10.1556/EuJMI.4.2014.1.2
80. Li J, Lu X, Sun Y, et al. A swimming pool-associated outbreak of pharyngoconjunctival fever caused by human adenovirus type 4 in Beijing, China. *Int J Infect Dis*. 2018;75:89–91. doi:10.1016/j.ijid.2018.08.009
81. Vieira AC, Höfling-Lima AL, Mannis MJ. Ocular rosacea: a review. *Arq Bras Oftalmol*. 2012;75(5):363–369. doi:10.1590/s0004-27492012000500016
82. Arman A, Demirseren DD, Takmaz T. Treatment of ocular rosacea: comparative study of topical cyclosporine and oral doxycycline. *Int J Ophthalmol*. 2015;8(3):544–549. Published 2015 Jun 18. doi:10.3980/j.issn.2222-3959.2015.03.19
83. Korting HC, Schöllmann C. Tetracycline actions relevant to rosacea treatment. *Skin Pharmacol Physiol*. 2009;22(6):287–294.
84. van Zuuren EJ. Rosacea. *New England J Med*. 2017;377(18):1754–1764.
85. Mohamed-Noriega K, Mohamed-Noriega J, Valdés-Navarro MA, Cuervo-Lozano EE, Fernández-Espinosa MC, Mohamed-Hamsho J. Conjunctival infection with Chlamydia trachomatis in sexual partners of patients with adult inclusion conjunctivitis. *Int Ophthalmol*. 2015;35(2):179–185. doi:10.1007/s10792-014-9930-z
86. Yang EB, Oetting TA. Adult Chlamydial Conjunctivitis: 23-year-old male with 6-week duration of red eyes. *EyeRounds.org*. February 28, 2007; Available from: http://www.EyeRounds.org/cases/68-Adult-Chlamydial-Conjunctivitis-Red-Eyes-Chronic.htm
87. Martin J, Kopplin L, Costakos D. Syphilitic interstitial keratitis treated with topical tacrolimus. *Am J Ophthalmol Case Rep*. 2021;23:101175. Published 2021 Jul 22. doi:10.1016/j.ajoc.2021.101175
88. Shoughy SS. Topical tacrolimus in anterior segment inflammatory disorders. *Eye Vis*. 2017;4:7. Published 2017 Mar 9. doi:10.1186/s40662-017-0072-z
89. Vemuganti GK, Murthy SI, Das S. Update on pathologic diagnosis of corneal infections and inflammations. *Middle East Afr J Ophthalmol*. 2011;18(4):277–284. doi:10.4103/0974-9233.90128
90. Alhassan MB, Rabiu M, and Agbabiaka IO. Interventions for Mooren's ulcer. *Cochrane Database Syst Rev*. 2014;1:1–15.
91. de Paula FH, Khairallah CG, Niziol LM, Musch DC, Shtein RM. Diffuse lamellar keratitis after laser in situ keratomileusis with femtosecond laser flap creation. *J Cataract Refract Surg*. 2012;38(6):1014–1019. doi:10.1016/j.jcrs.2011.12.030
92. Aristeidou A, Taniguchi EV, Tsatsos M et al. The evolution of corneal and refractive surgery with the femtosecond laser. *Eye and Vis* 2015;2:12. https://doi.org/10.1186/s40662-015-0022-6
93. Wilson SE. Biology of keratorefractive surgery- PRK, PTK, LASIK, SMILE, inlays and other refractive procedures. *Exp Eye Res*. 2020;198:108136. doi:10.1016/j.exer.2020.108136
94. Spadea L, Giovannetti F. Main complications of photorefractive keratectomy and their management. *Clin Ophthalmol*. 2019;13:2305–2315. Published 2019 Nov 27. doi:10.2147/OPTH.S233125
95. Chan AT, Ulate R, Goldich Y, Rootman DS, Chan CC. Terrien marginal degeneration: clinical characteristics and outcomes. *Am J Ophthalmol*. 2015;160(5):867–872.e1. doi:10.1016/j.ajo.2015.07.031
96. Zicari AM, Capata G, Nebbioso M, et al. Vernal Keratoconjunctivitis: an update focused on clinical grading system. *Ital J Pediatr*. 2019;45(1):64. Published 2019 May 21. doi:10.1186/s13052-019-0656-4
97. Azari AA, Arabi A. Conjunctivitis: a systematic review. *J Ophthalmic Vis Res*. 2020;15(3):372–395. Published 2020 Aug 6. doi:10.18502/jovr.v15i3.7456
98. Gokhale NS. Systematic approach to managing vernal keratoconjunctivitis in clinical practice: severity grading system and a treatment algorithm. *Indian J Ophthalmol*. 2016;64(2):145–148. doi:10.4103/0301-4738.179727
99. Deshmukh R, Reddy JC, Rapuano CJ, Vaddavalli PK. Phototherapeutic keratectomy: indications, methods and decision making. *Indian J Ophthalmol*. 2020;68(12):2856–2866. doi:10.4103/ijo.IJO_1524_20
100. Rao A, Sridhar U, Gupta AK. Amniotic membrane transplant with superficial keratectomy in superficial corneal degenerations: efficacy in a rural population of north India. *Indian J Ophthalmol*. 2008;56(4):297–302. doi:10.4103/0301-4738.39664
101. Malta JB, Soong HK. Diamond burr superficial keratectomy in the treatment of visually-significant anterior corneal lesions. *Arq Bras Oftalmol*. 2008;71(3):415–418. doi:10.1590/s0004-27492008000300021
102. Rathi VM, Vyas SP, Sangwan VS. Phototherapeutic keratectomy. *Indian J Ophthalmol*. 2012;60(1):5–14. doi:10.4103/0301-4738.91335
103. Vega-Estrada A, Alio JL. The use of intracorneal ring segments in keratoconus. *Eye and Vis*. 2016;3:8.
104. Bautista-Llamas MJ, Sánchez-González MC, López-Izquierdo I, et al. Complications and explantation reasons in

intracorneal ring segments (ICRS) implantation: a systematic review. *J Refract Surg.* 2019;35(11):740–747. doi:10.3928/1081597X-20191010-02
105. Moshirfar M, Thomson AC, Ronquillo Y. Corneal endothelial transplantation. In: *StatPearls*. Treasure Island: StatPearls Publishing; July 28, 2021
106. Ross AR, Said DG, Colabelli Gisoldi RAM, Nubile M, El-Amin A, Gabr AF, Abd Ed-Moniem M, Mencucci R, Pocobelli A, Mastropasqua L, Dua HS. Optimizing pre-descemet endothelial keratoplasty. *J Cataract Refract Surg.* 2020;46(5):667–674.
107. Parker JS, Dockery PW, Melles GRJ. Bowman layer transplantation: a review. *Asia-Pacific J Ophthalmol.* November–December 2020;9(6):565–570
108. Singh R, Gupta N, Vanathi M, Tandon R. Corneal transplantation in the modern era. *Indian J Med Res.* 2019;150(1):7–22. doi:10.4103/ijmr.IJMR_141_19
109. Wagoner MD, Ba-Abbad R, Al-Mohaimeed M, Al-Swailem S, Zimmerman MB; King Khaled Eye Specialist Hospital Corneal Transplant Study Group. Postoperative complications after primary adult optical penetrating keratoplasty: prevalence and impact on graft survival. *Cornea.* 2009;28(4):385–394. doi:10.1097/ICO.0b013e31818d3aef

Chapter 6
DIAGNOSES OF THE ANTERIOR CHAMBER, ANGLE STRUCTURES, AND CILIARY BODY

Chapter Outline

DOI: 10.1201/9781003255598-6

Anterior Chamber and Aqueous Humor

Review of Clinical Anatomy (See Also Chapter 8)

1. Boundaries
   a. Anterior: posterior cornea
   b. Posterior: front surface of iris and lens
   c. Peripheral: anterior chamber angle
2. Deepest portion is central (approximately 3 mm) and shallowest is periphery at iris insertion
3. Volume of aqueous is approximately 0.2 mL
4. Aqueous humor helps maintain intraocular pressure, and aids in metabolism of crystalline lens and nutrition of cornea
   a. Formed by secretion of ciliary processes and diffusion of nonpigmented epithelium
   b. Low in protein content
   c. Leaves eye through trabecular meshwork, canal of Schlemm, and into vortex veins at approximately 2 mL/min

I. Background Information on Uveitis[1–3]

A. Definition

1. Inflammation of all or part(s) of the uveal tract
2. Parts include iris, ciliary body, and choroid
3. Associated tissues, such as cornea, vitreous, and retina, may also be involved

B. Classification

1. Clinical
   a. Acute uveitis (versus chronic or recurrent uveitis)
      i. Important clinical management consideration
      ii. Sudden onset
      iii. Associated with moderate to severe pain
      iv. Expected duration of 6 to 12 weeks or less (with or without therapy)
   b. Chronic uveitis (versus acute or recurrent uveitis)
      i. Usually slow, insidious development
      ii. Usually lasting greater than 6 weeks (even with therapy)

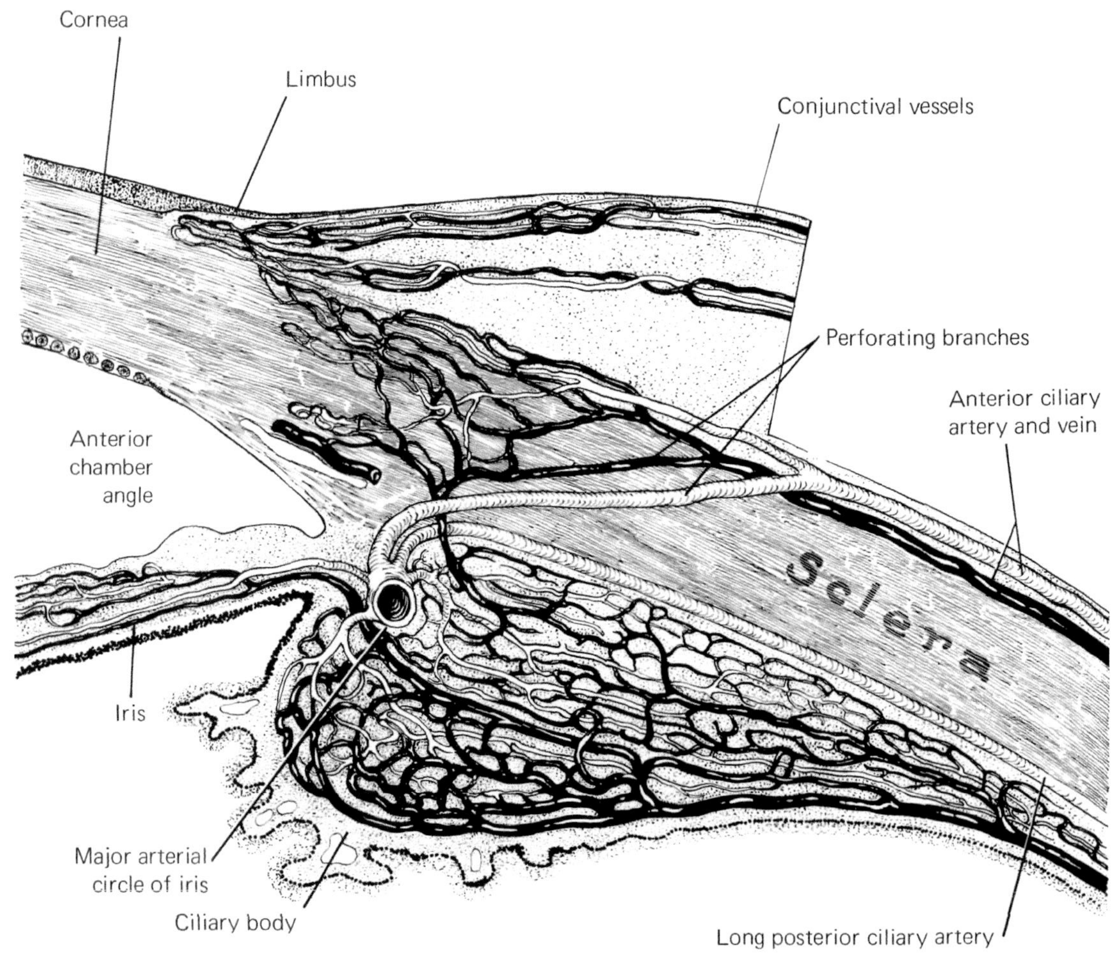

FIGURE 6.A Anterior chamber angle of the anterior segment.

ii. Usually unresponsive or poorly responsive to topical therapy, often to oral therapy as well
iii. Generally associated with posterior, disseminated, and granulomatous forms (see below)

c. Recurrent uveitis (versus acute or chronic)
i. First and second presentations (less than 6 to 12 weeks) considered acute
ii. Third (acute) presentation reclassifies condition as recurrent uveitis requiring complete medical evaluation
iii. Varies in response to topical and oral therapy
iv. Associated with all forms of uveitic syndromes

2. Anatomical classification
a. Anterior (main category considered in this chapter and most prevalent in clinical practice)
i. Iritis
- Inflammation of iris
- Usually acute
ii. Iridocyclitis
- Inflammation of iris and ciliary body
- Most common form of acute anterior uveitis
b. Intermediate or pars planitis
i. Also termed cyclitis or peripheral uveitis
ii. Inflammation of ciliary body or pars plana area
c. Posterior uveitis (almost always chronic)
d. Disseminated or diffuse uveitis (always chronic)

3. Pathological classification
a. Granulomatous
i. Tends to produce mutton fat keratic precipitates (KP) and iris nodules
ii. Frequently chronic, but could vary
b. Nongranulomatous
i. Usually acute but may be recurrent or chronic
ii. May produce fine KPs or none at all

C. Incidence and Prevalence of Uveitis (How Much?)

1. Generally stated at about 15 per 100,000 population

a. $\dfrac{\text{Drawing population}}{100{,}000} \times 15 =$ Potential number of uveitic cases in your community (a)

b. $\dfrac{\text{Number of active patient files}}{100{,}000} \times 15 =$ Potential number of active uveitic cases among your patients (b)

c. $\dfrac{\text{Number of active patient files}}{\text{Drawing population}} \times 100 =$ Your practice's % of community eyecare (c)

d. $([a] \times [c]) + b =$ Potential number of active uveitic presentations to your practice (d)

e. 80% of (d) = Approximate number of active uveitis cases among your patients

2. About 80% (12 of 15) are anterior uveitis
3. Calculations for primary eye care practices

D. Epidemiology and Demography (Who, When, and Where?)

1. Age distribution
a. Important clinical diagnostic consideration
b. Most prevalent from ages 20 to 50
c. Highly diagnostic in childhood and adolescence up to ages 15 to 20
d. Uncommon as primary diagnosis beyond age 70

2. Sex distribution
a. Greater in males due to trauma, ankylosing spondylitis, and Reiter's syndrome
b. Granulomatous type greater (two times) in females due to sarcoidosis
c. Childhood uveitis greater in females due to Still's disease (chronic juvenile idiopathic arthritis, greater in young girls)

3. Race
a. Related to uveitis syndromes
b. Caucasians have higher frequency of ankylosing spondylitis, reactive arthritis (Reiter's syndrome), and other HLA-B27 diseases
c. Black patients have a significantly higher rate of sarcoidosis (10 to 15 times greater) than general population
i. Especially Black females
ii. Especially in the southeastern United States
d. Asian patients have highest frequency of Vogt–Koyanagi–Harada syndrome and Behçet's syndrome
e. Mediterranean races have a higher frequency of Behçet's syndrome

4. Geography
a. Again, relative to uveitic-related diseases of a specific region
b. Always consider sarcoid in southeastern-American, Swedish, and Norwegian patients
i. Interestingly, sarcoid is not common (in any race) in the South Pacific
ii. Virtually nonexistent in South African Black patients
c. Vogt–Koyanagi–Harada syndrome and Behçet's syndrome most prevalent in Asian patients

5. Other factors
a. Increased frequency in "type A" (highstrung) personalities
i. Stress increases risk of uveitis
ii. Especially pars planitis
b. Hazardous occupations, sports, avocations increase risk of traumatic uveitis

E. Etiology

1. Exogenous (external) causes
a. Unknown (most common), over 50% idiopathic
b. Trauma
c. Ocular infection (e.g., syphilis, tuberculosis, Lyme disease, herpetic virus, etc.)
d. Allergic reactions

2. Endogenous (internal) causes
a. Unknown (most common)
b. Systemic diseases
c. Drug induced (e.g., Bisphonates for osteoporosis, Tumor necrosis factor-alpha inhibitors such as

etanercept and adalimumab used to treat rheumatoid arthritis, ankylosing spondylitis, inflammatory bowel disease, and psoriasis

d. Immunologic factors
   i. HLA-B27
      - Most common noninfectious etiology of anterior uveitis
      - Up to 50% of all acute and recurrent iritis cases

3. Anterior chamber associated immune deviation (AC AID)
   a. The very complex "immune-privileged" response involved with the iris and ciliary body
   b. Believed to be an evolutionary (teleologic) adaptation of the body to protect the eye from intraocular antigens
   c. Three elements involved
      i. Suppression (deviation) of T_{dh} (T_{regs}) cells of the delayed (type IV) hypersensitivity response (cell-mediated immune reaction) by special T-suppressor cells from the spleen
      ii. Preservation of humoral immunity (lymphokines) to stimulate B cell antibodies and cytotoxic T cell activity
      iii. Primed cytotoxic T cells (from spleen) induce cytotoxic immunity
   d. Potential benefits from ACAID ("values privilege")
      i. Delayed hypersensitivity (T_{dh} cell-mediated) reactions are destructive to the eye and difficult to control (e.g., chronic uveitis). Thus, their suppression (deviation) in the eye may be beneficial
      ii. The preserved antibodies and cytotoxic responses in ACAID provide forms of protection well tolerated by the eye
   e. Potential risks from ACAID (is "immune privilege" really a value?)
      i. Lack of delayed hypersensitivity leaves the eye vulnerable to pathogens that are generally eliminated by T_{dh} (T_{regs}) lymphocytes
         - Malignant cells
         - Herpes simplex virus
      ii. ACAID increases the potential for an "autoimmune cycle" associated with intraocular antigens (e.g., retinal S antigen)
4. More specific and extensive coverage of etiologies under "Assessment"

II. Primary Care of Acute Anterior Uveitis (AAU)[4–8] (See Also Chapter 8)

Subjective

- Presenting symptoms range from none to severe
  1. Range of symptoms is not necessarily directly proportional to severity of uveitis
  2. Many times, chronic granulomatous uveitis presents with little to no symptomatology
  3. Conversely, acute, or recurrent iridocyclitis (mild to moderate) may be excruciatingly painful and debilitating
- Pars planitis generally has little or no symptoms and must be diagnosed objectively
- However, anterior uveitis (iritis and iridocyclitis) has such clear-cut, predictable symptoms that the diagnosis can almost be made based on subjective symptomatology alone
- Classic symptom pattern
  1. A deep, boring pressure-type pain
     a. Usually reported as "in or behind" the eyeball
     b. Headache-type pain around the eye
     c. Patient denies or minimizes surface irritation, foreign-body sensation, burning, or itching
     d. Topical anesthetic does not relieve the pain
     e. Lid usually spasms or closes due to the pain
     f. When uveitis is associated with other conditions (e.g., trauma), try to elicit the "quality" of the pain (as well as quantity) to confirm uveitic component
  2. Photophobia ranges from mild to severe
     a. Patient may flinch slightly to bright light or may require lights to be diminished or put out because of pain
     b. Lid(s) may show increased blink rate, winking, or complete spastic closure
     c. More severe photophobia usually produces difficulty in slit-lamp examination especially during anterior chamber evaluation for cells and flare
  3. Vision is usually variable, depending on degree and type of uveitic presentation
     a. Ranges from normal to hazy in acute or recurrent anterior uveitis (AAU) and pars planitis
     b. Chronic uveitis usually produces more haziness and blurring of vision in spite of minimal discomfort (versus AAU)
     c. Increased discomfort with near (accommodation) vision often reported
  4. Hyperlacrimination ranges from watery sensation to glassy appearance to frank tearing and epiphora
     a. Important to note that no other form of discharge is associated with uveitis (pure inflammation)
     b. Important in differential diagnosis
     c. Any mucoid or purulent discharge should be considered a potential additional associated disease entity
- Beyond straightforward entering symptoms, the most important part of the uveitic workup is the subjective *history* and *risk factors*
  1. Age
     a. The key initial diagnostic milestone
     b. Narrows differential etiologies to highest risk possibilities of greatest frequency (Tables 6.1 and 6.2)
  2. Sex
     a. Further narrows high-risk possibilities between women and men
     b. Always compare risk factors in history
  3. Race
     a. Black patients have a distinct increased risk (10 times greater) for sarcoidosis (especially young females)
     b. Caucasian and Asian patients have varying predispositions to certain human leukocytic antigen (HLA) diseases
  4. Habitation
     a. Where does the patient live?
     b. Where was the patient born and raised?

TABLE 6.1 Risk Factors Associated with Anterior Uveitis Presentations by Age

	Less Than 20 Years Old		20 to 50 Years Old		Greater Than 50 Years Old	
Clinical Diagnosis	**Primary Care[a] (%)**	**Referral Clinics[b] (%)**	**Primary Care[a] (%)**	**Referral Clinics[b] (%)**	**Primary Care[a] (%)**	**Referral Clinics[b] (%)**
Unknown	~25	~40	>50	>35	>40	>30
Trauma	~50	—	~30	~10	~30	~10
Pars planitis	~20	~15	~10	>10	>1	<5
Sarcoidosis	<1	~4	~3	~3	—	<3
Adult rheumatoid arthritis	—	—	~2	~15	~15	>20
Juvenile ideopathic arthritis (JIA)	~1	~30	—	~2	—	—
Other human leukocytic antigen (HLA) dystrophy	—	~2	~2	~3	~1	<2
Fuchs' heterochromic iridocyclitis	~1	~6	~1	>10	~1	~2
Infection	~1	~2	~1	~10	~10	~18
Gastrointestinal disease	<1	<1	<1	~2	~2	~10

[a] Catania.
[b] Specialists.

TABLE 6.2 Rank Order by Age of Common Anterior Uveitis Etiologies

Age of Patient (yr)	Etiology	Rank Order of Primary Care Risk Factors
Less than 20	• Trauma	1
	• Unknown	2
	• Pars planitis	3
	• Infection	4
	• Juvenile idiopathic arthritis	5
	• Fuchs' heterochromic iridocyclitis	6
	• Sarcoidosis	7
	• Gastrointestinal disease	8
20 to 50	• Unknown Trauma	2
	• Pars planitis	3
	• Sarcoidosis	4
	• Human leukocytic antigen (HLA)	5
	• Infection	6
	• Fuchs' heterochromic iridocyclitis	7
	• Gastrointestinal disease	8
Greater than 50	• Unknown	1
	• Trauma	2
	• Human leukocytic antigen (HLA)	3
	• Infection	4
	• Gastrointestinal disease	5
	• Fuchs' heterochromic iridocyclitis	6
	• Pars planitis	7

5. Cohabitation
   a. Does patient live with someone?
   b. How long has patient lived with person(s)?
   c. Ocular and general health and well-being of cohabitants?
6. Sexual history
   a. Is patient sexually active?
   b. Any recent changes in sexual partners?
   c. Active or history of venereal disease?
   d. Exposure to any known venereal disease patients?
7. Personal history
   a. Diet
   b. Vocation
   c. Avocation
   d. Travel (risk of exposure to foreign disease)
   e. Medical and family history
   f. Active medications (or habitual drug use)
   g. Allergies or atopias
   h. Pets
8. Ocular history
   a. Disease, injury, or surgery (what and when?)
   b. Family history of ocular disease
   c. Previous uveitis (or history or symptoms of uveitis) as far back as the patient can recall (for recurrent possibilities)
9. Systemic disease
   a. Carefully assess direct or indirect possibilities of high-risk uveitic diseases or syndromes (see Table 6.8)
   b. Question patient for diagnosed history of such conditions or signs and symptoms of such conditions
10. Onset of current ocular signs and symptoms

a. As exact a starting point as possible
b. Consider duration as criteria for diagnosis of acute versus chronic uveitis

- Significant diagnostic indicators
  1. These include the most important differential diagnostic clinical criteria in uveitis (acute versus chronic versus recurrent)
     a. Onset, duration, and frequency
        i. Conditions lasting less than 12 weeks are usually acute
        ii. Conditions lasting greater than 6 to 12 weeks are usually chronic
        iii. More than two episodes (total, in either eye) constitutes recurrent uveitis
     b. Response to standard therapies
        i. Acute conditions will respond in 6 to 12 weeks or less
        ii. Most frequently, acute (and many recurrent) conditions will respond to topical medications alone
        iii. In a limited number of cases, oral medications may be required
     c. Recurrence
        i. Exacerbation on discontinuation of medication (after appropriate course) is indicative of potential chronicity and possible endogenous (systemic) cause
        ii. History of recurrent episodes separated by variable time intervals can occur unilaterally, bilaterally, or in alternating eyes
        iii. Clinical guidelines
           - Fewer than three recurrences with negative history and risk factors: assume acute
           - Three or more recurrences with or without positive history: assume recurrent uveitis
     d. Bilateral presentations
        i. Usually highly suggestive if endogenous and chronic uveitis response
        ii. Granulomatous bilateral uveitis is almost certainly systemically related
     e. Alternating eye recurrences
        i. Effectively, a combination of points c and d above
        ii. A history revealing uveitis in one eye followed by a recurrence in the opposite eye can be thought of as a "bilateral" condition
     f. Systemic history
        i. The presence of virtually any systemic diseases should be considered, confirmed, or ruled out as contributing to an ocular manifestation
        ii. Suspicious signs and symptoms of systemic disease should also be considered relative to an ocular manifestation
        iii. All systemic conditions directly associated with uveitis (with or without other "significant indicators") must be documented and considered in the differential diagnosis of a concomitant (or previous) uveitis (acute, chronic, or recurrent)

Objective

(See also Appendix 2)

- Visual acuity (VA)
  1. May remain as normal 20/20
  2. Moderate reduction: 20/25 to 20/60
  3. Severe reduction: 20/60 to 20/400
  4. Higher-risk reductions: less than 20/200
  5. Accommodation (near VA) usually moderately reduced and painful
  6. General "haziness" usually reported
- Eyelid signs (Figure 6.1)
  1. Blepharospasms
     a. Secondary to photophobia
     b. Unilateral uveitis can produce a bilateral response
  2. Congestion and edema
     a. Usually mild to moderate
     b. Erythema (redness) absent or mild
     c. Any pain on palpation is result of pressure on globe itself
  3. Pseudoptosis
- Conjunctiva
  1. Pink or purplish circumcorneal (perilimbal) flush
  2. Circumcorneal hyperemia (flush) usually produces a deep (scleral or episcleral) radiating vessel pattern (versus superficial, irregular conjunctivitis pattern), with injection decreasing further away from the limbus (versus conjunctivitis increasing superficial bulbar hyperemia towards the cul-de-sac) (Figures 6.2 and 6.3)
  3. Circumcorneal flush may be 360° or sectional (Figure 6.4)
     a. Usually never much less than 90°
     b. Any amount from 90° to 360° possible
  4. Cul-de-sacs in uveitis are white and quiet
- Cornea
  1. Epithelial edema
     a. Frequently present in acute presentations
     b. Microcystic edemas usually present in chronic (or advanced endothelial KP) cases
  2. Band keratopathy may develop in recurrent or advanced, chronic cases (e.g., Still's triad in JIA of uveitis, cataract, and band keratopathy)
  3. Stromal edema

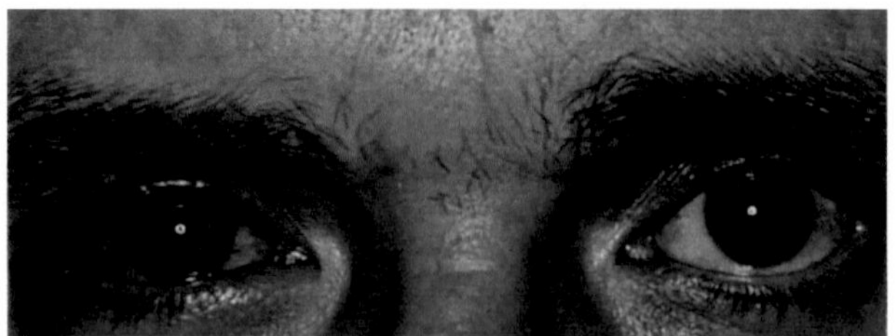

FIGURE 6.1 **Acute anterior uveitis (AAU)** gives a characteristic patient presentation of unilateral, subjective dull, aching ("headache-like") pain, and photophobia, with objective signs of pseudoptosis, circumcorneal flush, and hyperlacrimation.

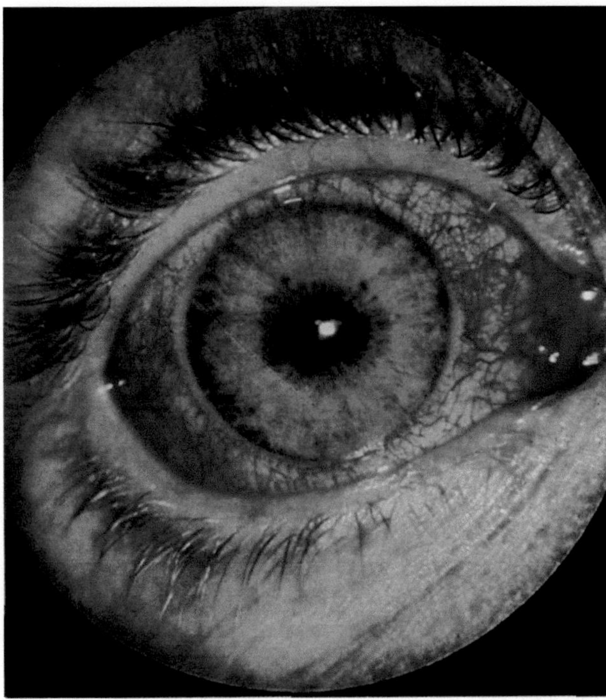

FIGURE 6.2 **Anterior uveitic inflammation** is characterized by superficial and deep, dilated vessels in a radiating pattern around the cornea (circumcorneal flush), with decreasing intensity away from the limbus versus conjunctivitis, which shows increasing superficial bulbar hyperemia towards the cul-de-sac. (See also Figure 6.3.)

   a. Present in acute (hot) presentations
   b. Present with dense KP
   c. Present in advanced and chronic cases
4. Striate keratitis
   a. Usually in advanced and chronic conditions
   b. Usually secondary to stromal edema
5. Keratic precipitates (KP)
   a. Fine
      i. Whitish-gray fibrin or epithelioid cells adherent to posterior cornea
      ii. Discrete small to medium-size dots (always less than 0.5 mm)
      iii. Apparent three-dimensional appearance (as if raised off posterior corneal surface)
      iv. Usually take days to form and weeks or months (or never) to disappear
      v. Old KPs usually flatten first and then disappear
   b. "Mutton fat" KP (Figure 6.5)
      i. Synonymous with chronic granulomatous types
      ii. Large, flat, confluent looking KP
      iii. Greasy, waxy, grainy-appearing surfaces
      iv. Accumulate pigment with age
      v. Usually do not disappear completely (as fine KP)
   c. Pigmented KP
      i. May be diffuse in AAU

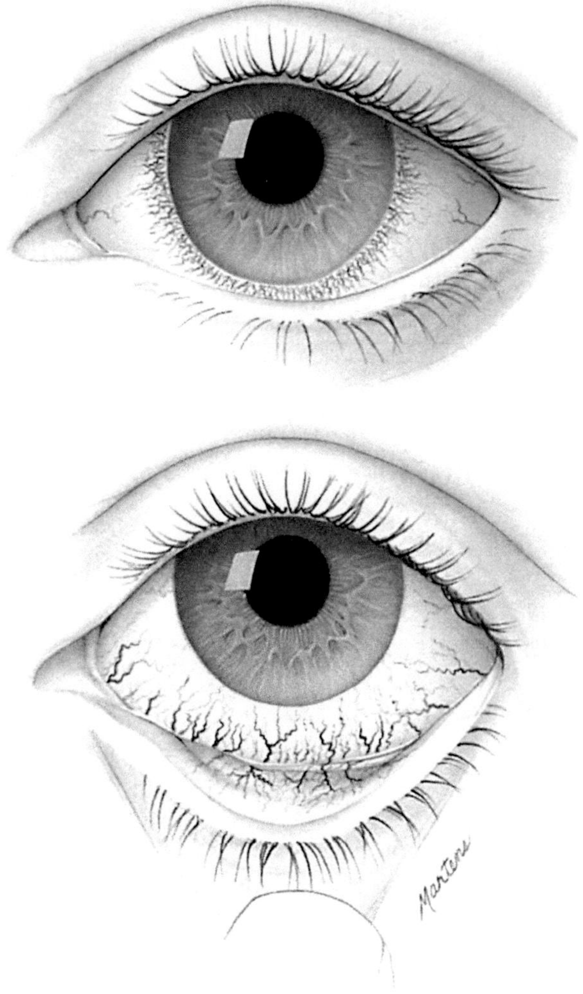

FIGURE 6.3 **Circumcorneal flush (above) versus bulbar conjunctival hyperemia (below).** Note the radiating circumcorneal appearance versus the random, irregular conjunctival pattern.

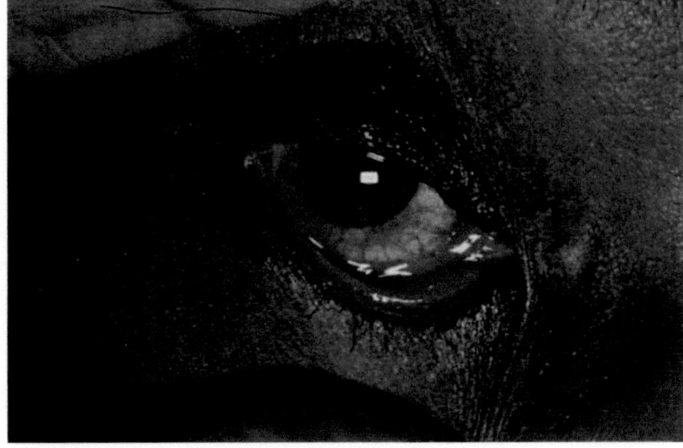

FIGURE 6.4 **Circumcorneal flush** in anterior uveitis may be 360° around the cornea or, as illustrated in this left eye, may be only partial with greatest involvement inferiorly and inferotemporally.

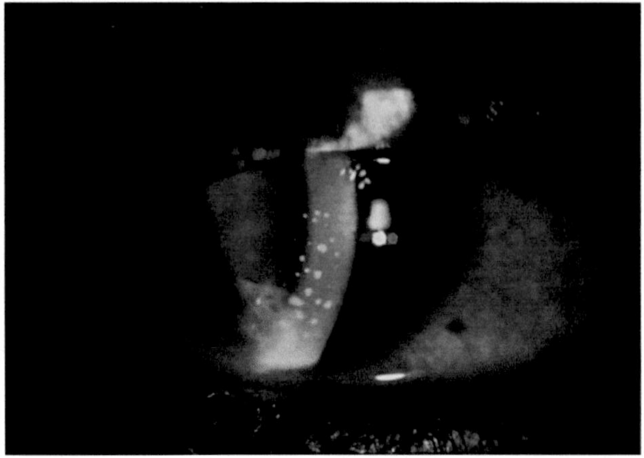

FIGURE 6.5 **Mutton fat keratic precipitates (KP)** are large, waxy accumulations on the posterior cornea of white blood cells and epithelioid cells present in the aqueous most commonly in chronic, granulomatous uveitis.

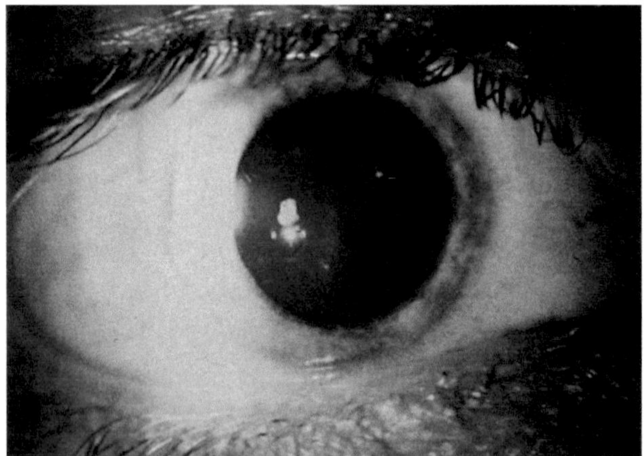

FIGURE 6.6 **Kruckenberg's spindle** is a vertically oriented accumulation ("spindle") of pigmented cells on the inferior half of the posterior corneal surface produced by upward convection currents in the aqueous humor. Prominent differential diagnostic considerations include recurrent uveitis and pigment dispersion syndrome.

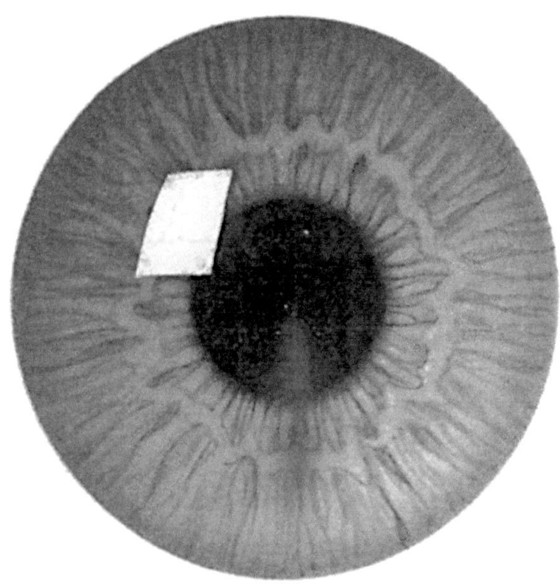

FIGURE 6.7 **Krukenberg's spindle** without visible base (Arlt's triangle; see also Figure 6.8).

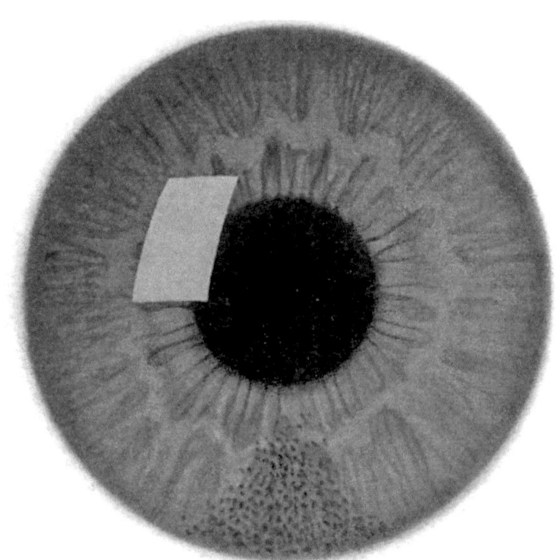

FIGURE 6.8 **Arlt's triangle** with wide inferior portion narrowing to superior apex created by upward convection currents in the anterior chamber aqueous.

- ii. Most often aqueous convection currents produce vertically oriented configurations called Krukenberg's spindle or Arlt's triangle (both with base down and apex up) on inferior posterior corneal surface (Figures 6.6 through 6.9)

6. Other endothelial changes (e.g., guttata) infrequent

- Anterior chamber
  1. Cells in the aqueous (classic uveitic sign; Figures 6.10 and 6.11)
     a. Usually white blood cells (WBC), abnormal in aqueous, leak from the ciliary body
     b. Red blood cells (RBC) or pigment cells may also be seen (less common than WBC)
     c. Usually move in slow upward direction
     d. Best viewing technique
        - i. Good slit lamp is essential
        - ii. Dark (black) room
        - iii. Dilated pupil makes ideal backdrop for best viewing
        - iv. Direct illumination with approximately 45° to 60° viewing angle
        - v. A 3- to 4-mm vertical beam at inferior cornea with small portion over iris and balance over pupil
        - vi. Beam width should be about 1 to 2 mm wide
        - vii. Focus beam first clearly on corneal surface
        - viii. With a "joystick," move back slowly to clear focus on anterior lens capsule

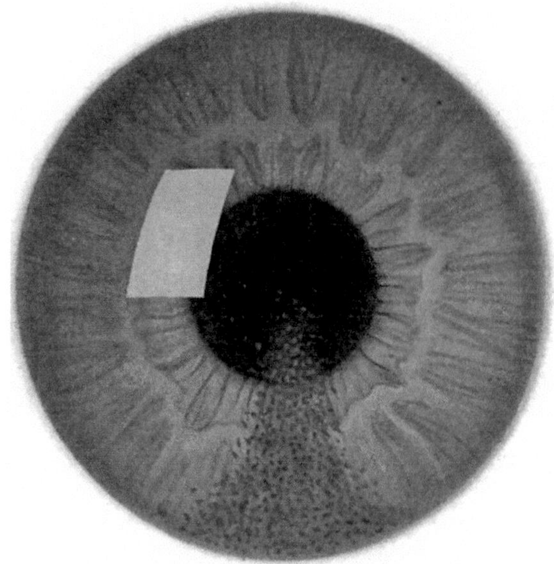

FIGURE 6.9 Arlt's triangle with Krukenberg's spindle found in recurrent or classic uveitis syndromes.

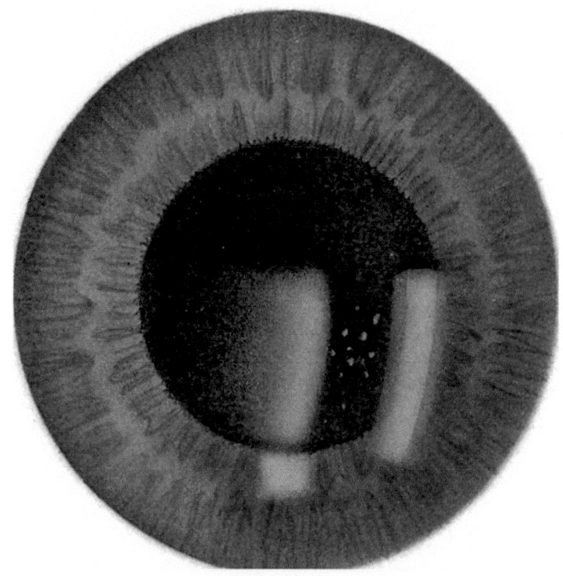

FIGURE 6.11 Aqueous cell (white blood cells) visible in the anterior chamber and graded (relatively) on a 1 to 4+ scale (see also Table 6.3).

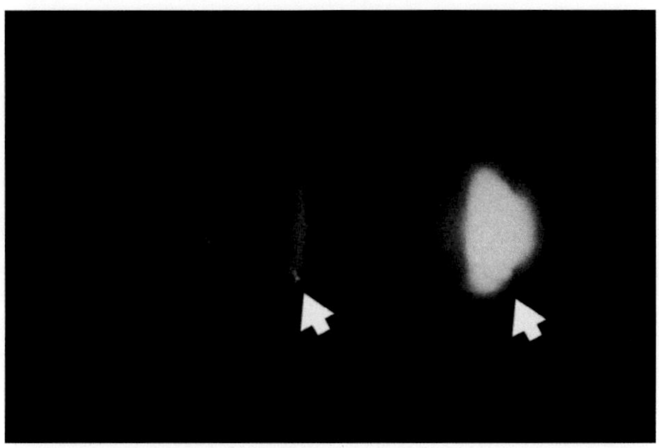

FIGURE 6.10 Cells and flare in the anterior chamber aqueous in anterior uveitis. The slit-lamp biomicroscope is focused on the turbid aqueous in the illuminated beam between the bright out-of-focus corneal image (right arrow) and the dull out-of-focus anterior crystalline lens surface (left arrow).

ix. Repeat refocusing from lens to cornea to lens two or three times to get feel of full distance of excursion with joystick
x. After two or three times, move only half-full distance from cornea to lens and hold
xi. Both cornea and lens capsule should be out of focus
xii. Optically "black" space between out of focus cornea and lens images will be clear, focus on aqueous
xiii. Concentrate your view on optically black space and watch for "cells" moving through field of view in a slow, upward (or irregular) motion
xiv. Compare lighter backdrop of iris with darker pupil backdrop for lighter and darker cells.

TABLE 6.3 Relative Grading of Cells[a]

Grade	Aqueous Finding
0–1+	1–5 cells in 30–60 sec
1–2+	5–10 cells in beam at once
2–3+	Cells scattered throughout beam
3–4+	Dense cells in beam

[a] In 2-mm-wide × 4-mm-high beam.

xv. Take at least 30 to 60 seconds or longer in suspect eyes (Table 6.3)

2. Flare in the aqueous (Figure 6.12)
   a. Caused by protein leaking from iris (triggered by prostaglandins)
   b. Produces an optically impure (versus black, clear) aqueous
   c. Slit-lamp examination procedure is same as described for cells
   d. Flare appears as turbidity or haziness in the aqueous
      i. Tyndall (Brownian movement) effect described in textbooks is difficult to appreciate
      ii. Best approach is to view many optically pure aqueous media first (in normal patients) and then flare will be comparatively obvious
      iii. Also, compare aqueous bilaterally in unilateral uveitis cases (for comparison)
   e. Flare is usually greater and more persistent in chronic granulomatous uveitis
      i. Often persists indefinitely
      ii. May also persist as "trace" flare in AAU (Table 6.4)
3. Hypopyon (endophthalmitis)
   a. Dense accumulation of WBC, usually polymorphonuclear cells (PMN), in severe acute uveitis

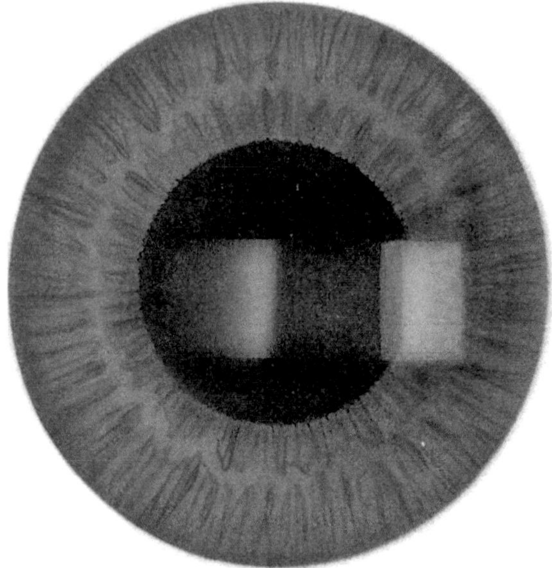

FIGURE 6.12 **Aqueous flare** (protein) visible in the anterior chamber and graded (relatively) on a 1 to 4+ scale (see also Table 6.4).

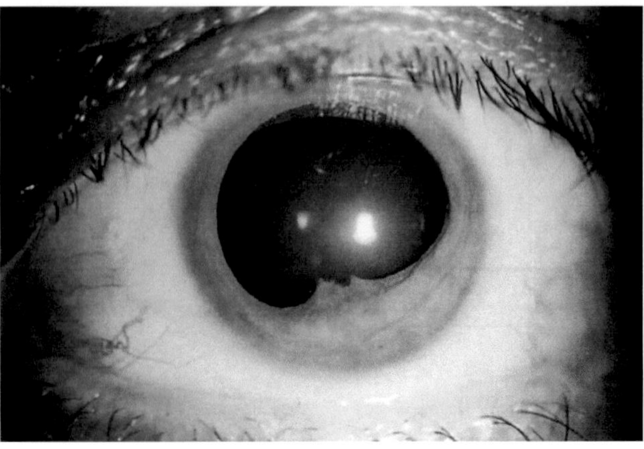

FIGURE 6.13 **Posterior synechiae** or fibrous adhesions of the pupil border or posterior iris to the anterior lens capsule. This case of adhesions at the inferior border of a dilated pupil in a patient with a history of recurrent anterior uveitis produces an irregular pupil shape (corectopia).

TABLE 6.4 **Relative Grading of Flare**[a]

Grade	Aqueous Finding
0–1+	Trace flare (by bilateral comparison)
1–2+	Obvious presence (by comparison)
2–3+	Hazy aqueous
3–4+	Dense haze or plasmoid aqueous

[a] In 2-mm-wide × 4-mm-high beam.

   b. Gravity produces inferior pooling and fluid level (straight top) in anterior chamber
   c. Make certain to rule out infectious keratitis or endophthalmitis (i.e., corneal ulcer synonymous with hypopyon)
4. Plasmoid aqueous (plastic iritis)
   a. Dense accumulation of flare or fibrin cells producing translucent to cloudy or opaque strands and sheets with small to large lumps (coagulates) of proteinous material in the anterior chamber
   b. Usually in severe acute uveitis and diabetic postop patients
   c. Cells move sluggishly (if at all) through thick cloudy aqueous
   d. Often associated with trauma
   e. Easily mistaken for lens material from assumed ruptured lens capsule (especially with history of blunt trauma)
5. Synechiae
   a. Anterior (peripheral)
      i. Fibrous adhesions between peripheral cornea and iris
      ii. Not as common as posterior synechiae
   b. Posterior (Figure 6.13)
      i. Fibrous adhesions between iris (usually at or just behind pupillary border or on posterior surface of iris surface) and anterior lens capsule
      ii. Form readily in heavy flare, chronic and recurrent AAU
      iii. May occur in conjunction with iris nodules
      iv. Sometimes mistaken for persistent pupillary membranes
         - Membranes come off collarette
         - Membranes are nonfibrous
      v. Seclusio pupillae (immobile pupil) is 360° posterior synechiae usually in chronic uveitis)

- Iris
  1. Atrophy in prolonged chronicity and certain specific recurrent forms (e.g., Fuchs' heterochromic iridocyclitis)
     a. Produces transillumination defects
     b. May produce decrease in iris pigment (Fuchs' heterochromic iridocyclitis)
  2. Granulomas
     a. Fleshy, whitish-pink, slightly vascularized mass
     b. Usually larger than other iris nodules
     c. Pupil border, anterior surface of iris or angle locations
     d. Nodules common in sarcoid (especially at angle location)
        i. Busacca nodules
           - Whitish-yellow lumps away from pupil border
           - Internal iris stroma
           - Always associated with granulomatous uveitis
        ii. Koeppe nodules
           - Most common nodule in uveitis
           - Round or oval solid tissue (cellular aggregates) masses
           - Located at pupil border in varying sizes
           - May accumulate pigmentation over time
  3. Swelling (or "boggy") iris
     a. Loss of iris crypt definition

b. Smooth velvety surface appearance
c. Usually associated with dense flare

- Pupil
  1. Reactions range from normal to sluggish
  2. Usually, but not always, miotic in acute presentations
  3. Frequent corectopia (irregular pupil shape, undilated or on dilation) secondary to posterior synechiae
  4. Fixed pupils may occur with advancing complications or chronicity
     a. Seclusio pupillae
     b. Iris bombe (seclusio with iris bowing anteriorly; see Figure 6.19)
     c. Secondary glaucomas
- Intraocular pressure (IOP)
  1. Usually reduced by 3 to 6 mm (as compared with contralateral eye) in early stages of acute presentations due to ciliary body hypotony (reduced aqueous production)
     a. Prolonged hypotony in chronic conditions could potentiate phthisis bulbi
     b. Chronic IOP below 5 mm Hg are at risk
  2. IOP may increase in untreated acute or chronic forms because of angle (trabecular) congestion reducing outflow (see also Glaucoma Chapter 8)
     a. Also consider iatrogenic, steroid-related increase in IOP
     b. Monitor IOP frequently
  3. Acute glaucoma (Posner–Schlossman syndrome or glaucomatocyclitic crisis; Figure 6.14)
     a. IOP increases to greater than 30 mm Hg
     b. Total congestion of trabecular meshwork due to inflammatory debris
  4. Chronic glaucoma
     a. High risk in prolonged uveitis
     b. Multiple-angle etiologies
     c. Seclusio pupillae
- Crystalline lens
  1. Epicapsular stars or pigment debris may occur in acute or chronic cases
     a. Frequently associated with posterior synechiae
     b. Clumps of pigment may persist

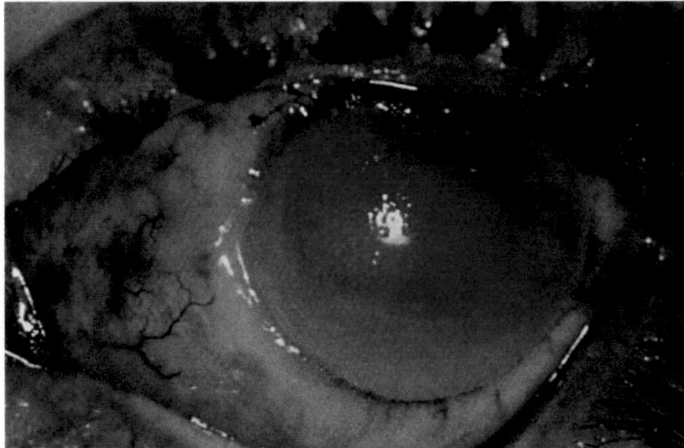

FIGURE 6.14 **Acute angle closure glaucoma** can mimic ("masquerade") as severe anterior uveitis with dense corneal edema. A definitive differentiating feature will always be intraocular pressure (IOP), that is significantly raised in acute angle closure glaucoma and reduced in anterior uveitis.

  2. Posterior subcapsular cataracts most common in prolonged recurrent and chronic endogenous forms
     a. May be associated with long-term steroids (oral or topical) in treatment
     b. Also associated with Fuchs' heterochromic recurrent iridocyclitis
  3. Mature cataracts usually limited to advanced rheumatoid cases (e.g., Still's disease)
- Vitreous
  1. Anterior and retrolental (Berger's) space
     a. Observable with direct slit-lamp illumination
     b. Cells appear adherent to vitreous strands (usually greater inferiorly)
     c. Strands may be broad and dense
  2. Posterior
     a. Must be viewed with Hruby, Goldman, or Volk 78 or 90D lens
     b. Involvement called vitritis and associated with posterior, chronic, endogenous uveitic syndromes
- Posterior globe (retina, choroid, optic nerve)
  1. Peripheral retinal involvements associated with intermediate uveitis or pars planitis ("snowballing" on pars plana)
  2. Posterior involvements are always diagnostic of advanced peripheral uveitis (pars planitis) or a chronic uveitic syndrome (Tables 6.5 and 6.8)

Assessment

(See also Appendix 3)

- Carefully examine subjective and objective presentations
- Rule out primary anterior segment ocular diseases and masquerade syndromes that mimic anterior uveitis (Table 6.6)
- Try "Henkind" test (easy, but not always accurate, i.e., beware of false-negative results)
  1. Occlude involved eye while shining light in contralateral (opposite) pupil
  2. Indirect (consensual) pupillary reflex should produce pain in occluded (involved) eye if uveitis present
- Consider significant indicators for acute versus recurrent versus chronic anterior uveitis
  1. Onset and duration (6 to 12 weeks or less = acute)
  2. Response to standard therapies (within 6 to 12 weeks = acute)
  3. Recurrences (2 = acute; 3 = recurrent potential)
  4. Unilateral and nongranulomatous = acute
  5. Bilateral = chronic potential
  6. Alternating eye recurrences (bilateral = recurrent or chronic)
  7. Granulomatous = chronic (probably)
  8. Systemic history (positive = chronic or recurrent potential) (Tables 6.7 and 6.8).
     a. Consider obvious categories
     b. Beware of "masquerade syndromes" (e.g., MS)
- Consider intermediate uveitis (pars planitis)
  1. Subjective
     a. Children and young adults (16 to 21)
     b. Gradual, insidious development
     c. May give history of previous anterior uveitis
  2. Objective
     a. Mild to moderate blurred vision

TABLE 6.5 Objective (Physical) Findings in Anterior Uveitis[a]

Clinical Classification	Objective (Physical) Findings	Acute and Recurrent	Chronic	Intermediate Uveitis (Pars Planitis)	Nongranulomatous	Granulomatous
Vision	20/20 (normal)	X		X	X	
	20/25 to 20/60	X		X	X	
	20/60 to 20/200		X			X
	Hiqh risk (<20/400)		X			X
	Painful accommodation	X			X	
Lids and conjunctiva	Blepharospasm	X			X	
	Lid congestion/edema	X			X	
	Circumcorneal flush	X	X		X	X
Cornea	Epithelial edema	X	X		X	X
	Band keratopathy		X			X
	Stromal edema/striae		X			X
	Fine keratitic precipitates	X			X	
	Pigmented keratitic precipitates	X	X		X	X
	Mutton fat keratitic precipitates		X			X
Anterior chamber	Cells and flare	X	X		X	X
	Hypopyon		X		X	X
	Plasmoid aqueous	X			X	
Iris	Posterior synechiae	X	X		X	X
	Iris atrophy		X		X	X
	Granulomas		X		X	X
	Busacca nodule		X			X
	Koeppe nodule		X		X	X
	Swelling		X			X
Pupil	Sluggish	X	X	X	X	X
	Miosis	X			X	
	Corectopia	X	X		X	X
	Fixed (nonreactive)		X		X	X
Intraocular pressure	Reduced	X			X	
	Chronic hypotony		X		X	X
	Increasing	X	X		X	X
	Acute glaucoma	X	X		X	X
	Chronic glaucoma		X	X	X	X
Lens	Capsule pigment	X	X		X	X
	Posterior subcapsular		X		X	X
	Mature cataract		X			X
Vitreous posterior chamber	Anterior vitreous cells			X		
	Posterior vitreous cells		X			X
	Peripheral retinal exudation			X		
	Posterior retinal involvement		X	X		X

[a] By clinical classification.

b. Mild to moderate photophobia
c. Vitreous floaters usually reported
d. Occasional exudates and/or peripheral anterior synechiae in anterior angle (viewed by gonioscopy)
e. Few cells visible in anterior chamber with moderate to abundant cells in the anterior vitreous
c. Fundus examination may reveal retinal edema, cystoid macula edema (CME), and retinal phlebitis
g. Most prominent posterior finding is inferior, inflammatory exudates over the pars plana region ("snowbanking")

3. Assessment
   a. Etiology unknown
   b. Rule out systemic causes (particularly sarcoidosis, Behçet's syndrome, and syphilis)
   c. Beware of "masquerade syndromes" (e.g., MS)
4. Plan
   (See "Plan" following and also Appendix 6)
   a. Mild: oral or depot steroids
   b. Moderate: oral or depot steroids
   c. Severe: vitrectomy, oral steroids (pulse dosages), or immunosuppressive drugs (e.g., cyclophosphamide, chlorambucil, cyclosporine, methotrexate)
5. Follow-up
   a. Course usually chronic and long term
   b. Prognosis on vision and resolution usually based on degree of involvement (lesser degree = better prognosis)
   c. Fluorescein angiography for retinal or macula complications
   d. Other complications include cataracts, glaucoma, and related inflammatory sequalae

TABLE 6.6 Differentiating Primary Anterior Segment Diseases from Anterior Uveitis

Condition	Common Findings	Compared with Anterior Uveitis
Conjunctivitis		
Subjective	• No pain	• Pain and photophobia
Objective	• Discharge • Hyperemia greater farther from limbus	• No discharge • Circumcorneal (perilimbal) flush
Episcleritis		
Subjective	• No photophobia	• Photophobia
Objective	• Hyperemic sector decreasing toward limbus • Clear chamber	• Hyperemic greatest at limbus • Cells and flare
Keratitis		
Subjective	• Superficial pain • Pain relieved with topical anesthetic	• Deep pain • No relief with topical anesthetic
Objective	• Corneal staining	• No direct corneal involvement
Scleritis		
Subjective	• General malaise	• No systemic symptoms (in acute form)
Objective	• Deep injection all the way to fornices (secondary uveitis common)	• Injection (circumcorneal) decreasing toward fornices
Acute glaucoma		
Subjective	• Sudden visual acuity decrease	• Insidious visual acuity reduction
Objective	• Increased intraocular pressure with corneal edema	• Decreased (acute) intraocular pressure with clear cornea
Masquerade syndromes		
Retinoblastoma	• Posterior lesion	• No posterior involvement
Leukemia	• Positive systemic and laboratory complete blood count	• No systemic involvement
Intraocular foreign body	• Contributory history	• Secondary
Malignant melanoma	• Posterior lesion	• No posterior involvement
Retinal detachment	• Fundus finding	• Secondary
Retinitis pigmentosa	• Fundus finding	• Secondary
Lymphoma	• Positive systemic and laboratory	• Secondary
Multiple sclerosis	• Neurological signs	• No neurological signs

[a] By selected subjective and objective findings.

TABLE 6.7 Summary of Subjective Symptoms and Objective Signs in Acute, Recurrent, and Chronic Anterior Uveitis

	Acute or Recurrent	Chronic
Subjective	• Usually moderate to severe	• Usually mild to moderate
	• Rapid onset	• Slow, insidious development
	• Mild to moderate haziness or visual acuity reduction	• Moderate to severe "haziness" or visual acuity reduction
	• Moderate to severe dull, aching pain, usually reported in or behind eye	• Mild to moderate pain response (sometimes no pain at all)
	• Distinctly photophobic	• Mild photophobia
	• Presentations <3 times (acute)/>2 times (recurrent)	• Remissions and exacerbations
	• Responsive to therapy in 6 to 12 weeks	• Poor response to therapy, usually >12 weeks
	• No systemic history (acute)	• Frequent systemic history
Objective	• Usually unilateral	• Bilateral or changing eyes
	• Lid congestion	• No lid involvement
	• Moderate circumcorneal flush	• Mild circumcorneal flush
	• Fine keratic precipitates	• Mutton fat keratic precipitates (granulomatous)
	• Cells and flare	• Cells and flare
	• Posterior synechiae (fresh)	• Dense synechiae (fibrous)
	• Occasional boggy iris	• Iris nodules and granulomas
	• Occasional miotic pupil	• Occasional fixed pupil
	• IOP reduced	• Frequent secondary glaucoma
	• No vitreoretinal complications	• Frequent vitreoretinal involvement
	• Minimal potential for complications	• Greater potential for complications

TABLE 6.8 Summary of Anterior Uveitis

	Age			Presentation						Etiology		Likely Gender		Laterality		Degree			Complication Potential		Prognosis		
Cause of Anterior Uveitis	<20	20–50	>50	Acute/ Recurrent	Chronic	Nongranulomatous	Granulomatous	Anterior	Posterior	Exogenous	Endogenous	Male	Female	Unilateral	Bilateral	Mild	Moderate	Severe	Low	High	Good	Guarded	Poor
Adult rheumatoid disease		X	X	X		X		X			X			X			X		X		X		
Ankylosing spondylitis		X		X		X		X			X	X			X		X	X	X		X		
Behçet's syndrome		X			X	X	X	X			X	X	(X)		X			X		X		X	
Crohn's disease		X			X	X		X			X	X			X		X		X		X		
Fuchs' heterochromic	X	X			X	X		X			X			X			X			X	X		
Glaucomatocy clitic		X	X	X		X		X		X				X			X	X		X		X	
Infectious disease				X		X		X		X				X		X	X		X		X		
Juvenile rheumatoid arthritis (JRA)	X				X	X		X			X		X		X			X		X			X
Juvenile xanthogranuloma (JXG)	X			X			X	X			X				X		X	X			X		
Keratouveitis		X	X	X		X		X		X				X			X				X		
Lens induced			X	X			X	X		X				X				X		X			X
Mononucleosis		X		X		X		X			X				X	X	X		X		X		
Pars planitis (intermediate uveitis)	X	X			X	X			X						X	X	X		X		X		
Reiter's syndrome		X		X		X		X			X	X			X		X		X		X		
Sarcoidosis		X			X		X	X	X		X				X		X	X		X		X	
Sclerouveitis			X	X		X		X		X				X				X		X			X
Subacute sclerosing panencephalitis	X			X		X		X			X			X			X	X		X		X	
Sympathetic ophthalmia					X		X	X	X		X				X			X		X		X	
Syphilis		X		X	X		X	X	X		X				X		X	X		X		X	
Trauma				X		X		X		X				X					X		X		
Tuberculosis		X			X		X	X	X		X				X		X		X			X	
Ulcerative colitis		X	X		X	X		X			X	X			X		X		X		X		
Unknown		X		X		X		X		X	X								X		X		
Vogt–Koyanagi–Harada syndrome		X			X	X	X	X	X		X				X	X	X			X		X	

- Consider major risk factors
  1. Age
  2. Race
  3. Sex
  4. Geographic considerations
  5. Other factors
- Consider risk factors by age of presenting patient (see Tables 6.1 and 6.2)
- Attempt to differentiate exogenous from endogenous causes
  1. Exogenous causes
     a. Unknown
     b. Trauma
     c. Infection
     d. Drug induced (toxic)
     e. Allergic response
     f. Keratitis (prostaglandins)
     g. Surgery
  2. Endogenous causes
     a. Unknown
     b. HLA antigens
     c. Sarcoidosis
     d. Granulomatous disease
     e. Infections
     f. Phacoantigenic
     g. Sympathetic ophthalmia
- Consider and compare all clinical signs and symptoms (subjective and objective), risk factors, epidemiology, and (most important) significant indicators, and assess the following:
  1. Anterior versus posterior (or disseminated)
  2. Acute versus chronic
     a. More or less than 6 to 12 weeks
     b. First, second, third (or greater) presentation(s)
  3. Granulomatous versus nongranulomatous
  4. Exogenous versus endogenous etiology
  5. Mild, moderate, or severe degree
  6. Risk of complications

a. Low
b. High
7. Prognosis
a. Good
b. Guarded
c. Poor

Plan: Acute Anterior Uveitis

(See also Appendices 4 and 6 and Tables 6.11 and 6.14)

Goals in treating anterior uveitis
1. Protect vision
2. Reduce tissue changes (e.g., KPs, cells, and flare)
3. Reduce scarring potential (e.g., synechiae)
4. Reduce pain
5. And "Above all, do no harm" (Hippocrates)
Always make sure that any known cause of a uveitic response is treated and managed in conjunction with the uveitis (the eye) itself

Therapeutic agents used for anterior uveitis
1. Topical agents (Table 6.9)
a. Mydriatic and cycloplegic agents
i. Avoid atropine due to pupil immobilization effect for prolonged period increasing risk of synechiae
ii. Conversely, atropine, may be useful in some situations and may be the only cycloplegic available at the pharmacy
• Intensely severe presentations
• Prolonged therapies
• Noncompliant patients
• Intense flare
iii. Homatropine 5% (difficult to get in United States)
iv. Cyclopentolate 0.5–2%
v. Scopolomine (no longer available in United States) may have a more positive effect on dark-skinned and Black patients
b. Anti-inflammatory agents and steroids
c. Antibiotics (when indicated)
2. Oral agents
a. Steroids (usually prednisone)
b. Nonsteroidal anti-inflammatory drugs (NSAIDs)
i. Aspirin
ii. Ibuprofen
iii. Naproxen
3. Other agents
a. Injectable (depot) steroids
b. Cytotoxic agents
c. Anticancer (immunosuppressive agents)

• Nontherapeutic therapies
1. Hot packs (for ciliary muscle spasm pain)
2. Dark glasses (for photophobia and dilation)
3. Temporary plus for near work (due to cycloplegia)
• Mild presentations (cells and flare: trace to 1+; no KP)
1. Therapy optional (depending on symptoms)
2. 1% tropicamide or 5% homatropine bid to tid
3. Oral ibuprofen (1200 to 1600 mg/day)
4. Cold packs q3–4h
5. RTC 48 hours, or PRN if worsening
6. Reassure patient
• Moderate presentations (cells and flare: 1 to 3+ and KPs)
1. 1% Cyclogyl (Cyclopentolate 1%) tid to qid or 1% atropine bid
2. 1% prednisolone q2–3h or Difluprednate 0.05% q4h
a. Use FML (fluorometholone) or 0.5% Loteprednol if there is a direct or family history of glaucoma
b. Always shake steroid suspensions thoroughly before use (and instruct patient on such)
2. Oral ibuprofen (1600 to 2400 mg/day; rule out contraindications)
3. Cold packs q3–4h
4. Dark glasses
5. Temporary plus for near work (optional for needs)
6. Counsel and advise patient carefully
a. Especially on nature, severity, and probable duration of pain
b. Explain medications
i. Their use
ii. Their side effects (near blur, dilation)

TABLE 6.9 Common Topical Agents Used in Anterior Uveitis Therapy

Generic Name	Sample Brand(s)	Concentration (%)	Duration	Potential Risks
Mydriatic/Cycloplegics				Angle closure (remote)
Atropine	Generics	0.5, 1, 2	7–14 days	Atropine toxicity
Cyclopentolate	Cyclogyl	0.5, 1, 2	6 to 12 hr	Angle closure (remote)
Phenylephrine	Generics	2.5, 10	4–8 hr	Cardiovascular (remote)
Tropicamide	Mydriacyl	0.5, 1	3–6 hr	Angle closure (remote)
Steroids			Dosage	Increased intraocular pressure, PSC, HSV
Dexamethasone	Generics	0.1	q 4 h for 1+ to 2+ AAU q 2 h for > 2+ AAU	Increased intraocular pressure, HSV, PSC (remote)
Difluprednate	Durezol	0.05	q 4 h for 1+ to 2+ AAU q 2–3 h for > 2+ AAU	Increased IOP, HSV, PSC (remote)
Fluorometholone	FML	0.1	q 4 h for 1+ to 2+ AAU q 2 h for > 2+ AAU	Increased IOP, HSV, PSC (remote)
Loteprednol	Lotemax, Inveltys	0.5, 1	q 2–3 h for 1+to 2+ AAU q 1–2 h for > 2+ AAU	Increased IOP (remote), HSV, PSC (remote)
Prednisolone	Pred Forte	1.0	q 2–3 h for 1+ to 2+ AAU	
	Omnipred	1.0	q 1–2 h for > 2+ AAU	Increased IOP, HSV, PSC (remote)

Abbreviations: PSC, posterior subcapsular cataract; HSV, herpes simplex virus.

TABLE 6.10 **Clinical Degree of Acute Anterior Uveitis**

Mild	Moderate	Severe
• Mild to moderate symptoms • Visual acuity 20/20 to 20/30 • Superficial circumcorneal flush • No keratic precipitates • Trace to 1+ cells and flare • Intraocular pressure reduced <4 mm Hg	• Moderate to severe symptoms • Visual acuity from 20/30 to 20/100 • Deep circumcorneal flush • Scattered keratic precipitates • 1–3+ cells and flare • Miotic, sluggish pupil • Mild posterior synechiae • Intraocular pressure reduced from 3–6 mm Hg • Mild iris swelling • Anterior vitreous cells	• Moderate to severe symptoms • Visual acuity ≤20/100 • Deep circumcorneal flush • Dense keratic precipitates 3–4+ cells and flare • Sluggish or fixed pupil • Posterior synechiae (fibrous) • Boggy iris (no crypts) • Raised intraocular pressure • Moderate to heavy anterior cells

TABLE 6.11 **Acute Anterior Uveitis: Treatment and Follow-Up**

A. Mild uveitic therapy
  1. Optional (depending on symptoms)
  2. 1% mydriacyl or 5% homatropine (bid to tid)
  3. Oral aspirin or ibuprofen
  4. Cold compresses
  5. Return to clinic 48 hr (or PRN if worsening)

B. Refer to nonophthalmological physician for systemic evaluation (with significant indicators)

C. Moderate uveitic therapy
  1. 1% Cyclogyl tid to qid
  2. 1% prednisolone q3–4h or Difluprednate 0.05% q4h
     a. Use fluorometholone (FML) or loteprednol if direct or family history of glaucoma
     b. Shake steroid suspensions well before using
  3. Oral aspirin (400 mg qid) or ibuprofen, (2 tabs q4h)
  4. Cold compresses
  5. Dark glasses
  6. Plus, for near (optional)
  7. Advise patient carefully (e.g., pain, course, compliance)
  8. Return to clinic 48 hr (or PRN if necessary)

D. Heavy uveitic therapy
  1. 1% Cyclogyl tid to qid
  2. 1% prednisolone q1 or q2h or Difluprednate 0.05% q2 to q3h
  3. Oral aspirin (400 mg q4h) or ibuprofen (2 tabs q3–4h)
  4. Cold compresses (q2–3h)
  5. Dark glasses
  6. Plus, for near (optional)
  7. Advise patient carefully
  8. Return to clinic 24 hr

E. Refer to ophthalmologist for possible depot or oral steroid therapy

F. Counsel, educate, advise patient regarding potential recurrent or chronic uveitis syndromes, and dismiss (PRN)

Note: Giving letter code to be used with Table 6.14.

    c. Discuss disease and its clinical course
  7. Return to clinic (RTC) in 48 hours
     a. PRN (or phone) after 24 hours, if symptoms worsen
     b. May get worse before getting better
     c. Should stabilize with medications within 48 to 72 hours

- Severe presentations (cells and flare >3+ with KPs)
  1. 5% homatropine or Cyclopentolate 1% tid to qid or 1% atropine bid-tid
  2. 1% prednisolone q1–2h or Difluprednate 0.05% q2–3h (see "Moderate Presentations" regarding Loteprednol)
  3. Oral ibuprofen (1600 to 2400 mg/day)
  4. Cold packs q2–3h
  5. Dark glasses
  6. Temporary plus for near work (optional for needs)
  7. Counsel and advise (see "moderate presentation")
  8. RTC 24 hours (Tables 6.10 and 6.11)
- Intermediate uveitis (pars planitis) presentations (see also Assessment)
  1. Mild to moderate presentations should be treated with oral or depot steroids
  2. Moderate to severe presentations usually produce posterior or disseminated uveitis and may require advanced therapies by skilled uveitic specialist and medical co-management
  3. No topical therapies are indicated in pars planitis
  4. RTC 3 to 5 days for reevaluation
  5. Often require long-term, low-grade chronic management care

Follow-Up (Table 6.12)

- Mild presentations
  1. RTC 48 hours (or PRN) is usually valuable

TABLE 6.12 Acute Anterior Uveitis: Follow-Up Protocol (by Degree of Presentation)

Mild Presentations
- 48 hr or PRN
- PRN if no medication provided
- Phone call valuable in PRN or no show
- If worsening, initiate or upgrade therapy

Moderate Presentations
- Compare subjective and objective findings at 48 hr
- Check intraocular pressure (for steroid responders)
- Should be no worse or better (count keratic precipitates)
- If worsening
  - Question compliance
  - Check dilation
  - Increase dosages
  - Return to clinic 24 hr
- If stabilizing
  - Continue medication for approximately 1 week, then taper steroids
  - Return to clinic 3–5 days
  - Return to clinic 3–5 days after medication discontinued

Severe Presentations
- Compare subjective and objective findings at 24 hr
- Check intraocular pressure (for steroid responders and secondary glaucomas)
- May be worse than initial presentation (count keratic precipitates)
- Continue all medication or increase steroids to q1h
- Reassure and reinstruct
- Return to clinic 24 hr
- If stabilizing return to clinic 48 hr
- If worsening after 3–5 days, depot or oral steroids may be indicated

    a. 48 hours RTC if medications provided
    b. PRN if mild or no medications prescribed
  2. If appointment scheduled, do not be surprised of "no show" (owing to complete resolution)
    a. Especially very mild cases
    b. Phone call follow-up is always appreciated
  3. If condition worsens, initiate, or increase therapy to "moderate presentation" level
- Moderate presentations
  1. On 48-hour return compare subjective and objective signs and check IOP for steroid responders
    a. If positive, discontinue (D/C) steroids; if ketone (e.g., prednisolone) based switch to ester (e.g., loteprednol) based
    b. Treat glaucoma, if no IOP reduction in 48 to 72 hours or if IOP greater than 30 mm Hg
  2. Uveitis should be no worse or better
    a. Sometimes it is difficult to assess change based on cells and flare alone
    b. Try quantifying (counting) KPs in given area on first visit and recount same area in follow-up (Figure 6.15)
      i. Increased count: uncontrolled condition
      ii. Stable count: controlled condition
  3. If condition is worsening
    a. Question compliance
    b. Check dilation
      i. May want to increase potency of dilator from shorter-acting to longer-acting drug (e.g., 1% tropicamide to 5% homatropine)
      ii. Also increase dosage (to q2–3h)
    c. Increase steroid dosage to q1–2h
    d. RTC 24 hours

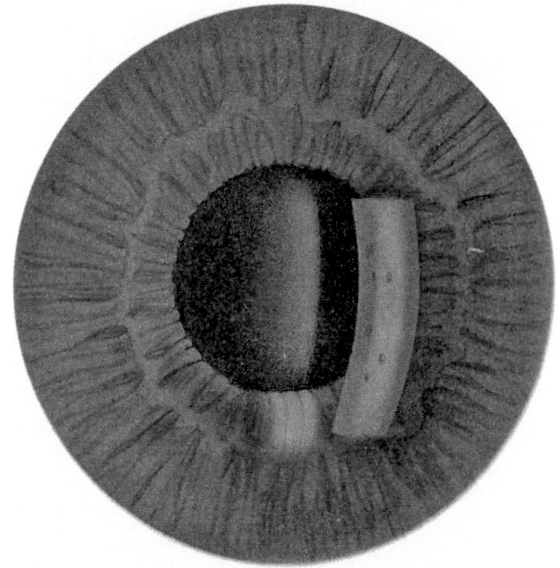

FIGURE 6.15 Keratic precipitates can be counted (six in this view) and used to monitor the progress of anterior uveitis. Beam size (height and width) and position on cornea must be kept constant at each visit for maximal accuracy.

  4. If condition is stable (usually the case)
    a. Continue all medications
      i. Never D/C steroids sooner than 7 to 10 days
      ii. Maintain dilation for 5 to 7 days (minimum)
    b. RTC 3 to 4 days (check IOP)

i. Dilation can be discontinued (tapering optional)
ii. Always taper steroids
- Use any gradual decrease, taking about 4 to 6 days or longer
- Suggest decreasing existing dose by one per day to zero
- Whatever, keep instructions simple

5. See patient once again about 3 to 5 days after all medications have been discontinued
6. Trace cells and flare may persist (sometimes indefinitely)

- Severe presentations
  1. On 24-hour return, compare findings from initial visit (check IOP)
  2. Flare and cells may often appear worse
  3. Count KP for baseline (see "Moderate Presentations" and Figure 6.15)
  4. If plasmoid aqueous developing (or more likely, still present from initial visit), increase steroids to every hour
  5. Otherwise, reassure patient (regarding pain and likely improvement), continue all medications, and RTC 24 hours
  6. On return visit, look for signs of stabilization
     a. Cells and flare holding
     b. KP count stable
     c. Any plasmoid aqueous dissolving
     d. Subjective pain diminishing
  7. Attempt to break any posterior synechiae with strong pupil dilators
     a. If synechiae unresponsive to dilation efforts (multiple dilators every 15 minutes for 1 to 2 hours), monitor patient closely during 6- to 12-week follow-up period
     b. Chronic synechiae increase the risk of follow-up complications (increased IOP, recurrences)
     c. YAG laser may be useful in breaking pupillary or peripheral synechiae
  8. RTC 48 hours on stabilization
  9. If condition is still progressive beyond 3 to 5 days, depot or oral steroids may be indicated
     a. Also, reassess your diagnosis at this point (e.g., acute versus chronic, exogenous versus endogenous)
     b. Consider co-management of oral steroid therapies with patient's primary physician
- Potential complications (Table 6.13)
  1. Steroid induced (iatrogenic)
     a. Increased IOP (steroid responders)
     b. Infectious reactions (especially HSV epithelial keratitis)
     c. Posterior subcapsular cataracts (with extended or oral steroids)
  2. Band keratopathy
  3. Intractable synechiae (e.g., seclusio pupillae: 360°)
  4. Secondary glaucomas
     a. Acute (Posner–Schlossman syndrome)
     b. Chronic
  5. Cataracts
  6. Chronic corneal edema
  7. Chronic KP formations
  8. Bullous keratopathy

TABLE 6.13 Anterior Uveitis: Complications

- Steroid induced (iatrogenic)
  - Increased intraocular pressure (steroid responder)
  - Infectious reactions (especially HSV epthelial keratitis)
  - Posterior subcapsular cataracts
- Band keratopathy
- Intractable synechiae (e.g., seclusio pupillae)
- Secondary glaucomas (e.g., Posner–Schlossman)
- Cataracts
- Chronic corneal edema
- Chronic keratic precipitates formations
- Bullous keratopathy
- Chronic cells and flare (anterior chamber and vitreous)
- Posterior involvements
- Optic nerve damage
- Phthisis bulbi

  9. Chronic cells and flare (anterior chamber or vitreous)
  10. Posterior changes
      a. Macula edema
      b. Retinal detachment
  11. Optic nerve damage
  12. Phthisis bulbi
- Prognosis
  1. Evaluation should be based on presentation and diagnosis) (Tables 6.8 and 6.14)
     a. Degree of presentation
     b. Acute versus chronic
     c. Nature of etiologic cause (if determined)
  2. Advise, educate, and counsel patient carefully

III. Chronic Anterior Uveitis[9]

A. General Considerations

1. Terminology
   a. Granulomatous
      i. Refers to small collections of modified macrophages or histiocytes surrounded by lymphocytes (giant cells)
      ii. Associated systemic granulomatous diseases
      - Tuberculosis
      - Sarcoidosis
      - Syphilis
      - Cat-scratch fever
      - Fungal infections

   b. Autoimmune
      i. Tissue injury associated with humoral or cell-mediated responses to body constituents
      ii. Hypersensitivity reactions are immune responses that injure the host by four types (Table 6.15; see also Chapter 2)

   c. Human leukocytic antigen (HLA)
      i. On the surface of nucleated cells
      ii. Important in tissue transplantation and diagnosis of certain diseases
      iii. More than 50 diseases are directly associated with a particular HLA antigen
      - HLA-B27
      - Ankylosing spondylitis
      - Reactive arthritis (Reiter's syndrome)
      - Crohn's disease

TABLE 6.14 Anterior Uveitis Management (by Age of Presentation)

Age at Presentation (yr)	Rate of Recurrence	Degree of Disease	Initial Therapy[a]	Follow-Up Care[a]: Response in Less Than 6 to 12 Weeks	Follow-Up Care[a]: Response in Greater Than 6 to 12 Weeks
Less than 20	First occurrence	• Mild	A	F	B[b]
		• Moderate	C	F	B[b]
		• Severe	D	F	B[b]
	Second occurrence	• Mild	A	F	B[b]
		• Moderate	C	F	B[b]
		• Severe	D	F	B[b]
	Third occurrence or significant indicators	• Mild	A, B[b]	—	—
		• Moderate	C, B[b]	—	—
		• Severe	D, B, E	—	—
From 20 to 50	First occurrence	• Mild	A	F	B[b]
		• Moderate	C	F	B[b]
		• Severe	D	F	B, E
	Second occurrence	• Mild	A	F	E
		• Moderate	C	F	E
		• Severe	D	F	B, E
	Third occurrence or significant indicators	• Mild	A, B	F[b]	E
		• Moderate	C, B[b]	—	—
		• Severe	C, B, E	—	—
Greater than 50	First occurrence	• Mild	A	F	B[b]
		• Moderate	C	F	B[b]
		• Severe	D	F	B, E
	Second occurrence	• Mild	A	F	B[b]
		• Moderate	C, B	F[b]	B[b]
		• Severe	D, B, E	—	—
	Third occurrence or significant indicators	• Mild	A, B	F[b]	B, E
		• Moderate	C, B[b]	F[b]	B, E
		• Severe	D, B, E	—	—

[a] Refer to Table 6.11 for letter code.
[b] Occurrence of any progressive ocular complications at this point indicates treatment E in Table 6.11.

TABLE 6.15 The Four Types of Hypersensitivity Reactions

Type	Manifestation	Immune Mechanism	Ocular Example
I	Immediate	IgE	Atopic iritis from allergy to shellfish
II	Cytotoxicity	IgG, IgM, ± complement	Microbial iritis involved in pathogenesis of uveitis
III	Immune complex	Igg, IgM, + complement	Autoimmune lens induced sympathetic ophthalmia
IV	Cell mediated	Sensitized T lymphocytes	Possible chronic uveitic relationship

[a] Traditional categories; see also Chapter 2.

- Ulcerative colitis
- HLA-B5
- Behçet's syndrome
- HLA-Dw4
- Rheumatoid arthritis

2. Specific diagnosis of cause
   a. Made in about 10% to 12% of all cases
   b. Therefore, therapy is specific for only 10% to 12% of cases
   c. Remaining (90%) therapy is empiric and general
3. Diagnostic workup for cause
   a. Expensive, with literally hundreds of tests available and payoff on most limited
   b. The more common causes of anterior uveitis make up most of the 10% to 12% definitive diagnosed cases
   c. Most anterior uveitis looks alike, irrespective of cause
4. Pathophysiology
   a. Prostaglandins
   b. Hypersensitivity reactions (immune responses)
   c. Human leukocytic antigens (HLA) related

B. Clinical Medicine (See Also Chapter 9)

1. Preliminary systemic evaluation by primary eye practitioner before referral for complete medical workup
2. Referral to physician for uveitic workup should be as specific as reasonably possible based on ocular impressions, suspicions, and preliminary systemic evaluation
   a. Consider patient's primary physician as potential coordinator of medical and laboratory workup

   b. Specialist may be consulted if no primary or family physician indicated by patient and preliminary systemic evaluation produces high index of suspicion in specific organ system or pathophysiological area (e.g., gastrointestinal, rheumatoid, infectious)
      i. Internist (internal medicine)
      ii. Rheumatologist

Subjective

- History most important part of evaluation
- Careful review of systems to elicit specific associated symptoms (including but not limited to)
  1. Joint problems
  2. Stiffness
  3. Lower back pain
  4. Past medical illnesses
  5. Family medical history
  6. Infectious conditions
  7. Urinary tract problems (e.g., infection)
  8. Trauma

Objective

- Slit-lamp examination and dilated fundus examination
- Blood tests
  1. Venereal Disease Research Laboratory (VDRL)
  2. Fluorescein treponema absorption (FTA-ABS)
  3. Complete blood count (CBC)
  4. WBC
  5. Electrolytes (increased calcium)
- Radiological studies
  1. Chest radiograph (x-ray)
  2. Tuberculosis
  3. Sarcoid
  4. Sacroiliac (S-1) joint film (for men)
- Skin tests: purified protein derivative (PPD)
- Other tests
  1. Angiotensin-converting enzyme (ACE)
  2. Antinuclear antigens (ANA)
  3. Biopsy of conjunctiva
  4. Enzyme-linked immunosorbent assay (ELISA)
  5. Fixation reaction
  6. Histoplasmin complement
  7. HLA typing
  8. Rheumatoid factor
  9. Sedimentation rate
  10. Toxoplasmin dye test
  11. Kveim test

Assessment

(See also Appendix 3)

- Chronic nongranulomatous
  1. Exogenous
     a. Trauma
        i. Sterile inflammation following penetrating injury from small foreign body with resultant decomposing tissue
        ii. Secondary to viral introduction at time of intraocular injury
     b. Postsurgical
  2. Endogenous
     a. Unknown (most frequent)
     b. Ocular
        i. Pars planitis (intermediate uveitis)
        ii. Fuchs' heterochromic iridocyclitis
        iii. Posner–Schlossman glaucomatocyclitic crisis
     c. Infection
        i. Herpes simplex
        ii. Herpes zoster
        iii. Rubeola
        iv. Subacute sclerosing panencephalitis (SSPE)
     d. Systemic
        i. Reactive arthritis (Reiter's syndrome)
        ii. Behçet's syndrome
        iii. Arthritides
        iv. Ankylosing spondylitis
        v. Juvenile idiopathic arthritis (JIA)
        vi. Regional enteritis (Crohn's disease)
        vii. Ulcerative colitis
        viii. Whipple's disease (extremely rare)
- Chronic granulomatous
  1. Infectious
     a. Tuberculosis (TB)
     b. Syphilis
     c. Leprosy
     d. Mycotic
     e. Parasitic
  2. Noninfectious
     a. Sarcoidosis
     b. Juvenile xanthogranuloma (JXG)
     c. Vogt–Koyanagi–Harada syndrome
     d. Sympathetic ophthalmitis
     e. Phacoanaphylactic

C. Specific Diseases

1. Ankylosing Spondylitis[5,10,11]

a. Pathophysiology
   i. Chronic proliferative inflammation of joint capsules and intervertebral ligaments
   ii. Arthritic syndrome
   iii. 25–35% will have acute anterior uveitis
b. Physical
   i. Limitation of motion of lumbar spine
   ii. Lower back pain with morning stiffness
   iii. Limitation of chest expansion (late in disease)
c. Radiology
   i. Calcification of sacroiliac joint (Figure 6.16)
   ii. "Bamboo spine"
d. Diagnosis
   i. History
   ii. Clinical examination
   iii. Males four times more frequent than females in severe forms
   iv. 80% HLA-B27 positive (10% in normal population)
e. Treatment
   i. Local steroid injection
   ii. Nonsteroidals
      - NSAIDs
      - Tumor necrosis factor inhibitors
      - Biologic immunosuppressants (e.g., secukinumab or ixekizumab)
      - Sulfasalazine
f. Ocular
   i. Related to duration of disease: 50% occur after 15 years of disease

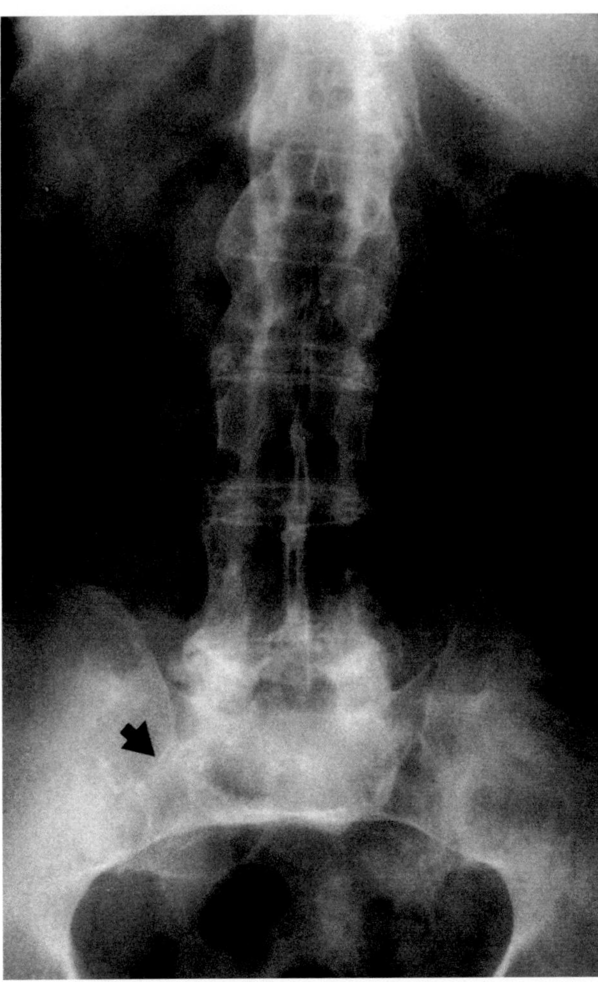

FIGURE 6.16 **Ankylosing spondylitis** is a rheumatoid disease causing chronic lower back pain as a result of bony ankylosis of the sacroiliac joints, best diagnosed by sacroiliac (SI) joint x-rays revealing ossification and calcification of the joint (arrow). This disease is a notorious cause of chronic and recurrent uveitis.

ii. Anterior uveitis usually unilateral

g. Course
   i. Mild cases often undiagnosed
   ii. Disease progressive in severe forms

2. *Behçet's Syndrome*[12]

a. Etiology
   i. Proposed viral etiology with many immunological features
   ii. Associated with HLA-B5, 70% of the time
b. Epidemiology
   i. Young adults
   ii. Greater in Asian patients
   iii. Women two times more frequent than men
c. Clinical
   i. Recurrent oral ulcerations (aphthous type)
   ii. Genital ulcerations
   iii. Uveitis and cutaneous vasculitis
   iv. Phlebitis
   v. Aneurysms
   vi. Meningoencephalitis
   vii. Synovitis
d. Diagnosis
   i. Recurrent oral aphthous ulcers plus any two additional associated signs (above)
e. Treatment
   i. Steroids
   ii. Immunosuppressives (e.g., Interferon alpha, adalimumab, or infliximab)
   iii. No treatment is curative
f. Course
   i. Often unrelenting
   ii. Visual prognosis is poor

3. *Crohn's Disease (Regional Enteritis)*[13–15]

a. Epidemiology
   i. Usually 20- to 30-year range
   ii. Males greater than females
b. Clinical
   i. Chronic diarrhea, abdominal pain, fever, malnourishment, fatigue, and weight loss
   ii. Relapsing granulomatous inflammatory disorder affecting any portion of gastrointestinal tract
   iii. Most common site is terminal ileum or colon
c. Diagnosis
   i. History
   ii. Imaging studies (e.g., colonoscopy, endoscopy, CT, MRI)
   iii. "String sign" on barium enema
   iv. Intestinal biopsy
   v. Must rule out ulcerative colitis
d. Treatment
   i. Enteral (liquid diet) and Parenteral (IV) nutrition used in conjunction with other therapies to ensure proper nutrition
   ii. Medical
      - Steroids used to treat flare-ups
      - Immunomodulators (e.g., thiopurines and methotrexate)
      - Biologics such as adalimumab (Humira), vedolizumab (Entyvio), ustekinumab (Stelara)
      - Azothriopine combined with anti-TNF alpha (e.g., infliximab)
   iii. Surgical
      - Resection of diseased section of tract
      - Significant percentage of patients require surgery
e. Ocular
   i. Symptomatic anterior uveitis in up to 17% of cases
   ii. Asymptomatic forms rare
f. Course
   i. Classically recurs and remits
   ii. Occasionally it remits permanently
   iii. Usually chronic and progressive
   iv. Complications
      - Metabolic disturbances
      - Hemorrhage
      - Perforation of tract
      - Adhesions
      - Peritonitis
      - Abscesses
      - Fistulas
   v. Unlike ulcerative colitis, Crohn's disease presents no increased risk for cancer

4. *Fuchs' Heterochromic Iridocyclitis*[16]

a. Etiology: possible inflammatory process involving rubella
b. Incidence: 2 to 3% of all uveitis
c. Clinical
  i. 90% unilateral
  ii. Asymptomatic, mild inflammatory syndrome
  iii. Floaters common presenting symptom
  iv. Syndrome
    - Recurrent chronic anterior uveitis
      – Fine KPs
      – Abnormal angle vessels
    - Heterochromia (loss of iris pigment) more noticeable with a light iris
    - Cataract
    - Glaucoma (occasionally)
e. Treatment
  i. Standard anterior uveitic therapy
  ii. Treat complications appropriately
  iii. Associated glaucomas are difficult to control

5. *Glaucomatocyclitic Crisis (Posner–Schlossman Syndrome)*[17]

a. Etiology: unknown
b. Clinical
  i. Recurrent chronic unilateral anterior uveitis with pain in young adults with markedly elevated IOP
  ii. Patients complain of halos around lights, blurred vision, and mild discomfort
c. Diagnosis
  i. Acute glaucoma
  ii. Open angles
  iii. Anterior chamber reaction
d. Treatment
  i. Topical treatment for uveitis
  ii. IOP control
e. Course
  i. Each episode can last for hours or months
  ii. Condition typically involves males 20 to 50 years old

6. *Juvenile Idiopathic Arthritis (JIA)*[18–20] *(Originally Juvenile Rheumatoid Arthritis)*

a. Epidemiology
  i. Children
  ii. Females four times greater than males
b. Pathophysiology
  i. Chronic synovial inflammation
  ii. Erosion of articular cartilage
c. Clinical
  i. Ocular involvement most common (30%) in mono- and oligoarticular types
  ii. Joints
    - Swollen, stiff, warm, and tender
    - Limited range of motion
  iii. Still's ocular triad
    - Iridocyclitis
      – Acute or chronic
      – Symptomatic or asymptomatic
    - 70% of patients reduce to 20/200 over 10 to 20 years with disease
    - Eyes often remain white
      – Band keratopathy
      – Uveitis
      – Cataract
d. Diagnosis
  i. No specific test available
  ii. Some non-specific tests
    - Rheumatoid factor
    - ANA
    - HLA typing
  iii. Rule out joint infection, malignancy, trauma, and avascular necrosis
  iv. Should have minimum of 6 weeks of chronic observed synovitis
e. Treatment
  i. Standard therapy for uveitis
  ii. If long-term topical steroids needed for inflammation control consider switching to systemic methotrexate or TNF alpha inhibitors (e.g., adalimumab and infliximab) to reduce steroid ocular side effects
  iii. NSAIDs, disease modifying antirheumatic drugs (DMARDs), and/or biologics for arthritis
f. Course
  i. Arthritis prognosis is guarded
  ii. Ocular prognosis is poor

7. *Juvenile Xanthogranuloma (JXG)*[21]

a. Etiology: unknown
b. Clinical: dermatological disease in children
c. Diagnosis: biopsy
d. Ocular
  i. Anterior uveitis
  ii. Iris nodule
  iii. Glaucoma
  iv. Spontaneous hyphema
e. Treatment
  i. Standard and supportive uveitic therapies
  ii. Monitor for secondary glaucoma

8. *Intermediate Uveitis (Pars Planitis)*[22,23]

a. Etiology: unknown
b. Incidence
  i. 10% of all uveitis
  ii. 70% bilateral
c. Clinical
  i. Minimal symptoms such as floaters, blurry vision
  ii. Vitreous cells and opacities (anteriorly, behind crystalline lens)
  iii. Inflammatory cells can spill over into anterior chamber
  iv. "Snowballs" → larger inflammatory collections
  v. "Snowbanking" → white exudates on the inferior pars plana
  vi. Possibly cystoid macula edema
  vii. Vision may reduce to 20/40 or less
d. Treatment (see also "Acute Uveitis, Plan")
  i. Standard topical therapy rarely useful
  ii. Periocular (subtenon)/intraocular and/or oral steroids
  iii. Immunomodulatory agents (e.g., methotrexate, azathioprine, and cyclosporine)
  iv. Anti-tumor necrosis factor agents or biologicals
  v. Cryotherapy or indirect laser photocoagulation to the peripheral retina can be done.
  vi. Par plana vitrectomy
e. Course
  i. Can remit and exacerbate
  ii. Severe cases can be unrelenting

9. *Reactive Arthritis (Reiter's Syndrome)*[24]

a. Etiology → autoimmune reaction triggered by infection
   i. Enteritis or urethritis symptoms precedes arthritis by 3 days to 6 weeks
   ii. Post-venereal exposure usually chlamydia
   iii. Post-dysentery cause is Shigella, Salmonella, and Campylobacter
b. Clinical
   i. Triad (syndrome)—majority of patients do not present with classic triad
      - Arthritis (usually monoarticulate, especially knee and ankle)
      - Urethritis
      - Conjunctivitis
   ii. Other findings
      - Anterior uveitis
      - Genitourinary (e.g., nongonococcal urethritis, cervicitis, prostatitis, circinate balanitis)
      - Mucosa and skin (e.g., nail dystrophy, oral ulcers, keratodermic blenorrhygicum)
c. Diagnosis
   i. Any two of the triad warrant presumptive diagnosis for syndrome
   ii. Anterior uveitis usually present
d. Ocular
   i. Conjunctivitis or uveitis present in at least 30% of syndrome
   ii. Conjunctivitis may be mild and self-limiting or severe with secondary inflammatory iridocyclitis
   iii. Cataracts and cystoid macular edema complications
e. Treatment
   i. Oral antimicrobial treatment with active infection
   ii. NSAIDs
   iii. Disease-modifying antirheumatic drugs (DMARDs), methotrexate, and biologics if no response to NSAIDs
f. Course
   i. Usually prolonged course of remissions and exacerbations
   ii. Occasionally resolves spontaneously

10. *Rheumatoid Arthritis*

a. Incidence of anterior uveitis in patients with rheumatoid arthritis (RA) parallels that of the general population
b. Uveitis not considered a specific part of disease

11. *Sarcoidosis*[25,26]

a. Etiology: unknown
b. Ocular epidemiology
   i. Peaks between 20 to 30 and 50 to 60 years of age
   ii. More likely to present in African Americans than Caucasians
c. Clinical
   i. Multisystem disorder
   ii. Granulomatous disease
   iii. Noncaseating epithelioid tubercles
   iv. Pulmonary node(s) most common
d. Diagnosis (Figure 6.17)
   i. Diagnosis of exclusion
   ii. Lymph node (or tissue) biopsy (e.g., conjunctiva)
   iii. Kviem test: granulomatous response to an intradermal injection of a suspension of sarcoid tissue extract in individuals with sarcoidosis.

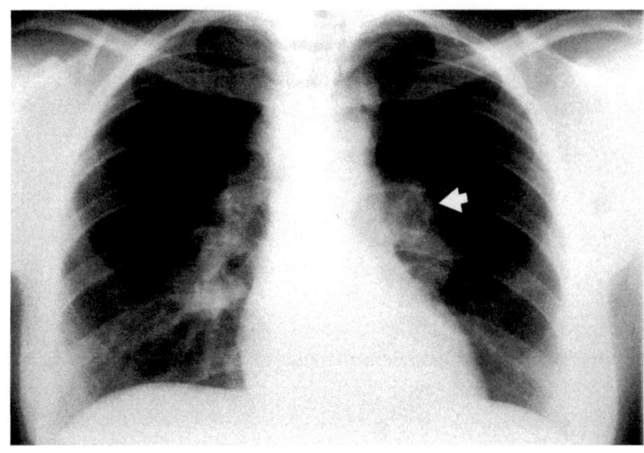

FIGURE 6.17 **Sarcoidosis** is a granulomatous disease of unknown etiology, with its greatest incidence in young Black females, in the southeastern gulf states in the United States, and in Sweden. It can be diagnosed by chest x-ray (hilar adenopathy, at arrow) and recurrent or chronic uveitis.

   iv. Hilar (lung) adenopathy on chest radiograph
e. Ocular
   i. Any part (anterior to posterior) of eye or adnexa may be involved
      - Most common ocular manifestations are uveitis, dry eye (keratoconjunctivitis sicca), and conjunctival nodules (granulomas)
      - If multiple ocular sites are involved, sarcoid consideration should be high
   ii. Ocular involvement from 25% to 50% of cases
f. Treatment
   i. Nonsteroidals
   ii. Steroids
   iii. Systemic immunosuppressants and biologics
g. Course
   i. Highly variable
   ii. If only benign hilar adenopathy, 80% remission rate

12. *Syphilis*[27–30]

a. Etiology
   i. *Treponema pallidium* infection
   ii. Congenital or acquired
b. Clinical
   i. "Great mimicker" (highly variable signs and symptoms imitating many different disease conditions)
   ii. Acquired and congenital
   iii. Primary, secondary, and tertiary involvement
c. Diagnosis
   i. Clinical suspicion
   ii. Mostly men
   iii. Diagnostic tests
      - Direct detection methods
         - Polymerase Chain Reaction (PCR)
         - Darkfield Microscopy
         - Direct Fluorescent Antibody Testing
      - Serological (Blood) Tests
         - First Test for treponemal specific antibodies
            - FTA-ABS and Enzyme immunoassays
            - If positive (indicates a recent or remote infection), proceed to Second Test

- Second Test for nontreponemal antibodies (to confirm active infection)
  - Reactive rapid plasma reagin (RPR) and VDRL

iv. Hutchinson's triad
- Leucitic interstitial keratitis (90% of all interstitial keratitis)
- Notched and enamel hypoplasia of incisor teeth
- Eighth nerve deafness

v. May have flattened nasal bridge

d. Ocular
i. Any part (anterior to posterior) of eye or adnexa may be involved
ii. Anterior or posterior uveitis
- Posterior uveitis and panuveitis are the most common

iii. Interstitial keratitis
iv. Argyll Robertson pupil
v. Chorioretinitis ("salt and pepper fundus")

e. Treatment
i. Intramuscular penicillin or oral doxycycline (if allergic)
ii. Steroids (oral and topical) for uveitis and interstitial keratitis

f. Course
i. Progressive, if it is not medically treated
ii. Often produces permanent damage and (if not treated) death

13. *Tuberculosis (TB)*[31]

a. Etiology
i. Mycobacterium tuberculosis infection
ii. Granulomatous disease

b. Clinical
i. Only 10% of infected patients are symptomatic
ii. New infections most prevalent in developing countries
iii. Leading cause of infectious morbidity and mortality worldwide

c. Diagnosis
i. Chest radiography
ii. PPD (Tuberculin skin testing)
iii. Interferon-release gamma assay

d. Ocular
i. Any part (anterior to posterior) of eye or adnexa may be involved
ii. Anterior, intermediate, posterior uveitis (posterior most frequent), panuveitis
iii. Ocular TB may be present without signs of pulmonary TB
iv. Unsure if ocular TB due to direct infection or hypersensitivity reaction

e. Systemic treatment
i. Isoniazid
ii. Ethambutol
iii. Rifampin
iv. Pyrazinamide

14. *Ulcerative Colitis*[32–34]

a. Epidemiology
i. Equal frequency in males and females
ii. Greater in white patients than Black patients
iii. Familial incidence is 15%

b. Clinical
i. Abdominal discomfort, cramping, increased frequency of bowel movements and bloody diarrhea
ii. Inflammatory disease of mucosa and submucosa of the colon
iii. Frequent relapses
iv. Recurrence risk always present

c. Diagnosis
i. History
ii. Endoscopy, colonoscopy, sigmoidoscopy
iii. CT, MRI, x-rays
iv. Blood and stool studies
v. Differential considerations
- Dysentery
- Crohn's disease
- Diverticulitis
- Cancer of the colon

d. Ocular
i. Episcleritis, scleritis, and uveitis most common ocular manifestations
ii. Patients with accompanying arthritis have a much higher incidence of anterior uveitis

e. Treatment
i. Aminosalicylates (e.g., mesalamine) used for mild to moderate disease
ii. Steroids for flare-ups
iii. Immunosuppressants and biologics for moderate to severe disease
iv. Colon resection for cases not responding to medical treatment

f. Complication
i. Chronic exacerbations
ii. Colon cancer expected in 10% of patients with disease for 10 years or more

D. Systemic Management Considerations

(See also Appendix 6)

1. Immediate considerations in chronic anterior uveitis
   a. Ongoing suspicion of cause
   b. Early recognition of complications
   c. Management and co-management
      i. Reinstitution of uveitic therapies
      ii. Preliminary systemic evaluation
      iii. Referral to appropriate ophthalmic or medical specialist for more extensive diagnostic evaluation
2. Long-term management considerations for the primary eye practitioner in management of chronic anterior uveitis
   a. Continued monitoring and recognition of exacerbation
   b. Prevention and maintenance of controllable and treatable complications
   c. Close monitoring and maintenance of visual needs
   d. Continued coordination of care with specialists
3. Management responsibilities of co-managing ophthalmic or medical specialist(s)
   a. Ongoing monitoring of systemic condition and any potential complications
   b. Management of immunosuppressive therapies and associated risks and complications
   c. Continued communication with patient's primary eye care practitioner

Anterior Chamber Angle Structures (Anterior to Posterior), Iris, Ciliary Body, and Crystalline Lens

Review of Clinical Anatomy (See Also Glaucoma Chapter 8)

1. Anterior chamber angle structures and ciliary body
   a. Schwalbe's line is a demarcation line between posterior cornea (Descemet's membrane) and trabecular meshwork
   b. Trabecular meshwork encircles the anterior chamber
      i. Composed of uveal and corneoscleral portion
      ii. Filters aqueous humor en route to the canal of Schlemm
      iii. Innervated by sympathetic and parasympathetic fibers of the autonomic nervous system and from trigeminal nerve (cranial nerve V)
   c. Canal of Schlemm is a channel within the trabecular meshwork
      i. Connects with venous system through 25 to 30 collector channels anastomosing in deep scleral plexus
      ii. Drains aqueous into anterior ciliary and episcleral veins
   d. Scleral spur attaches sclera to ciliary muscle
   e. Ciliary body extends from scleral spur to ora serrata
      i. Uveal portion adjacent to sclera includes
         - Suprachoroid (lamina fusca)
         - Ciliary (smooth) muscle innervated by short ciliary branches of inferior division of cranial nerve III
           – Longitudinal fibers (Brucke muscle) to open canal of Schlemm
           – Circular fibers to relax zonules (accommodation)
           – Radial fibers (continuous with circular fibers)
           – Blood vessel layer contains major arterial circle
         - Connective tissue splitting Bruch's membrane (lamina basalis choroideae)
      ii. Epithelial portion adjacent to the posterior chamber includes
         - Pars plicata (corona ciliaris) or ciliary processes of fingers of tissue covered by nonpigmented epithelium continuous with sensory retina
         - Pars plana (orbicularis ciliaris) adjacent to retina terminating in a toothed, scalloped margin (ora serata) with corresponding connections to each ciliary process
           – Aqueous humor and hyaluronic acid secreted by processes through epithelium to posterior chamber
           – Flows out of posterior chamber through zonules and pupil into anterior chamber
           – Small amounts flow into vitreous chamber
      iii. Nerve supply

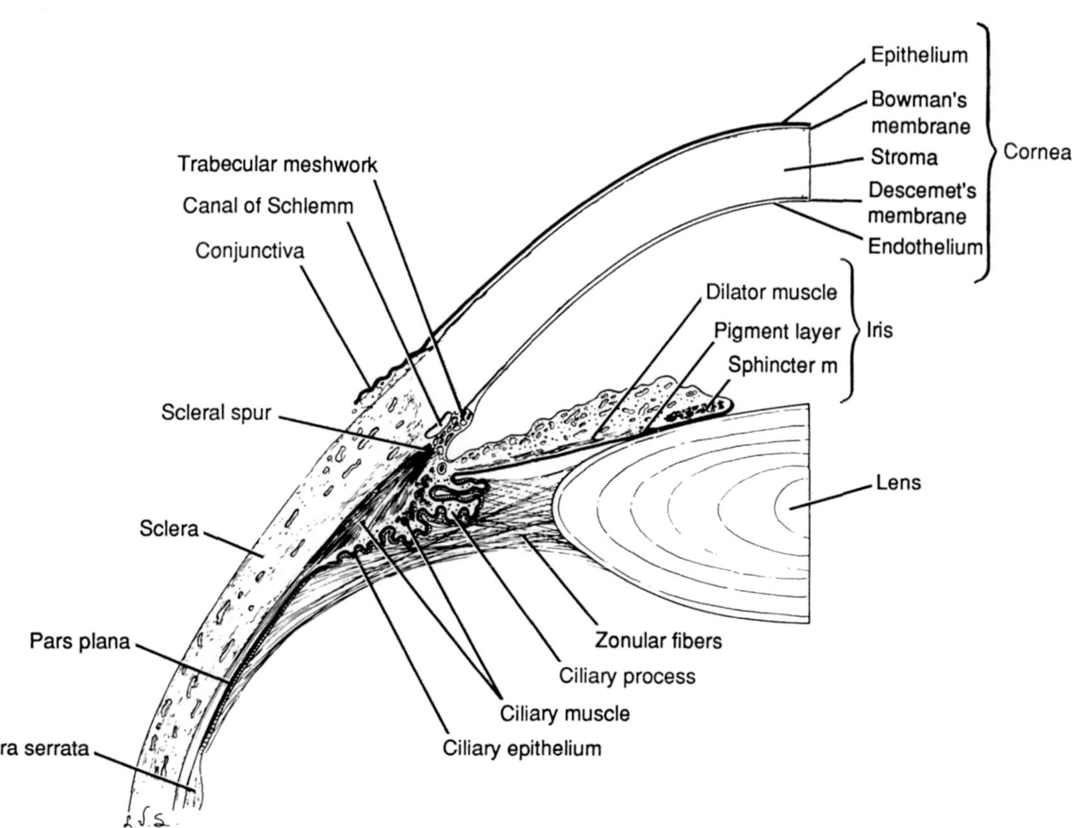

FIGURE 6.B The anatomy of the anterior chamber angle and surrounding structures.

- Motor supply to ciliary muscle from oculomotor (cranial nerve III)
- Postganglionic parasympathetic fibers synapse in ciliary ganglion and distributed by short ciliary nerves

2. Iris
   a. Structural characteristics
      i. Anterior most part of uveal tract of middle tunic (choroid, ciliary body, iris)
      ii. Central opening (pupil) slightly nasal to anterior
      iii. Inserts at base of ciliary body and rests on the lens
      iv. Central, pupillary zone and peripheral, ciliary zone joined by minor vascular circle with the pupillary zone relatively flat and ciliary zone marked with radial ridges (crypts)
      v. Two layers
         - Anterior and posterior stroma
           – Anterior contains radiating vessels from major arterial circle of iris and enmeshed chromatophores (melanin) within collagen fibrils
           – Posterior contains more elastic fibers and less chromatophores and blood vessels
         - Iris pigmented epithelium with two layers of cells
           – Anterior layer intermingles with dilator pupillae muscle (absent in radial sphincter region)
           – Posterior layer cells covered (on lenticular side) with basement membrane continuous with ciliary body; may also produce a pigment frill around pupil; rich in melanin
      vi. Muscles
         - Sphincter pupillae (smooth) muscle in pupillary zone of iris stroma around pupil
         - Dilator (smooth) muscle located between stroma and posterior layer of iris pigmented epithelium extending from ciliary body to sphincter muscle
   b. Nerve supply
      i. Motor supply
         - Dilator muscle innervated by sympathetic fibers of long ciliary nerves
         - Sphincter muscle innervated by parasympathetic fibers of oculomotor (cranial nerve III) that synapse in the ciliary ganglion and distribute with short ciliary nerves
         - Sympathetics to iris arteries carried through short ciliary nerves
      ii. Sensory innervation supplied by short and long ciliary nerves
   c. Vascular supply
      1. Radial vessels in the stromal layer created by two long posterior ciliary arteries and seven anterior ciliary arteries from the major arterial circle in the ciliary body
      ii. Vessels radiate towards pupillary margin and anastomose at the collarette minor vascular circle of the iris
      iii. Drainage is through the vortex veins
3. Crystalline lens
   a. Structural characteristics
      i. Biconvex, transparent structure behind iris and pupil and anterior to shallow depression (lenticular fossa) in vitreous face
      ii. Held in position by suspensory ligaments called zonules inserting anterior and posterior to lens equator
      iii. Lens forms fibers throughout life with old fibers compressed in nucleus
      iv. Three structural components
         - Capsule around entire lens, which is smooth, acellular serving as an anterior basement membrane for underlying lens epithelium and posterior basement membrane for cell nuclei
         - Lens epithelium with elongated nucleii (fibers) extending to posterior capsule
           – As cells mature, they lose their nuclei which harden and compress into lens nucleus
           – These cells begin to form largest portion of cells with aging
         - Lens substance
           – Cortex of newly formed soft lens fibers (nuclei)
           – Nucleus (central) of increasingly dense, hardening older lens fibers
      v. Zonules are modified collagen fibrils
         - Attach to nonpigmented epithelium between ciliary processes and to lens capsule
         - Attachment zone on the lens extends about 2 mm in front of the equator and 1 mm behind

I. Irritations and Injuries

A. Angle Recession

Refer to "Hyphema" in this chapter, under "Objective" in the "SOAP" section.

B. Contusive (Blunt) Trauma

1. Produced by direct, contrecoup, or contusive injuries
2. Clinical results of trauma to iris and ciliary body
   a. Angle recession
   b. Cyclodialysis
   c. Hyphema
   d. Iridodialysis
   e. Iridoschisis
   f. Iritis
   g. Pigmentary disturbances
   h. Sphincter pupillae rupture (miosis or mydriasis)
   i. Vossius ring (pigment on anterior lens capsule)

C. Hyphema[35,36] (See Also Chapter 8)

Background Information

- Accumulation of whole red blood in the anterior chamber (Figure 6.18)
  1. Usually less than one-third of chamber involved
  2. Most common involvement is inferior (owing to gravitational effect)
- Contusive injury most common cause
  1. Medical conditions can increase risk
     a. Leukemia

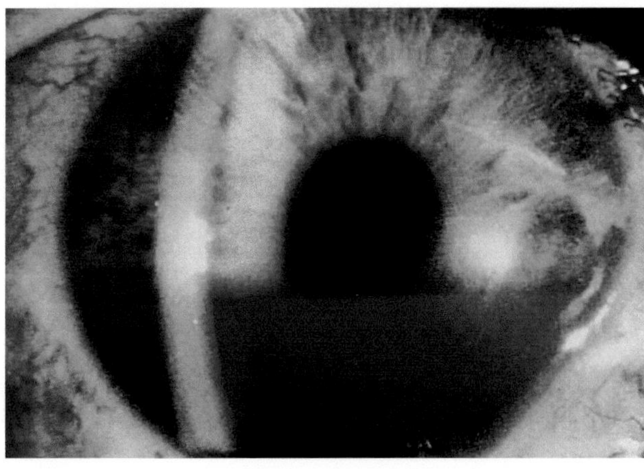

FIGURE 6.18 Hyphema is the accumulation of whole red blood in the anterior chamber, usually secondary to contusive (blunt) injury. Intensity may range from red blood cells in the aqueous (microhyphema), to blood levels (approximately 4 mm in this patient), to a chamber filled with blood ("eight-ball hyphema").

  b. Hemophilia
  c. Von Willebrand
  d. Sickle cell
  e. Iris neovascularization secondary to diabetes
  f. Anticoagulate drugs
- Microhyphema: diffuse RBC in anterior chamber
- "Eight-ball" hemorrhage: anterior chamber completely filled with whole red blood
- Important clinical statistics regarding risk of hyphema (excluding microhyphema, which has low risks for glaucoma or rebleed)
  1. Approximately 5% develop secondary glaucoma
  2. Approximately 25% rebleed (increasing risk of secondary glaucoma)
  3. Approximately 30% have temporary IOP incrrease during acute phase (first 5 to 7 days)
  4. Approximately 75% demonstrate some degree of recession or rupture of iris root (increasing risk of secondary glaucoma)

Subjective

- Usually history of blunt trauma associated
  1. Racket sport injuries (ball or racket)
  2. Hockey injuries (puck or stick)
  3. Fists
  4. High-speed projectile (e.g., paint ball, car airbags)
- More common in children (through teenage years)
- Vision widely variable based on degree of blood
  1. May be normal (in microhyphema)
  2. May be hazy (in aqueous clouded with blood)
  3. Variable degrees of reduction, depending on blood level
  4. Light perception (LP) to no light perception (NLP) in "eight-ball" hemorrhage
- Pain varies from mild to severe
  1. Relative to uveitic reaction
  2. Relative to acute IOP increases
- Frequently an unexplainable drowsiness (somnolence) is reported or demonstrated during acute phase
  1. Especially in children
  2. Not necessarily proportional to degree of blood
  3. Produces suspicion of neurological complications, especially when hyphema is associated with head trauma

Objective

(See also Appendix 2)

- Injured eyes usually have all findings associated with blunt trauma to the lids, conjunctiva, and cornea
- Anterior chamber appearance varies with amount, position, and degree of accumulated blood
  1. Least degree is microhyphema with discrete RBC seen with slit lamp in anterior chamber
  2. Blood may produce a red haze to the aqueous with increasing amounts (but not enough for a level)
  3. Free blood clots may be seen fixed or floating in the aqueous
     a. May be seen floating anywhere in chamber, but usually greatest in inferior chamber
     b. May be fixed anywhere
        i. Iris stromal surface
        ii. Chamber angle
        iii. Corneal endothelial surface
  4. Most typically, blood accumulates inferiorly with a distinct blood level visible without instrumentation
     a. This is the superior level of the inferior blood accumulated pool (from gravitational effects on the loose RBC in the aqueous)
     b. Occasionally coagulates and may produce an irregular (versus straight) line
  5. Classification by amount of blood in chamber
     a. Microhyphema: circulating red blood cells in aqueous
     b. Grade 1: layered blood occupying less than one-third anterior chamber
     c. Grade 2: layered blood filling one-third to one-half of anterior chamber
     d. Grade 3: layered blood filling one half to less than total volume of anterior chamber
     e. Grade 4: a total clotted mass of blood filling the entire anterior chamber
  6. Anterior chamber completely filled with blood is called an "eight-ball" hemorrhage
     a. Ominous appearance of blackish-purplishred anterior chamber
     b. Iris, pupil aperture, angle, and red reflex (with ophthalmoscope) are not visible
        i. Slit-lamp examination demonstrates clear or edematous cornea anterior to dense blood mass
        ii. Fundus examination (even with pupil dilation) is impossible and must be postponed
           - If posterior damage is feared (with blunt trauma), B-scan ultrasonography may be indicated
           - Foreign-body concerns may indicate ultrasonography or computerized tomography (CT)
     c. "Eight-ball" hemorrhages often produce small to extensive peripheral anterior synechiae after reabsorption

- On reabsorption of major portion of blood, gonioscopy may reveal varying degrees of angle recession or rupture of the iris root (see also Figure 6.21)
  1. Usually appears as black strip or elongated whole at base of iris (between ciliary body and trabeculum)
  2. Recession may be small (<10°) or large (up to 360°)
  3. Degree of hyphema need not be proportional to amount of recession or rupture
  4. The greater amount of recession, the greater the risk of secondary glaucoma
     a. Recessions greater than 180° pose an extremely high risk (about 75%) for secondary glaucoma
     b. May occur as long as 10 to 15 years after injury
     c. Thus, unilateral contusive injury (with angle recession, diagnosed or undiagnosed) should be considered the leading cause of any unilateral glaucoma at any time in life
- IOP varies during acute phase
  1. Often (30%) raised dramatically (>35 mm Hg) because of acute congestion from anterior chamber blood
  2. Infrequently reduced because of ciliary body hypotony
- Pupil size, shape, and reactions may vary during acute phase
  1. Normal
  2. Corectopia (irregular shape)
  3. Sluggish or no reactions
  4. Miosis (due to accompanying uveitis)
- Rebleeds usually occur during the first 2- to 5-day period following initial bleed (or rebleed)
  1. Rebleeds are usually worse than original presenting hyphema
  2. Almost always occur before seventh day after first bleed

Assessment

- Rule out other associated tissue damage (e.g., intraocular foreign body, orbital compartment syndrome = rapid rise in intraorbital pressure due to hemorrhaging secondary to trauma or surgery and causes ischemia of optic nerve and vision loss) in cases of contusion injury
- Rule out neurological complications in cases associated with unexplained somnolence
- In children, rule out underlying risks
  1. Juvenile xanthogranuloma (recurrent spontaneous hyphema)
  2. Retinoblastoma (microhyphema)
- Rule out herpes simplex uveitis (usually microhyphema)
- Spontaneous hyphemas may be idiopathic or systemically related

Plan: Hyphema

(See also Appendix 6)

- Reduce all ambulatory activity to a minimum
  1. Noncompliant patients should be hospitalized for 5- to 7-day period during resolution
  2. Rate of rebleeds no greater with minimal activity versus strict bed rest
  3. Sedation not indicated in ambulatory patient
- Apply unilateral shield over involved eye
  1. Bilateral shielding proven to be of no value
  2. Rate of rebleeds same with unilateral or bilateral
- Have patient sleep with head raised 30° to 45°
  1. Lowers venous pressure to reduce IOP
  2. Promotes more rapid blood resorption
- Topical or oral steroids not indicated unless required for treatment of associated anterior uveitis
- OTC analgesic for pain management (aspirin contraindicated!!)
- Pupil dilation is optional
  1. Varied opinions on value in reducing re bleeds or enhancing resorption
  2. Atropine (0.5% bid) has shown some value in reducing rebleeds
- If IOP raised, used topical and oral antiglaucoma agents
  1. Anticoagulants also valuable with increased IOP
  2. Need for rapid reabsorption (to reduce angle congestion) essential
- Antifibrinolytic agents have proved useful in reducing rate of rebleeds (controversial)
  1. Oral aminocaproic acid, 50–100 mg/kg body weight (not to exceed 30 g/day) qid for 5 days
  2. Contraindicated in renal disease
  3. May cause nausea and vomiting
  4. No effect on final visual acuity
- Surgical intervention should be avoided in patients with less than 50% hyphema or complicated cases
  1. Corneal blood staining
     a. "Eight-ball" (total) hyphema lasting longer than 7 days with normal IOP, or
     b. After 5 days if IOP exceeds 35 mm Hg
  2. Anterior chamber wash out surgery to prevent optic atrophy for total hyphema
     a. After 7 days if IOP exceeds 25 mm Hg or
     b. After 2 days if IOP exceeds 60 mm Hg

Follow-Up

- Patient must be seen daily for close monitoring during first 5 to 7 days
  1. Visual acuities
  2. Slit-lamp examination
  3. IOP by applanation tonometry
  4. Monitoring of corneal clarity (regarding blood staining)
  5. Size of hyphema
  6. Compliance with instructions (regarding activities)
- Rebleeds will almost always occur before seventh day
  1. On rebleed, all management steps must be reinstituted as from day number 1
  2. Prognosis with rebleeds worsens (e.g., regarding risk of secondary glaucoma, corneal blood staining)
- Corneal blood staining is produced by entrance of hemoglobin and hemosiderin into corneal stroma
  1. Primary causes
     a. Duration of blood exposure 6 to 7 days or more
     b. Greater than 50% hyphema (of anterior chamber)
     c. Corneal endothelial defect(s)
     d. Increased IOP (drives blood into stroma)
  2. Staining may (or may not) clear within months to years
     a. Often a residual posterior corneal line results (at site of blood level)
     b. Most resultant corneal stains are mild
     c. Greater at periphery

- Optic atrophy may result from severe acute or uncontrolled secondary glaucomas
- Generally, most mild hyphemas run a 5- to 7-day course and resolve without complications
    1. More severe involvements (e.g., 50%, rebleeds) may produce permanent damage and ongoing glaucoma problems
    2. All (mild through severe) hyphemas should be managed as lifelong risk factors for glaucoma
        a. IOP in involved eye may rise anytime in life
        b. Advise patient and recheck annually

II. Noninflammatory Conditions

A. Aniridia[37,38]

1. Congenital absence of iris or small 360° stump of iris base
2. Usually associated with other congenital anomalies
    a. Sensory nystagmus
    b. Lens opacities and dislocations
    c. Retinopathies
    d. Mental retardation
    e. Neurological disorders
3. Visual prognosis usually poor
    a. Foveal hypoplasia
    b. Optic nerve hypoplasia
    c. Glaucoma
    d. Cataract
    e. Keratopathy due to limbal stem cell failure
4. Best diagnosed by slit lamp and gonioscopy
5. Increased risks
    a. Corneal pannus
    b. Secondary glaucoma
        i. Drops ineffective
        ii. Surgery may not be effective
6. May be associated with Wilms' tumor (Miller's syndrome)
7. Condition generally produces difficult management problems

B. Atrophies

1. Aging

a. Thinning of iris stroma with flattening of architecture
    i. Disappearance of crypts (especially at pupillary zone)
    ii. Sphincter becomes more visible (brownish)
    iii. Pupillary ruff appears eroded
b. Miosis and pupillary immobility often present

2. Essential Iris Atrophy[39]

a. Usually white females at 30 to 40 years of age
b. Unilateral condition
c. Development of through-and-through iris holes (pseudopolycoria)
d. Progresses over a 1- to 3-year period
e. Pupil distortion and displacement caused by peripheral anterior synechiae
f. Complications
    i. Secondary glaucoma
    ii. Corneal edema
    iii. Pain
    iv. Reduced vision
g. Mimics Chandler's syndrome
    i. Corneal endothelial changes
    ii. Iris atrophy
    iii. Milder glaucoma

3. Iridoschisis[40]

a. Bilateral in patients over 65 years of age
b. Anterior iris stroma splits into fibers (with associated blood vessels versus persistent pupillary membranes), with one end remaining attached to iris and other floating freely in anterior chamber ("shredded wheat" appearance)
c. Significant (50%) risk of primary angle closure glaucoma
d. Monitor closely

4. Secondary Atrophies

a. Glaucomatous
b. Ischemic
c. Neurogenic (syphilitic)
d. Postinflammatory
e. Posttraumatic

C. Coloboma[41,42]

1. Autosomal-dominant hereditary trait
2. Unilateral or bilateral incomplete closure (cleft)
3. Keyhole pupil (down to ciliary body) at inferior 6-o'clock position (slightly medialward)
4. May cause photophobia and visual distortion
    a. Treatment options
        i. Tinted or opaque contact lenses
        ii. Artificial prosthetic iris
5. May be associated with other colobomas
    a. Choroid
    b. Retina
    c. Optic nerve

D. Configurations of the Iris

1. Corectopia

a. Irregularly shaped pupil(s)
b. Variable causes (see Appendix 2)

2. Iris Bombe[43]

a. Iris bowed anteriorward from posterior 360° synechiae at pupillary border (Figure 6.19)
b. Usually secondary to anterior segment inflammation (seclusio pupillae)
c. Results in secondary glaucoma

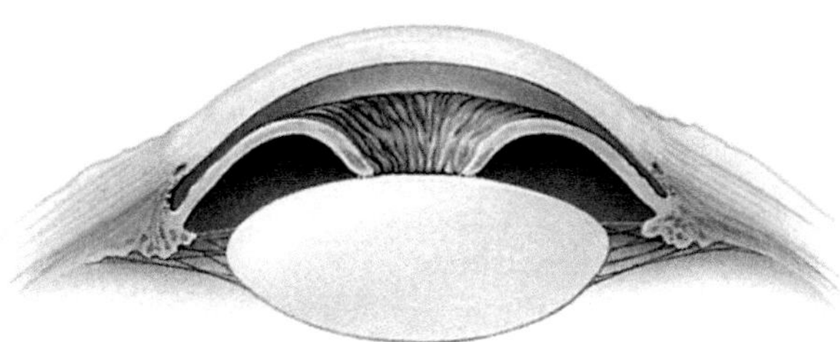

FIGURE 6.19 **Iris bombe** in chronic anterior uveitis is usually a product of 360° posterior synechiae (seclusio pupillae).

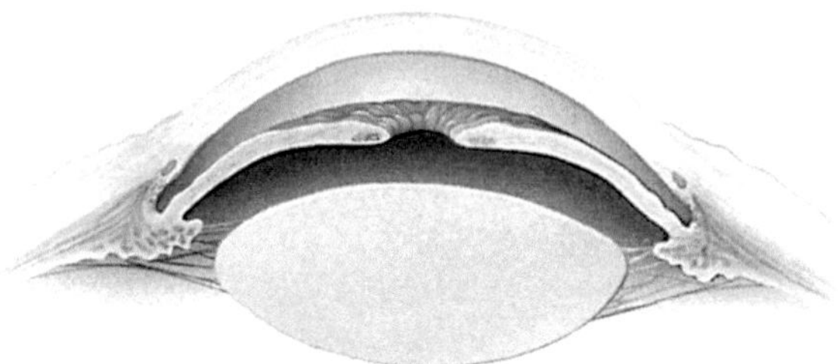

FIGURE 6.20 **Plateau iris** represents an anterior insertion of the iris root to the ciliary body with retention of a deep central anterior chamber and narrowed anterior chamber angles.

3. *Plateau Iris*[44]

a. Anterior insertion of iris on ciliary body with deep anterior chamber (Figure 6.20)
b. Frequent cause of angle closure

4. *Polycoria*[45]

a. Multiple pupillary apertures within single iris
b. Variable causes (see Appendix 2)
c. See "Coloboma" for contact lens treatment options

E. Cysts[46]

1. Uncommon, unilateral, multiple cysts of iris or ciliary body
2. Majority of cases diagnosed by 1 year of age, can grow over time
3. Peripheral and usually inferotemporal
4. Produce "bumpy," irregular peripheral iris surface or abrupt, localized bulge(s)
5. Need to differentiate from melanomas which are usually inferior, with corectopia, and/or diffuse iris elevation
6. May block trabeculum and raise IOP
7. Pupil dilates normally (versus masses)
8. Best viewed through gonioscopy
9. Treatable with laser therapy, fine needle aspiration, and surgical excision
10. Cysts may be secondary
    a. Intraocular surgery
    b. Pharmaceutical agents (e.g., phospholine iodide)

F. Iridodialysis[47]

1. Disinsertion of iris base from ciliary body (Figure 6.21) usually after blunt or penetrating trauma
2. Produces irregular iris configurations and pseudopolycoria
3. Common in large hyphemas
4. Increased risk of glaucoma
5. No treatment indicated in absence of symptoms (e.g., diplopia, photophobia)

G. Iridodonesis

1. Tremulous (quivering or shaky) iris
2. Multiple causes
    a. Rupture of zonules
    b. Dislocation of crystalline lens
    c. Marfan's syndrome
    d. Megalocornea

H. Iridoschisis

Refer to Atrophies.

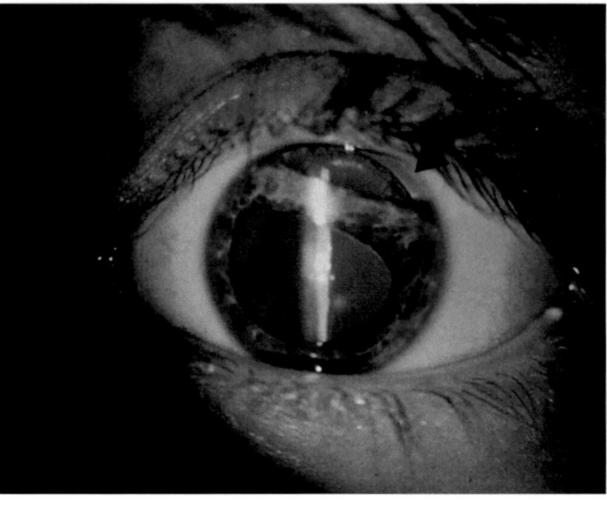

FIGURE 6.21 **Iridodialysis** is a rupture of the iris from its root frequently resulting from contusive (blunt) injury. Note the edge of the crystalline lens (arrow) in this large superior tear.

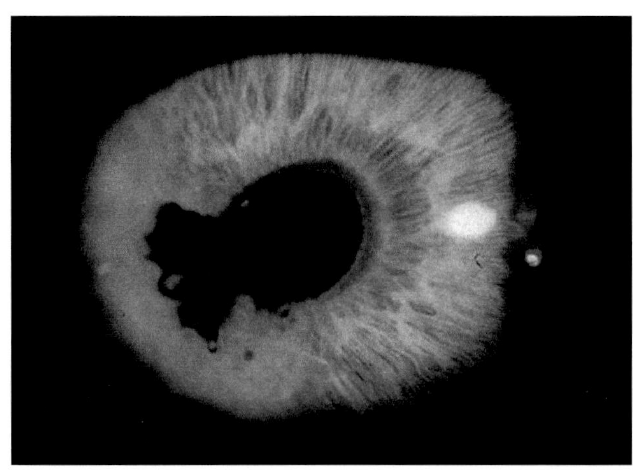

FIGURE 6.22 **Iris melanoma** at the iris pupil border producing an irregularly shaped pupil (corectopia).

I. Masses and Neoplasias

1. Amyloidosis
2. Brushfeld's spots (e.g., Down syndrome)[48]
3. Granulomas
4. Hemangiomas
5. Iris nevus (Cogan–Reese) syndrome
6. Juvenile xanthogranuloma (nevoxanthoen dothelioma)
7. Leiomyoma (neoplastic)
8. Leukemia (neoplastic)
9. Lymphoma (neoplastic)
10. Medulloepitheliomas
11. Melanomas (neoplastic; Figure 6.22), uncommon
12. Metastatic tumors (neoplastic), rare compared to choroid melanoma
13. Neurilemmomas
14. Neurofibromas (Lisch nodules)
15. Nevi (iris freckles)
16. Reactive lymphoid hyperplasia
17. Reticulum cell sarcoma (neoplastic)
18. Retinoblastoma (neoplastic)

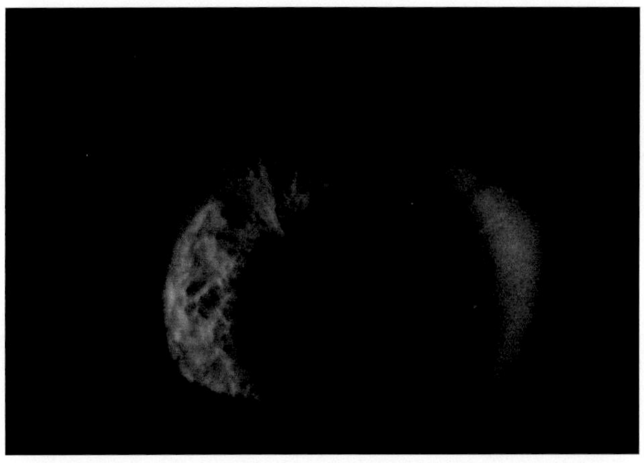

FIGURE 6.23 **Persistent pupillary membrane** is an embryologic strand originating from the iris collarette and frequently adhering (in this figure) to the anterior lens surface. It is differentiated from posterior synechiae by its origin (collarette versus posterior iris or border) and an elastic nature versus fibrous strands in posterior synechiae.

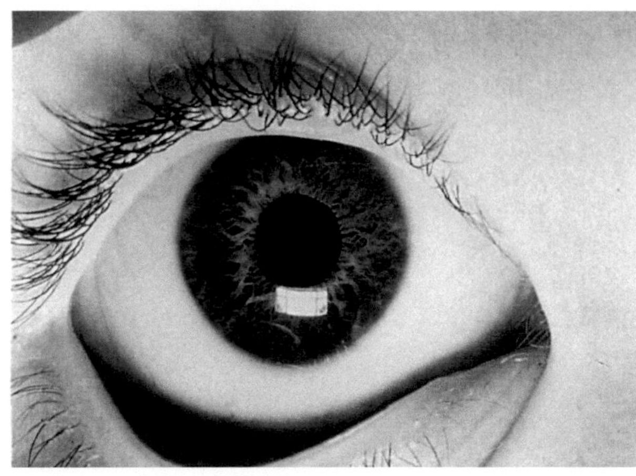

FIGURE 6.24 **Iris heterochromia** segment in the superior nasal quadrant of a left iris. Heterochromia may be unilaterally segmental or involving the complete iris, when it may produce bilaterally different colored irides (heterochromia iridium). In bilateral situations, Fuchs' heterochromic iridocyclitis or intraocular foreign body (in the darker pigmented eye) should be considered.

J. Persitent Pupillary Membrane(s) or Remant(s)[49]

1. Fine avascular threads, often pigmented (less than iris stroma; Figure 6.23)
2. May be single threads, branched, or meshwork
3. One end attached to iris collarette and other end loose or attached to pupil, iris stroma (elsewhere), or anterior lens capsule
4. Rather common (especially in children)
5. May break with pupil dilation (pharmaceutically induced or natural), trauma, spontaneously, and so forth; disappear or persist
6. No treatment indicated unless severe enough to significantly to block the pupil and potentially induce amblyopia
7. No increased risks

K. Pigmentation Variations

(Little to no iris pigmentation = "blue eyes." Increasing iris pigmentation = "green" to "hazel" to "brown" eyes.)

1. Albinism[50]

a. Oculocutaneous albinism
   i. Sex-linked recessive trait (female carrier, males affected)
   ii. Normal skin and hair pigmentation
   iii. Deficient ocular pigmentations with iris transillumination defects
   iv. Poor visual acuity
b. Tyrosinase-negative oculocutaneous albinism
   i. Complete pigment deficiency (skin, hair, and eyes)
   ii. Marked iris transillumination defects
   iii. Poor visual prognosis
      - Serious visual reduction
      - Nystagmus
      - High myopia
      - Severe photophobia
c. Tyrosinase-positive oculocutaneous albinism
   i. Milder form of complete albinism
   ii. Skin, hair, and eyes have mild pigmentation that may increase with age
   iii. Visual prognosis is better than negative form

2. Heterochromia (Variations in Pigmentation)[51]

a. Irregular unilateral or bilateral distribution (Figure 6.24)
b. In absence of pathology, may be isolated genetic abnormality or autosomal dominant genetic trait
c. Occasional wedge-shaped sectors of hyper or hypopigmentation
   i. Sectorial heterochromia (heterochromia iridis)
d. "Heterochromia iridium": condition in which the pigment of one iris is completely different from that of the opposite iris
e. Pathological causes
   i. Fuchs' heterochromic iridocyclitis
   ii. Intraocular foreign-body hemosiderosis
   iii. Intraocular neoplasias

3. Nevus (Iris Freckle)

a. Hyperpigmented spot on iris stroma, common
b. May be flat or raised
c. Creates no distortions to iris architecture, pupil or on pupil dilation (versus melanoma)
d. Slight increased risk of melanoma (iris or choroid)
e. Monitor for changes and photodocument (if possible)
f. No treatment indicated

III. Inflammatory Conditions

A. Iridocyclitis

Refer to "Acute Anterior Uveitis."

B. Iritis

Refer to "Acute Anterior Uveitis."

C. Rubeosis Iridis[52]

1. Proliferation of neovascular network on anterior surface of iris and anterior chamber angle
2. Circumferential pattern with greatest concentration of vessels at pupillary zone and angle

3. Leads to fibrovascular peripheral anterior synechiae secondary glaucoma (resistant to treatment)
4. Multiple causes
   a. Diabetes mellitus
   b. Ocular inflammation
   c. Intraocular tumors (with necrosis)
   d. Neovascular glaucoma
   e. Vascular occlusive disease
   f. Ocular ischemic syndrome

References

1. Duplechain A, Conrady CD, Patel BC, Baker S. Uveitis. In: *StatPearls*. Treasure Island: StatPearls Publishing; February 25, 2021.
2. Harthan JS, Opitz DL, Fromstein SR, Morettin CE. Diagnosis and treatment of anterior uveitis: optometric management. *Clin Optom*. 2016;8:23–35. Published 2016 Mar 31. doi:10.2147/OPTO.S72079
3. Keino H, Horie S, Sugita S. Immune privilege and eye-derived T-regulatory cells. *J Immunol Res*. 2018;2018:1679197. Published 2018 May 20. doi:10.1155/2018/1679197
4. de Groot-Mijnes JD, de Visser L, Zuurveen S, et al. Identification of new pathogens in the intraocular fluid of patients with uveitis. *Am J Ophthalmol*. 2010;150(5):628–636. doi:10.1016/j.ajo.2010.05.015
5. Biggioggero M, Crotti C, Becciolini A, Miserocchi E, Favalli EG. The management of acute anterior uveitis complicating spondyloarthritis: present and future. *Biomed Res Int*. 2018;2018:9460187. Published 2018 Oct 14. doi:10.1155/2018/9460187
6. Islam N, Pavesio C. Uveitis (acute anterior). *BMJ Clin Evid*. 2010;2010:0705. Published 2010 Apr 8.
7. Mahabadi N, Kim J, Edens MA. Iritis. In: *StatPearls*. Treasure Island: StatPearls Publishing; July 15, 2021.
8. Babu K, Mahendradas P. Medical management of uveitis: current trends. *Indian J Ophthalmol*. 2013;61(6):277–283. doi:10.4103/0301-4738.114099
9. Sen HN, Larson TA, Meleth AD, Smith WM, Nussenblatt RB. Subconjunctival sirolimus for the treatment of chronic active anterior uveitis: results of a pilot trial. *Am J Ophthalmol*. 2012;153(6):1038–1042. doi:10.1016/j.ajo.2011.12.018
10. Wenker KJ, Quint JM. Ankylosing spondylitis. In: *StatPearls*. Treasure Island: StatPearls Publishing; July 16, 2021.
11. Ward MM, Deodhar A, Gensler LS, et al. Update of the American college of rheumatology/spondylitis association of America/spondyloarthritis research and treatment network recommendations for the treatment of ankylosing spondylitis and nonradiographic axial spondyloarthritis. *Arthritis Care Res*. 2019;71(10):1285–1299. doi:10.1002/acr.24025
12. Hatemi G, Seyahi E, Fresko I, Talarico R, Hamuryudan V. One year in review 2019: Behçet's syndrome. *Clin Exp Rheumatol*. 2019;37 Suppl 121(6):3–17.
13. Veauthier B, Hornecker JR. Crohn's disease: diagnosis and management. *Am Fam Physician*. 2018;98(11):661–669.
14. Caio G, Lungaro L, Caputo F, et al. Nutritional treatment in Crohn's disease. *Nutrients*. 2021;13(5):1628. Published 2021 May 12. doi:10.3390/nu13051628
15. Porter RJ, Kalla R, Ho GT. Ulcerative colitis: recent advances in the understanding of disease pathogenesis. *F1000Res*. 2020;9:F1000 Faculty Rev-294. Published 2020 Apr 24. doi:10.12688/f1000research.20805.1
16. Moshirfar M, Villarreal A, Ronquillo Y. Fuchs uveitis syndrome. In: *StatPearls*. Treasure Island: StatPearls Publishing; July 7, 2021.
17. Huq M, Sanan N, Daniels P, Hostoffer R. Posner–Schlossman syndrome in common variable immunodeficiency. *Case Rep Ophthalmol Med*. 2020;2020:8843586. Published 2020 Oct 15. doi:10.1155/2020/8843586
18. Angeles-Han ST, Ringold S, Beukelman T, et al. 2019 American College of rheumatology/arthritis foundation guideline for the screening, monitoring, and treatment of juvenile idiopathic arthritis-associated uveitis. *Arthritis Care Res*. 2019;71(6):703–716. doi:10.1002/acr.23871
19. Ringold S, Angeles-Han ST, Beukelman T, et al. 2019 American College of rheumatology/arthritis foundation guideline for the treatment of juvenile idiopathic arthritis: therapeutic approaches for non-systemic polyarthritis, sacroiliitis, and enthesitis. *Arthritis Care Res*. 2019;71(6):717–734. doi:10.1002/acr.23870
20. Parker DM, Angeles-Han ST, Stanton AL, Holland GN. Chronic anterior uveitis in children: psychosocial challenges for patients and their families. *Am J Ophthalmol*. 2018;191:xvi–xxiv. doi:10.1016/j.ajo.2018.03.028
21. Meyer P, Graeff E, Kohler C, Munier F, Bruder E. Juvenile xanthogranuloma involving concurrent iris and skin: clinical, pathological and molecular pathological evaluations. *Am J Ophthalmol Case Rep*. 2017;9:10–13. Published 2017 Sep 23. doi:10.1016/j.ajoc.2017.09.004
22. Babu BM, Rathinam SR. Intermediate uveitis. *Indian J Ophthalmol*. 2010;58(1):21–27. doi:10.4103/0301-4738.58469
23. Ozdal PC, Berker N, Tugal-Tutkun I. Pars planitis: epidemiology, clinical characteristics, management and visual prognosis. *J Ophthalmic Vis Res*. 2015;10(4):469–480. doi:10.4103/2008-322X.176897
24. Cheeti A, Chakraborty RK, Ramphul K. Reactive arthritis. In: *StatPearls*. Treasure Island: StatPearls Publishing; March 7, 2021.
25. Klein JT, Horn TD, Forman JD, Silver RF, Teirstein AS, Moller DR. Selection of oligoclonal V beta-specific T cells in the intradermal response to Kveim-Siltzbach reagent in individuals with sarcoidosis. *J Immunol*. 1995;154(3):1450–1460.
26. Pasadhika S, Rosenbaum JT. Ocular sarcoidosis. *Clin Chest Med*. 2015;36(4):669–683. doi:10.1016/j.ccm.2015.08.009
27. Koundanya VV, Tripathy K. Syphilis ocular manifestations. In: *StatPearls*. Treasure Island: StatPearls Publishing; February 14, 2021.
28. Etheridge T, Bowen RC, Raven M, Snow KB, Urban AW, Chang JS. Ocular syphilis: clinical manifestations and treatment course. *WMJ*. 2019;118(4):191–195.
29. Pessoa L, Galvão V. Clinical aspects of congenital syphilis with Hutchinson's triad. *BMJ Case Rep*. 2011;2011:bcr1120115130. Published 2011 Dec 21. doi:10.1136/bcr.11.2011.5130
30. Henao-Martínez AF, Johnson SC. Diagnostic tests for syphilis: new tests and new algorithms. *Neurol Clin Pract*. 2014;4(2):114–122. doi:10.1212/01.CPJ.0000435752.17621.48
31. Shakarchi FI. Ocular tuberculosis: current perspectives. *Clin Ophthalmol*. 2015;9:2223–2227. Published 2015 Nov 26. doi:10.2147/OPTH.S65254
32. Malik TF, Aurelio DM. Extraintestinal manifestations of inflammatory bowel disease. In: *StatPearls*. Treasure Island: StatPearls Publishing; March 6, 2021.
33. Troncoso LL, Biancardi AL, de Moraes HV Jr, Zaltman C. Ophthalmic manifestations in patients with inflammatory bowel disease: a review. *World J Gastroenterol*. 2017;23(32):5836–5848. doi:10.3748/wjg.v23.i32.5836
34. Ungaro R, Mehandru S, Allen PB, Peyrin-Biroulet L, Colombel JF. Ulcerative colitis. *Lancet*. 2017;389(10080):1756–1770. doi:10.1016/S0140-6736(16)32126-2
35. Gharaibeh A, Savage HI, Scherer RW, Goldberg MF, Lindsley K. Medical interventions for traumatic hyphema. *Cochrane Database Syst Rev*. 2013;12(12):CD005431. Published 2013 Dec 3. doi:10.1002/14651858.CD005431.pub3
36. Gragg J, Blair K, Baker MB. Hyphema. In: *StatPearls*. Treasure Island: StatPearls Publishing; June 29, 2021.
37. Tripathy K, Salini B. Aniridia. In: *StatPearls*. Treasure Island: StatPearls Publishing; February 14, 2021.
38. Hingorani M, Hanson I, van Heyningen V. Aniridia. *Eur J Hum Genet*. 2012;20(10):1011–1017. doi:10.1038/ejhg.2012.100

39. Meirelles SH, Barreto AS, Buscacio ES, Shinzato E, Patrão LF, de Oliveira Silva MS. Retinitis pigmentosa with concomitant essential iris atrophy and glaucoma: case report. *Clin Ophthalmol.* 2015;9:2139–2145. Published 2015 Nov 26. doi:10.2147/OPTH.S75384
40. Pieklarz B, Grochowski ET, Saeed E, Sidorczuk P, Mariak Z, Dmuchowska DA. Iridoschisis: a systematic review. *J Clin Med.* 2020;9(10):3324. Published 2020 Oct 16. doi:10.3390/jcm9103324
41. Zerkaoui N. Colobome irien bilatéral [Bilateral iris coloboma]. *Pan Afr Med J.* 2018;30:1. Published 2018 May 2. doi:10.11604/pamj.2018.30.1.14505
42. Vegunta S, Patel BC. Optic nerve coloboma. In: *StatPearls.* Treasure Island: StatPearls Publishing; July 1, 2021.
43. Ikegawa W, Suzuki T, Namiguchi K, Mizoue S, Shiraishi A, Ohashi Y. Changes in anterior segment morphology of Iris Bombe before and after laser peripheral iridotomy in patients with uveitic secondary glaucoma. *J Ophthalmol.* 2016;2016:8496201. doi:10.1155/2016/8496201
44. Bourdon H, Aragno V, Baudouin C, Labbé A. Iridoplasty for plateau iris syndrome: a systematic review. *BMJ Open Ophthalmol.* 2019;4(1):e000340. Published 2019 Sep 22. doi:10.1136/bmjophth-2019-000340
45. Sherman SW, Canestraro J, Bogomolny D, Marr B. Relief of symptomatic pseudo-polycoria due to iris biopsy using a daily contact lens. *Am J Ophthalmol Case Rep.* 2021;22:101084. Published 2021 Apr 1. doi:10.1016/j.ajoc.2021.101084
46. Konopińska J, Lisowski Ł, Mariak Z, Obuchowska I. Clinical features of Iris cysts in long-term follow-up. *J Clin Med.* 2021;10(2):189. Published 2021 Jan 7. doi:10.3390/jcm10020189
47. Huang JY, Liu YL, Huang YC, Lin CP. A novel technique for closed-chamber iridodialysis repair. *Taiwan J Ophthalmol.* 2019;10(3):208–211. Published 2019 Aug 8. doi:10.4103/tjo.tjo_26_19
48. Postolache L, Parsa CF. Brushfield spots and Wölfflin nodules unveiled in dark irides using near-infrared light. *Sci Rep.* 2018;8(1):18040. Published 2018 Dec 21. doi:10.1038/s41598-018-36348-6
49. Lee HJ, Kim JH, Kim SJ, Yu YS. Long-term lens complications following removal of persistent pupillary membrane. *Korean J Ophthalmol.* 2018;32(2):103–107. doi:10.3341/kjo.2017.0069
50. Federico JR, Krishnamurthy K. Albinism. In: *StatPearls.* Treasure Island: StatPearls Publishing; August 28, 2020.
51. Rennie IG. Don't it make my blue eyes brown: heterochromia and other abnormalities of the iris. *Eye.* 2012;26(1):29–50. doi:10.1038/eye.2011.228
52. Niestrata-Ortiz M, Li JP, Davies N. Rubeosis iridis in patients with diabetes: not forgetting oculoischaemic syndrome as a differential. *BMJ Case Rep.* 2014;2014:bcr2014207236. Published 2014 Nov 17. doi:10.1136/bcr-2014-207236

Chapter 7
PRE- AND POSTOPERATIVE MANAGEMENT OF CATARACT AND REFRACTIVE SURGERY PATIENTS

Chapter Outline

DOI: 10.1201/9781003255598-7

Section 1: Cataract Surgery

I. Common Types of Cataracts[1]

A. Nuclear sclerotic (NS) cataracts
   1. This is the most common form of cataract
   2. It begins at the nucleus of the lens (the central zone)
   3. Nuclear sclerotic cataracts progress slowly, often developing over years
   4. They begin with a gradual hardening and yellowing ("brunescence") of the nucleus that spreads to other layers of the lens as it progresses
   5. An interesting fact about this type of cataract is as it progresses it creates a phenomenon known as Second Sight
      a. Second Sight creates a temporary improvement in close-up (near-sight) vision as the lens swells adding plus power
      b. However, as the cataract progresses this temporary vision improvement (at distance and near) diminishes
   6. As nuclear sclerotic cataracts progress, vision becomes worse overall

B. Cortical cataracts
   1. Start from the outermost layer of the lens (reverse of the nuclear type)
   2. Progressing opacities create "spokes" that lead from the outer zones of the lens centrally toward the nucleus
   3. Symptoms of this cataract are blurred vision, difficulty with glare, and changes in both contrast and depth perception
   4. Hyperopic shift common
   5. Higher risk of development with diabetes

C. Posterior subcapsular cataracts (PSCs)
   1. First noticeable changes occur in night vision (diminution and glare)
   2. Subsequently, increased difficulty with near vision
   3. This type of cataract develops quickly, typically over months not years
   4. Increased risk for development with:
      a. Diabetes
      b. Extreme nearsightedness
      c. Use of steroids (recreational or as part of medical treatment)

II. Cataract Surgical Procedures (Lensectomy)[2–4]

A. Two types of lensectomy (lens extraction)
   1. Intracapsular or small incision cataract extraction (SICS)
      a. Small incision (sometimes double incision) to accommodate surgical instruments and phacoemulsification (ultrasound liquification and aspiration) probe
      b. Most common type of cataract procedure
   2. Extracapsular (ECCS)
      a. Large incision
      b. Lens cortex and nucleus extracted in one piece
      c. Done only when phacoemulsification not sufficient to disassemble nucleus (e.g., mature and hypermature cataracts)

B. Surgical procedure (lensectomy) options
   1. Standard IOL procedure
      a. Keratotomy (keratolimbal incision done with scalpel and/or scissors to provide an entry port)
      b. Inject viscoelastic into anterior chamber (sodium hyaluronate or other methylcellulose substances to protect corneal endothelium and maintain chamber depth)
      c. Anterior capsulorhexis (opening in the anterior capsule create with forceps)
      d. Nuclear disassembly ("laser phacofragmentation," a chopping technique to fracture nucleus)
      e. Phacoemulsification (ultrasound liquification and aspiration)
      f. Insertion of IOL into capsular bag/sac (usually preloaded in inserter)
      g. After IOL unfolds, rotate and center the optic
      h. Close keratotomy (sutureless or interrupted sutures)
      i. Astigmatic (arcuate) keratotomy (AK) are arcuate incisions at the steepest meridians of a regular or oblique astigmatic cornea, performed, if necessary, immediately or 2 to 3 months post-op to reduce ("relax") induced irregular meridional curvature:
         i. Arcuate incisions are made with a scalpel, usually to ¾ to ⅞ corneal thickness
         ii. Incisions can be made most accurately with a femtosecond laser
   2. Femtosecond laser procedure
      a. The femtosecond laser is an infrared laser with a wavelength of 1053 nm
      b. As opposed to excimer laser's ultraviolet photoablation of tissue, femtosecond lasers photodisrupt tissue with a pulse duration of 10 to 15 seconds (<1 picosecond) which creates a 1μ cavitation bubbles that expand and separate (cut) tissue layers, completely eliminating collateral tissue damage to create a precise dissection
      c. Under computer control, cavitation bubbles are applied at a rate of > 30,000 per second in any direction to produce linear, horizontal, vertical, diagonal, curved incisions which replace (with maximal accuracy) steps in the lensectomy
      d. Traditional use of scalpel, scissors, probes (for keratotomies and capsulorhexis) at 80μ to 100μ blade accuracy replaced with 5μ to 8μ femtosecond accuracy
      e. Nuclear disassembly (laser phacofragmentation) done at >43% reduction in energy and 51% reduction in endothelial cell loss[5]
      f. Some of the most popular femtosecond lasers for lensectomy (and for corneal refractive surgery, discussed later in this chapter) include:
         i. *iLASIK IntraLase* (Johnson & Johnson Vision)
         ii. *Femto LDV* (Ziemer Ophthalmic Systems)
         iii. *Victus* (Bausch + Lomb)
         iv. *VisuMax* (Carl Zeiss Meditec AG)

III. Intraocular Lens Implants (IOL, *aka* Pseudophakia) Options (*Circa* 2022)

A. Intraocular lens (IOL) options[6]
   1. Monofocal IOLs
      a. Unilateral (for congenital or traumatic cataracts)

TABLE 7.1 **Effects of Spherical Aberrations (SA) in Presbyopia and Pseudophakia**

	Distance Vision		Intermediate and Near Vision
	Photopic	**Mesopic/ Scotopic**	
<SA	• Image quality improves • Depth of focus reduced	Image quality improves due to no significant reduction in contrast sensitivity	Decreased depth of focus reduces function
>SA	• Image quality slightly reduced • Increased depth of focus inproves range	Measurable reductions (MTF) due to reduced contrast sensitivity	Increased depth of focus increases range and function

Pseudo-accommodating (*multifocal*) and accommodating IOL Options

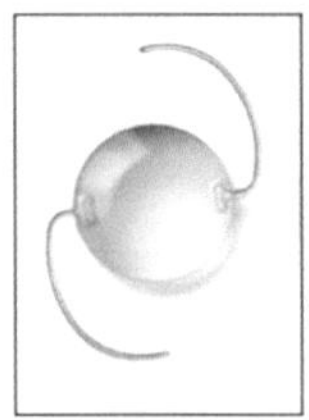

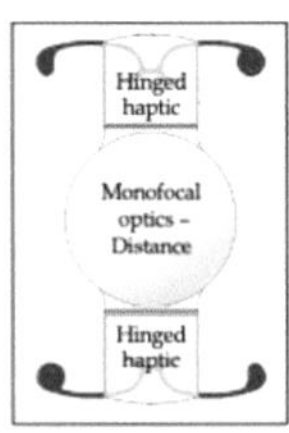

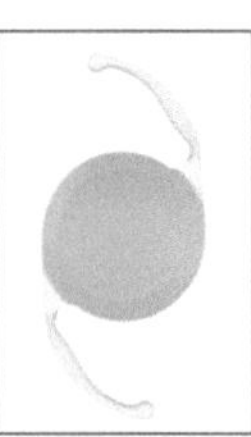

Tecnis®* 9000** Acrylic Zonale by AMO — ***ReStor® Acrylic Diffractive by Alcon — ***Crystalens®*** Translational Silicone by B&L — ***AcrySof® IQ*** PanOptix® Trifocal by Alcon

FIGURE 7.1 Pseudo-accommodating (multifocal) and accommodating IOL options: the 4 principle "premium IOLs" (as they're referred to) include the distant-dominant *Tecnis* 9000 by J&J; the near dominant, diffractive *ReStor* by Alcon; the translational (accommodative) *Crystalens* by B&L; and the *Acrysof IQ PanOptix* trifocal by Alcon.

b. Bilateral (to eliminate need for spectacles)
c. Monovision (for presbyopia)
   i. Needs thorough explanation and adaptable patient
   ii. Best candidates previous monovision patients (CL or specs)
   iii. Best option, "modified" monovision (versus full add power) at ~1.00 to 1.25 D, non-dominant eye
d. Aspherics (to reduce positive spherical aberrations—see Table 7.1)
   i. e.g., B&L *Sofport*
e. Torics (for post-op astigmatism ≥0.75 D)

2. Multifocal (*aka* presbyopic correcting) IOLs (Figure 7.1)
   a. Pseudo-accommodating (bifocal or trifocal design)
      i. e.g., Alcon *ReStor* (Near dominant optics)
      ii. e.g., J&J (formerly AMO) *Tecnis* (Distance dominant optics)
      iii. Trifocal (e.g., Alcon *PanOptic*)[7,8]
         - Multifocal trifocal refractive/diffractive optics
         - Intermediate (+1.65) and near (+2.35) at the corneal plane
         - Aspheric apodized optics reduces halos and glare
3. Extended depth of focus
   a. Tecnis *Symfony*
4. Accommodative (translational design) IOL
   a. *Crystalens*, B&L (most popular)
   b. Bihinged moveable optic
5. Aspherics (many multifocal IOLs have aspheric optics)
6. Torics (many multifocal IOLs have toric designs as well)
7. Phakic IOLs (see refractive lens exchange with natural lens below)
8. Other international and less popular IOLs
   a. ACOR IOLs ("Piggybacked" multifocal/monofocal IOLs)
   b. DualOptics IOL ("Piggyback" system in animal studies)
   c. HumanOptics Akkommodative 1CU (injected hydrophilic)
   d. Light Adjustable IOL (animal studies on molecular lens)
   e. Medennium SmartLens (thermodynamic hydrophilic)
   f. QuestVision FlexiOptic (haptic contoured to capsule bag)
   g. Sarafarazi Elliptical Accommodating IOL (B&L)
   h. Membrane Lens (anterior phakic IOL by Nordan)
   i. Visiogen Synchrony IOL (dual anterior/posterior optics)
   j. Vivarte Baikoff IOL (by Ciba)

B. Refractive lens exchange (RLE)[9]
1. Definition: removal of the crystalline lens in a clear state and its replacement with a specialized intraocular lens to create an optimal refractive condition
2. Synonyms:
   a. Clear lensectomy
   b. Refractive lensectomy
   c. Clear lens exchange
   d. Lens-based refractive surgery
3. High hyperopic procedures (to eliminate need for heavy spectacle lenses)
4. High myopic procedures (to reduce or eliminate the need for spectacles)
5. Phakic IOLs (IOL with natural lens), see also Figures 7.3 and 7.4 and Appendix 5
   a. *Verisyse* J&J (anterior chamber IOL) (Internationally, *Artisan* by OPHTEC)[10]
   b. *Visian* Staar ICL (Implantable Collamer Lens)[11], posterior chamber—in sulcus
   c. Other international and less popular phakic IOLs

Anterior Chamber	Posterior Chamber
Acrysof, Alcon	*PRL*, Ciba
GBR, IOL Tech	
Kelman Duet, Tekia	
MemoryLens, Ciba	
NewLife, IOL Tech	
NuVita, B&L	
ThinOptX	

IV. Preoperative Cataract Evaluation (and Patient Selection Criteria)[12]

A. Subjective presentation
1. History
   a. Slowly progressive reduction in vision (distance and/or near)
   b. No significant ocular, medical, or medication contributing history, although often patients (particularly aging) will be on topical or oral medication(s) which may be directly or indirectly associated with cataract development
   c. No active retinal or optic nerve diseases or disorders
2. Symptoms
   a. Poor vision (distance [≤20/40] and/or near [≤J3 to J4])
   b. Significant reduction in night vision (or dim illumination)
   c. Halos around lights (spherical aberrations [see Table 7.1])
   d. Glare, flare and/or distorted lights at night (coma)
   e. Overall reduction in night vision and contrast sensitivity
   f. Monocular "double vision"
   g. Apparent improvement in near vision ("second sight" with NS)
   h. Frequent prescription changes
   i. Quantitative and qualitative vision loss is relative to patients' subjective perceptions of loss and must be weighed in surgical considerations.

B. Objective examination
1. Rule out (R/O) all active ocular pathology
2. Do BIO (binocular indirect ophthalmoscopy)
   a. R/O and/or diagram any fundus abnormalities
   b. R/O any macular abnormalities
      i. Cystoid macular edema
      ii. Macular degeneration
3. Slit-lamp biomicroscopic examination (SLE)
   a. Rule out (R/O) or document significant corneal endothelial dropout or guttata
   b. Identify zone(s) of lenticular opacities (see "Common Types of Cataracts" above)
   c. Lenticular changes generally graded as 1+ to 4+ or hypermature
4. Take precise measurements of constricted (miotic) and dilated (scotopic) pupils

C. Referral criteria (see Table 7.2)
1. Physical findings should be consistent with significant subjective symptoms:
   a. Observable lens opacities >1+ to 2+
   b. Distance vision ≤ 20/40 and/or near vision ≤ J3 to J4
   c. Contrast sensitivity (glare testing or Brightness Acuity Test [BAT]) with ≥ 2-line reduction in visual acuity
2. Final decision based mostly on patient's subjective presentation (patients have varying visual needs and personal assessments of their visual function and this must be considered in final decision to refer for surgery)
3. Best to ask two simple questions for patients considering multifocal IOLs:
   a. "This new procedure may create persistent halos around lights at night that the brain adapts to quickly. Would that bother you?"
   b. "Would you accept the probable use of reading glasses for certain limited conditions?"
4. For refractive lens exchange—RLE (with clear lens for refractive or cosmetics purpose)[13]
   a. +0.25 to +8.00 D hyperopic/presbyopes (with corneal cylinder less than 2 to 3 D)
   b. Very high myopes (> −6 to 8.00 D)
   c. Patients with significant higher order aberrations (HOAs) measured by wavefront aberrometry and contrast sensitivity difficulties
   d. Patient should be seeking less dependence on multifocal spectacles or contact lenses (for HOA and/or cosmetic reasons)
   e. Patient should demonstrate an adaptable personality
   f. Benefits of RLE versus corneal refractive procedures
      i. Decreased induction of higher order aberrations
      ii. Eliminate the risk of corneal ectasia
      iii. Provide better uncorrected VAs than laser refractive procedures for higher myopes and hyperopes
      iv. Eliminates accommodation in non-presbyopes with phakic IOLs (replaced by pseudoaccommodating IOLs or near spectacle Rx)
      v. Reduced retinal detachment risk in myopes (versus aphakia)
   g. Contraindications
      i. Demanding night vision needs
      ii. Extended night driving (e.g., truck driver, etc.)
      iii. Immobile or small, fixed pupils (can be pre-treated with laser pupilloplasty [?])
      iv. Corneal cylinder greater than 2 to 3 D (would require bioptic procedure)
      v. Low to moderate myopes
      vi. Extreme dry eye signs and symptoms
      vii. Personality disorders
      viii. Patients experiencing "life-altering" times

D. General multifocal IOL recommendations and considerations (to patient and surgeon)
1. *Distance oriented* (e.g., sports, driving) patients:
   a. With smaller pupils: Distance dominant IOL
   b. With larger pupils: Distance or near dominant IOL
2. *Near oriented* (e.g., reading, sewing) patients:
   a. With smaller pupils: Near dominant IOL
   b. With larger pupils: Distance or near dominant IOL

TABLE 7.2 **Presbyopic Correcting IOLs**

Positives (Pros)	Negatives (Cons)
• Only effective distance & near vision correction without glasses, bifocals or multifocal contact lenses • Proven safe and effective outpatient refractive surgical procedure • Provides sharp distance, intermediate and near vision without full time use of glasses • Eliminates the need for bifocals • Permanently eliminates the risk of cataract formation • Reversible to monofocal intraocular lens, if necessary (must be within 3 to 6 months minimum) • Comparable cost to other refractive procedure (e.g., Lasik, PRK, Lasck)	• Produces some halos around lights (greatest in dim illumination) • Intraocular surgery risks including infection, edema, retinal detachment • Part time use of near or distance glasses in some lighting conditions • Requires a 3 to 6 month period of adaptation to *"new visual system"* • Not advisable for patients with very demanding visual needs at night • Not advisable for certain conditions including some nearsighted patients • Partial coverage by private insurance and Medicare for cataract patients (no coverage for cosmetic procedures)

3. Patients with small, immobile pupils:
    a. Monofocal (*mononvision*)
    b. Accommodating IOL
4. Present positive and negative (pro and con) considerations of presbyopic correcting IOLs (Table 7.2)

E. Patient counseling (explanation of procedure, reassurance, and Q&A)
1. Risks of cataract surgery (to be discussed with surgeon)
    a. Anesthesia risks
    b. Surgical risks
    c. Cost considerations
2. Eye with lesser vision is done first
3. About a 2-week interval between eyes although increasing literature supporting same day bilateral procedures[14]
4. Always done as out-patient procedure *(will need a driver)*
5. *Always* request the earliest time (surgeons are notorious for falling behind)

V. Intraoperative Considerations[15]

A. Pre-op timeframe, about 30 to 45 mins
B. Anesthesiologist does history first
C. Usually intravenous (IV) sedation (relaxed but not sleeping)
D. Gurney trip to the operating room or (if femtosecond laser to be used) laser room and then operating room
E. You are conscious during the procedure:
1. Unless you request otherwise; or
2. Persistent movement (eye or body)

F. Total procedure time (barring complications) usually 10 to 15 mins., often less than 10 minutes
G. Recovery room time usually 30 to 60 mins. (longer if necessary)
H. Standard postoperative follow-up schedule: 24 hrs; 2 wks; 3 months
I. Patient must be advised that they will be experiencing a "new visual system" and early symptomatology will represent a period of adaptation

VI. Postoperative IOL Management (Table 7.3)

A. Clinical Management (SOAP Format with Display Icons)

Subjective (MONO, MF, RLE day #1, #14, #30 to 90 post-op);

Objective (MONO, MF, RLE day #1, #14, #30 to 90 post-op);

Dx **Assessment** (MONO, MF, RLE day #1, #14, #30 to 90 post-op);

℞ **Plan** (MONO, MF, RLE day #1, #14, #30 to 90 post-op);

Follow-Up (MONO, MF, RLE after day #1, #14, #30 to 90 post-op);

Urgencies and Emergencies

B. Post-Op Return Visit (RV) Routine Schedule

1. Day #1 post-op
2. Day #14 post-op
3. Day #30 to #90 post-op

C. Step-by-Step Post-Op SOAP Management by Type of IOL and Visit Schedule

1. Steps and clinical findings vary slightly for each type of IOL and their respective visits. Use specific section below [MONO, MF or RLE] for the IOL type you are managing
2. **Subjective** and ***Urgencies and Emergencies*** categories are similar for all IOL categories with limited additions for some IOL types. Thus, generic **Subjective** and ***Urgencies and Emergencies*** categories are presented immediately below which apply to all IOL SOAP outlines:

Subjective (General questions directly below plus any additional items in specific SOAP note)

Questions to ask:

- "How are you feeling today?" Any residual effects from the anesthesia?
- If the patient is taking any oral meds, "Are you experiencing any adverse reactions?"
- "Have you had any issues or discomfort in the operated eye?"
- "Have you (or a caregiver) been able to instill the eyedrops effectively?"
- Rule out any significant ocular surface irritation and/or any uveitic (deep) pain
- "Have you noticed any significant changes (better or worse) in your vision?"
    - Blurring (intermittent, decreasing, increasing, constant, progressing)

TABLE 7.3 Postoperative Care for IOL Patients: Routine Care and Potential Complications

POSTOPERATIVE CARE FOR IOL PATIENTS		
ROUTINE CARE (Minimum [required by Medicare modifiers] 3 visits over 3-month post-op period)		
Clinical Tests	**Normal Findings**	**Action (if any required)**
> Patient interview	Comfortable and acceptable BCVA (D/N)	
> Pinhole vision	≥20/30	Recheck in 2 weeks if ≤ 20/40
> Keratometry	Clear mires	Artificial tears if mires distorted
> Refraction (NO AUTO REFRACTOR!)	Start with Ks and push plus	Repeat at each post-op visit (3)
> BCVA – Distance	≥20/40	Repeat at each post-op visit (3)
>BCVA – Near (with dist. correction)	≥ J4 at intermediate and near distances	Repeat at each post-op visit (3)
> Cornea (SLE)	Mid edema at week 1	(See "Potential Complications" below if needed)
> Anterior Chamber (SLE)	Trace cells and flare up to month 1	(See "Potential Complications" below if needed)
> Pupil and iris (SLE)	PERRLA and pupil size relative to SXs	(See "Potential Complications" below if needed)
> IOL (SLE)	Centered and proper ant/Post. orientation	(See "Potential Complications" below if needed)
> Retina/Macula	Same as pre-operative status	(See "Potential Complications" below if needed)
> ONH (90 D)	Same as pre-operative status	(See "Potential Complications" below if needed)
> IOP (T_A)	Same range as pre-operative IOP	(See "Potential Complications" below if needed)
> Wave front aberrometry (optional)	Perform if BCVA ≤ 20/40	Phone consult with surgeon if HOAs ≥ 0.4μ *RMS*

POTENTIAL COMPLICATIONS	
Patient Complaint or Abnormal Finding	**Action (If Any Required)**
> Blurred distance vision (gradual onset)	Recheck refraction (especially cyl)/Add or increase artificial tears
> Blurred near vision (gradual onset)	Recheck refraction (especially cyl)/Add or increase artificial tears
> Best correctable distance vision < 20/40	Hard CL over refraction. If no improvement, phone consult with surgeon
> Sudden blur or loss of vision	IOP, SLE, BIO, 90 D and phone consult or refer to surgeon
> Ocular surface pain or irritation	SLE and treat appropriately
> Acute surface inflammation (≥ 2+ redness)	Topical steroid QID for 48 hours. If no improvement, refer to surgeon
> Leaking keratotomy incision (+ Seidel sign)	Refer to surgeon for suture repair
> Deeper intraocular pain (uveitic type)	SLE, BIO and phone consult or refer to surgeon (STAT if endophthalmitis)
> Hyphema (free RBCs or accumulated blood level)	Refer to surgeon STAT
> Posterior capsular fibrosis reducing visual acuity	If BCVA ≤ 20/40, refer to surgeon for possible YAG capsulotomy
> Decentered, tilted or luxated IOL	Refer to surgeon
> Gradual, insidious rise in IOP	Phone consult with surgeon
> Acute rise in IOP (See Chapter 8, Section III G. 2.)	Refer to surgeon STAT
> CME	Refer to surgeon

    – Spherical aberrations (halos, glare, photophobia, etc.) (see Table 7.1)
    – Dysphotopsias (arcs or streaks of light)
- Assess subjective complaints relative to pupil diameter and advise on lighting adjustments (increased) for halos and distance vision

Urgencies and Emergencies **(General findings directly below plus any additional items in specific SOAP note)**

(Check Section D, "Potential Postoperative Complications" below and Table 7.3 and Appendix 5 for additional potential postoperative complications, their clinical effects, and corrective actions.)

ASAP or STAT referral to surgeon for:

- Leaking keratotomy or AK incision with Seidel sign after 14 days
- Increasing inflammation (redness) greater than 2 to 3+ or endophthalmitis
- Flat anterior chamber
- Excess lens fragments in anterior chamber
- Deep intraocular (uveitic type) pain in the post-op eye
- Hyphema (free RBCs in aqueous or accumulated blood level in chamber)
- Acute increase in IOP: usually severe eye pain with nausea and vomiting

MONOFOCAL (MONO) IOL DAY #1 POST-OP SOAP[16]

(Some surgeons prefer to see the patient on Day #1 post-op)

Subjective Monofocal (MONO) Day #1

Questions to ask: (See generic **Subjective** page 292)

Objective Monofocal (MONO) Day #1

Perform the following tests and evaluate results based on Table 7.3:

- Pinhole distance vision: Goal @ 20/20 to 20/40
- Uncorrected distance vision expectations (fair to good)
  - > Near with monovision should be fair to good
- Keratometry mires or topography should be clear and undistorted
- Refraction or over-refraction (NO AUTOREFRACTOR!)
  > Start with +0.75 fog
  - > Push plus and min. cyl.
- BCVA—distance: Should be about equal to pinhole vision with or without overcorrection
- BCVA—near (without plus overcorrection): Goal @ J2 to J6
- Cornea (SLE): > document any epithelial defect (SPK or abrasions)
  - > Diagram any endothelial irregularities (striae, folds, guttata as compared to pre-examination documentation)
  - > Check keratotomy incision for leakage (use NaFl burping)
    - – Anesthetize cornea with proparacaine and instill NaFl
    - – Apply slight pressure on the cornea with a blunt instrument just outside the incision and observe any aqueous outflow from the wound noted by NaFl streaming (Seidel sign)
    - – Rule out ocular hypotension with T_A
- If astigmatic keratotomy (AK) was performed immediately (or later) after surgery, check arcuate incisions with Seidel sign (see above) for any leakage (produced by a full-thickness versus partial incision)
- Anterior chamber (SLE): > chamber (and angle) should be deep
  - > May see some WBCs but should not see RBCs (hyphema)
  - > Small amount(s) of lens fragments
- Pupil and Iris (SLE): > should have PERRLA
  - > Iris should be clear of any blood and note if intraoperative iridotomy was performed
- IOL (SLE)
  - > IOL should be centered in pupillary zone, perhaps with edge(s) observable in dim illumination (scotopic pupil)
  - > Distinctly observable lens edge (i.e., in pupillary zone) indicates a dislocated IOL and may require surgical relocation or replacement
- Ocular surface may demonstrate inconsequential subconjunctival hemorrhage and/or hyperemia (post-op effect) but not > 1 to 2+
- Retina /Macula (BIO): retina should be at pre-operative condition and macula should demonstrate a foveal reflex
- ONH (90 D): should be flat and C/D consistent with preoperative status
- IOP (T_A): Should be normal to slightly raised (< 4 mm Hg)
  - > Rule out steroid-induced raised IOP
- Wavefront aberrometry (optional): HOA values should be ≤ 0.4*s* RMS

Assessment Monofocal (MONO) Day #1

Dx Diagnostic considerations based on subjective (**S**) and objective (**O**) information

- Assuming subjective (**S**) responses and all clinical findings (**O**) within normal limits (WNL), the post-op eye should be considered stable and recovering well
- Any actions and/or adjustments in response to clinical findings from subjective (**S**) and/or objective (**O**) above should be conducted per Table 7.3

Plan Monofocal (MONO) Day #1

Provide necessary care for any positive clinical findings from **S**, **O**, and **A** per Table 7.3:

- Reassure patient of positive response to surgery and recovering well
- Strongly advise use of artificial tears daily (q ≥ 4 h or greater)
- Ask patient if they have any questions
- Advise on likelihood of minor changes in vision (positive or negative)
- If Seidel sign present with any corneal incisions, report to surgeon and monitor at 14-day visit for closure
- In case of flat anterior chamber, refer back to surgeon
- In case of acute inflammation ≥ 2+, consult with surgeon for treatment approach
- For hyphema (whole blood in anterior chamber), refer to surgeon
- For microhyphema (RBCs in anterior chamber), recheck in 3 to 5 days
- Explain the phenomenon of "neuroadaptation" to the patient regarding the likelihood of some visual perceptual variations from their pre-op visions:
  - > "You're adjusting to a 'new visual system'"
  - > "Your brain will adapt through a process called 'neuroplasticity'"
  - > "During this process you will experience variable vision"
  - > Depending on individuals, duration lasts from weeks to (sometimes) years
  - > This is extremely valuable counseling for short- and long-term reassurance
- With any abnormal or suspicious **S** and/or **O** findings, reschedule accordingly
- If patient comfortable and **S** and **O** findings WNL, schedule Day #14 RV

Follow-Up Monofocal (MONO) from Day #1 to #14

Advise patient to contact you immediately if:

- Red or increasingly irritated eye(s) not responding to artificial tears
- Acute and/or increasing pain in the post-op eye
- Sudden loss of vision

Urgencies and Emergencies Monofocal (MONO) from Day #1 to #14

(Check Section D, "Potential Postoperative Complications" below and Table 7.3 and Appendix 5 for additional potential postoperative complications, their clinical effects, and corrective actions.)

ASAP or STAT referral to surgeon for:
(See generic ***Urgencies and Emergencies*** page 293)

MONOFOCAL (MONO) IOL DAY #14 POST-OP SOAP

(RV may be adjusted per Day #1 findings and instructions)

Subjective (MONO) Day #14

Questions to ask: (See generic **Subjective** page 292)

Objective (MONO) Day #14

Perform the following tests and evaluate results based on Table 7.3:

- Pinhole vision: Goal @ 20/20 to 20/40
- Uncorrected distance vision expectations—should be good:
  > If monovision, near vision should be good to excellent
- Keratometry mires or topography should be clear and undistorted
- Refraction (NO AUTO REFRACTOR!): Establish final near (dist. if necessary) Rx
- Cylinder error ≥ 0.75 may cause vision reduction and/or subjective complaints
- BCVA—Distance: > Should be correctable (w/o Rx) to @ 20/20 to 20/30
  > Refract through hard contact lens if BCVA < 20/30
- BCVA—Near (with dist. correction if needed): Goal @ J1 to J3
- Cornea (SLE): > Document any epithelial defect (SPK or abrasions)
  > Recheck and compare (to Day #1) any endothelial irregularities
- Confirm elimination of any Seidel signs observed at Day #1
- Anterior chamber (SLE): chamber (and angle) should remain deep and clear
- Pupil and Iris (SLE): > should have PERRLA
  > Iris should be clear of any blood and note (and diagram?) if intraoperative iridotomy was performed
- IOL (SLE)
  > IOL should remain centered in the pupillary zone as from Day #1
  > Lens tilt or dislocation (luxation) will produce irregular astigmatism and reduced vision
- Retina/Macula (BIO): retina should be at pre-operative condition and macula should continue to demonstrate a foveal reflex
- ONH (90 D): Should be flat and C/D consistent with pre-operative status
- IOP (T_A): Should be back to pre-op level
- Rule out steroid-induced raised IOP
- Wavefront aberrometry (optional): Consider HOA levels if BCVAs are reduced

Assessment Monofocal (MONO) Day #14

Dx Diagnostic considerations based on subjective (**S**) and objective (**O**) information

- Assuming subjective responses and all clinical findings within normal limits (WNL), the post-op eye should be considered stable and recovering well
- Any actions and/or adjustments in response to clinical findings from subjective (**S**) and/or objective (**O**) above should be conducted per Table 7.3

Plan Monofocal (MONO) Day #14

℞ Provide necessary care based on Table 7.3

- Reassure patient of positive post-op progress
- Strongly advise use of artificial tears daily (q ≥ 4 h or greater)
- If irregular astigmatism from lens tilt or dislocation is significant, refer to surgeon for possible lens manipulation
- Ask patient if they have any questions
- With any abnormal or suspicious **S** and/or **O** findings, reschedule accordingly
- If patient comfortable and **S** and **O** findings WNL, schedule Day #30 to #90 RV

Follow-Up Monofocal (MONO) from Day #14 to #30 to #90

Advise patient to contact you immediately if:

- Acute and/or increasing pain in the post-op eye
- Sudden loss of vision

Urgencies and Emergencies Monofocal (MONO) from Day #14 to #30 to #90

(Check Section D, "Potential Postoperative Complications" below and Table 7.3 and Appendix 5 for additional potential postoperative complications, their clinical effects, and corrective actions.)

ASAP or STAT referral to surgeon for:
(See generic ***Urgencies and Emergencies*** page 293)

MONOFOCAL (MONO) IOL DAY #30 TO #90 POST-OP SOAP (SEE ALSO TABLE 7.3)

(RV may be adjusted per Day #14 findings and instructions)

Subjective Monofocal (MONO) Day #30 to #90

(See generic **Subjective** page 292 plus additional questions below)

Questions to ask:

- Ask about neuroadaptative progress

Objective Monofocal (MONO) Day #30 to #90

Perform the following tests and evaluate results based on Table 7.3:

- Uncorrected distance vision expectation (should be excellent, i.e., 20/20):
  - > With monovision: intermediate good; near may need low powered plus correction
- Refraction: over-refraction (over uncorrected or spectacle corrected) if VA reduced
- Cylinder error ≥ 0.75 may cause vision reduction and/or subjective complaints
- BCVA—distance: probable best final vision
- BCVA—near (with distance correction): probable best final vision
- Cornea (SLE): check carefully for posterior capsular opacification (PCO) or fibrosis (Figure 7.2) refer to surgeon for YAG capsulotomy if vision significantly reduced
- Possible non-specific ocular surface inflammation
- ONH (90 D): reconfirm foveal reflex
- IOP (T_A): should be at pre-operative level
- Wavefront aberrometry (optional): only if significant higher order aberrations (spherical aberrations [subjective halos, glare, see Table 7.1, coma, 4th order astigmia [distortion])

Assessment Monofocal (MONO) Day #30 to #90

Dx Diagnostic considerations based on subjective (**S**) and objective (**O**) information

- Assuming subjective responses and all clinical findings within normal limits (WNL), the post-op eye should be considered stable and recovering well
- Any actions and/or adjustments in response to clinical findings from subjective (**S**) and/or objective (**O**) above should be conducted per Table 7.3

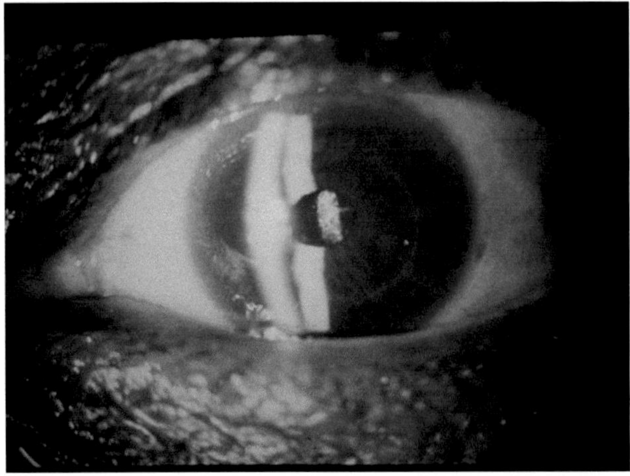

FIGURE 7.2 Posterior capsular fibrosis (or opacification): after 3 to 6 months (generally), fibrosis develops centrally (~25% of cases) on the posterior capsule causing the patient to reports an insidious reduction in vision (≤ 20/30) greater at distance. An Nd:YAG laser is used to perform a posterior capsulotomy.

Plan (MONO) Day #30 to #90

℞ Provide necessary care based on Table 7.3:

- Advise patient of final visual acuities (distance and near)
- Prescribe final near and distance (if necessary) Rx (bifocal preferable)
- Ask about neuroadaptative progress
- Advise on continued use of artificial tears daily (tid to qid)
- In case of ocular surface inflammation, treat appropriately with antibiotic and steroid
- Ask patient if they have any questions
- If patient comfortable and **S** and **O** findings WNL, schedule routine RV

Follow-Up Monofocal (MONO) after Day #30 to #90

Advise patient to contact you immediately if:

- Red or increasingly irritated eye(s) not responding to artificial tears
- Acute and/or increasing pain in the post-op eye
- Any sudden or insidious changes in vision
- Sudden or increasing flashes and/or floaters in field of vision
- Any questions?

Urgencies and Emergencies Monofocal (MONO) after Day #30 to #90

(Check Section D, "Potential Postoperative Complications" below and Table 7.3 and Appendix 5 for additional potential postoperative complications, their clinical effects, and corrective actions.)

ASAP or STAT referral to surgeon for:
(See generic ***Urgencies and Emergencies*** page 293)

MULTIFOCAL (MF AND ACCOMODATING IOL) DAY #1 POST-OP SOAP[17]

(See also Table 7.3 and Appendix 5)
(Some surgeons prefer to see the patient at Day #1 post-op)

1. Pseudo-accommodating (AMO *Tecnis*, Alcon *ReStor, Panoptix*, et al.)
2. Accommodating (translational design; B&L *Crystalens*, et al.)

Subjective (MF AND Accommodating IOL) Day #1

(See generic **Subjective** page 292 plus additional questions below)

Questions to ask:

- Are you able to read small print with good lighting (newspaper, books, labels, etc.)?
- Do you have to adjust your head position in any way to see up close (e.g., read)?

Objective (MF and Accommodating IOL) Day #1

Perform the following tests and evaluate results based on Table 7.3:

- Pinhole vision: Goal @ 20/20 to 20/60
- Uncorrected vision expectations
  - > *ReStor*: distance—fair; near—fair to good (fair intermediate with *PanOptix*)
  - > *Tecnis*: distance—variable; near—fair to good
  - > *Crystalens*: poor to fair due to cycloplegia
- Keratometry mires or topography should be clear and undistorted
- Refraction or over-refraction (NO AUTO REFRACTOR!); > Start at +0.75 fog
  - > Push plus & min. cyl.
- Don't prescribe corrective lenses at this visit
- BCVA—distance: should be about equal to pinhole vision
- BCVA—near (with dist. overcorrection if needed): Goal @ J3 to J8 (may be reading through distance segment?)
- Cornea (SLE): > document any epithelial defect (SPK or abrasions)
  - > Diagram any endothelial irregularities (striae, folds, guttata as compared to pre-examination documentation)
  - > Check keratotomy incision for leakage (use burping with NaFl)
    - – Anesthetize cornea with proparacaine and instill NaFl
    - – Apply slight pressure on the cornea with a blunt instrument just outside the incision and observe any aqueous outflow from the wound noted by NaFl streaming (Seidel sign)
    - – Rule out ocular hypotension with T_A
- If astigmatic keratotomy (AK) was performed immediately (or later) after surgery, check arcuate incisions with Seidel sign (see above) for any leakage produced by a full-thickness versus partial incision
- Anterior chamber (SLE): > chamber (and angle) should be deep and clear
  - > May see some WBCs but should not see RBCs (hyphema)
  - > Small amount(s) of lens fragments
- Pupil and Iris (SLE)
  - > Should have PERRLA
  - > Iris should be clear of any blood and note if intraoperative iridotomy was performed
- IOL (SLE)
  - > IOL should be centered in the pupillary zone, perhaps with edge(s) observable in dim illumination (dilated pupil)
  - > Distinctly observable lens edge (i.e., in pupillary zone) indicates a dislocated IOL and may require surgical relocation or replacement
  - > Crystalens optic should demonstrate a slight vaulting posteriorward
- Ocular surface may demonstrate inconsequential subconjunctival hemorrhage and/or hyperemia (post-op effect) but no > 1 to 2+
- Retina/macula (BIO): retina should be at pre-operative condition and macula should demonstrate a foveal reflex
- ONH (90 D): should be flat and C/D consistent with pre-operative status
- IOP (T_A): should be normal to slightly raised (< 4 mm Hg)
  - > Rule out steroid-induced raised IOP
- Wavefront aberrometry (optional): HOA values should be ≤ 0.4*s* RMS

Assessment (MF and Accommodating IOL) Day #1

Dx Diagnostic considerations based on subjective (**S**) and objective (**O**) information

- Assuming subjective responses and all clinical findings within normal limits (WNL), the post-op eye should be considered stable and recovering well
- Any actions and/or adjustment in response to clinical findings from subjective (**S**) and/or objective (**O**) above should be conducted per Table 7.3

Plan (MF and Accommodating IOL) Day #1

℞ Provide necessary care for any positive clinical findings from **S**, **O**, and **A** above per Table 7.3:

- Reassure patient of positive response to surgery and recovering well
- If Seidel sign present with any corneal incisions, report to surgeon and monitor at 14-day visit for closure
- Strongly advise the use of artificial tears daily (q ≥ 4 h or greater)
- Explain any issues related to adjustment to distance and near IOL segments patient may have reported in subjective (**S**)
- Recommend accommodative push-up exercises for improved distance to near translation with accommodative IOL (*Crystalens*)
- Advise on likelihood of transition from distance to near will take some time
- Reassure on continued adaptation to multifocal effects
- Ask patient if they have any questions
- Advise on likelihood of minor changes in vision (positive or negative)
- In case of acute inflammation ≥ 2+, contact surgeon for advice
- For hyphema (whole blood in anterior chamber), refer to surgeon
- For microhyphema (RBCs in anterior chamber), recheck in 3 to 5 days
- Explain the phenomenon of "neuroadaptation" to the patient regarding the likelihood of some visual perceptual variations from their pre-op visions, especially when transitioning from distance to near vision:
  - > "You're adjusting to a 'new visual system'"
  - > "Your brain will adapt through a process called 'neuroplasticity'"
  - > "During this process you will experience variable vision"
  - > Depending on individuals, duration lasts from weeks to (sometimes) years
  - > This is extremely valuable counseling for short- and long-term reassurance
  - > Substantial and/or continuing complaints of halos and/or night driving glare may be ameliorated with brimonidine (*Alphagan*), combined carbachol and brimonidine (*Brimochol*), or 0.5% to 1.25% Pilo (*Vuity*) qd and auto dome light; Alphagan *preferred drug due to least side effects*

- With any abnormal or suspicious **S** and/or **O** findings, reschedule accordingly
- If patient comfortable and **S** and **O** findings WNL, schedule Day #14 RV

Follow-Up (MF and Accommodating IOL) from Day #1 to #14

Advise patient to contact you immediately if:

- Red or increasingly irritated eye(s) not responding to artificial tears
- Acute and/or increasing pain in the post-op eye
- Sudden loss of vision

Urgencies and Emergencies (MF and Accommodating IOL) from Day #1 to #14

(Check Section D, "Potential Postoperative Complications" below and Table 7.3 and Appendix 5 for additional potential postoperative complications, their clinical effects, and corrective actions.)

ASAP or STAT referral to surgeon for:
(See generic ***Urgencies and Emergencies*** page 293)

MULTIFOCAL (MF AND ACCOMMODATING IOL) DAY #14 POST-OP SOAP

(See also Table 7.3 and Appendix 5)
(RV may be adjusted per Day #1 findings and instructions)

Subjective (MF and Accommodating IOL) Day #14

(See generic **Subjective** page 292 plus additional questions below)

Questions to ask:

- "Have you been adapting well to the multifocal optics effects?"
- "Have you noticed any significant changes (better or worse) in your distance and/or near vision?"
- Transition from distance to near vision improving?

Objective (MF and Accommodating IOL) Day #14

Perform the following tests and evaluate results based on Table 7.3:

- Pinhole vision: Goal @ 20/20 to 20/40
- Uncorrected vision expectations
  - > *ReStor:* distance—should be good; near—fair to good (good intermediate with *PanOptix*)
  - > *Tecnis:* distance—fair to good (still variable); near—fair to good (variable)
  - > *Crystalens:* distance—good to excellent; near—fair to good (variable)
- Keratometry mires or topography should be clear and undistorted
- Refraction (NO AUTO REFRACTOR!): consider near (distance if necessary) Rx but don't prescribe anything at this visit (temporary distance Rx if absolutely necessary)
  - > Don't let mutlifocals "suck up minus or cyl!"
  - > Leave them at most plus for best VA
- Cylinder error ≥ 0.75 may cause vision reduction and/or subjective complaints
- BCVA—distance: > should be correctable (w/o Rx) to @ 20/20 to 20/40
  - > Refract through hard contact lens if BCVA < 20/40
- BCVA—near (with dist. correction if needed): Goal @ J2 to J5
- With *Crystalens*, if VAs and refraction don't correlate well or if near VA is < J3, do cycloplegic refraction
- Cornea (SLE)
  - > Document any epithelial defect (SPK or abrasions)
  - > Recheck and compare (to Day #1) any endothelial irregularities
- Confirm elimination of any Seidel signs observed at Day #1
  - > Anterior chamber (SLE): chamber (and angle) should remain deep and clear
- IOL (SLE)
  - > Lens tilt or dislocation (luxation) will produce irregular astigmatism and reduced vision
  - > *Crystalens* vault should be reconfirmed
- Pupil and Iris (SLE): > should have PERRLA
  - > Iris should be clear of any blood and note (and diagram?) if intraoperative iridotomy was performed
- IOL (SLE): IOL should remain centered in the pupillary zone as from Day #1
- Possible non-specific ocular surface inflammation
- Retina /Macula (BIO): retina should be at pre-operative condition and macula should continue to demonstrate a foveal reflex
- ONH (90 D): should be flat and C/D consistent with pre-operative status
- IOP (T_A): should be back to pre-op level
  - > Rule out steroid-induced raised IOP
- Wavefront aberrometry (optional): consider HOA levels if BCVAs are reduced

Assessment (MF and Accommodating IOL) Day #14

Dx Diagnostic considerations based on subjective (**S**) and objective (**O**) information

- Assuming subjective responses and all clinical findings within normal limits (WNL), the post-op eye should be considered stable and recovering well
- Any actions and/or adjustment in response to clinical findings from subjective (**S**) and/or objective (**O**) above should be conducted per Table 7.3

Plan (MF and Accommodating IOL) Day #14

Provide necessary care based on Table 7.3:

- Reassure patient of positive post-op progress
- Ask about neuroadaptative progress
- If irregular astigmatism from lens tilt or dislocation is significant, refer to surgeon for possible lens manipulation
- Ask about multifocal optics adjustment (i.e., distance to near transition, etc.)
- Strongly advise the use of artificial tears daily (q ≥ 4 h or greater)

- In case of ocular surface inflammation, treat appropriately with antibiotic and steroid
- Accommodative (pushup, "tromboning") exercises may enhance near vision
- Ask patient if they have any questions
- With any abnormal or suspicious **S** and/or **O** findings, reschedule accordingly
- If patient comfortable and **S** and **O** findings WNL, schedule Day #30 to #90 RV

Follow-Up (MF and Accommodating IOL) from Day #14 to #30 to #90

Advise patient to contact you immediately if:

- Red or increasingly irritated eye(s) not responding to artificial tears
- Acute and/or increasing pain in the post-op eye
- Sudden loss of vision

Urgencies and Emergencies (MF and Accommodating IOL) from Day #14 to #30 to #90

(Check Section D, "Potential Postoperative Complications" below and Table 7.3 and Appendix 5 for additional potential postoperative complications, their clinical effects, and corrective actions.)

ASAP or STAT referral to surgeon for:

(See generic ***Urgencies and Emergencies*** page 293)

MULTIFOCAL (MF AND ACCOMMODATING IOL) DAY #30 TO #90 POST-OP SOAP

(See also Table 7.3)

(RV may be adjusted per Day #14 findings and instructions)

Subjective (MF and Accommodating IOL) Day #30 to #90

(See generic **Subjective** page 292 plus additional questions below)

Questions to ask:

- "Are you comfortable with your multifocal (bi- or trifocal) vision?"
- Ask about neuroadaptative progress

Objective (MF and Accommodating IOL) Day #30 to #90

Perform the following tests and evaluate results based on Table 7.3:

- Uncorrected vision expectations
  - > *ReStor*: distance—good to excellent; near—good (good intermediate with *PanOptix*)
  - > *Tecnis*: distance—good to excellent; near—fair to good (variable)
  - > *Crystalens*: distance—good to excellent; near—fair to good (variable)
- Refraction: > over-refraction (over uncorrected or temporary lens correction)
  - > Prescribe final (maximum plus) spectacle Rx if indicated (single vision or bifocal)
- BCVA—distance: probably best final vision
- BCVA—near (with dist. correction): probably best final vision
- Cornea (SLE)
  - > Check for posterior capsular opacification (PCO) or fibrosis
  - > Mild to moderate PCO may reduce multifocal optics significantly
  - > Refer to surgeon for YAG capsulotomy if PCO significant and/or reducing vision
- ONH (90 D): reconfirm foveal reflex
- IOP (T_A): should be at pre-operative level
- Wavefront aberrometry (optional): only if significant higher order aberrations; (spherical aberrations [subjective halos, glare, see Table 7.1], coma, 4th order astigmia [distortion])

Assessment (MF and Accommodating IOL) Day #30 to #90

Dx Diagnostic considerations based on subjective (**S**) and objective (**O**) information

- Assuming subjective responses and all clinical findings within normal limits (WNL), the post-op eye should be considered stable and recovering well
- Any actions and/or adjustment in response to clinical findings from subjective (**S**) and/or objective (**O**) above should be conducted per Table 7.3

Plan (MF and Accommodating IOL) Day #30 to #90

℞ Provide necessary care based on Table 7.3:

- Advise patient of final visual acuities (distance and near)
- Prescribe final near and distance (if necessary) Rx (bifocal preferable)
- Ask about neuroadaptative progress
- Explain that adjustment(s) to multifocal optics (e.g., head positioning, etc.) will become the subconscious norm
- Advise on continued use of artificial tears daily (tid to qid)
- Ask patient if they have any questions
- If patient comfortable and **S** and **O** findings WNL, schedule routine RV

Follow-Up (MF and Accommodating IOL) after Day #30 to #90

Advise patient to contact you immediately if:

- Red or increasingly irritated eye(s) not responding to artificial tears
- Acute and/or increasing pain in the post-op eye
- Any sudden or insidious changes in vision
- Sudden or increasing flashes and/or floater in field of vision
- Any questions?
  - > Possible late developing fibrosis (PCO) will begin to reduce vision (distance and near) and patient will need posterior capsule YAG capsulotomy

Urgencies and Emergencies (MF and Accommodating IOL) after Day #30 to #90

(Check Section D, "Potential Postoperative Complications" below and Table 7.3 and Appendix 5 for additional potential postoperative complications, their clinical effects, and corrective actions.)

ASAP or STAT referral to surgeon for:
(See generic ***Urgencies and Emergencies*** page 293)

REFRACTIVE LENS EXCHANGE (RLE) IOL DAY #1 POST-OP SOAP[9,17]

(Some surgeons prefer to see the patient at 24 hours post-op)

1. High hyperopes (> +6 to +8 D) pseudophakic lens exchange
2. High myopes (> −6 to −8 D) natural lens removal
3. Phakic IOLs (IOL with natural lens), see also Figures 7.3 and 7.4
   a. *Verisyse* (anterior chamber lens) for −5.00 to −20.00 myopia
   b. *Visian* ICL (Implantable Collamer Lens), a posterior chamber (in sulcus) for −3.00 to −23.00 myopia

Subjective (RLE) Day #1

Questions to ask: (See generic **Subjective** page 292)

Objective (RLE) Day #1

Perform the following tests and evaluate results based on Table 7.3:

- Pinhole distance vision: Goal @ 20/20 to 20/40
- Uncorrected vision expectations (depending on procedure)

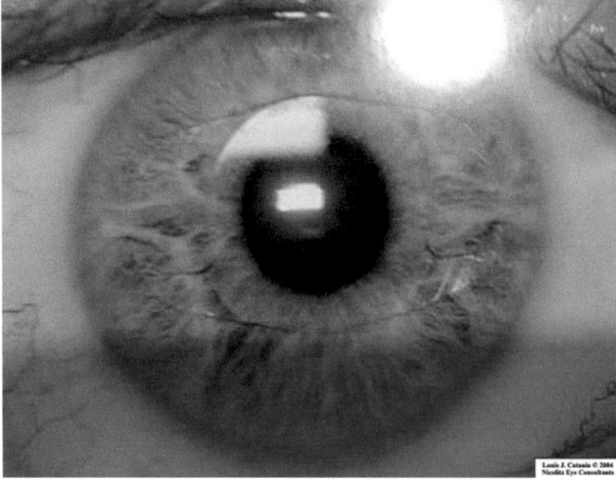

FIGURE 7.3 *Verisyse* anterior chamber phakic IOL by J&J (International: *Artisan* by Ophtec) for use in refractive lens exchange (RLE): this phakic IOL corrects higher degrees of myopia (≥ 10 D) while retaining the natural crystalline lens (for retinal security). It is attached to the mid iris stroma by haptic enclavation.

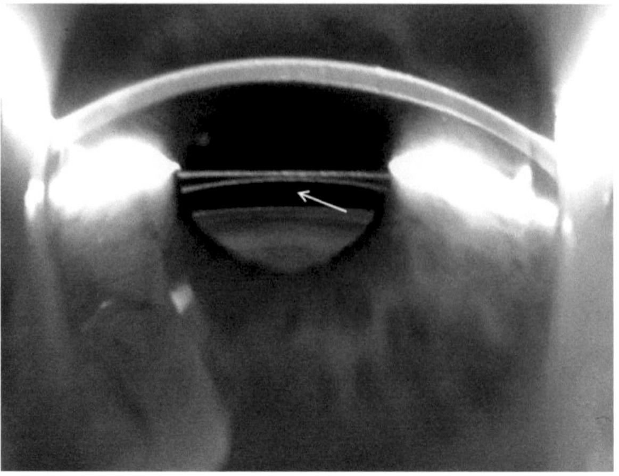

FIGURE 7.4 Visian posterior chamber phakic IOL by Staar for use in refractive lens exchange (RLE): This phakic IOL is implanted in the sulcus of the lens chamber anterior to the natural crystalline lens. It is critical that the posterior surface of the IOL remains "vaulted" approximately 0.5 to 1.0 mm (< 0.5 risks anterior lens capsule touch and secondary opacification and > 1.0 risks narrowing anterior angle). This photo demonstrates the use of Scheimpflug imaging to compare vault to corneal thickness (~0.5 mm).

  > Anterior chamber IOL (*Verisyse*): distance—Should be good (depending on corneal clarity); near—fair to good (depending on corneal clarity) (non-presbyope)
  > Posterior chamber IOL (*Visian ICL*): distance—should be good; near—fair to good (non-presbyope)
- Keratometry mires or topography should be clear and undistorted
- Refraction or over-refraction (NO AUTO REFRACTOR!); > Start at +0.75 fog
- Push plus & min. cyl.
- BCVA—distance: should be about equal to pinhole vision with or without overcorrection
- BCVA—near (non-presbyope): Goal @ J2 to J4
- Cornea (SLE): > cornea may show slight haze (edema, especially with *Verisyse*)
  > Document any epithelial defect (SPK or abrasions)
  > Check keratotomy incision for leakage (use NaFl burping)
    – Anesthetize cornea with proparacaine and instill NaFl
    – Apply slight pressure on the cornea with a blunt instrument just outside the incision and observe any aqueous outflow from the wound noted by NaFl streaming (Seidel sign)
    – Rule out ocular hypotension with T_A
- If astigmatic keratotomy (AK) was performed at immediately (or later) after surgery, check arcuate incisions with Seidel sign (see above) for any leakage (produced by a full-thickness versus partial incision)
- Anterior chamber (SLE)
  > Chamber (and angle) should be deep and clear
  > May see few WBCs but should not see RBCs (hyphema)
- Pupil and Iris (SLE)
  > Should have PERRLA
  > Iris should be clear of any blood and note if intraoperative iridotomy was performed

- IOL (SLE)
  - > Posterior chamber IOLs should be centered in the pupillary zone with lens edge(s) occasionally visible at the dilated pupil border
  - > *Verisyse* (anterior chamber lens) should be centered over the pupil (Figure 7.3) with the optic and enclavated haptics attached to mid-iris stroma clearly observable
  - > With anterior chamber IOL (*Verisyse*) diagram any endothelial irregularities (striae, folds, guttata as compared to pre-examination documentation)
  - > With posterior chamber IOL (*Visian ICL*) measure separation ("vault") between posterior lens surface and natural lens. Should be at least 0.5 mm which can be approximated by the thickness of the corneal optical section parallelpiped at 30° to 45° (Figure 7.4)
  - > Vault less than 0.5 mm = risk of lenticular touch and resultant hazing
  - > Vault greater than 1.5 mm = risk of narrow angle (anterior iris pressure)
  - > Use Scheimpflug imaging to approximate the vault by comparing it to the corneal thickness (~ 0.5 mm)
- Ocular surface may demonstrate inconsequential subconjunctival hemorrhage and/or hyperemia (post-op effect) but no > 1 to 2+
- Retina /Macula (BIO): retina should be at pre-operative condition and macula should demonstrate a foveal reflex
- ONH (90 D): should be flat and C/D consistent with preoperative status
- IOP (T_A): should be normal to slightly raised (< 4 mm Hg)
- > Rule out steroid-induced raised IOP
- Wavefront aberrometry (optional): HOA values should be ≤ 0.4*s* RMS

Assessment (RLE) Day #1

Dx Diagnostic considerations based on subjective (**S**) and objective (**O**) information

- Assuming subjective responses and all clinical findings within normal limits (WNL), the post-op eye should be considered stable and recovering well
- If corneal endothelium compromised with *Verisyse* IOL, corneal thickness and edema must be monitored closely
- If *Visian ICL* vault is less than 0.5 mm, monitor anterior surface of natural lens closely
- Any actions and/or adjustment should be conducted per Table 7.3

Plan (RLE) Day #1

℞ Provide necessary care for any positive clinical findings from **S**, **O**, and **A** above per Table 7.3:

- Reassure patient of positive response to surgery and recovering well
- Strongly advise the use of artificial tears daily (q ≥ 4 h or greater)
- Ask patient if they have any questions
- Advise on likelihood of minor changes in vision (positive or negative)
- If Seidel sign present with any corneal incisions, report to surgeon and monitor at 14-day visit for closure
- In case of ocular surface inflammation, treat appropriately with antibiotic and steroid
- For hyphema (whole blood in anterior chamber), refer to surgeon
- For microhyphema (RBCs in anterior chamber), recheck in 3 to 5 days
- Explain the phenomenon of "neuroadaptation" to the patient regarding the likelihood of some visual perceptual variations from their pre-op visions
  - > "Your adjusting to a 'new visual system'"
  - > "Your brain will adapt through a process called 'neuroplasticity'"
  - > "During this process you will experience variable vision"
  - > Depending on individuals, duration lasts from weeks to (sometimes) years
  - > This is extremely valuable counseling for short- and long-term reassurance
- With any abnormal or suspicious **S** and/or **O** findings, reschedule accordingly
- If patient comfortable and **S** and **O** findings WNL, schedule Day #14 RV

Follow-Up (RLE) from Day #1 to Day #14

Advise patient to contact you immediately if:

- Acute and/or increasing pain in the post-op eye
- Sudden loss of vision
- Instruct patient to report any "hazy" vision (due to corneal edema)

Urgencies and Emergencies (RLE) from Day #1 to #14

(Check Section D, "Potential Postoperative Complications" below and Table 7.3 and Appendix 5 for additional potential postoperative complications, their clinical effects, and corrective actions.)

ASAP or STAT referral to surgeon for:

(See generic ***Urgencies and Emergencies*** page 293 plus additional items below)

- Increasing hazy and/or reduced vision (from corneal endothelial compromise)
- Dislocation of anterior chamber IOL (*Verisyse*)

REFRACTIVE LENS EXCHANGE (RLE) IOL DAY #14 POST-OP SOAP[9]

(RV may be adjusted per Day #1 findings and instructions)

Subjective (RLE) Day #14

Questions to ask: (See generic **Subjective** page 292)

Objective (RLE) Day #14

Perform the following tests and evaluate results based on Table 7.3:

- Pinhole vision: Goal @ 20/20 to 20/40
- Uncorrected vision expectations (depending on procedure)

  - > Anterior chamber IOL (*Verisyse*): distance—should be good; near (non-presbyope)—good
  - > Posterior chamber IOL (*Visian ICL*): distance—should be good; near (non-presbyope)—good
- Keratometry mires or topography should be clear and undistorted
- Refraction (NO AUTO REFRACTOR!): establish final near (dist. if necessary) Rx
- BCVA—distance: > Should be correctable (w/o Rx) to @ 20/20 to 20/30
  - > Refract through hard contact lens if BCVA < 20/30
- BCVA—near (with distance correction if needed): Goal @ J1 to J3
- Cornea (SLE): > Document any epithelial defect (SPK or abrasions)
  - > Recheck and compare (to Day #1) any endothelial irregularities
- Anterior chamber (SLE): chamber (and angle) should remain deep and clear
- Confirm elimination of any Seidel signs observed at Day #1
- Pupil and Iris (SLE)
  - > Should have PERRLA
  - > Note any increase in corneal edema (from *Verisyse*)
  - > Confirm stable iris attachment with *Verisyse*
  - > Iris should be clear of any blood or infiltrates
- IOL (SLE): IOL should remain centered in the pupillary zone as from Day #1
- Retina/macula (BIO): retina should be at pre-operative condition and macula should continue to demonstrate a foveal reflex
- ONH (90 D): should be flat and C/D consistent with pre-operative status
- IOP (T_A): should be back to pre-op level
- > Rule out steroid-induced raised IOP
- Wavefront aberrometry (optional): consider HOA levels if BCVAs are reduced

Assessment (RLE) Day #14

Dx Diagnostic considerations based on subjective (**S**) and objective (**O**) information

- If corneal endothelium compromised with *Verisyse* IOL has increased, consider referring patient back to surgeon for possible lens removal
- If *Visian ICL* vault continues to be less than 0.5 mm, continue to monitor natural lens closely

Plan (RLE) Day #14

℞ Provide necessary care based on Table 7.3:

- Reassure patient of positive post-op progress
- Ask about neuroadaptative progress
- Strongly advise the use of artificial tears daily (q ≥ 4 h or greater)
- In case of ocular surface inflammation, treat appropriately with antibiotic and steroid
- With corneal endothelium compromise (with *Verisyse*) reschedule within 14 days for reassessment; lenticular changes can wait for routine 30 days
- Ask patient if they have any questions
- With any abnormal or suspicious **S** and/or **O** findings, reschedule accordingly
- If patient comfortable and **S** and **O** findings WNL, schedule Day #30 to #90 RV

Follow-Up (RLE) from Day #14 to #30 to #90

Advise patient to contact you immediately if:

- Red or increasingly irritated eye(s) not responding to artificial tears
- Acute and/or increasing pain in the post-op eye
- Sudden loss of vision
  - > Instruct patient to report any "hazy" vision (due to corneal edema)

Urgencies and Emergencies (RLE) from Day #14 to #30 to #90

(Check Section D, "Potential Postoperative Complications" below and Table 7.3 and Appendix 5 for additional potential postoperative complications, their clinical effects, and corrective actions.)

ASAP or STAT referral to surgeon for:

(See generic ***Urgencies and Emergencies*** page 293 plus additional items below)

- Dislocation of anterior chamber IOL (*Verisyse*)
- Increasing hazy and/or reduced vision (from corneal endothelial compromise)

REFRACTIVE LENS EXCHANGE (RLE) IOL DAY #30 TO #90 POST-OP SOAP

(RV may be adjusted per Day #14 findings and instructions)

Subjective (RLE) Day #30 to #90

(See generic **Subjective** page 292 plus additional questions below)

Questions to ask:

- Ask about neuroadaptative progress

Objective (RLE) Day #30 to #90

Perform the following tests and evaluate results based on Table 7.3:

- Uncorrected vision expectations (depending on procedure)
  - > Anterior chamber IOL (*Verisyse*): distance—should be excellent; near—good) (non-presbyope)
  - > Posterior chamber IOL (*Visian* ICL): distance—should be excellent; near—good) (non-presbyope)
- Refraction: over-refraction (over uncorrected or spectacle corrected) if VA reduced
- BCVA—distance: probable best final vision
- BCVA—near (with dist. correction): probable best final vision
- Cornea (SLE): should be in pre-operative state

- Evaluate progress of any corneal endothelial compromise from *Verisyse*
- Evaluate progress of anterior lenticular surface with *Visian ICL*
- ONH (90 D): reconfirm foveal reflex
- IOP (T_A): should be at pre-operative level
- > Rule out steroid-induced raised IOP
- Wavefront aberrometry (optional): only if significant higher order aberrations; (spherical aberrations [subjective halos, glare, see Table 7.1], coma, 4th order astigmia [distortion])

Assessment (RLE) Day #30 to #90

Dx Diagnostic considerations based on subjective (**S**) and objective (**O**) information

- Assuming subjective responses and all clinical findings within normal limits (WNL), the post-op eye should be considered stable and recovering well
- Any actions and/or adjustment in response to clinical findings from subjective (**S**) and/or objective (**O**) above should be conducted per Table 7.3

Plan (RLE) Day #30 to #90

℞ Provide necessary care based on Table 7.3:

- Prescribe near (or bifocal) Rx
- Advise patient of final visual acuities (distance and near)
- Ask about neuroadaptative progress
- Advise on continued use of artificial tears daily (tid to qid)
- If corneal endothelium seriously compromised (≥ 2+) with *Verisyse* IOL and/or has increased within 14- to 30-day period, refer patient back to surgeon for possible lens removal
- Ask patient if they have any questions
- If patient comfortable and **S** and **O** findings WNL, schedule routine RV

Follow-Up (RLE) after Day #30 to #90

Advise patient to contact you immediately if:

- Red or increasingly irritated eye(s) not responding to artificial tears
- Acute and/or increasing pain in the post-op eye
- Any sudden or insidious changes in vision
- Sudden or increasing flashes and/or floaters in field of vision
- Any questions?

Urgencies and Emergencies (RLE) after Day #30 to #90

(Check Section D, "Potential Postoperative Complications" below and Table 7.3 and Appendix 5 for additional potential postoperative complications, their clinical effects, and corrective actions.)

ASAP or STAT referral to surgeon for:

(See generic ***Urgencies and Emergencies*** page 293 plus additional item below)

- Sudden decrease in vision and hazy vision if patient with endothelial compromise not referred back to surgeon

D. Potential Postoperative Complications, Clinical Effects, and Corrective Actions with Intraocular Lenses (IOLs)[18] (See Also Table 7.3 and Appendix 5)

1. For monofocal and multifocal IOLs:

Complication	Clinical Effect, and Corrective Action
Lens tilt, decentered or dislocated.	Irregular astigmatism (higher order aberration); Consider lens manipulation or removal
Ocular surface infection.	Acute conjunctivitis with or without discharge; Treat with antibiotic and steroid
Acute inflammation (Uveitis)	Red, deep pain with ant. chamber cells and flare. Consult with surgeon and treat according to advice
Hyphema	Red blood (whole or cells) in anterior chamber; Monitor microhyphema (cells) and refer
Posterior capsule opacification (PCO)	Insidious reduction in vision after 3 to 6 months; Perform posterior YAG laser capsulotomy
Rise in intraocular pressure (IOP)	Angle block or closure if acute; Refer for surgical amelioration
Cystoid macula edema (CME)	Insidious reduction in vision after one month; consider NSAID or steroid intervention
Increased risk of retinal detachment	Associated mostly with higher myopia; Laser pretreat or retinal referral if detached

2. For *Crystalens* (all mono/multifocal complications, plus):

Reduced or no IOL translocation	Reduction or loss of near correction; Cycloplege and accommodative pushups
Anterior shift of IOL optic	Increase in myopic refraction; Attempt IOL manipulation and cycloplege

3. For refractive lens exchange (RLE) phakic IOLs (all mono/multifocal, plus):

Acute rise in IOP with *Verisyse*	Angle blocked by lens haptics; Refer for surgical amelioration
Endothelial loss with *Verisyse*	Corneal edema and reduction in vision; Consider lens removal and corneal rehab.
Lenticular touch with *Visian*	Lens opacities resulting in visual reduction; Consider lens removal, lensectomy and IOL
Pupillary block with *Visian*	Insidious rise in intraocular pressure (IOL); Surgically release or remove IOL and treat IOP

E. Options for Post-Lensectomy "Absolute Presbyopia"

1. Near spectacle correction
   a. With monofocal IOL
      1) Single vision: full distance over-refraction plus +2.50 to 3.00 D or based on near working distance
      2) Bifocal: full distance over-refraction and +2.50 to 3.00 D or based on near working distance
   b. With multifocals and RLE
      1) Single vision: full distance over-refraction plus +1.25 to 2.50 D (max.)

2) Bifocal: full distance over-refraction and +1.25 to 2.50 D add (max.)
2. Miotics (for chronic symptoms of spherical aberrations and coma)[19]
 a. Optional alternative to near Rx for monofocal, multifocal, RLE
 b. *Alphagan* (brimonidine tartrate) qd; preferred drug due to least side effects
 c. Pilocarpine drops, 1.25% qd (*Vuity*) FDA approved, November 2021
  1) Adjust concentration based on resultant pupil size (2 to 3 mm ideal)
  2) Slight burning sensation on instillation
 d. Combined carbachol and brimonidine (*Brimochol*) qd

Section 2: Corneal Refractive Surgery

I. General Patient Section

A. Myopia
1. Also known as nearsightedness or shortsightedness
2. Most common (and best) candidates for corneal refractive surgery
3. Levels of myopia in minus (–) diopters (D) according to the National Institutes of Health:
 a. Mild myopia: 0 D to –1.5 D
 b. Moderate myopia: from –1.5 D to –6.0 D
 c. High myopia: –6.0 D or greater
 d. Pathological myopia occurs with more than –8.0 D associated with higher frequency, greater risk of retinal disease, cataract, and glaucoma

B. Hyperopia
1. Also known as farsightedness or hypermetropia
2. More common in aging and presbyopia
3. Levels of hyperopia in plus (+) diopters (D) according to the National Institutes of Health
 a. Low hyperopia: +2.00 D or less
 b. Moderate hyperopia: from +2.25 to +5.00 D
 c. High hyperopia: +5.25 D or greater
4. Due to a more aspheric cornea (oblate and thus > higher order aberrations), the quality of hyperopic corneal refractive surgery tends to be slightly less than myopic correction:
 a. However, from their lifelong, pre-procedure compromised visual quality, hyperopes tend to tolerate some compromises in corneal refractive procedure's quality of vision
 b. This is *not the case* with myopes who demand the greatest quality of vision possible

C. Astigmatism
1. Meridional curvature (cylinder) can occur in the cornea (corneal astigmatism) or on the anterior surface of the crystalline lens (lenticular astigmatism). This is an important consideration in the selection and postoperative management of corneal refractive procedures
2. Levels of astigmatism are another important factor in corneal refractive surgery
 a. Mild astigmatism: < 1.00 D
 b. Moderate astigmatism: 1.00 to 2.00 D
 c. High astigmatism: 2.00 to 4.00 D
 d. Extreme astigmatism: > 4.00 D

D. Epithelial basement membrane disorder (EBMD) (see also Chapter 5)
1. Also known as "map, dot, fingerprint dystrophy" due to its appearance in the epithelium and its frequent pattern of corneal dystrophy (i.e. bilateral, centrally located, single layer involvement)
2. This condition is included with corneal refractive procedures due to one of EBMD's most effective treatments (in later stages), "excimer laser phototherapeutic keratectomy (PTK)"
3. The basic histopathology of EBMD includes a multilaminated epithelial basement membrane producing weak columnar epithelial cell adhesions and disrupted epithelial hemidesmosomes and anterior stromal anchoring fibrils
4. This weakened adhesion of epithelial cells on the corneal surface leading to significant discomfort, pain, and increased risk of infection (through loss of an intact epithelial barrier)
5. EBMD also produces the painful condition of recurrent corneal erosion (RCE)

II. Corneal Refractive Technologies

A. Lasers
1. Excimer ("excited dimer") laser[20]
 a. Excimer is a gas laser (argon and fluorine, ArFl) that emits an intense, albeit cold, pulse of ultraviolet (UV) light energy of 193 nanometer (*nm*) wavelength
 b. This light energy breaks the carbon bonds of cells and effectively vaporizes (photoablates) corneal stromal tissue:
 c. The laser beam delivery to the cornea is either as a "flying spot" (adjustable from 0.6 to 2.0 mm spot size), a scanning slit (overlapping small spots), or wavefront-guided, all 3 systems providing rapid ablation speeds of 2 to 4 seconds per diopter (based on spot size, pulse energy, and tracking systems)
 d. The photoablation produces a change in shape of the corneal stromal surface and a resultant change in refractive power (myopic reduction with central ablation and flattening and hyperopic reduction with peripheral ablation and central steepening)
 e. Excimer lasers used in corneal refractive procedures (top 5 *circa* 2022)
  i. *Allegretto WAVE Eye-Q* Excimer Laser System (Alcon)
  ii. *VISX STAR S4* IR Excimer Laser System (Johnson & Johnson)
  iii. *MEDITEC MEL 80* Excimer Laser System (Zeiss)
  iv. *TECHNOLAS 217Z* Zyoptix System (Bausch + Lomb)
  v. *Nidek EC-5000 CX3* (Nidek)
2. Femtosecond (FS) laser[21]
 a. The femtosecond laser is an infrared laser with a wavelength of 1053nm
 b. As opposed to excimer laser ultraviolet photoablation of tissue, femtosecond lasers photodisrupt tissue with a pulse duration of 10–15

seconds (< 1 picosecond) which creates a 1μ cavitation bubbles that expand and separate (cut) tissue layers, completely eliminating collateral tissue damage to create a precise dissection

c. Under computer control, cavitation bubbles are applied at a rate of > 30,000 per second in any direction to produce linear, horizontal, vertical, diagonal, curved incisions which replace (with maximal accuracy) use of blade-cutting instruments (e.g., scalpel, scissors, etc.) which cut at 80 to 100μ accuracy versus 5 to 8μ femtosecond accuracy

d. Femtosecond lasers used corneal refractive procedures (*circa* 2022)
   i. *iLasik IntraLase* (Johnson & Johnson)
   ii. *Femtec* (20/10 Perfect Vision, Heidelberg, Germany)
   iii. *Femto LDV* (Ziemer Ophthalmic Systems, Port, Switzerland)
   iv. *VisuMax* (Carl Zeiss Meditec AG, Jena, Germany)
   v. *WaveLight FS200* (Alcon Laboratories Inc, Ft Worth, Texas)
   vi. *VICTUS* (Bausch & Lomb, Rochester, NY)
   vii. *LenSx* (Alcon Laboratories Inc, Ft Worth, Texas)

e. In corneal refractive surgery, the precise cutting ability of the femtosecond laser provides for "bladeless" procedures with greater precision accuracy

f. The primary use of the femtosecond laser in corneal refractive procedures is the creation of the flap in LASIK and epi-LASIK procedures (see Microkeratomes below)

g. Corneal refractive procedures in which the femtosecond laser is used include:
   i. Laser-assisted in situ keratomileusis (LASIK)
   ii. Astigmatic (arcuate) keratotomy (AK)
   iii. Small incision lenticule extraction (SMILE)
   iv. Intrastromal corneal ring segments (ICRS) (*aka* Intacs)

h. Notwithstanding the value of the femtosecond laser in the above presented corneal refractive procedures, its most valuable function in refractive surgery may be its role as a microkeratome in the LASIK and LASEK procedures

B. Microkeratome[22]
   1. Mechanical microkeratome
      a. Mechanical microkeratomes use an oscillating-blade system that docks to a suction ring (producing an increase in IOP up to 45 mm Hg) to create a corneal lamellar flap
      b. Produces meniscus shaped flap with risk of buttonhole effect (too thin centrally) and induced refractive variable
      c. Given blade-cutting accuracy (+/− 80 to 100μ), flap thickness is usually calibrated at a maximum of ~150 micron (μ) to insure minimum 50% resultant corneal center thickness after flap creation and ablation for the refractive errors
         i. The photoablation process ablates (removes) tissue at ~0.50μ per pulse (varies slightly with laser energies and types)
         ii. Remember, 1μ = 1 one-thousandth of a millimeter or 1000μ = 1 mm)
         iii. The average central corneal thickness = ~0.5 to 0.55 mm or 500 to 550μ
         iv. A general rule is to never thin corneas with photoablation procedures (ablated tissue plus flap thickness) by more than 50% or ≤ 250 to 275μ (or best, based on the patient's pachymetry) beyond which the risk of thinning (ectasia) increases significantly
         v. Photoablation by 6.5-mm excimer laser beam diameter (to accommodate an average mid-dilated pupil) will yield a refractive shift of ~1 D per ~20 pulses
         vi. Thus, a photoablation of a −8 D myopic with a 500μ corneal center thickness using a mechanical microkeratome at a 150μ flap thickness would yield a resultant post ablation corneal center thickness of ~270μ (500μ – 150μ flap – 8 D × 20 pulses × 0.50μ per pulse or 80μ = 270μ)
         vii Given a range of 80 to 100μ blade accuracy produces a resultant risk of corneal ectasia
         viii. > 10 to 12 D (> 200 to 240μ) begin to approximate the safe limits of PRK and must always be considered in patient selection
   2. Femtosecond laser microkeratome
      a. Given the calculations described immediately above and given femtosecond cutting accuracy of 5 to 8μ, perhaps the greatest advantage of the femtosecond laser is its ability to cut thin flats accurately at ≤ 100μ
      b. Such accuracy allows for the safe creation of flaps…
         i. In thin corneas
         ii. In steep corneas
         iii. In high refractive errors
      c. It produces a more uniform thickness across the flap
      d. Planar flap (versus meniscus shape with mechanical microkeratome) insures most accurate refractive result
      d. It produces more predictable hinge lengths
      e. The steep side-cuts by the laser provide improved flap realignment

III. Procedure Options

A. Radial keratotomy (RK)[23]
   1. Procedure developed in the 1970s using radial incisions (from 4 to 32) in the peripheral cornea to "relax" tension and flatten the central cornea to reduce myopia
   2. The long-term results (through early 1990s) proved to be a disaster with weakened corneas resulting in irreversible corneal hazing, scarring, and poor quality vision (lower and higher order aberrations)
   3. The procedure has been virtually eliminated from refractive surgery and replaced by excimer laser surface photoablation and LASIK procedures
   4. No need for any additional pre-, intra- or postoperative discussion on this procedure.

B. Phototherapeutic keratectomy (PTK)[24]

1. Per the histopathology of the epithelial basement membrane (described in I. D. 3. above) a very shallow photoablation (≤ 50μ) of the anterior stromal surface (including Bowman's membrane) will remove the weakened stromal anchoring fibrils and allow (hopefully) stronger regenerated fibrils to ameliorate the EBMD and RCE
2. Hemidesmosomes also regenerate to add to epithelial adherence to stroma
3. As a therapeutic treatment, further discussion on this procedure can be found in Chapter 5, "Diagnoses of the Cornea"

C. Photorefractive keratectomy (PRK)[25] (see also Section V. A.) (Figure 7.5)

1. PRK is the application of an excimer laser to photoablate the corneal surface to adjust the curvature to correct a refractive error (myopia, hyperopia, astigmatism and mixed astigmatism):
    a. For review of excimer laser technology, see Section II. A. 1.
    b. For a step-by-step description of the excimer laser surface photoablation procedure, see Section V. A.
2. Photoablation of the central cornea reduces corneal convexity (flatter) and shorter axial length producing a reduction in myopia
3. Photoablation of the peripheral cornea steepens the surface convexity and increases axial length, producing a reduction in hyperopia
4. Meridional ablation (at the axis of the corneal cylinder) produces a reduction in the corneal cylinder (but does not influence lenticular cylinder and thus, resultant refractive cylinder)
    a. Pre-operatively, the amount of cylinder between cornea and total refractive cylinder (corneal plus lenticular) resolves the degree of astigmatism produced by the lens
    b. This resultant degree of lenticular astigmatism provides a calculated amount of astigmatic corneal ablation needed to correct the resultant refractive astigmatism
5. Surface ablation complications
    a. Dense anterior stroma (for increased corneal surface protection) produces a more intense immune response than deeper ablations (see LASIK procedure)
    b. Increased immune response can produce corneal haze and steepening curvature
    c. Also, immune response can produce increased central corneal curvature with resultant refractive regression (towards myopia)
    d. Retreatment indicated for increased reduction in acuity from hazing by ≥ 2 lines of vision reduction or myopic shift of ≥ 0.75 D
6. FDA refractive correction range approvals for excimer laser photoablation vary according to instrument model (Top 5 in 2021)
    a. *Allegretto WAVE Eye-Q*: > Myopia up to –7.00 D and up to 3.00 D astigmatic component
        i. Not approved for hyperopia
    b. *AMO VISX*: > Myopia less than –14.00 D with astigmatism between 0.50 and –5.00 D (with eye tracker)
        i. Hyperopia between +0.50 and +5.00 D with astigmatism up to 3.00 D
    c. *MEDITEC MEL 80*: > Myopia less than or equal to –7.00 D with astigmatism less than or equal to –3.00 D
        i. Hyperopia less than or equal to +5.00 D with astigmatism of less than or equal to 3.00 D
    d. *TECHNOLAS 217Z*: > Myopia from less than –11.00 D with astigmatism less than 3.00 D
        i. Hyperopia between 1.00 and 4.00 D with astigmatism up to 2.00 D
    e. *Nidek EC-5000 CX3*: > Myopia from –1.00 to –14.00 D with astigmatism less than or equal to 4.00 D
        i. Hyperopia between +0.50 and +5.00 D with astigmatism from 0.50 to 2.00 D
7. Laser application methods include:
    a. Broad-beam, scanning-slit
    b. Flying-spot systems
    c. Wavefront guided:
        i. Uses corneal wavefront aberrometry mapping to improve correction of higher order aberrations (HOAs)
        ii. More likely reduces induced HOAs (versus existing HOAs), particularly spherical aberration, to produce improved vision
    d. Eye-tracking technology allows the beam to remain centered on the pupil in the presence of small ocular movements

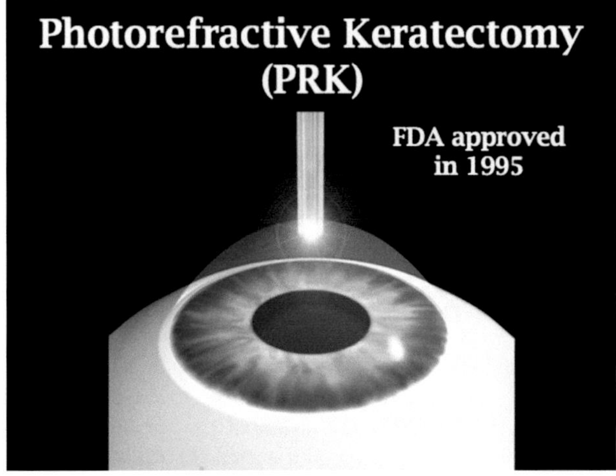

FIGURE 7.5 Photorefractive keratectomy (PRK): This original corneal laser refractive surgery procedure uses the excimer laser to centrally (for myopia) photoablate the anterior corneal stroma after removal of the surface epithelium. The procedure is similar to phototherapeutic keratectomy which removes anterior stromal scars and weakened anterior stromal fibers and hemidesmosomes in the treatment of epithelial basement membrane disorders.

D. LASIK[26] (femtosecond and excimer laser intrastromal ablation) (see also Section V, B) (Figure 7.6)

1. Laser-assisted in situ keratomileusis (LASIK) is a corneal lamellar refractive procedure

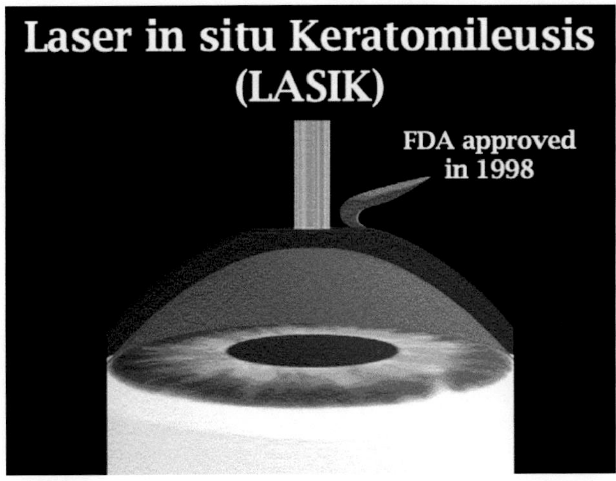

FIGURE 7.6 Laser in situ keratomileusis (LASIK): this procedure (FDA approved in 1998) proved to be a preferred corneal laser refractive procedure because of its sparing of epithelial denuding and its deeper stromal ablation (reducing myopic regression). The procedure involved cutting a corneal (anterior stromal) flap of ~150μ with a mechanical or femtosecond microkeratome and then photoablating the deeper (less reactive) corneal stroma.

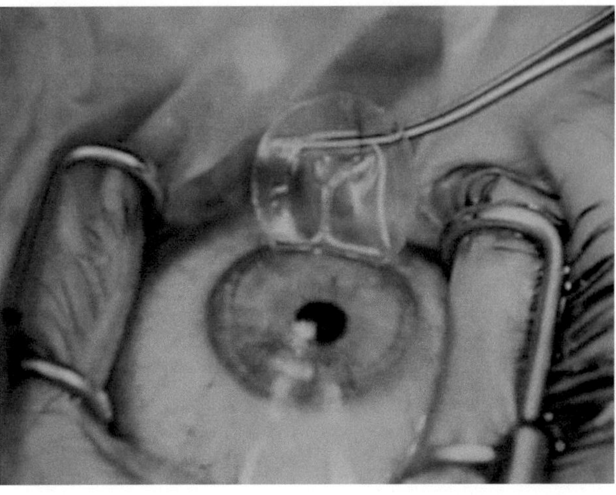

FIGURE 7.7 Corneal flap lifted: after mechanical microkeratome or photodissection with the femtosecond laser, the corneal flap is lifted with forceps to expose the mid stroma for ablation with the excimer laser. Flaps can be cut substantially thinner (≤ 100μ) with the computer-controlled femtosecond laser which cuts a planar versus a meniscus shaped flap (greater risk of a "buttonhole" complication).

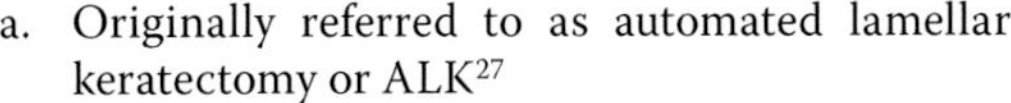

a. Originally referred to as automated lamellar keratectomy or ALK[27]
b. The original ALK procedure was performed with a double pass of a mechanical microkeratome:
    i. The first pass is the creation of a flap (described above under Section II, B, 1: "Mechanical Microkeratome")
    ii. After the flap was created, the microkeratome was recalibrated for a second pass over the intrastromal surface (the "power cut") producing a lenticle and resultant flattening of the corneal curvature for a refractive adjustment
    iii. The power adjustment was modulated by the thickness of the lenticle
    iv. After the second pass, the flap was laid back over the stromal surface
c. LASIK differs from original ALK and surface ablation procedures (PRK, LASEK, and epi-LASIK) in 2 ways:
    i. It uses a single cut of a microkeratome (mechanical or femtosecond laser [II, B] – laser being the preferred method) to create a flap of combined epithelial and anterior stromal tissue, exposing an anterior stromal bed (depth dependent on the depth of the tissue dissection)
    ii. Lifting of the flap allows for photoablation of deeper corneal stroma by an excimer laser to alter the curvature of the cornea to produce a refractive change (Figure 7.7)

2. Creation of a LASIK flap by the femtosecond laser produces minimal epithelial disturbance and resultant patient discomfort
3. More so, deeper photoablation of the stroma produces less immune response than surface ablation (greater immune protection on surface tissue) and thus, less likelihood of regression (myopic shift) and possible corneal haze (see "Surface Ablation Regression" page 306)
4. Absence of corneal haze or myopic regression in LASIK (deep ablation) precludes the need for retreatment unless significant initial undercorrection
5. FDA laser approval ranges for LASIK correction are similar to those for PRK (surface ablation) (see Section III. B. 2. [Prescription Ranges] directly above)
6. Based on the amount of post-procedure induced astigmatism, an astigmatic (arcuate) keratotomy (AK, *aka* limbal relaxing incisions—procedure description in Section V. D. below) can be performed immediately after the procedure (while the patient is still on the table) or at an indefinite later date

E. LASEK[28] (laser-assisted sub-epithelial keratomileusis) Uses the femtosecond laser (or a mechanical microkeratome or an "epikeratome" that uses a blunt oscillating blade) to create a single layer flap by scoring the epithelial surface, applying dilute ethanol alcohol to loosen the epithelium from the anterior stroma and then, peeling the epithelial layer back for anterior stromal (including Bowman's layer) photoablation by the excimer laser
1. After all epithelial refractive procedures (PRK, LASEK, and Epi-LASIK) a soft lens is applied to the eye for at least 48 to 72 hours
2. As described above, the anterior stromal surface is slightly more immune responsive than deeper stroma (more immune protection) and thus, tends to produce a greater response to photoablation "insult"

3. However, less cutting of deep stromal tissue (as in LASIK) reduces the increase in stromal nerve disturbance and resultant dry eye symptoms
4. And foremost, the thin epithelial flap reduces the risk of corneal ectasia in thin corneas
5. Based on the amount of post-procedure astigmatism measured by keratometry immediately after the procedure, an astigmatic keratotomy (AK, *aka* limbal relaxing incisions—procedure description in Section V. D. below) can be performed immediately after the procedure (while the patient is still at the laser) or at a later date

F. Epi-LASIK[29]
1. Similarly to LASEK, Epi-LASIK creates an epithelial flap through dilute ethanol alcohol softening of the epithelial layer, but without scoring the layer with a femtosecond laser
2. Rather than creating an epithelial flap, anterior stroma is exposed by pushing the epithelial cells to the side with a blunt probe to expose the Bowman's layer and anterior stromal surface for photoablation by the excimer laser
3. After photoablation, the epithelial cells are either replaced or discarded
4. As stated above, after all epithelial refractive procedures (PRK, LASEK, and Epi-LASIK) a soft lens is applied to the eye for at least 24 hours
5. And again, this procedure reduces the ectasia risk in thin corneas
6. Based on the amount of post-procedure induced astigmatism, an astigmatic keratotomy (AK, *aka* limbal relaxing incisions—procedure description in Section V. D. below) can be performed immediately after the procedure (while the patient is still on the table) or at an indefinite later date

G. Astigmatic (or arcuate) keratotomy[30] aka limbal relaxing incisions (LRI)
1. Limbal relaxing incisions in astigmatic (arcuate) keratotomy (AK) are incisions made in the paracentral cornea to change its curvature to reduce or eliminate corneal astigmatism
2. The incisions are placed just inside the vascular limbal arcade in one or both hemi-meridians of the steepest astigmatic power to flatten the curvature and modify low to moderate degrees of astigmatism
3. Arcuate incisions in the paracentral cornea at the steepest meridians of the meridional or oblique (astigmatic) cornea can be performed, if necessary, immediately post-op or 2 to 3 months afterward to reduce astigmatism
4. They can be used with surface ablation or intrastromal keratoplasties

H. Other intracorneal therapeutic procedures (see "Common Corneal Surgical Procedures" in Chapter 5)
1. Full-thickness penetrating keratoplasty (PK, *aka* corneal transplant)
2. Partial penetrating keratoplasty
3. Deep anterior lamellar keratoplasty (DALK)
4. Endothelial keratoplasty (EK)
5. Pre-Descemet's EK (PDEK)
6. Descemet's stripping EK (DSEK)
7. Descemet's membrane EK (DMEK)
8. Bowman membrane transplant (BMT)

I. Epikeratoplasty (*Epikeratophakia*)[31]
1. This procedure uses a donor lamellar corneal lenticule which is sutured onto the host cornea after removal of the epithelium to provide refractive power change
2. The edge of the lenticule is placed into a shallow lamellar dissection, then tucked under and sutured to the peripheral cornea
3. The procedure yielded considerable complications and has effectively been abandoned as a refractive surgery option

J. Laser thermal keratoplasty (LTK)[32] (see also Section V, below)
1. This technique steepens the central corneal curvature by means of heat-induced shrinkage of collagen fibers in the midperiphery of the cornea
2. Treatment is applied by a noncontact thulium or holmium laser
3. The amount of refractive change depends on a number of variables including the total amount of energy delivered, number of pulses, pulse energy, spot size, and optical zone
4. The procedure is limited to mild to moderate farsightedness
5. Presbyopic correction possible with monovision approach

K. Conductive keratoplasty (CK)[32] (see also Section V, below)
1. Conductive keratoplasty uses a contact probe to deliver radio frequency energy by inserting the tip sequentially in multiple locations of the paracentral cornea
2. The energy produces shrinkage of collagen lamellae that leads to steepening of the central cornea
3. FDA approval for patients aged 40 years or older
   a. For the temporary reduction of 0.75 to 3.25 D of hyperopia
   b. For treatment of presbyopia, with a spherical equivalent of 0.75 to 3.00 D and 0 to 0.75 D of astigmatism
4. All refractive measurements are specified as being obtained under cycloplegia
5. Presbyopic correction possible with monovision approach

L. Small incision lenticule extraction (SMILE)[33] (see Section V, below)
1. This intracorneal procedure is used mostly in higher refractive errors (not hyperopic) with thin corneas
2. The *SMILE* procedure uses the *VisuMax* femtosecond laser to create a lenticule of stromal tissue which is then removed through a side port incision (also made with the femto laser)
3. Removal of the lenticule reshapes the cornea to correct the myopic refractive error
4. FDA approved for myopia from $\geq$ 1.00 D plus astigmatism up to 6.00 D and, if $\geq$ −8.00 D astigmatism to be $\leq$ −0.50 D:

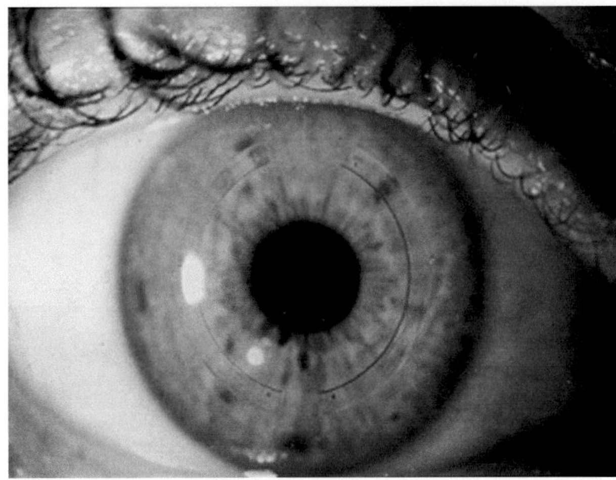

FIGURE 7.8 Intrastromal corneal ring segments: these intrastromal PMMA, semicircular rings (150 mm length) are implanted into anterior stromal channels (created by hand or, more accurately, a femtosecond laser) in the midperipheral cornea to flatten the curvature, correcting myopia, myopic astigmatism, reduce higher order aberrations and most valuably, stabilizing keratoconic and other ectatic corneas.

a. Approval limited to *VisuMax* (*Meditec* Zeiss) femtosecond Laser
b. Commercial name for procedure: *Relex Smile* by *MedRx*

M. Intrastromal corneal ring segments (ICRS)[34] (Intacs by *Refractec*) (see also Section V, below and Figure 7.8)
1. Intrastromal corneal ring segments (ICRS) (Intacs) are circular, PMMA ring segments of 150° arc with variable lengths and thicknesses (to vary flattening of the cornea)
2. FDA approved for the correction of −1.00 to −3.00 D of spherical equivalent at the spectacle plane, with 0 to 1.00 D of astigmatism and irregular astigmatism
3. Intrastromal channels (2) are created manually or with femtosecond laser
4. Ring segments are threaded into each lamellar channels
5. The technology is used for keratoconus and some other corneal ectasia conditions (e.g., pellucid marginal degeneration, LASIK-induced ectasia)
6. In 2004, the FDA approval of ICRS (Intacs) was extended to include treatment of corneal ectasias including keratoconus with central corneal thickness > 450μ
7. Using the ICRS technology alone and in combination with contact lenses has also proven valuable in stabilization and improved visual correction of keratoconic and other ectatic corneal conditions
   a. Visual correction varies with keratoconus and ectatic conditions
   b. Gas permeable (GP) lenses frequently required post-procedure

IV. Preoperative Examination[35] (See Also Tables 7.4 and 7.5)

A. Subjective considerations
1. Assess patient's reasons for considering refractive surgery:
   a. Cosmetic ("no more glasses")
   b. Recreational (contact sports, camping, hunting, etc.)
   c. Occupational (first responders, outdoor tasks, etc.)
2. Does the patient have realistic goals and expectations?
3. Does the patient understand and accept the associated risk?
4. Is the patient stable, mature, and prepared to accept the responsibilities associated with the refractive surgery process?
5. Does the patient have realistic expectations regarding resulting vision and its potential limitations?
6. Obtain a complete medical history for any refractive surgery contraindications
   a. Current and past ocular or medical conditions (e.g., HSV, diabetes)
   b. Current medications (e.g., corticosteroids)
   c. Allergies, past and present
   d. Of principal interest, active or uncontrolled diabetes
   e. Pregnancy and nursing mothers
   f. See also Table 7.4 and Table 7.5
7. Rule out (through history and full examination) any active or chronic ocular disease, especially macular degeneration and contact lens history

B. Objective examination
1. Discontinue contact lens wear: 4 weeks for GPHCL; 2 weeks for SCL
   a. Do second set of measurements (refraction and keratometry) 1 week after discontinued CL wear
   b. If GPHCL history greater than 5 years, best to do an additional set of measurements one week after second set to establish stable refraction and Ks
   c. "Stable" readings means refractions vary by less than 0.50 diopter and Ks less than 0.50 D change
2. If stable, proceed with required measurements for refractive surgery
   a. Uncorrected vision
   b. Corrected vision
   c. Ocular dominance (especially if considering monovision)
   d. Manifest refraction
      i. Cycloplegic refraction in hyperopes
      ii. Differential between manifest and cycloplegic should not exceed 0.75 D
      iii. If so, instruct on accommodation relaxing techniques (pushups, etc.)
   e. Wavefront aberrometry

TABLE 7.4 Corneal Refractive Instruments and Procedures: Advantages and Disadvantages

	Advantages	Disadvantages
Microkeratomes		
Mechanical microkeratome	For use in photorefractive keratectomy	Potential for uneven flap thickness
	Creates a secure epithelial flap	Risk of corneal perforation (e.g., buttonhole)
	Fast, comfortable procedure for patient	IOP increase ≥ 65 mm Hg
	Suction for IOP increase short (3–5 secs.)	May disturb weak epithelium
	Better in cases requiring new (second) flap	Meniscus (thin center) flap vs. planar flap
	Shorter suction time safer in glaucoma	Risk of increased HOA induction
	Less risk of inflammation (DLK)	+/– 80 to 100μ vs. +/– 5μ accuracy with laser
Femtosecond (FS) laser	For use in LASIK procedure	Requires full femtosecond laser instrument
	Computerized flap accuracy	Requires precise suction ring placement
	Uniform flap thickness to within ~5μ	Risk of corneal edema
	Precise edge architecture	Post procedure photophobia reported
	IOP increase ≥ 25 mm Hg	Suction for IOP increase ~15 to 20 seconds
	Precise flap diameter and hinge placement	Increased time—less patient cooperation
Lasers		
Excimer laser	Laser used for corneal photoablation	Thins the cornea increasing risk of ectasia
	Photoablation highly accurate (± 0.25 D)	Induces some higher order aberrations
		Epithelial discomfort with surface ablation
Femtosecond (FS) laser	For use in LASIK procedure	Need for IOP increase (≥ 25 mm Hg)
	Provides deep stromal bed photoablation	Requires separate laser platform
	Computer accuracy down to 5 to 8μ	Requires precise suction ring placement
	Cuts precise flap (epithelial and stromal)	Usually additional cost to patient
	Less flap complications	Can produce increased light sensitivity
	Greater control over flap parameters	Issues (above) re: femto microkeratome
	Ability to cut thinner flaps for higher Rx	
	Used in intracorneal procedures	
Refractive Procedures		
Photorefractive keratectomy	Excellent results for all refractive errors	Post-op discomfort from epithelial removal
(PRK)	Safe procedure for thin corneas (<500μ)	Bandage contact lens or eye patch required for 1 to 5 days post-op
	No flap cutting means less dry eye	Possible regression from surface ablation
	No flap means no flap complications	Requires a few weeks of post-op meds
Laser in situ keratomileusis	Excellent results from deep stromal bed	Creation of flap includes flap risks (above)
LASIK	Painless (no epithelial disturbance)	Increased lamellar inflammation (DLK)
	Bladeless procedure with laser accuracy	Slight increased risks with thin corneas
	Computer accuracy for all dissections	Risk of dry eye due to nerve cuts with flap
	Excellent results for all refractive errors	Risk of epithelial ingrowth (under flap)
	No risk of refractive regression	Rx enhancements require lifting flap
	Flap creation safe and effective	Extended risk of flap dislodgement
Laser epithelial keratomileusis	Better procedure for thin corneas	Some post-op discomfort (temporary)
LASEK	Minimal risk of flap dislodgement	Post-op soft lens bandage may be required
	Less risk of post-op dry eye	Risk of epithelial flap wrinkling/dislodging
		Slower epithelial healing due to alcohol
		Risk of Rx regression with surface ablation
Epithelial LASIK	Safer procedure for thin corneas	Some post-op discomfort (temporary)
Epi-LASIK	Minimal risk of flap dislodgement	Post-op soft lens bandage may be required
	Less risk of post-op dry eye	Risk of epithelial flap wrinkling/dislodging
		Risk of Rx regression with surface ablation
Intracorneal Procedures		
Auto lamellar keratoplasty	Effective for higher degrees of myopia	Risks of mechanical keratome (see above)
(ALK)	No laser preparation required	Results not as predictable as LASIK
	Refractive results are immediate	Risk of induced astigmatism
Laser thermal keratoplasty	For mild to moderate farsightedness	Variable refractive results
(LTK)	Procedure done within seconds	Some discomfort after procedure
	Minimally invasive as non-contact laser	Remaining peripheral ring-shaped scar
		Possibility of induced astigmatism
		Refractive regression and retreatment likely
Conductive keratoplasty	For mild to moderate farsightedness	Variable refractive results
(CK)	Use radiofrequency vs. heat energy	Some discomfort after procedure

(*Continued*)

TABLE 7.4 (CONTINUED) **Corneal Refractive Instruments and Procedures: Advantages and Disadvantages**

	Advantages	Disadvantages
	Procedure done within seconds	Remaining peripheral spot scars
	Minimally invasive using a probe	Possibility of induced astigmatism
		Refractive regression and retreatment likely
SMILE	No regression with intrastromal lenticle	For nearsightedness only
(Small incision lenticule extraction)	No need for flap and flap complications	Must have ≤ 0.50 D corneal cylinder if ≥ −8
	Less dry eye from less corneal incisions	Increased surgical risks
	No need for excimer laser photoablation	Any post-op corrections must be PRK
Corneal rings	Excellent procedure for keratoconus	Requires a skilled ophthalmic surgeon
(Intacs)	Safe and effective (with skilled surgeon)	Needs central corneal thickness ≥ 450μ
	Stabilizes cones in keratoconus	Surgical complications always possible
	Reduces refractive errors and HOA	Post-op ring migration possible

   f. Keratometry (remember total refractive astigmatism minus corneal astigmatism [cylinder] equals lenticular astigmatism and must be compensated for in corneal refractive surgery)
   g. Corneal topography/tomography
   h. Pachymetry (corneal thickness should be ≥ 500μ)
   i. Corneal white to white measurements
   j. Scotopic pupil size
   k. Photopic pupil size
   l. Brow and orbit description
      i. Enophthalmos
      ii. Exophthalmos (proptosis)
      iii. High or low brow
   m. Slit-lamp biomicroscopic examination
   n. Dilated fundus examination (rule out diabetic retinopathy and macular degeneration)

C. Procedure selection and recommendations
   1. Patient selection based on advantages and disadvantages listed in Table 7.4
   2. Recommended procedure based on Subjective Considerations (above) and indications and contraindications listed in Table 7.5

D. Patient counseling (explanation of procedures; reasons for recommended procedure; instructions; Q&A)
   1. Explain clinical findings as they relate to refractive surgery options
   2. Describe the various refractive procedure options based on the refractive error
   3. Discuss strengths and weaknesses and indications and contraindications for each procedure (see Tables 7.5)
   4. Make your recommendation of optimal procedure for the patient
   5. Provide step-by-step explanation of the selected procedure (see Section V, A, below)
   6. Enumerate the potential risks and complications of the selected procedure (see Table 7.6 for surface ablation and Table 7.7 for stromal ablation below):
      a. Explain temporary discomfort (1 to 5 days) after PRK (or PTK) procedure and use of soft lens bandage or pressure patch and pain medications
      b. Possibility of less than perfect (20/20) result with any procedure
      c. Possibility of "hazy vision" immediately after surgery, lasting for days to weeks
      d. Neuroadaptation process (adjusting to "new vision") can last for weeks to months
      e. Halos and glare (greater at night) lasting weeks to months, but almost always resolving (through neuroplasticity)
         i. If scotopic pupil ≥ corneal ablation zone, halos and spherical aberrations will persist
         ii. See miotic discussion page 304
      f. Need for spectacle correction (or enhancement procedure) if resultant vision is < 20/40
      g. Possibility of an under- or overcorrection based on individual eye response
      h. Explain presbyopia and the fact that near vision not corrected with refractive surgery:
         i. Monovision treatment (undercorrecting one eye [~1.00 D] for near vision) and educate on need for near spectacles as presbyopia progresses
         ii. Has minimal to no negative effects on distance vision
         iii. Slight reduction binocular vision and stereopsis
         iv. Also mention the option of refractive lens exchange and phakic IOLs
      i. Discuss possible post-procedure discomfort and pain medications with surface ablation (PRK)
      j. Possible post-op procedural complications after LASIK or LASEK (flap)
         i. Dry eye symptoms
         ii. Epithelial ingrowth (requiring lifting of flap and removal of cells)
         iii. Wrinkling of the flap (requiring smoothing procedure)
         iv. Dislodgement of the flap (requiring lifting and replacement)
         v. Hinge defect and loss of flap (resultant epithelial regrowth and slight refractive alteration)
   7. Discuss post-op visits and medications schedule
   8. The time involved for visual recovery for the recommended procedure (i.e., discuss temporary hyperopic shift for the first 2–3 months after PRK treatment)

TABLE 7.5 **Corneal Refractive Procedures: Indications and Contraindications**

	Indications	Contraindications
Microkeratomes		
Mechanical microkeratome	• Cuts flap in intrastromal keratomileusis • Can be used in LASIK procedure • Used in cases requiring new (second) flap	• Risk of uneven flap thickness • Greater risks with thin corneas • Increased risks with weak epithelium • Slight increased risk in glaucoma patients
Femtosecond (FS) laser	• For use in LASIK and LASEK procedure • Cuts flaps in intrastromal keratomileusis • Used in penetrating keratoplasty • Creates tunnels for intracorneal rings • Used in lensectomy (cataract surgery)	• Sight increased risk in glaucoma patients • Increased risk in poor corneal endothelium • Patient compliance with laser procedure
Lasers		
Excimer laser	• Laser used for corneal photoablation • Corrects myopia up to 12 Diopters • Corrects hyperopia up to 6 Diopters • Corrects astigmatism up to 6 Diopters	• Thins cornea (increases risk of ectasia) • Patients with higher order aberrations • Deep cornea stromal scarring
Femtosecond (FS) laser	• For use in LASIK procedure • Better in thin corneas • Better in higher refractive errors (≥ 6 D) • SMILE: myopia up to 12 Diopters • SMILE: astigmatism up to 6 Diopters (myopia ≤ −8 D) • Used in intracorneal procedures	• Issues (above) re: femto microkeratome
Refractive Procedures		
Photorefractive keratectomy (PRK)	• Excellent results for all refractive errors • Safe procedure for thin corneas (< 500μ) • Better in dry eyes (less nerve cutting) • Corrects myopia up to 12 Diopters • Corrects hyperopia up to 6 Diopters • Corrects astigmatism up to 6 Diopters	• Patients with cataracts • Patients with macular degeneration • Any active eye disease • Active or uncontrolled diabetes • Active pregnancy or nursing mother
Laser in situ keratomileusis LASIK (aka Automated Lamellar keratoplasty, see ALK below)	• Better in corneas >500μ • Better in higher refractive errors (≥ 6 D) • Corrects myopia up to 12 Diopters • Corrects hyperopia up to 6 Diopters • Corrects astigmatism up to 6 Diopters	• See femtosecond contraindications above • Patients with cataracts • Patients with macular degeneration • Any active eye disease • Active or uncontrolled diabetes • Active pregnancy or nursing mother • Risk of dry eye due to nerve cuts with flap
Laser epithelial keratomileusis LASEK	• Better procedure for thin corneas • Better in dry eyes (no stromal cutting) • Corrects myopia up to 12 Diopters • Corrects hyperopia up to 6 Diopters • Corrects astigmatism up to 6 Diopters	• See femtosecond contraindications above • Patients with cataracts • Patients with macular degeneration • Any active eye disease • Active or uncontrolled diabetes • Active pregnancy or nursing mother • Moderate to advanced EBMD • Increased patient discomfort • Increased epithelial healing time • Risk of regression (from surface ablation)
Epithelial LASIK Epi-LASIK	• Safer procedure for thin corneas • Better in dry eyes (no stromal cutting) • Corrects myopia up to 12 Diopters • Corrects hyperopia up to 6 Diopters • Corrects astigmatism up to 6 Diopters	• Patients with cataracts • Patients with macular degeneration • Any active eye disease • Active or uncontrolled diabetes • Active pregnancy or nursing mother • Moderate to advanced EBMD • Increased patient discomfort • Increased epithelial healing time • Risk of regression (from surface ablation)
Intracorneal Procedures		
Auto lamellar keratoplasty (ALK)	• Same indications as LASIK (above) • Effective for higher degrees of myopia	• Risks of mechanical keratome (see above) • Results not as predictable as LASIK • Risk of induced astigmatism • Patients with cataracts

(*Continued*)

TABLE 7.5 (CONTINUED) **Corneal Refractive Procedures: Indications and Contraindications**

	Indications	Contraindications
		• Patients with macular degeneration • Any active eye disease • Active or uncontrolled diabetes • Active pregnancy or nursing mother
Laser thermal keratoplasty (LTK)	• For mild to moderate farsightedness • Minimally invasive as non-contact laser	• Variable refractive results • Some discomfort after procedure • Remaining peripheral ring-shaped scar • Possibility of induced astigmatism • Refractive regression and retreatment likely • Patients with cataracts • Patients with macular degeneration • Any active eye disease • Active or uncontrolled diabetes • Active pregnancy or nursing mother
Conductive keratoplasty (CK)	• For mild to moderate farsightedness • Minimally invasive procedure	• Variable refractive results • Remaining peripheral spot scars • Possibility of induced astigmatism • Refractive regression and retreatment likely • Patients with cataracts • Patients with macular degeneration • Any active eye disease • Active or uncontrolled diabetes • Active pregnancy or nursing mother
SMILE (Small incision lenticule extraction)	• For nearsightedness only • Corrects from 1 to 10 diopters of myopia • Femtosecond laser required • Need corneal thickness ≥ 500μ • Must have ≤ 0.50 D corneal cylinder if ≥ −8 D	• See femtosecond contraindications above • Patients with cataracts • Patients with macular degeneration • Any active eye disease • Active or uncontrolled diabetes • Active pregnancy or nursing mother
Corneal rings (Intacs)	• Procedure for keratoconus • Reduces refractive errors and some HOAs	• Needs central corneal thickness ≥ 450μ • See femtosecond contraindications above • Patients with cataracts • Patients with macular degeneration • Any active eye disease • Active or uncontrolled diabetes • Active pregnancy or nursing mother

TABLE 7.6 **Potential Complications Associated with Excimer Laser Corneal Surface Photoablation (PRK/PTK)**

Complication	Management
• Artifact reduction of measured IOP (due to corneal thinning: consider nomogram adjustment)	• Monitor IOP at every visit
• Corneal ectasia	• Monitor pachymetry and keratometry
• Corneal haze or scarring (early or delayed onset)	• Top. steroids q4h (min.) to resolution
• Corneal infiltrates or ulceration (sterile or microbial)	• Implement corneal ulcer protocol
• Corneal melting or perforation	• Refer to surgeon (STAT)
• Corticosteroid-induced complications (e.g., increased IOP, glaucoma, cataract)	• D/C steroid and treat increased IOP
• Decreased contrast sensitivity	• Reassure on gradual improvement
• Decreased corneal sensitivity	• R/O early herpes simplex keratitis
• Development or increased dry eye symptoms	• Heavy lubrication (ongoing)
• Induced regular or irregular astigmatism	• Refer to surgeon for possible retreat or AK
• Loss of BCVA	• Reassure on improvement and possible treatment enhancement
• Need for reading correction	• Prescribe near Rx
• Partial regression of effect	• Monitor and possible retreatment if VA significantly reduced
• Ptosis	• Reassure on improvement—beyond 6 months consider blepharoplasty
• Reactivation of HSV keratitis	• HSV treatment protocol
• Recurrent corneal erosion	• Soft lens corneal bandage and possible PTK
• Symptomatic undercorrection or overcorrection	• Refer to surgeon for treatment enhancement
• Visual aberrations, including glare or starburst/halo effect, especially at night	• Sunglasses, lighting, and possible Alphagan drops

TABLE 7.7 **Potential Complications Associated with LASIK, LASEK, Epi-LASIK, Lamellar Procedures**

Complication	Management
• Artifact reduction of measured IOP (due to corneal thinning: consider nomogram adjustment)	• Monitor IOP at every visit
• Corneal ectasia (progressive corneal steepening)	• Monitor pachymetry and corneal topography
• Corneal haze or scarring (early or delayed onset)	• Top. Steroids q4h (min.) to resolution
• Corneal infiltrates, ulceration (sterile or microbial)	• Implement corneal ulcer protocol
• Corneal melting, perforation (sterile or microbial)	• Refer to surgeon (STAT)
• Corticosteroid-induced complications (e.g., ocular hypertension, glaucoma, cataract)	• D/C steroid and treat increased IOP
• Decreased contrast sensitivity	• Reassure on gradual improvement
• Decreased corneal sensitivity	• R/O early herpes simplex keratitis
• Deep lamellar keratitis (DLK)	• Mild to mod.: Heavy steroids (q2–4h) Severe: Lift flap, irrigate and heavy steroids
• Development, exacerbation of dry eye symptoms	• Heavy lubrication (ongoing)
• Epithelial ingrowth (epithelial cells under flap)	• Lift flap and debride the interface
• Flap necrosis	• Refer to surgeon for flap removal
• Induced regular or irregular astigmatism	• Refer to surgeon for possible retreat or AK
• Interface debris	• Lift flap and remove
• Loss of BCVA	• Reassure on improvement and possible treatment enhancement
• Partial regression of effect	• Monitor and possible retreatment if VA significantly reduced
• Persistent flap edema	• Topical steroid drops and hypertonic saline
• Premature need for reading correction	• Prescribe near Rx
• Pressure-induced sterile (stromal) keratitis (PISK)	• Do not use (or d/c) topical steroids; Treat with IOP lowering meds
• Ptosis	• Reassure on improvement – beyond 6 months consider blepharoplasty
• Rainbow glare associated with femtosecond laser	• Transient LASIK phenomenon from light scatter; PTK on the posterior flap surface may help
• Reactivation of HSV keratitis	• HSV treatment protocol
• Recurrent corneal erosion	• Soft lens corneal bandage and possible PTK
• Striae (microstriae and macrostriae)	• Refer to surgeon for flap lift and hydration; "ironing" with sponge or heated spacula; suturing
• Symptomatic undercorrection or overcorrection	• Refer to surgeon for treatment enhancement
• Transient-light sensitivity associated with femtosecond laser	• Aggressive steroids to reduce inflammation
• Traumatic flap dislocation	• Reposition or refer to surgeon for removal
• Visual symptoms, including glare or starburst/halo effect, especially at night	• Sunglasses, lighting and possible Alphagan drops
• Worsening corneal stromal dystrophy	• Depending on degree, corneal transplant may be indicated

V. Intraoperative Operations

A. Excimer laser corneal surface ablation (PRK)[25,35] (see also Section III, B)
   1. The corneal epithelium is removed to expose the stromal surface
   2. Stromal surface ablation compared to intrastromal (LASIK) ablation:
      a. Ablation of intrastromal tissue is preferable to surface stromal ablation (PRK) because of a less pronounced immune response
      b. Such an immune response is responsible for a transient corneal haze and for refractive regression in surface ablation as it tends to reestablish the steeper corneal curvature
   3. Epithelium recovers on the surface over a 24- to 72-hour post-op period

B. Laser-assisted in situ keratomileusis (LASIK)[26,35]
   1. Keratomileusis (reshaping of the cornea) using a femtosecond (FS) laser and an excimer laser for intrastromal photoablation is referred to as LASIK. The step-by-step procedure is as follows
      a. A corneal flap is created by applying the FS laser suction ring onto the surface of the cornea to stabilize the eye and slightly raise the pressure to provide a firm, consistent corneal curvature upon which the laser beam is applied
         i. A computerized FS program for cutting the flap provides for precise diameter measurement (usually the diameter of a mid-dilated pupil) and the dissection (photodisruption) of a horizontal cleavage plane
         ii. A vertical or angled cleavage plane flap as the flap's edge with a calculated hinge width (uncut edge) and the flap is folded back

   b. The intrastromal bed is photoablated with the excimer laser (with little to no immune response from the intrastromal tissue) and the flap is folded back down over the reshaped cornea with no sutures required
2. Laser-assisted sub-epithelial keratomileusis (LASEK)[28,35]
   a. In this procedure the femtosecond laser dissects (scores) just the epithelial layer (versus a deeper stromal cut in LASIK)
   b. Alcohol is then applied to the epithelium which loosens its adherence to the anterior stroma which allows the surgeon to push the epithelium to the side with a blunt probe and expose the anterior stromal surface
   c. After the exposed anterior stroma is photoablated with the excimer laser, the epithelial flap is pulled back over the anterior stroma surface and smoothed
   d. Besides reducing the discomfort of epithelial disturbance (e.g., PRK), this LASEK procedure is valuable in very thin corneas where a 100μ (LASIK) flap plus ablation depth might present the risk of a resultant corneal ectasia
3. Epi-LASIK (epithelial flap with excimer ablation)[29,35]
   a. Similarly to LASEK, epi-LASIK is characterized by an epithelial flap rather than the full-thickness stromal flap
   b. In epi-LASIK, an epithelial flap is created by the use of an applanating microkeratome (epi-keratome) that flattens the corneal surface
   c. An instrument (epithelial separator) that has an oscillating plastic blade with a thin blunt edge separates and lifts the epithelial flap
   d. After excimer surface stromal ablation, the epithelial cells are either replaced or discarded achieving all the benefits described (above) for LASEK

C. Astigmatic (or arcuate) keratotomy[30,35]: *aka* Limbal relaxing incisions (LRI)
1. If the corneal cylinder (astigmatism) is too high a degree for effective photoablation (≥ 4 to 6 D) and/or if corneal cylinder is induced by PRK or LASIK procedure, the meridional or oblique corneal curvatures can be modified by "limbal relaxing incisions" (LRI) or a procedure referred to as astigmatic keratotomy (AK)
2. Arcuate incisions are made with a scalpel, usually to ¾ to ⅞ corneal thickness and of a calculated arc length (AK nomogram) up to 60°
3. These AK incisions can also be made (more accurately) with a femtosecond laser

D. Other intracorneal procedures (see also Section III, G)
1. Laser thermal keratoplasty (LTK)[32,35]
   a. This procedure is limited to mild to moderate farsightedness
   b. Uses a thulium laser to apply pulses of laser light in ring formation to the corneal periphery
   c. The thermal energy is applied through a non-contact laser beam which delivers 16 spots (2 concentric circles)
   d. The heat generated shrinks the peripheral collagen fibers steepening the shape of the central corneal correcting up to ~2.50 D of hyperopia
   e. Leaves a peripheral ring-shaped scar which maintains the refractive adjustment
   f. Overcorrection made in initial treatment to allow for regression (accuracy of final result variable)
   g. Astigmatism cannot be corrected and there is a risk of induced astigmatism
   h. Treatment procedure accomplished in seconds
2. Conductive keratoplasty (CK)[32,35]
   a. This is a similar procedure to LTK for mild to moderate hyperopia without astigmatism
   b. Radiofrequency energy (350–400 kHz) within peripheral corneal stroma to a depth of 500 μm is delivered to multiple locations on the cornea by a probe (by *Refractec*) which shrinks the collagen and steepens the central cornea
   c. Depending on number of spots (based on corrective power nomogram), procedure is completed in under one minute
   d. Spot scars remain in paracentral cornea and regression is common
3. Small incision lenticule extraction (SMILE)[33,35] (*Relex Smile* by *MedRx*)
   a. An alternative to LASIK surgery for the correction of nearsightedness is another stromal lamellar procedure using the *VisuMax* femtosecond laser (Carl Zeiss Meditec)
   b. The femtosecond incisions consist of four separate cuts
      i. Posterior cut (creates posterior side of lenticule)
      ii. Side cut (creates outline for the lenticule)
      iii. Cap cut (for anterior surface of lenticule)
      iv Side cut (creates opening port incision for lenticule extraction)
   c. These cuts are completed in succession in the integrated procedure
   d. The lenticule is subsequently extracted by the surgeon through the opening incision and discarded
   e. With the lenticule removed, the shape of the cornea is altered (flattened), correcting nearsightedness
4. Intrastromal corneal ring segments (ICRS)[34,35], Intacs (see also III, H, 7)
   a. ICRS segments (2) are small PMMA (polymethyl methacrylate) devices originally developed and approved by FDA (1999) for flattening central cornea through paracentral corneal traction to correct nearsightedness
   b. Femtosecond laser produce photodisruption (cavitation) tunnels in the paracentral cornea at a depth of 70% to 80% of pachymetry with radial incisions at the end of each tunnel into which ICRS segments are inserted
   c. The flattening effects have now been shown to reduce keratometric readings in keratoconus (see Chapter 5) resulting in better corrected visual acuities, stabilization of the central corneal cone, and reduction of induced higher order aberrations (HOAs)

VI. Postoperative (SOAP) Management[36] (See Also Tables 7.6 and 7.7)

A. Post-Op Visit Schedule (Assuming Normal, Expected Results)

PRK/PTK	LASIK/LASEK/ Epi-LASIK	Intracorneal Procedures
Day #1, #3 to #5	Day #1; Week #1 to #2	Day #1; Week #1 to #2
Month #1, #3 to #6	Month #1, #3 to #6	Month #1, #3 to #6

B. Subjective and Urgencies and Emergencies Categories

Subjective and ***Urgencies and Emergencies*** categories are similar for all refractive procedures with limited additions for some procedures. Thus, generic **Subjective** and ***Urgencies and Emergencies*** categories are presented immediately below which apply to all IOL SOAP outlines

Subjective (General questions directly below plus any additional items in specific SOAP note)

ⓘ Questions to ask:

- "Have you (or your caregiver) been instilling your eyedrops as instructed?"
- "Have you had any significant issues or discomfort in your eyes?"
- "Have you noticed any significant changes (better or worse) in your vision?"
  - Blurring (intermittent, decreasing, increasing, constant, progressing)
  - Spherical aberrations (halos, glare, etc.) see Table 7.1
- Dysphotopsias (arcs or streaks of light)
- Assess subjective complaints relative to corneal clarity and pupil diameter (advise on lighting adjustments if halos reported)

Urgencies and Emergencies **(General findings directly below plus any additional items in specific SOAP note)**

(Check Section D, "Potential Postoperative Complications" and Table 7.3 for additional potential postoperative complications, their clinical effects, and corrective actions.)

ASAP or STAT referral to surgeon for:

- Increasing ocular surface inflammation greater than 2 to 3+
- Insidious vision reduction with no improvement over 24 hours
- Sudden loss of vision
- Increasing red eye with/or deep, uveitic pain or endophthalmitis

C. SOAP for Photorefractive Keratectomy (PRK) (Excimer Surface Ablation) and Phototherapeutic Keratectomy (PTK)

PRK/PTK DAY #1 AND #3 TO #5 POST-OP SOAP

(Some surgeons prefer to see the patient at Day #1 post-op)

Subjective (PRK/PTK) Day #1 and #3 to #5

ⓘ Questions to ask: (See generic **Subjective** page 316)

Objective (PRK/PTK) Day #1 and #3 to #5

Perform the following tests:

- Day #1 leave bandage contact lens in place barring any suspicious findings (e.g., infection); remove at Day #3 to #5
- Pinhole distance vision: Goal @ 20/20 to 20/40
- Uncorrected distance vision expectations (fair to good):
  - > Near with monovision should be fair to good
- Keratometry mires or topography should be clear and undistorted
- Refraction (optional day #1)
- BCVA—distance: Should be about equal to pinhole vision with or without overcorrection;
- BCVA—near (with plus correction if presbyopic): Goal @ J2 to J4
- Cornea (SLE): > Document (diagram) post-op epithelial defect
  - > Diagram any endothelial irregularities (striae, folds, guttata as compared to pre-examination documentation)
  - > If AK performed, check incisions for leakage (produced by a full-thickness versus partial incision)
- Anterior chamber (SLE): > chamber (and angle) should be deep and clear
  - > May see trace cells, no RBCs (hyphema)
- Pupil and Iris (SLE): > should have PERRLA
- Ocular surface may demonstrate inconsequential subconjunctival hemorrhage and/or hyperemia (post-op effect) but not > 1 to 2+
- Retina/macula (BIO): retina should be at pre-operative condition and macula should demonstrate a foveal reflex
- IOP (T_A): defer tonometry at Day #1 and #3 to #5)

Assessment (PRK/PTK) Day #1* and *#3 to #5

Dx Diagnostic considerations based on subjective (**S**) and objective (**O**) information

- Noteworthy findings to document at Day #1 and #3 to #5 visits:
  - > Rule out corneal ectasia
  - > Corneal haze: 0 to 1+ = Iris features clear and visible
    - 1 to 3+ = Iris features cloudy

> 3 to 4+ = Iris features barely visible or obscured
> Focal corneal infiltrate(s): rule out corneal ulcer (sterile or infectious?)
> Diffuse stromal infiltrates = Deep lamellar keratitis (DLK)
> Decreased contrast sensitivity
> Decreased corneal sensitivity: look for other herpetic signs
> Development or increased dry eye symptoms: Instruct on frequent use of tears
> Induced regular or irregular astigmatism
> Loss of BCVA: Do nothing on Day #1 and #3 to #5
> Need for reading correction: Provide temporary readers
> Partial regression of effect: Do nothing on Day #1 and #3 to #5
> Ptosis: reassure on likelihood of improvement
> Reactivation of HSV keratitis
> Recurrent corneal erosion: Consider soft lens bandage
> Symptomatic undercorrection or overcorrection: Do nothing on Day #1 and #3 to #5
> Visual aberrations, including glare or starburst/halo effect, especially at night: Recommend maximum lighting (dome light in car and consider 0.5% to 1.25% Pilo bid [*Vuity*], combined carbachol and brimonidine [*Brimochol*], or *Alphagan* [*preferred due to least side effects*])

Plan (PRK/PTK) Day #1 and #3 to #5

℞ Provide necessary care for any positive clinical findings from **S**, **O**, and **A** above per Table 7.6:

- Leave bandage lens in place for the first 3 to 5 days
- If corneal epithelium is not sufficiently regenerated after 48 hours, reapply bandage lens for additional 24 to 48 hours
- Reassure patient that procedure was a success and things are progressing well
- Wear your sunglasses when you are outside during daylight hours for comfort and for optimal results
- DO NOT rub your eyes or squeeze your eyelids tightly
- Try to sleep as much as possible for the first 24 hours after surgery
- No strenuous physical activity for the first week following surgery
- DO NOT swim for 4 weeks following surgery
- OK to shower or bath but avoid getting water in your eye for 2 weeks following surgery
- Try to stay away from smoky or dusty rooms or areas with chemical vapors
- DO NOT wear makeup or apply lotions for the first 2 weeks following surgery
- DO NOT drive or operate machinery while taking narcotic pain medications (if prescribed)
- Plan on 1 to 2 days before returning to work (may be longer in some cases)
- Some of your eyedrops may sting or cause temporary blurred vision
- Maintain your usual diet and medications
- Drink plenty of water
- Use the medications prescribed as directed
- Expect your vision to fluctuate and be blurry for several days
- Explain the phenomenon of "neuroadaptation" to the patient regarding the likelihood of some visual perceptual variations from their pre-op visions:
  > "You're adjusting to a 'new visual system'"
  > "Your brain will adapt through a process called 'neuroplasticity'"
  > "During this process you will experience variable vision"
  > Depending on individuals, duration lasts from weeks to (sometimes) months
  > This is extremely valuable counseling for short- and long-term reassurance
- With any abnormal or suspicious **S** and/or **O** findings, reschedule accordingly
- Strongly advise the use artificial tears daily (q ≥ 4 h or greater)
- Ask patient if they have any questions
- If patient comfortable and **S** and **O** findings WNL, schedule Month #1 to #3 RV

Follow-Up (PRK/PTK) from Day #1, #3 to #5 to 1- until 3-month visit

Advise patient to contact you immediately if:

- Red or increasingly irritated eye(s) not responding to artificial tears
- Acute and/or increasing pain in eye(s)
- Any sudden or insidious changes in vision
- Sudden or increasing flashes and/or floaters in field of vision
- Any questions?

Urgencies and Emergencies (PRK/PTK) Day #1 and #3 to #5

(Check Table 7.6 for additional potential postoperative complications, their clinical effects, and corrective actions.)

ASAP or STAT referral to surgeon for:

(See generic ***Urgencies and Emergencies*** page 316 plus additional items below)

- Corneal haze (3 to 4+): iris features barely visible or obscured
- Infectious corneal infiltrate(s)
- Deep lamellar keratitis, Grade 3+

PRK/PTK MONTH #1 AND #3 TO #6 POST-OP SOAP

Subjective (PRK/PTK) Month #1 and #3 to #6

ⓘ Questions to ask: (See generic **Subjective** page 316)

Objective (PRK/PTK) Month #1 and #3 to #6

Perform the following tests:

- Uncorrected vision, distance (goal: 20/20) and near (goal J1 to J2)

- Keratometry or topography (optional): Should be clear and undistorted
- Refraction (any shift towards myopia?)
- BCVA—distance: should be about equal to pinhole vision with or without overcorrection
- BCVA—near (with plus correction if presbyopic): Goal @ J1 to J2
- Cornea (SLE): > epithelial defect should be closed completely and non-staining or mild SPK; > stroma should 0 to 1+ haze
  - > Diagram any endothelial irregularities (striae, folds, guttata as compared to pre-examination documentation)
  - > Anterior chamber (SLE): > chamber (and angle) should be deep and clear
- Pupil and Iris (SLE): > should have PERRLA
- Ocular surface should be white and quiet
- Retina/Macula (BIO): retina should be at pre-operative condition and macula should demonstrate a foveal reflex
- IOP (T_A): should be normotensive
  - > Rule out steroid-induced raised IOP

Assessment (PRK/PTK) Month #1 and #3 to #6

Dx Diagnostic considerations based on subjective (**S**) and objective (**O**) information

- Noteworthy findings to document at Month #1 and #3 to 6:
  - > Rule out corneal ectasia
  - > Corneal haze: 0 to 1+ = Iris features clear and visible
    - – 1 to 3+ = Iris features cloudy
  - > 3 to 4+ = Iris features barely visible or obscured
  - > Focal corneal infiltrate(s): rule out corneal ulcer (sterile or infectious?)
  - > Diffuse stromal infiltrates = Deep lamellar keratitis (DLK)
  - > Decreased contrast sensitivity
  - > Development or increased dry eye symptoms: Instruct on frequent use of tears
  - > Loss of BCVA: careful refraction
  - > Need for reading correction: prescribe final near correction for presbyopes
  - > Partial regression of effect: monitor unless uncorrected VA below 20/30
  - > Ptosis: reassure on possible improvement or refer for blepharoplasty
  - > Symptomatic undercorrection or overcorrection: consider PRK enhancement or prescribe distance or bifocal correction
  - > Visual aberrations, including glare or starburst/halo effect, especially at night: recommend maximum lighting (dome light in car and consider 0.5% or 1.25% Pilo bid [*Vuity*], combined carbachol and brimonidine [*Brimochol*], or *Alphagan* [*preferred due to least side effects*])

Plan (PRK/PTK) Month #1 and #3 to #6

℞ Provide necessary care for any positive findings from **S**, **O**, and **A** above per Table 7.6:

- Strongly advise the use artificial tears daily (q ≥ 4 h or greater)
- Ask patient if they have any questions
- With any abnormal or suspicious **S** and/or **O** findings, reschedule accordingly
- Visual aberrations, including glare or starburst/halo effect, especially at night: recommend maximum lighting (dome light in car and consider 0.5% or 1.25% Pilo bid [*Vuity*], combined carbachol and brimonidine [*Brimochol*], or *Alphagan* [*preferred due to side effects*])
- If patient comfortable and **S** and **O** findings WNL, schedule routine 6 to 12 months

Follow-Up (PRK/PTK) Month #1 and #3 to #6

Advise patient to contact you immediately if:

- Red or increasingly irritated eye(s) not responding to artificial tears
- Acute and/or increasing pain in eye(s)
- Any sudden or insidious changes in vision
- Sudden or increasing flashes and/or floater in field of vision
- Any questions?

Urgencies and Emergencies (PRK/PTK) Month #1 and #3 to #6

(Check Table 7.6 for additional potential postoperative complications, their clinical effects, and corrective actions.)

ASAP or STAT referral to surgeon for:

(See generic ***Urgencies and Emergencies*** page 316)

D. LASIK, LASEK, Epi-LASIK

1. LASIK (laser in situ keratomileusis) for myopia, hyperopia, and compound astigmatism
2. LASEK (Femto epithelial flap with excimer laser surface ablation)
3. Epi-LASIK (epikeratome epithelial flap with excimer laser surface ablation)

LASIK, LASEK, EPI-LASIK DAY #1 POST-OP SOAP

(Some surgeons prefer to see the patient at Day #1 post-op)

Subjective (LASIK, LASEK, Epi-LASIK) Day #1

(See generic **Subjective** page 316 plus additional item below)

ⓘ Questions to ask:

- Occasional reference to "light streaks" (probably glare after a blink)

Objective (LASIK, LASEK, Epi-LASIK) Day #1

Perform the following tests:

Noteworthy findings to document at Day #1:

- If bandage contact lens was used, remove it for corneal examination
- Pinhole distance vision: Goal @ 20/20 to 20/40
- Uncorrected distance vision expectations (fair to good)
- Near with monovision should be fair to good

- Keratometry mires or topography will appear moderately improved over pre-operative appearance
- Refraction (optional Day #1)
- BCVA—distance: should be about equal to pinhole vision with or without overcorrection
- BCVA—near (with plus correction if presbyopic): Goal @ J2 to J4
- Cornea (SLE): > document (diagram if necessary) corneal flap, edges, and interface
  - > For LASIK: flap and edges should be flat with clear interface
  - > For LASEK/Epi-LASIK: mild to moderate epithelial staining with flat edges and clear interface with no epithelial cells or debris
    - Diagram any endothelial irregularities (striae, folds, guttata as compared to pre-examination documentation)
    - If AK performed, check incisions for leakage (produced by a full-thickness versus partial incision)
- Anterior chamber (SLE): > chamber (and angle) should be deep and clear
  - > May see trace cells, no RBCs (hyphema)
- Pupil and Iris (SLE): > should have PERRLA
- Ocular surface may demonstrate inconsequential subconjunctival hemorrhage and/or hyperemia (post-op effect) but not > 1 to 2+
- Retina/macula (BIO): retina should be at pre-operative condition and macula should demonstrate a foveal reflex
- IOP (T_A): defer tonometry at Day #1

Assessment (LASIK, LASEK, Epi-LASIK) Day #1

Dx Diagnostic considerations based on subjective (**S**) and objective (**O**) information:

Noteworthy findings to document at Day #1:

- Corneal ectasia (progressive corneal steepening): Monitor
- Corneal haze: consider steroid q4h if haze > 1 to 2 +
- Corneal haze and diffuse infiltration: > 0 to 1+ = iris features clear and visible
- > 1 to 3+ = iris features cloudy: Steroid drops q4h; 3 to 4+ = iris features barely visible or obscured: DLK, see below
- Focal corneal infiltrate(s): rule out corneal ulcer (sterile or infectious?): monitor
- Corneal ulceration superficial or under flap (sterile or microbial): STAT referral to surgeon for flap lift and treatment
- Corneal melting, perforation (sterile or microbial): STAT referral to surgeon
- Decreased contrast sensitivity
- Decreased corneal sensitivity: rule out herpes simplex keratitis
- Deep lamellar keratitis (DLK): 1 to 2 +: steroid drops q4h
- 2 to 3 +: steroid drops q2h
- 3 to 4 +: lift flap, irrigate, steroid drops q2h
- Development, exacerbation of dry eye symptoms
- Epithelial ingrowth: cells under flap: If ingrowth lifting flap edge and/or effecting vision (i.e., central flap zone), lift flap and debride with blade, peel with forceps, possibly Nd:YAG laser or mitomycin C or ethanol: 44% recurrence rate with any treatment
- Induced regular or irregular astigmatism: consider AK for regular astigmatism ≥ 0.75
- Significant interface debris: lift flap and irrigate interface

Plan (LASIK, LASEK, Epi-LASIK) Day #1

℞ Provide necessary care for any positive findings from **S**, **O**, and **A** above per Table 7.7:

- Reapply bandage contact lens only if corneal epithelium is significantly disrupted
- Reassure patient that procedure was a success and things are progressing well
- Wear your sunglasses when you are outside during daylight hours for comfort and for optimal results
- DO NOT rub your eyes or squeeze your eyelids tightly
- Try to sleep as much as possible for the first 24 hours after surgery
- No strenuous physical activity for the first week following surgery
- DO NOT swim for 4 weeks following surgery
- OK to shower or bath but avoid getting water in your eye for 2 weeks following surgery
- Try to stay away from smoky or dusty rooms or areas with chemical vapors
- DO NOT wear makeup or apply lotions for the first 2 weeks following surgery
- DO NOT drive or operate machinery while taking narcotic pain medications (if prescribed)
- Plan on 1 to 2 days before returning to work (may be longer in some cases)
- Some of your eyedrops may sting or cause temporary blurred vision
- Maintain your usual diet and medications
- Drink plenty of water
- Use the medications prescribed as directed
- Expect your vision to fluctuate and be blurry for several days
- Explain the phenomenon of "neuroadaptation" to the patient regarding the likelihood of some visual perceptual variations from their pre-op visions:
- "You're adjusting to a 'new visual system'"
- "Your brain will adapt through a process called 'neuroplasticity'"
- "During this process you will experience variable vision"
- Depending on individuals, duration lasts from weeks to (sometimes) months
- This is extremely valuable counseling for short- and long-term reassurance
- With any abnormal or suspicious **S** and/or **O** findings, reschedule accordingly
- Strongly advise the use artificial tears daily (q ≥ 4 h or greater)
- Ask patient if they have any questions
- If patient comfortable and **S** and **O** findings WNL, schedule Week #1 or #2 RV

Follow-Up (LASIK, LASEK, Epi-LASIK) Day #1

Advise patient to contact you immediately if:

- Red or increasingly irritated eye(s) not responding to artificial tears
- Acute and/or increasing pain in eye(s)

- Any sudden or insidious changes in vision
- Sudden or increasing flashes and/or floaters in field of vision
- Any questions?

Urgencies and Emergencies (LASIK, LASEK, Epi-LASIK Day #1)

(Check Table 7.7 for additional potential postoperative complications, their clinical effects, and corrective actions.)

ASAP or STAT referral to surgeon for:

(See generic ***Urgencies and Emergencies*** page 316 plus additional item below)

- Dislocated or traumatic amputated flap
- Insidious vision reduction with no improvement over 24 hours

LASIK, LASEK, EPI-LASIK WEEK #1 OR #2 POST-OP SOAP

Subjective (LASIK, LASEK, Epi-LASIK) Week #1 or #2

Questions to ask: (See generic **Subjective** page 316)

Objective (LASIK, LASEK, Epi-LASIK) Week #1 or #2

Perform the following tests:

Noteworthy findings to document at Week #1 or #2 visits:

- Pinhole distance vision: Goal @ 20/20 to 20/30
- Uncorrected distance vision expectations (good to excellent, i.e. 20/20)
- Near with monovision should be good
- Refraction (but do not prescribe)
- BCVA—distance: should be about equal to pinhole vision with or without overcorrection
- BCVA—near (prescribe plus correction if presbyopic): Goal @ J1 to J2
- Cornea (SLE): > document (diagram if necessary) corneal flap, edges and interface
  - > For LASIK: flap and edges should be flat with clear interface
  - > For LASEK/Epi-LASIK: mild epithelial staining with flat edges and clear interface with no epithelial cells or debris
    - – Diagram any endothelial irregularities (striae, folds, guttata as compared to pre-examination documentation)
- Anterior chamber (SLE): > chamber (and angle) should be deep and clear
- Pupil and Iris (SLE): > should have PERRLA
- Ocular surface may demonstrate inconsequential subconjunctival hemorrhage and/or hyperemia (post-op effect) but not ≤ 1 to 2+
- IOP (T_A): defer tonometry

Assessment (LASIK, LASEK, Epi-LASIK) Week #1 or #2

Dx Diagnostic considerations based on subjective (**S**) and objective (**O**) information

Noteworthy findings to document at week #1 or #2:

- Corneal haze: consider steroid q4h if haze > 1 to 2 +
- Corneal haze and diffuse infiltration: 0 to 1+ = iris features clear and visible
  - > 1 to 3+ = iris features cloudy: steroid drops q4h
  - > 3 to 4+ = iris features barely visible or obscured: DLK, see below
- Focal corneal infiltrate(s): rule out corneal ulcer (sterile or infectious?): monitor
- Corneal ulceration superficial or under flap (sterile or microbial): STAT referral to surgeon for flap lift and treatment
- Corneal melting, perforation (sterile or microbial): STAT referral to surgeon
- Deep lamellar keratitis (DLK): 1 to 2+: steroid drops q4h
  - > 2 to 3 +: steroid drops q2h
  - > 3 to 4 +: lift flap, irrigate, q2h
- Development, exacerbation of dry eye symptoms
- Epithelial ingrowth: cells under flap: if ingrowth lifting flap edge and/or effecting vision (i.e., central flap zone), lift flap and debride with blade, peel with forceps, possibly Nd:YAG laser or mitomycin C or ethanol: 44% recurrence rate with any treatment
- Interface debris: lift flap and irrigate interface

Plan (LASIK, LASEK, Epi-LASIK) Week #1 or #2

Rx Provide necessary care for any positive findings:

- Reassure patient that procedure was a success and things are progressing well
- Wear your sunglasses when you are outside during daylight hours for comfort and for optimal results
- DO NOT rub your eyes or squeeze your eyelids tightly
- DO NOT swim for 2 more weeks
- Try to stay away from smoky or dusty rooms or areas with chemical vapors
- Use the medications prescribed as directed to completion (usually ~2 weeks)
- Expect mild, occasional fluctuations in vision for a few more weeks
- Re-explain the phenomenon of "neuroadaptation" to the patient regarding the likelihood of some visual perceptual variations from their pre-op visions
  - > "You're adjusting to a 'new visual system'"
  - > "Your brain will adapt through a process called 'neuroplasticity'"
  - > "During this process you will experience variable vision"
  - > Depending on individuals, duration lasts from weeks to (sometimes) months
  - > This is extremely valuable counseling for short- and long-term reassurance
- With any abnormal or suspicious **S** and/or **O** findings, reschedule accordingly
- Strongly advise the use artificial tears daily (q ≥ 4 h or greater)

- Ask patient if they have any questions
- If patient comfortable and **S** and **O** findings WNL, schedule in 1 to 3 (to 6) months

Follow-Up (LASIK, LASEK, Epi-LASIK) Week #1 or #2

Advise patient to contact you immediately if:

- Red or increasingly irritated eye(s) not responding to artificial tears
- Acute and/or increasing pain in eye(s)
- Any sudden or insidious changes in vision
- Sudden or increasing flashes and/or floater in field of vision
- Any questions?

Urgencies and Emergencies (LASIK, LASEK, Epi-LASIK) Week #1 or #2

(Check Table 7.7 for additional potential postoperative complications, their clinical effects, and corrective actions.)

ASAP or STAT referral to surgeon for:

(See generic ***Urgencies and Emergencies*** page 316 plus additional items below)

- Dislocated or traumatic amputated flap
- Insidious vision reduction with no improvement over 24 hours

LASIK, LASEK, EPI-LASIK MONTH #1, #3 TO #6 POST-OP SOAP

Subjective (LASIK, LASEK, Epi-LASIK) Month #1, #3 to #6

(See generic **Subjective** page 316 plus additional item below)

Questions to ask:

- Arcs or streaks of light?

Objective (LASIK, LASEK, Epi-LASIK) Month #1, #3 to #6

Perform the following tests:

Noteworthy findings to document at Month #1, #3, or #6s:

- Uncorrected vision, distance (goal: 20/20 to 20/25) and near (goal: J1)
- Refraction (prescribe Rx, if distance ≤ 20/30)
- BCVA—near (prescribe plus correction if presbyopic): Goal @ J1 to J2
- Cornea (SLE): > Recheck corneal flap, edges and interface against Day #1 diagrams (or photos)
  - > For LASIK: flap and edges should be flat with clear interface
  - > For LASEK/Epi-LASIK: mild epithelial staining with flat edges and clear interface with no epithelial cells or debris
- Anterior chamber (SLE): > chamber (and angle) should be deep and clear
- Pupil and Iris (SLE)
  - > Should have PERRLA
- Ocular surface should be white and quiet
- IOP (T_A): should be approximately equal to pre-op pressures
  - > Rule out steroid-induced raised IOP

Assessment (LASIK, LASEK, Epi-LASIK) Month #1, #3 to #6

Dx Diagnostic considerations based on subjective (**S**) and objective (**O**) information

Noteworthy findings to document at Month #1, #3, and #6:

- Corneal haze: consider steroid q4h if haze > 1 to 2 +
- If focal corneal infiltrate(s), rule out corneal ulcer (sterile or infectious?): monitor
- Evaluate ocular surface for exacerbation of dry eye signs (and symptoms)
- Epithelial ingrowth: if documented but not treated at week # 1or #2, compare (from diagrams) if any progress. If so, consider treatment only if edge involved and/or visual disruption
- Interface debris: if significant, lift flap and irrigate interface
- Partial regression effect: if uncorrected VA ≤ 20/30, prescribe Rx
- Symptomatic undercorrection or overcorrection: consider re-ablation or prescribe distance or bifocal correction
- Visual aberrations, including glare or starburst/halo effect, especially at night: recommend maximum lighting (dome light in car and consider 0.5% or 1.25% Pilo bid [*Vuity*], combined carbachol and brimonidine [*Brimochol*], or *Alphagan* [*preferred due to least side effects*])

Plan (LASIK, LASEK, Epi-LASIK) Month #1, #3 to #6

Rx Provide necessary care for any positive findings:

- Strongly advise the use of artificial tears daily (bid to tid or greater)
- Need for reading correction: Prescribe final near correction for presbyopes
- Ask patient if they have any questions
- With any abnormal or suspicious **S** and/or **O** findings, reschedule accordingly
- Visual aberrations, including glare or starburst/halo effect, especially at night: Recommend maximum lighting (dome light in car and consider 0.5% or 1.25% Pilo bid [*Vuity*], combined carbachol and brimonidine [*Brimochol*], or *Alphagan* [*preferred due to side effects*])
- If patient comfortable and **S** and **O** findings WNL, schedule routine 6 to 12 months

Follow-Up (LASIK, LASEK, Epi-LASIK) Month #1, #3 to #6

Advise patient to contact you immediately if:

- Red or increasingly irritated eye(s) not responding to artificial tears
- Acute and/or increasing pain in eye(s)
- Any sudden or insidious changes in vision
- Sudden or increasing flashes and/or floater in field of vision
- Any questions?

Urgencies and Emergencies (LASIK, LASEK, Epi-LASIK) Month #1 to #6

(Check Table 7.7 for additional potential postoperative complications, their clinical effects, and corrective actions.)

ASAP or STAT referral to surgeon for:

(See generic ***Urgencies and Emergencies*** page 316 plus additional items below)

- Dislocated or traumatic amputated flap
- Insidious vision reduction with no improvement over 24 hours

E. Potential Complications Associated with LASIK, LASEK, EPI-LASIK, LAMELLAR Procedures

Loss of BCVA	Reassure on improvement and possible treatment enhancement
Partial regression of effect	Monitor and possible retreatment if VA significantly reduced
Persistent flap edema	Topical steroid drops and hypertonic saline
Premature need for reading correction	Prescribe near Rx
Pressure-induced sterile (stromal) keratitis (PISK)	Do not use (or d/c) topical steroids; Treat with IOP lowering meds
Ptosis	Reassure on improvement—beyond 6 months consider blepharoplasty
Rainbow glare associated with femtosecond laser	Transient LASIK phenomenon from light scatter; PTK on the posterior flap surface may help
Reactivation of HSV keratitis	HSV treatment protocol
Recurrent corneal erosion	Soft lens corneal bandage and possible PTK
Striae (microstriae and macrostriae)	Refer to surgeon for flap lift and hydration; "ironing" with sponge or heated spacula; suturing
Symptomatic undercorrection or overcorrection	Refer to surgeon for treatment enhancement
Transient-light sensitivity associated with femtosecond laser	Aggressive steroids to reduce inflammation
Traumatic flap dislocation	Reposition or refer to surgeon for removal
Visual symptoms, including glare or starburst/halo effect, especially at night	Sunglasses, lighting and possible Alphagan drops
Worsening corneal stromal dystrophy	Depending on degree, corneal transplant may be indicated

F. Thermal Keratoplasty Procedures

1. Laser thermal keratoplasty (LTK)
2. Conductive keratoplasty (CK)

LASER THERMAL AND CONDUCTIVE KERATOPLASTY PROCEDURES[37] (DAY #1 POST-OP SOAP)

(Some surgeons prefer to see the patient at Day #1 post-op)

Subjective (Laser Thermal and Conductive Keratoplasty) Day #1

(See generic **Subjective** page 316 plus additional item below)

Questions to ask:

- May be slight persisting foreign-body sensation

Objective (Laser Thermal and Conductive Keratoplasty) Day #1

Perform the following tests:

Noteworthy findings to document at Day #1 visits:

- Pinhole distance vision: Goal @ 20/20 to 20/40
- Uncorrected vision, distance expectation (variable)
- Uncorrected near vision should be ~J3 to J6 (variable) if presbyopic
- Keratometry mires or topography should be mild to moderately distorted
- Refraction (optional Day #1)
- BCVA—distance: should be about equal to pinhole vision with or without overcorrection
- BCVA—near (with plus correction if necessary): Goal @ J2 to J4
- Cornea (SLE): > document (diagram if necessary) appearance of peripheral cornea:
  - > Peripheral ring-shaped haze likely out to limbus with thermal keratoplasty
  - > Dense peripheral spots and haze with conductive keratoplasty
- Anterior chamber (SLE): > chamber (and angle) should be deep and clear
  - > May see trace cells, no RBCs (hyphema)
- Pupil and iris (SLE): > should have PERRLA
- Ocular surface may demonstrate inconsequential subconjunctival hemorrhage and/or hyperemia (post-op effect) but not > 1 to 2+
- Retina/macula (BIO): retina should be at pre-operative condition and macula should demonstrate a foveal reflex
- IOP (T_A): defer tonometry at Day #1

Assessment (Laser Thermal and Conductive Keratoplasty) Day #1

Dx Diagnostic considerations based on subjective (**S**) and objective (**O**) information

- Assuming subjective (**S**) responses and all clinical findings (**O**) within normal limits (WNL), the post-op eye should be considered stable and recovering well
- Any actions and/or adjustment in response to clinical findings from subjective (**S**) and/or objective (**O**) above should be conducted per Table 7.3

Plan (Laser Thermal and Conductive Keratoplasty) Day #1

Provide necessary care for any positive findings:

- Reassure patient that procedure was a success and things are progressing well
- Wear your sunglasses when you are outside during daylight hours for comfort and for optimal results
- DO NOT rub your eyes or squeeze your eyelids tightly

- DO NOT swim for 2 more weeks
- Try to stay away from smoky or dusty rooms or areas with chemical vapors
- Use the medications prescribed as directed to completion (usually ~2 weeks)
- Expect mild, occasional fluctuations in vision for a few more weeks
- If any abnormal or suspicious **S** and/or **O** findings, reschedule accordingly
- Strongly advise the use of artificial tears daily (q ≥ 4 h or greater)
- Ask patient if they have any questions
- If patient comfortable and **S** and **O** findings WNL, schedule in 1 to 2 weeks

Follow-Up (Laser Thermal and Conductive Keratoplasty) Day #1 to Week #1

Advise patient to contact you immediately if:

- Red or increasingly irritated eye(s) not responding to artificial tears
- Acute and/or increasing pain in eye(s)
- Any sudden or insidious changes in vision
- Sudden or increasing flashes and/or floater in field of vision
- Any questions?

Urgencies and Emergencies (Laser Thermal and Conductive Keratoplasty) Day #1

(Check Table 7.7 for additional potential postoperative complications, their clinical effects, and corrective actions.)

ASAP or STAT referral to surgeon for:
(See generic ***Urgencies and Emergencies*** page 316)

LASER THERMAL AND CONDUCTIVE KERATOPLASTY PROCEDURES (WEEK #1 OR #2 POST-OP SOAP)

Subjective (Laser Thermal and Conductive Keratoplasty) Week #1 or #2

Questions to ask: (See generic **Subjective** page 316)

Objective (Laser Thermal and Conductive Keratoplasty) Week #1 or #2

Perform the following tests:

- Pinhole distance vision: Goal @ 20/20 to 20/40
- Uncorrected vision, distance expectation (variable)
- Uncorrected near vision should be ~J2 to J4 (variable)
- Keratometry mires or topography will be mild to moderately distorted
- Refraction (prescribe on if distance vision ≤ 20/40)
- BCVA—distance: should be about equal to pinhole vision with or without overcorrection
- BCVA—near (with plus correction if necessary): Goal @ J1 to J2
- Cornea (SLE): > document (diagram if necessary) appearance of peripheral cornea:
  - > Peripheral ring-shaped haze likely out to limbus with thermal keratoplasty
  - > Dense peripheral spots and haze with conductive keratoplasty
- Anterior chamber (SLE): > chamber (and angle) should be deep and clear
  - > May see trace cells, no RBCs (hyphema)
- Pupil and iris (SLE)
  - > Should have PERRLA
- Ocular surface may demonstrate inconsequential subconjunctival hemorrhage and/or hyperemia (post-op effect) but not ≤ 1 to 2+
- Retina/macula (BIO): retina should be at pre-operative condition and macula should demonstrate a foveal reflex
- IOP (T_A): should be equal to pre-procedure IOP
  - > Rule out steroid-induced raised IOP

Assessment (Laser Thermal and Conductive Keratoplasty) Week #1 or #2

Dx Diagnostic considerations based on subjective (**S**) and objective (**O**) information

- Assuming subjective (**S**) responses and all clinical findings (**O**) within normal limits (WNL), the post-op eye should be considered stable and recovering well
- Any actions and/or adjustment in response to clinical findings from subjective (**S**) and/or objective (**O**) above should be conducted per Table 7.3
- Residual irregular astigmatism (may persist indefinitely)

Plan (Laser Thermal and Conductive Keratoplasty) Week #1 or #2

Rx Provide necessary care for any positive findings:

- Assuming subjective (**S**) responses and all clinical findings (**O**) within normal limits (WNL), the post-op eye should be considered stable and recovering well
- Any actions and/or adjustment in response to clinical findings from subjective (**S**) and/or objective (**O**) above should be conducted per Table 7.3

Follow-Up (Laser Thermal and Conductive Keratoplasty) Week #1 or #2

Advise patient to contact you immediately if:

- Red or increasingly irritated eye(s) not responding to artificial tears
- Acute and/or increasing pain in eye(s)
- Any sudden or insidious changes in vision
- Sudden or increasing flashes and/or floater in field of vision
- Any questions?

Urgencies and Emergencies (Laser Thermal and Conductive) Keratoplasty Month #1 to #6

(Check Table 7.7 for additional potential postoperative complications, their clinical effects, and corrective actions.)

ASAP or STAT referral to surgeon for:
(See generic ***Urgencies and Emergencies*** page 316)

LASER THERMAL AND CONDUCTIVE KERATOPLASTY PROCEDURES (MONTH #1, #3 TO #6 POST-OP SOAP)

Subjective (Laser Thermal and Conductive Keratoplasty) Month #1, #3 to #6

Questions to ask: (See generic **Subjective** page 316)

Objective (Laser Thermal and Conductive Keratoplasty) Month #1, #3 to #6

Perform the following tests:

- Uncorrected vision, distance expectation (variable)
- Uncorrected near vision should be ~ J1 to J2 (variable)
- Keratometry mires or topography will be mild to moderately distorted
- Refraction (prescribe only if distance vision ≤ 20/40)
- BCVA—distance: should be about equal to pinhole vision with or without overcorrection
- BCVA—near (with plus correction if necessary): Goal @ J1 to J2
- Cornea (SLE): > appearance of peripheral cornea should be resolved:
  - > Persistent peripheral ring-shaped haze likely with thermal keratoplasty
  - > Residual dense peripheral spots with conductive keratoplasty
- Anterior chamber (SLE): > chamber (and angle) should be deep and clear
- Pupil and iris (SLE): > should have PERRLA
- IOP (T_A): should be equal to pre-procedure IOP
  - > Rule out steroid-induced raised IOP

Assessment (Laser Thermal and Conductive Keratoplasty) Month #1, #3 to #6

Dx Diagnostic considerations based on subjective (**S**) and objective (**O**) information

- Assuming subjective (**S**) responses and all clinical findings (**O**) within normal limits (WNL), the post-op eye should be considered stable and recovering well
- Any actions and/or adjustment in response to clinical findings from subjective (**S**) and/or objective (**O**) above should be conducted per Table 7.3

Plan (Laser Thermal and Conductive Keratoplasty) Month #1, #3 to #6

Provide necessary care for any positive findings:

- Assuming subjective (**S**) responses and all clinical findings (**O**) within normal limits (WNL), the post-op eye should be considered stable and recovering well
- Any actions and/or adjustment in response to clinical findings from subjective (**S**) and/or objective (**O**) above should be conducted per Table 7.3
- Advise on long term (1 to 3 years) refractive regression and retreatment likely
- Possible residual irregular astigmatism and resultant visual reduction and aberrations (spherical and coma)

Follow-Up (Laser Thermal and Conductive Keratoplasty) Month #1, #3 to #6

Advise patient to contact you immediately if:

- Red or increasingly irritated eye(s) not responding to artificial tears
- Acute and/or increasing pain in eye(s)
- Any sudden or insidious changes in vision
- Sudden or increasing flashes and/or floaters in field of vision
- Any questions?

Urgencies and Emergencies (Laser Thermal and Conductive Keratoplasty) Month #1, #3 to #6

(Check Table 7.7 for additional potential postoperative complications, their clinical effects, and corrective actions.)

ASAP or STAT referral to surgeon for:
(See generic ***Urgencies and Emergencies*** page 316)

G. Other Intracorneal Procedures

1. Small incision lenticule extraction (SMILE)
2. Intrastromal corneal ring segments (ICRS) (Intacs by *Refractec*)

1. Small Incision Lenticule Extraction (SMILE)

(Follow same SOAP post-op protocol as outlined on page 316 for LASIK, LASEK, Epi-LASIK)

INTRASTROMAL CORNEAL RING SEGMENTS (ICRS)[38] INTACS

(See also "Intrastromal Corneal Rings" in Chapter 5 and Table 7.5)

(Some surgeons prefer to see the patient at Day #1 post-op)

Subjective (ICRS INTACS) Day #1

Questions to ask: (See generic **Subjective** page 316)

Objective (ICRS INTACS) Day #1

Perform the following tests:

- Pinhole distance vision: Goal @ 20/20 to 20/40
- Uncorrected distance vision expectations (poor to fair)
- Keratometry mires or topography will appear moderately distorted
- Refraction (optional Day #1)
- BCVA—distance: should be about equal to pinhole vision with or without overcorrection

- BCVA—near (with plus correction if presbyopic): Goal @ J2 to J4
- Cornea (SLE): > document (diagram if necessary)
  - > Corneal surface (epithelium) should be clear (slight SPK possible)
  - > Channels, incision apertures, and ring segments should be clear with mild to moderate surrounding edema
- Rule out
  - > Anterior chamber perforation
  - > Implant extrusion (through channel incisional aperture)
  - > Shallow ring positioning
  - > Corneal thinning over ring segments
- Anterior chamber (SLE)
  - > Chamber (and angle) should be deep and clear
  - > May see trace cells, no RBCs (hyphema)
- Pupil and iris (SLE): > should have PERRLA
- Ocular surface may demonstrate inconsequential subconjunctival hemorrhage and/or hyperemia (post-op effect) but not > 1 to 2+
- Retina/macula (BIO): retina should be at pre-operative condition and macula should demonstrate a foveal reflex
- IOP (T_A): defer tonometry at Day #1

Assessment (ICRS INTACS) Day #1

Dx Diagnostic considerations based on subjective (**S**) and objective (**O**) information

- Slight corneal ectasia possible over ring segments: monitor
- Any focal corneal infiltrate(s): rule out corneal ulcer (sterile or infectious?): monitor
- Decreased corneal sensitivity: rule out herpes simplex keratitis
- Channel incisional apertures should be flat and closed
- Keratometry may reveal induced regular or irregular astigmatism: monitor
- Channels, incision apertures, and ring segments should be clear with mild to moderate surrounding edema

Plan (ICRS INTACS) Day #1

℞ Provide necessary care for any positive findings:

- Reassure patient that procedure was a success and things are progressing well
- Explain that final refractive and visual result vary considerably
- Discuss likelihood of spectacle Rx or contact lenses (especially with keratoconus)
- Wear your sunglasses when you are outside during daylight hours for comfort and for optimal results
- DO NOT rub your eyes or squeeze your eyelids tightly
- No strenuous physical activity for the first week following surgery
- DO NOT swim for 4 weeks following surgery
- OK to shower or bath but avoid getting water in your eye for 2 weeks following surgery
- Try to stay away from smoky or dusty rooms or areas with chemical vapors
- Plan on 1 to 2 days before returning to work (may be longer in some cases)
- Some of your eyedrops may sting or cause temporary blurred vision
- Maintain your usual diet and medications
- Drink plenty of water
- Use the medications prescribed as directed
- Expect your vision to fluctuate and be blurry for several days
- With any abnormal or suspicious **S** and/or **O** findings, reschedule accordingly
- Strongly advise the use artificial tears daily (q ≥ 4 h or greater)
- Ask patient if they have any questions
- If patient comfortable and **S** and **O** findings WNL, schedule Week #1 or #2 RV

Follow-Up (ICRS INTACS) Day #1

Advise patient to contact you immediately if:

- Red or increasingly irritated eye(s) not responding to artificial tears
- Acute and/or increasing pain in eye(s)
- Any sudden or insidious changes in vision
- Sudden or increasing flashes and/or floater in field of vision
- Any questions?

Urgencies and Emergencies (ICRS INTACS) Day #1

(Check Table 7.5 for additional potential postoperative complications, their clinical effects, and corrective actions.)

ASAP or STAT referral to surgeon for:

(See generic ***Urgencies and Emergencies*** page 316 plus additional items below)

- Anterior chamber perforation from ring segment movement
- Implant extrusion (through channel incisional aperture)

INTRASTROMAL CORNEAL RING SEGMENTS (ICRS) INTACS (WEEK #1 OR #2 POST-OP SOAP)

Subjective (ICRS INTACS) Week #1 or #2

Questions to ask: (See generic **Subjective** page 316)

Objective (ICRS INTACS) Week #1 or #2

Perform the following tests:

- Pinhole distance vision: Goal @ 20/20 to 20/40
- Uncorrected distance vision expectations (fair to good)
- Keratometry mires or topography will appear moderately distorted
- Refraction (postpone prescribing unless uncorrected vision ≤ 20/40)

- BCVA—distance: should be about equal to pinhole vision with or without overcorrection
- BCVA—near (with plus correction if presbyopic): Goal @ J2 to J4
- Cornea (SLE): > document (diagram if necessary):
  - > Corneal surface (epithelium) should be clear (slight SPK possible)
  - > Channels, incision apertures, and ring segments should be clear with mild to moderate surrounding edema
  - > Small, fine, white deposits will begin to appear in the segment channels
- Rule out
  - > Anterior chamber perforation
  - > Implant extrusion (through channel incisional aperture)
  - > Shallow ring positioning
  - > Corneal thinning over ring segments
- Anterior chamber (SLE): > chamber (and angle) should be deep and clear
- Ocular surface may demonstrate inconsequential subconjunctival hemorrhage and/or hyperemia (post-op effect) but not > 1 to 2+
- IOP (T_A): defer or IOP should at pre-procedure levels
  - > Rule out steroid-induced raised IOP

Assessment (ICRS INTACS) Week #1 or #2

Dx Diagnostic considerations based on subjective (**S**) and objective (**O**) information

- Slight corneal ectasia possible over ring segments: monitor
- Channel incisional apertures should be flat and closed
- Keratometry may reveal induced regular or irregular astigmatism: monitor
- Fine, white corneal deposits in channels will create a light outline to the segments (within normal limits)

Plan (ICRS INTACS) Week #1 or #2

Provide necessary care for any positive findings:

- Reassure patient that procedure was a success and things are progressing well
- Explain that final refractive and visual result may continue to fluctuate
- DO NOT rub your eyes or squeeze your eyelids tightly
- Some of your eyedrops may sting or cause temporary blurred vision
- Maintain your usual diet and medications
- Use the medications prescribed as directed
- With any abnormal or suspicious **S** and/or **O** findings, reschedule accordingly
- Strongly advise the use of artificial tears daily (q ≥ 4 h or greater)
- With any abnormal or suspicious **S** and/or **O** findings, reschedule accordingly
- Visual aberrations, including glare or starburst/halo effect, especially at night: recommend maximum lighting (dome light in car and consider 0.5% to 1.25% Pilo bid [*Vuity*], combined carbachol and brimonidine [*Brimochol*], or *Alphagan* [*preferred due to least side effects*])
- If patient comfortable and **S** and **O** findings WNL, schedule routine 3- to 6-month RV
- Ask patient if they have any questions
- If patient comfortable and **S** and **O** findings WNL, schedule 3- to 6-month RV

Follow-Up (ICRS INTACS) Week #1 or #2

Advise patient to contact you immediately if:

- Red or increasingly irritated eye(s) not responding to artificial tears
- Acute and/or increasing pain in eye(s)
- Any sudden or insidious changes in vision
- Sudden or increasing flashes and/or floaters in field of vision
- Any questions?

Urgencies and Emergencies (ICRS INTACS) Week #1 or #2

(Check Table 7.5 for additional potential postoperative complications, their clinical effects, and corrective actions.)

ASAP or STAT referral to surgeon for:

(See generic ***Urgencies and Emergencies*** page 316 plus additional items below)

- Anterior chamber perforation from ring segment movement
- Implant extrusion (through channel incisional aperture)

INTRASTROMAL CORNEAL RING SEGMENTS (ICRS) INTACS (MONTH #3 TO #6 POST-OP SOAP)

Subjective (ICRS INTACS) Month #3 to #6

Questions to ask: (See generic **Subjective** page 316)

Objective (ICRS INTACS) Month #3 to #6

Perform the following tests:

- Pinhole distance vision: Goal @ 20/20 to 20/40
- Uncorrected distance vision expectations (fair to good)
- Keratometry mires or topography should moderately improve over pre-operative appearance
- Refraction (prescribe single vision or bifocals if uncorrected vision ≤ 20/40)
- BCVA—near (with plus correction if presbyopic): Goal @ J to J2
- Cornea (SLE): > document (diagram if necessary):
  - > Corneal surface (epithelium) should be clear
  - > Channels, incision apertures and ring segments should be clear with fine, while deposits forming outline of ring segments
- Rule out
  - > Anterior chamber perforation
  - > Implant extrusion (through channel incisional aperture)
  - > Shallow ring positioning
  - > Corneal thinning over ring segments

Assessment (ICRS INTACS) Month #3 to #6

Dx Diagnostic considerations based on subjective (**S**) and objective (**O**) information

- Slight corneal ectasia possible over ring segments: stable
- Channel incisional apertures should be flat and closed
- Keratometry mires (or topography) should be moderately improved over pre-operative appearance
- Fine, white corneal deposits in channels creating a light outline to the segments (within normal limits) should remain stable (have patient report any significant increase in density)

Plan (ICRS INTACS) Month #3 to #6

℞ Provide necessary care for any positive findings:

- Strongly advise the use artificial tears daily (bid to tid or greater)
- Prescribe final distance and near correction, if not done at 1- to 2-week visit
- Ask patient if they have any questions
- With any abnormal or suspicious **S** and/or **O** findings, reschedule accordingly
- Visual aberrations, including glare or starburst/halo effect, especially at night: recommend maximum lighting (dome light in car and consider 0.5% or 1.25% Pilo bid [*Vuity*], combined carbachol and brimonidine [*Brimochol*], or *Alphagan* [*preferred due to least side effects*])
- If patient comfortable and **S** and **O** findings WNL, schedule routine 6 to 12 months

Follow-Up (ICRS INTACS) Month #3 to #6

Advise patient to contact you immediately if:

- Red or increasingly irritated eye(s) not responding to artificial tears
- Acute and/or increasing pain in eye(s)
- Any sudden or insidious changes in vision
- Sudden or increasing flashes and/or floaters in field of vision
- Any questions?

Urgencies and Emergencies (ICRS INTACS) Month #3 to #6

(Check Table 7.5 for additional potential postoperative complications, their clinical effects, and corrective actions.)

ASAP or STAT referral to surgeon for:

(See generic ***Urgencies and Emergencies*** page 316 plus additional items below)

- Anterior chamber perforation from ring segment movement
- Implant extrusion (through channel incisional aperture)

References

1. Boyd K, Turbert D. What are cataracts? *AAO.Org*. EyeSmart; September 13, 2021.
2. American Academy of Ophthalmology. Accessed 1/20/2021. Cataract surgery (https://www.aao.org/eye-health/diseases/what-is-cataract-surgery).
3. American Optometric Association. Accessed 1/20/2021. Cataract (https://www.aoa.org/healthy-eyes/eye-and-vision-conditions/cataract?).
4. National Eye Institute. Accessed 1/20/2021. Cataract surgery (https://www.nei.nih.gov/learn-about-eye-health/eye-conditions-and-diseases/cataracts/cataract-surgery).
5. Lundstrom M, Behndig A, Kugelberg M. et al. Decreasing rate of capsule complications in cataract surgery: eight-year study of incidence, risk factors, and data validity by the Swedish National Cataract Register. *J Cataract Refract Surg.* 2011;37(10):1762–1767.
6. Thompson V. IOLs: Choosing the best implant for cataract surgery. *All About Vision*. September 2021. 2000–2022 AAV Media, LLC.
7. https://www.fda.gov/medical-devices/recently-approved-devices/alcon-laboratories-inc-acrysofr-iq-panoptixr-trifocal-intraocular-lens-model-tfnt00-and-acrysofr-iq.
8. https://www.ncbi.nlm.nih.gov/pmc/articles/PMC5472417/
9. Boxer Wachler BS. Refractive lens exchange (lens replacement surgery). *All About Vision*. September 2021. 2000–2022 AAV Media, LLC.
10. van Rijn G, Gaurisankar Z, Ilgenfritz AP, et al. Middle- and long-term results after iris-fixated phakic intraocular lens implantation in myopic and hyperopic patients: a meta-analysis. *J Cataract Refract Surg.* January 2020;46(1):125–137.
11. Patel AS, Baartman B, Taravella M, et al. *Implantable Collamer Lens. AAOphth EyeWiki*. October 5, 2021.
12. See CW, Mustafa I, Woreta FA. Preoperative evaluation for cataract surgery. *Curr Opin Ophthalmol.* January 2019;30(1):3–8.
13. Jonker SMR, Berendschot TTJM, Saelens IEY, Bauer NJC, Nuijts RMMA. Phakic intraocular lenses: an overview. *Indian J Ophthalmol.* 2020;68(12):2779–2796.
14. Masket S. Same day bilateral cataract surgery: Who benefits? *Ophthalmology.* January 01, 2021;128(1):11–12.
15. McGhee GNJ, Zhang J, Patel DV. A perspective of contemporary cataract surgery: the most common surgical procedure in the world. *J R Soc New Zealand.* 2020;50(2): 245–262.
16. Marchese A, Bandello F. Current challenges in the postoperative management of cataract surgery. *Touch Rev Ophthalmol.* 2021;15(1): 15–17. July 16 2021.
17. Salerno LC, Tiveron MC Jr, Alió JL. Multifocal intraocular lenses: types, outcomes, complications and how to solve them. *Taiwan J Ophthalmol.* 2017;7(4):179–184.
18. Randolph J, Miller K, Choi J, et al. Complications of cataract surgery. *AAOphth EyeWiki*. February 28, 2020.
19. Cimberle M. Treatment landscape for presbyopia evolving toward noninvasive options. *Ocular Surgery News*. September 22, 2021.
20. Pidro A, Biscevic A, Pjano MA, Mravicic I, Bejdic N, Bohac M. Excimer lasers in refractive surgery. *Acta Inform Med.* 2019;27(4):278–283.
21. Sioufi K, Zheleznyak K, MacRae S, et al. Femtosecond lasers in cornea & refractive surgery. *Exp Eye Res.* 2021;205:108477.
22. Xia LK, Yu J, Chai GR, Wang D, Li Y. Comparison of the femtosecond laser and mechanical microkeratome for flap cutting in LASIK. *Int J Ophthalmol.* 2015;8(4):784–790. Published 2015 August 18.
23. Tuteja SY, Rappama M. Radial Keratotomy. *N Engl J Med* 2019; 380:e4. DOI: 10.1056/NEJMicm1808841.
24. Deshmukh R, Reddy JC, Rapuano CJ, Vaddavalli PK. Phototherapeutic keratectomy: Indications, methods and decision making. *Indian J Ophthalmol.* 2020;68(12):2856–2866.
25. Cennamo, G., Menna, F., Sinisi, F. et al. Twenty-year follow-up of excimer laser photorefractive keratectomy: a retrospective observational study. *Ophthalmol Ther* 2020;9:917–927.
26. Kates MM, Tuli S. What is LASIK eye surgery? *JAMA.* 2020;324(8):815.
27. Azar DT. *Refractive Surgery* (2nd ed.). Philadelphia: Mosby/Elsevier; 2007.
28. Boxer Wachler BS. LASEK eye surgery: How it works. *All About Vision.* May 2021.
29. Taneri S, Kießler S, Rost A, Schultz T, Dick HB. Epi-Bowman keratectomy versus alcohol-assisted photorefractive keratectomy:

wound healing and complications. *Ther Adv Ophthalmol.* January 22, 2021;13:2515841420988215.
30. Sorkin N, Mimouni M, Santaella G. Comparison of manual and femtosecond astigmatic keratotomy in the treatment of postkeratoplasty astigmatism. *Acta Ophth.* 2021 August;99(5):461–574, e621-e776.
31. Jung, Yh., Kim, M.K. Clinical outcomes in post-epikeratophakic eyes after removal of epikeratoplasty lenticule. *BMC Ophthalmol.* 2021;21:350.
32. McDonald MB, Mychajlyszyn A, Mychajlyszyn D, et al. Advances in corneal surgical and pharmacological approaches to the treatment of presbyopia. *J Ref Surg.* June 01, 2021;37(S1):Online.
33. Ahmed AA, Hatch KM. Advantages of small incision lenticule extraction (SMILE) for mass eye and ear special issue. *Semin Ophthalmol.* 2020;35(4):224–231
34. Park SE, Tseng M, Lee JK. Effectiveness of intracorneal ring segments for keratoconus. *Curr Opin Ophthalmol.* July 2019;30(4):220–228.
35. Ambrósio R Jr. Preoperative assessment for risk management in corneal refractive surgery. *Eur Ophthal Rev.* 2019;13(1):17–8. Published Online: September 27th 2019.
36. Refractive Errors & Refractive Surgery Preferred Practice Pattern®: Care Process, Management. *2017 by the American Academy of Ophthalmology.* Published by Elsevier Inc. https://doi.org/10.1016/j.ophtha.2017.10.003.
37. Jayanegara, W. Management of refractive surgery in refractive abnormalities. *Bali J Ophthalmol.* 2020;3(2):99–106.
38. D'Oria F, Abdelghany AA, Ledo N, et al. Incidence and reasons for intrastromal corneal ring segment explantation. *Am J Ophthalmol.* 2021; 222:351–358.

Chapter 8
PRIMARY CARE DIAGNOSIS, TREATMENT, AND MANAGEMENT OF GLAUCOMA

Chapter Outline

DOI: 10.1201/9781003255598-8

Section 1: Background and Diagnosis

Review of Clinical Anatomy[1,2]

1. Anterior angle and aqueous in glaucoma (see Chapter 6, for related angle anatomy)
   a. Aqueous humor dynamics
      i. Ciliary body (CB)
         - Made up of ciliary muscle, vasculature, and pigmented/non-pigmented epithelium
         - Both parasympathetic and sympathetic innervation
         - Site of aqueous production in ciliary processes within pars plicata
           - Site of uveoscleral (unconventional) outflow (not pressure dependent)
             i. Aqueous ⇒ supraciliary space ⇒ inner scleral surface ⇒ scleral (emissarial) canals of vortex vein
             ii. Accounts for 10–30% of outflow
           - Aqueous provides nutrients to avascular structures in anterior segment and transports waste
           - Iris inserts into anterior CB
           - Vasculature from major circle of iris
             i. Separates the posterior and anterior chambers
             ii. Angle formed by the iris and the cornea
         - Inflow
           - Aqueous from CB ⇒ posterior chamber ⇒ around lens through pupil to anterior chamber ⇒ circulation via convection currents
             i. Aqueous entering anterior to scleral spur exits out conventional path
             ii. Aqueous entering posterior to scleral spur exits out uveoscleral path
           - Circadian rhythm of flow (not well understood) with 1.5 to 4.5 μL/min flow rate
           - 50% reduction in production during sleep
      ii. Limbus
         - Transition zone between the cornea and the sclera
         - Outflow
           - Site of trabecular (conventional) outflow (pressure dependent)
           - Trabecular meshwork (TM) ⇒ Schlemm's canal ⇒ collector channels ⇒ episcleral and conjunctival veins
           - IOP must be greater than episcleral venous pressure
             i. Episcleral venous pressure around 8–10 mm Hg
             ii. Accounts for 70–90% of outflow
         - Scleral spur
           - Collagen fibers that form a projection into the AC where CB attaches
         - TM made up of three layers—uveal and corneoscleral meshworks, and juxtacanalicular connective tissue
           - Greatest resistance to outflow is juxtacanalicular tissue
         - Schlemm's canal
           - Tube 190 to 350 μm in diameter at base of the scleral sulcus that drains aqueous
         - Schwabe's line
           - Transition zone between TM and cornea endothelium
2. Optic Nerve (ON) Cranial Nerve II
   a. Structural and functional characteristics
      i. Made up of the axons of the retinal ganglion cells (RGC) from the retina that converge at the optic disc, travel along the rim, out through the lamina cribosa in an organized arcuate pattern
         - Distribution of retinal nerve fibers (see Figure 8.1)
           - Fibers from nasal half of the retina travel to nasal disc straight-on or arc superiorly and inferiorly
           - Fibers from the macula to temporal disc are the papillomacular bundle
           - Fibers from the temporal retina travel to the disc as superior and inferior arcuate fibers with the horizontal raphe in between

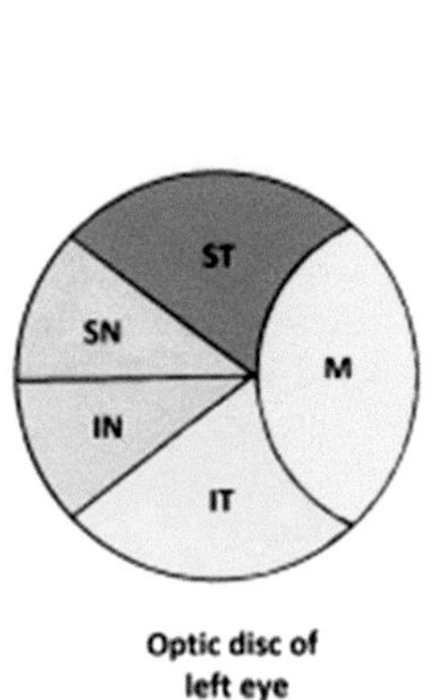

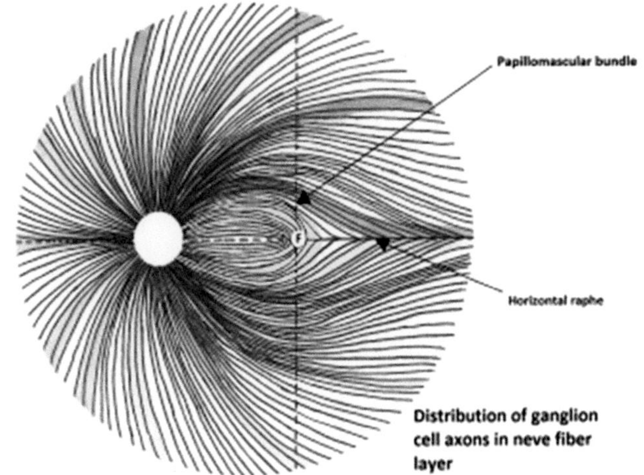

FIGURE 8.1 Organization of retinal ganglion cell axons. (*Source*: Reprinted from Danesh-Meyer HV, Yoon JJ, Lawlor M, Savino PJ. Visual Loss and Recovery in Chiasmal Compression. *Prog Retin Eye Res.* 2019;73:100765. November 2019. With permission from Elsevier.)

   ii. The right and left ON axon bundles unite forming the chiasm, where 50% of the axons cross to the contralateral side forming the optic tracts
   iii. The RGC axons in the optic tracts then synapse in the lateral geniculated nucleus where these neurons form the optic radiations and end by synapsing in the visual cortex
3. Optic Nerve Head (ONH) (see Figure 8.2)
   a. Extends from surface of retina to just posterior to lamina cribosa
      i. Depression in center of nerve = optic cup
         - Formed by axons turning to pass through the scleral foramen
         - Lighter color of cup due to visibility of lamina cribosa
         - Absence of retinal receptors at ONH causes a natural blind spot in visual field
      ii. Lamina cribosa
         - Inner surface of cup bottom (covers scleral foramen) made up of special connective tissue, elastic fibers, and astrocytes
         - Fenestrated (200–300 holes) where RGC axons and central retinal vein exit and central retinal artery enters
         - Barrier between inside of globe (higher pressure) and extra ocular cerebrospinal fluid space (lower pressure)
            – Abnormalities in this pressure gradient influence axoplasmic flow and retinal vein pressure
            – May contribute to thinning and backward bowing of lamina cribosa in glaucoma
         - Astrocytes provide connective tissue support
            – Least amount of support inferior and superior which is where glaucomatous changes often initially manifest
            – These axons correlate to arcuate and nasal visual fields (VF) where first sign of VF loss
   b. Disc and cup dimensions dependent on orientation, shape, and size of scleral foramen
      i. Large scleral foramen causes larger discs with corresponding cups
      ii. Oblique insertion yields tilted discs
      iii. Disc area 0.68 mm^2 to 4.42 mm^2 average 2.42 mm^2
      iv. Length average 1.5–2.0 mm
      v. These variabilities in disc/cup size and orientation must be considered when evaluating nerve for glaucoma
   c. Posterior ciliary arterioles are primary blood supply to ONH
      i. Gives neuro-retinal rim healthy orange/pink color
4. Visual pathway (see Figure 8.3)
   a. Retina
      i. 10 layers, each with distinct function (see above RGC for the purpose of this chapter)
      ii. Corresponding VF defect is central or peripheral in same eye as the abnormality
   b. Optic nerve
      i. VF loss from affected eye

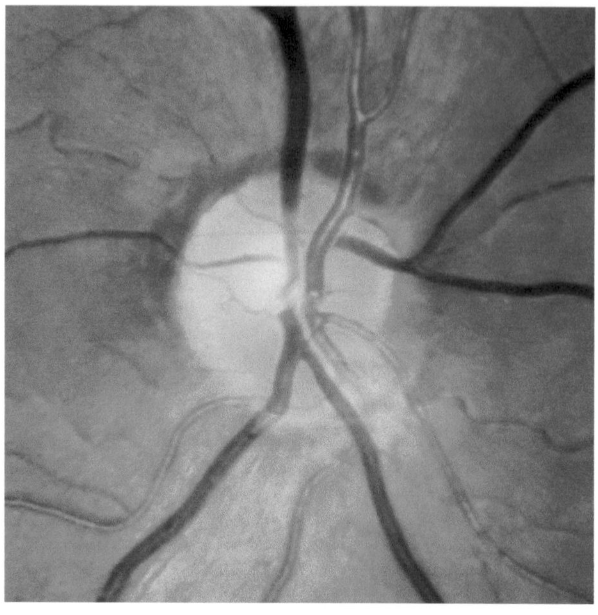

FIGURE 8.2 Normal appearing optic nerve.

         - E.g., right optic nerve lesion yields partial to total right eye blindness, but the left eye is unaffected
   c. Optic chiasm (behind and above pituitary stalk)
      i. Axons from the nasal half of each retina cross over to the contralateral optic tract
      ii. Axons from the temporal retina remain ipsilateral and cross over at the chiasm to join axons from the other eye on the opposite side of the brain
      iii. Bitemporal VF defect (partial to complete)
         - E.g., left eye cannot see left VF, right eye cannot see the right VF
         - Caution: defects here don't always give the textbook presentation and can be missed
   d. Optic tract (each hemisphere)
      i. Left-axons from the left temporal and the right nasal retina
      ii. Right-axons from the right temporal and the left nasal retina
      iii. Some axons leave tract and project to the pretectum to regulate pupil function
         - Ipsilateral nasal field loss with contralateral temporal field loss = homonymous VF defect (partial to complete)
            – E.g., right optic tract lesion results in a left-sided VF loss for each eye
      iv. Supplied by anterior choroidal and posterior communicating arteries
   e. Lateral geniculate nucleus
      i. Located in thalamus, contains six layers of neurons
         - Magnocellular deepest two layers
            – Motion, depth perception, and contrast sensitivity

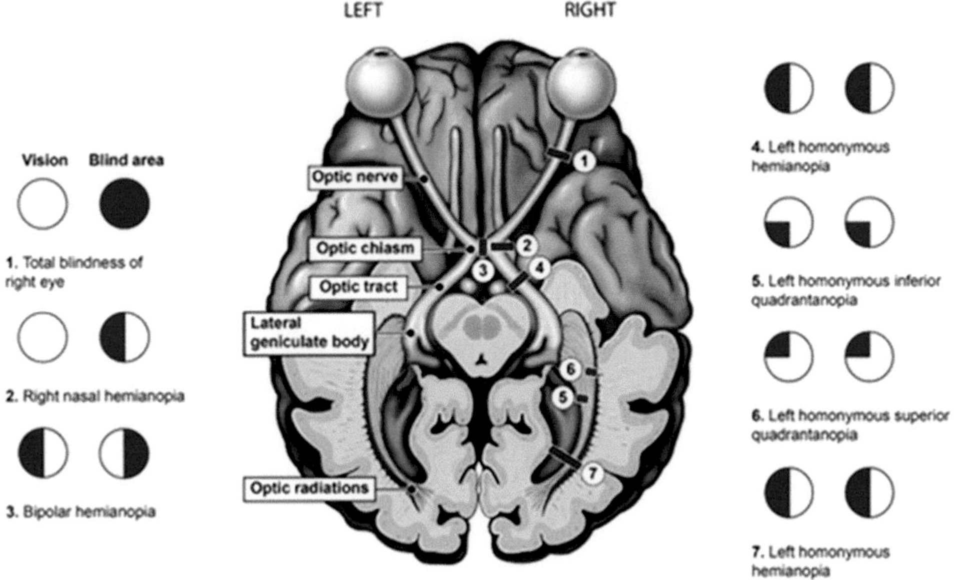

FIGURE 8.3 Illustration of the visual pathway and corresponding VF defects. (*Source*: Patel SC, Smith SM, Kessler AT, Bhatt AA. Imaging of the Primary Visual Pathway Based on Visual Deficits. *J Clin Imaging Sci* 2021;11:19. Copyright © 2021 Published by Scientific Scholar on behalf of *Journal of Clinical Imaging Science*.)

- Parvocellular upper four layers
  - Red/green color, fine spatial resolution
- Koniocellular: interspersed between M and P layers
  - Blue/yellow color

f. Optic radiations
   i. Divided into superior (dorsal) and inferior (Meyer's) loops
      - Meyer's loop = axons from inferior retina (superior VF) though temporal lobe
        - E.g., left temporal lobe lesion yields right homonymous superior quadranopsia (pie in the sky)
      - Dorsal loop = axons from superior retinal quadrants (inferior VF) through the parietal lobe
        - E.g., left parietal lobe lesion yields a right homonymous inferior quadranopsia (pie on the floor)

g. Visual cortex
   i. Located on both sides of calcarine sulcus of occipital lobe
   ii. VF deficits here yield contralateral homonymous hemianopsia with macular sparing
      - Central vision is often spared because of the double vascular supply from the middle and posterior cerebral artery

5. Pupillary reflex pathway (parasympathetic)
   a. RGCs ⇒ ON ⇒ chiasm ⇒ tract ⇒ splits off before the lateral geniculate nucleus to pretectal area of midbrain ⇒ projects bilaterally to Edinger–Westphal nucleus ⇒ CN III parasympathetic fibers ⇒ ciliary ganglion ⇒ sphincter pupillae
   b. Relative afferent pupillary defect (RAPD)
      i. Occurs if problem in retina or optic nerve anterior to chiasm
         - Most often indicates optic nerve disease

I. Current Concepts in Glaucoma

A. Background Information

1. Global incidence/prevalence (how much?)[3]
   a. 64.3 million people worldwide estimation
      i. Expected to 111.8 million by 2040
   b. Global prevalence 3.54%
      i. Primary open angle glaucoma (POAG) highest in Africa 4.2%
      ii. Primary angle closure glaucoma (PACG) highest in Asia 1.09%
2. United States incidence/prevalence
   a. Estimated 3.36 million by 2020 will have glaucoma with 50% unaware they have it[4]
   b. 1.9% in the United States[5]
3. Epidemiology and demography (who, when, and where?)[6]
   a. Race
      i. Black patients 6× more likely to develop POAG than white patients
         - Begins at an earlier age and more aggressive progression
         - Highest prevalence is in Nigeria
         - 3.4% prevalence in the United States[5]
      ii. Asians more likely to develop PACG
      iii. Hispanic or Latino ethnicity
         - 1.5% prevalence in the United States[5]
      iv. White patients 1.7% prevalence[5]
   b. Age
      i. Risk increases over 40 years old
   c. Sex
      i. Females > Males[5]
         - Only due to longer life expectancy of women, occurring at later age, otherwise no clear gender predilection[7]
         - Higher PACG in females compared to males
         - 2× higher incidence pigmentary glaucoma in men[8]

d. Genetics
   i. Family history[7]
      - 50% POAG patients have a positive family history
      - 9× greater risk of POAG if parents, sibling, or child with POAG
   ii. Changes or loss in the DNA sequences
      - Pseudoexfoliation glaucoma (PXF)
         – *LOXL1* with possible environmental factor[9]
      - Juvenile open angle glaucoma (JOAG)[10]
         – Mutations in *MYOC* coding for myocilin
         – 50% chance of inheriting the mutation (dominant inheritance)
      - Congenital glaucoma[11]
         – 2 gene mutations: *CYP1B1 LTBP2*
         – Autosomal recessive
e. Other risk factors[7]
   i. Myopia, hypotension, hypertension, trauma, obstructive sleep apnea, use of topical steroids, Pseudoexfoliation Syndrome (PXF), pigment dispersion syndrome (PDS), vasospasm (migraines, Raynaud's), and diabetes

4. Public health considerations
   a. Leading cause of blindness affecting quality of life
      i. 7.7 million worldwide have glaucoma induced moderate to severe vision loss[12]
   b. Challenges in blindness prevention/reduction[13]
      i. Underdiagnosed/advanced disease at time of diagnosis
      ii. Incorrect treatment/mismanagement (see "Treatment and Management" below)
         - Underestimation of severity of disease and rate of progression
         - Insufficient IOP lowering
         - Poor compliance and adherence
   c. Benefits of optometrists managing glaucoma patients
      i. Optometrists are primary eye care physicians medically trained to treat and manage glaucoma in the interest of public health
         - Access to optometrists greater than ophthalmologists
         - More cost-effective seeing optometrist as specialists often charge more than primary care providers
         - Intervention earlier in glaucoma continuum to thwart progression
         - Scope expansion increasing optometrist ability to manage glaucoma
            – Mild to moderate glaucoma managed therapeutically and with non-invasive laser procedures, in the wheelhouse of the profession of optometry
         - Reward and personal satisfaction in preventing vision loss over a patient's lifetime
            – Establish lifelong patient/doctor relationship
         - Growth of medical eye care practice allows optometrist to provide more professional services

B. Glaucomatous Process/Pathophysiology[14,15]

1. Progressive neurodegenerative disease resulting in retinal ganglion cell death (apoptosis) characterized by optic neuropathy and resultant VF loss
   a. Numerous contributing factors cause remodeling of the lamina cribrosa which causes disruption of axonal transport
      i. Nutrients must be delivered along the entire axon from the retina to the lateral geniculate body in the brain
      ii. Axonal transport is dependent on
         - Energy, oxygen, and glucose from normal blood flow
         - Disruption leads to ischemia, hypoxia, and RGC apoptosis
      iii. Historically glaucoma thought to be solely caused by elevated IOP >22 mm Hg [ocular hypertension (OHTN)], but many with OHTN do not develop glaucoma, and many with normal or low IOPs can have glaucomatous loss
         - Glaucoma can develop or progress at any IOP
         - Reduction of intraocular pressure is still the only proven method to halt or slow progression
         - Once apoptosis starts, neuronal damage continues even if causative agent controlled
            – The apoptotic environment is toxic to surrounding cells which causes apoptotic repetition for years
            – May explain why progression in some patients continues despite IOP lowering
   b. Contributory factors
      i. Elevated IOP/OHTN (>22 mm Hg)
         - Resistance in TM/conventional outflow pathway (see #2 below)
         - Thought to be principal factor in glaucomatous optic neuropathy
         - Elevated IOP, larger cups, and advancing age are associated with retinal vein occlusions[16]
      ii. Imbalance in translaminar pressure gradient between intracranial pressure (ICP) and IOP[17]
         - Average IOP = 16 mm Hg, average ICP = 12 mm Hg
            – Widening imbalance of this small pressure gradient from either elevation in IOP or decrease in ICP, could result in disruption of axonal transport ⇒ lamina cribrosa (LC) remodeling
         - Positional changes may also contribute to changes in translaminar pressure gradient[18,19]
      iii. Biomechanics/corneal hysteresis[20]
         - Hysteresis is a viscoelastic tissue property of ability of the cornea to absorb and dissipate energy
         - Cornea, sclera, and LC collagen formation are all derived from extracellular matrix coded by the same genes
         - A less rigid cornea (low hysteresis) could potentially have an LC that is less able to absorb IOP changes ⇒ remodeling of LC ⇒ excavation/cupping
            – Low corneal hysteresis is associated with visual field progression compared to CCT
            – Biomarker that has shown prediction of rate of progression as well as conversion to glaucoma
      iv. Central corneal thickness (CCT)
         - Thin CCT (<555 μm) 3× greater risk for progression to glaucoma in OHTN[21]

TABLE 8.1 **Differentiation of Glaucomatous versus Non-Glaucomatous Findings**

	Glaucoma	Non-Glaucoma
Age	Age >50 years	Age <50 years
Visual acuity	Slow loss—can have good central acuity until advanced	• Rapid decrease, worse than 20/40
Color vision loss	Only when advanced stage	Occurs early, rapid change
APD	Occurs if asymmetric or unilateral glaucoma	Always present
IOP	Can vary but more often >22 mm Hg	Within normal ranges <22 mm HG can mimick LTG
Visual field	Correlates to location and amount of rim loss—arcuate, nasal step, respects horizontal midline	Respects vertical midline but can be altitudinal if optic neuropathy like NAION
Optic nerve head	• Excavation of lamina • Vertical C/D ratio ≥ 0.6 • Cup asymmetry > 0.2 between eyes • Bayonetting or nasalization of vessels • Notching with focal rim loss	• Pallor in absence of cupping • Vessels centered in cup • Rim tissue present but pale—no longer pink

- Black patients have thinner CCT which can cause IOP to be underread by Goldmann tonometry[22]

v. Pro-inflammatory cytokines/oxidative stress[23]
- Glial production of tumor necrosis factor alpha (TNF-α) is a mediator for oxidative stress which leads to axonal disruption and neurodegeneration

vi. Autoimmune dysfunction[24]
- Elevated IOP allows T-cells that are pre-sensitized by exposure to commensal microbiota to pass through the blood–brain barrier into the retina where they initiate RGC degeneration

vii. Ocular perfusion pressure (OPP)/hemodynamics[25]
- Pressure where blood enters the eye
- Difference between blood pressure and IOP
- Elevated IOP causes mechanical compression that restricts blood flow and decreases perfusion
- Reduced ocular blood flow and insufficient autoregulation lead to ischemia and reperfusion damage RGC apoptosis
  - Ocular Perfusion Pressure = 2/3 [diastolic BP + 1/3(systolic BP – diastolic BP)] – IOP
  - OPP <56 mm HG is potential risk factor for glaucoma or progression[26]
- OPP is decreased if low BP, high IOP, or both
- Night IOP increases while diastolic BP decreases = lower OPP
  - Low BP is associated with development of NTG as well as progression[27]
  - BP meds should be taken in AM to avoid nocturnal dip in BP
  - Calcium channel blockers are associated with increased risk of glaucoma, especially amlodipine[28]

2. TM obstruction (see Section 1. a.)
   a. Outflow obstruction occurs due to increased stiffening and contraction of the juxtacanalicular tissue and inner wall of Schlemm's canal[29]
   b. Leads to elevated IOP which cascades into the glaucomatous processes described above
   c. Role of nitrous oxide[30]
      i. Important in rho kinase inhibition, which causes TM to relax, increasing permeability and outflow

TABLE 8.2 **Pneumonic for Remembering Non-Glaucomatous Optic Neuropathies (NIGHT TIC)**

Neuritis
Ischemic
Granulomatous
Hereditary
Toxic
Trauma
Irradiation
Compression

      ii. Decreased nitrous oxide activity in the TM, Schlemm's canal, and ciliary muscle have been found in patients with POAG which leads to TM stiffening

3. Normal (low) tension glaucoma (NTG/LTG)
   a. All above non-IOP contributing factors could help explain normal tension glaucoma
4. Differential diagnosis[31] (see Tables 8.1 and 8.2)
   a. Non-glaucomatous versus glaucomatous optic neuropathy
      i. Important to differentiate because other ON disorders can have similar findings to NTG
      ii. Neuroimaging indicated for associated non-glaucomatous findings
      iii. Non-glaucomatous mimickers
         - Anterior ischemic optic neuropathy (AION), hereditary optic neuropathy, compressive lesions, and demyelinating disease
         - Be careful! End-stage glaucoma can have pallor due to rim loss

II. Diagnosing Glaucoma

A. Standards of Care/Testing

1. Minimum testing to diagnose and treat glaucoma patients
   a. Best corrected visual acuity
   b. Pupillary reflexes
      i. Check for afferent pupillary defect (APD)
   c. Goldmann applanation is the gold standard of IOP acquisition in glaucoma and most accurate way to measure IOP[32]
      i. Non-contact tonometry is less accurate, and it should not be used when treating glaucoma

ii. Tonopen also is not as reliable as Goldmann but better than non-contact
    - May be better for astigmatism >3D, irregular corneas, or infection due to disposable latex covering
iii. Icare tonometer does not require anesthesia if patient allergic and has a disposable tip
    - Patient can self-check IOP at home
iv. Pascal dynamic contour tonometer – unaffected by CCT or biomechanics but IOP readings differ from Goldmann standards
v. Goldmann accuracy assumed CCT was constant at 520 μm[33]
    - IOP/CCT correction tables should not be used as there are other biomechanical influences
    - Just keep in mind that CCTs >600 μm may have IOPs that read higher than the real IOP and CCT <500 μm may read artificially lower than true IOP
vi. Must measure diurnal cure—AM and PM IOPs
vii. Accurate measuring important!
    - Instill right amount of dye
        - Too much dye makes thick mires causing the IOP reading to be overestimated
        - Too little dye makes thin mires causing the IOP reading to be underestimated
    - Make sure when sterilizing probe between patients, you allow it to dry so as not to cause corneal chemical burn
    - Patients should not be "squeezing" eyelids
    - Hold superior eyelid at brow and do not press on globe
    - Position patient so slit lamp is not pushing against chest or stomach
        - If overweight or also petite in stature, have patient sit at edge of exam chair, remove foot stool to drop knees
    - Tell patient to breathe and not hold breath—holding breath or straining can increase IOP
    - Calibrate probe every 6 months

d. Pachymetry
  i. Measure central corneal thickness (CCT) using ultrasound
    - Important to place pachymeter probe at the corneal apex where the cornea is the thinnest
  ii. One lifetime CCT measurement may not hold its accuracy if develops Fuchs' or has refractive surgery
    - Billable service usually one time

e. Evaluation of angle
  i. Van Herick
    - Gives rough initial estimate of angle but not equivalent or substitution of gonioscopy
    - Technique
        - Place slit-lamp beam at limbus approximately a 60° angle
        - Compare width of the corneal section to the width of the shadow adjacent to it
        - If same size, angle is open
        - If no shadow seen, angle is narrow
  ii. Gonioscopy
    - Definitive way to evaluate and visualize the angle
    - Uses mirrors to view angle indirectly
        - Goldmann 3-mirror lens, Zeiss 4-mirror lens
        - 4-mirror technique is preferred so angle is not inadvertently opened due to suctioning of 3-mirror to cornea
    - Technique
        - Anesthetize eye topically and set slit lamp at 10–25× magnification using short narrow vertical beam
        - Place 4 mirror squarely on corneal surface, taking care not to indent
        - Due to mirror use, remember that the angle that is viewed is 180° away from the mirror that is being used—looking through nasal mirror views temporal angle
        - Challenging to learn this but you must be able to evaluate the angle to know which type of glaucoma you are dealing with because treatments are different
        - You must gonio any patient suspicious for glaucoma
    - Good way to practice is to gonio four contact lens (CL) patients a day for 2 weeks
        - These patients hold their eyes open better and are used to having something on their cornea
    - You will see a lot of normal angles because many CL patients are myopes so you can recognize abnormal angles easier
  iii. Gonioscopically Normal Angle (see Figure 8.4)
    - Inferior angle is widest and most pigmented
    - Widest to narrowest structure visible: iris, ciliary body (CB), scleral spur (SS), nonpigmented and pigmented trabecular meshwork (TM), and Schwalbe's line (SL)
        - Use mnemonic "**I C**an **S**ee **T**he **L**ine" to remember widest to narrowest structures seen **Iris** ⇒ **CB** ⇒ **SS** ⇒ **TM** ⇒ **SL**
    - Iris
        - Contour should be regular and fairly flat
    - CB
        - Darkest taupe-colored band between the scleral spur and iris root
    - SS
        - Internal extension of the sclera
        - Appears as white stripe between CB and TM
    - TM
        - Pigmentation variation can be normal finding but uniform in appearance

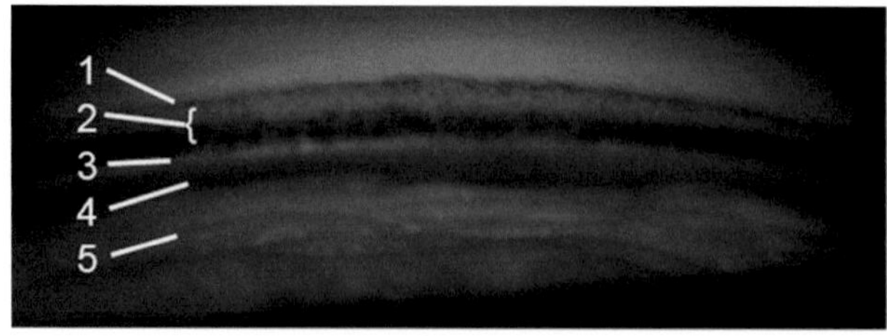

FIGURE 8.4 Gonioscopic view of the angle. (*Source*: By Snoop—Own work, CC BY-SA 3.0 de, https://commons.wikimedia.org/w/index.php?curid=32169453.)

- Anterior non-pigmented and posterior pigmented portions
- Pigmented TM is where filtration occurs to Schlemm's canal

• SL
- Peripheral termination of Descemet's membrane
- If prominent, called posterior embryotoxon

• Iris Processes
- Iris projections that extend from iris to CB or SS
- Found in 35% of normal eyes[34]
- Also associated with Axenfeld–Rieger syndrome

f. Gonioscopic grading of the angle
   i. Three grading systems: Scheie, Shaffer, and Spaeth
      • These systems help clinicians evaluate angle for openness and risk of closure utilizing structures seen/not seen, the degree of angle width, amount of angle pigment, synechiae, indentation, and iris insertion/contour
      • Over the years, I combined the best pearls from all three systems relying most on Schaffer system when grading
         - Evaluating for peripheral anterior synechiae, pigment, iris contour, and indentation if narrow (see Table 8.3 and Figure 8.5)

TABLE 8.3 Muckley's Gonioscopy Grading System

Structure Seen	Degree Open	Grade	Closure Risk
Iris/CB	35°–45°	4	Improbable
SS	25°–35°	3	Improbable
TM	15°–25°	2	Possible
SL	0°–15°	1	Highly probable/closed

Notes: Iris Contour: Flat, Convex, Concave, Plateau.
Grade Pigment: Grade 0 (lightest) to 4 (darkest).
Note presence of peripheral anterior synechiae (PAS).
Note structure seen in parenthesis if indentation performed.

FIGURE 8.5 Muckley's documentation of angle structures seen in gonioscopy.

g. Schaffer (system): based on angular width between cornea and iris
   i. Grade 4: 35–45° closure improbable
   ii. Grade 3: 20–35° closure improbable
   iii. Grade 2: 10–20° closure possible
   iv. Grade 1: <10° closure probable
   v. Slit: shallow some areas closed
   vi. Grade 0: 0° closed 360°

h. Biomicroscopy
   i. Evaluate all structures/layers of anterior segment carefully looking for glaucoma-related abnormalities such as pseudoexfoliation (PXF), pigmentary dispersion syndrome (PDS), trauma, and other iris and lens abnormalities such as heterochromia, iris strands/hypoplasia with posterior embryotoxon (Axenfeld–Rieger), neovascularization, mature cataract, or lens dislocation

i. Fundus exam (see Figure 8.6)
   i. Critically evaluate the disc (see Section B. 5., "Analysis and Abnormalities")
      • Look at overall size of disc: is it small, average, large, or anomalous?
      • Slit-lamp estimation of disc size
         - Using vertical light scale on slit lamp, measure the disc size in mm
         - Multiply that measurement by the corrective value below
         - Volk 66D has no corrective value
         - Volk 78D × 1.11 (mm)
         - Volk 90D and Super field × 1.33 (mm)
         - High myopia, fundus lenses underestimate, and hyperopia leads to an overestimation
      • Look at the rim—**most important area to look at!**
         - Rim width is the distance between the border of disc and the position of blood vessel bending
         - Healthy pink or pallor?
         - Any focal areas of rim loss (notching)

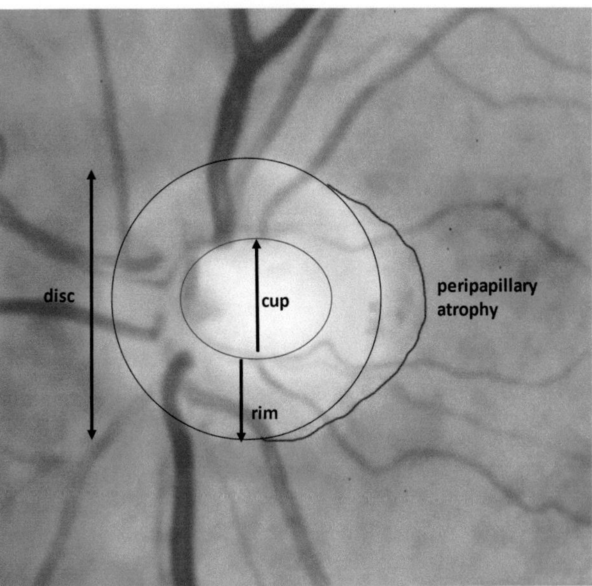

FIGURE 8.6 Evaluation of the optic nerve for glaucoma.

- Thinning especially inferior or superior?
- Hemorrhage? Drance?
- Assess cup
  - High individual variability
  - Should not enlarge over time unless glaucomatous process
  - Larger horizontally than vertically, (opposite of the disc)
  - Size of cup is function of disc size and width of rim
  - Whether cups are big or little has no importance if you have healthy rim tissue
- Document any peripapillary atrophy (PPA)
  - Beta zone: central PPA closest to nerve were atrophy of retinal pigment epithelium: possibly suggestive glaucoma
  - Alpha zone: located peripheral to beta zone away from the nerve where retinal pigmented epithelium is hyper- or hypopigmented: more common in normal eyes

ii. Evaluate retinal nerve fiber layer (RNFL)
- Very challenging to see
  - Try using red-free filter
  - Look at the borders of the blood vessels: if sharp, then there is less NFL overlying them

j. Disc documentation

i. Photography
- Helpful in diagnosing and evaluating for progression
  - New baselines need established when advanced imaging technology evolves
  - Photography technology remains stable over years and photos can easily be compared
  - Photos can show notching, pallor, Drance hemes, PPA better than advanced imaging techniques
  - Can utilize stereo or non-stereo photography
  - Less expensive than advanced imaging machines

ii. Documentation in record
- Disc size
  - Large/average/small is sufficient
- Cup to disc ratio
- Rim findings
- Note PPA and RNFL abnormalities

k. Visual field (VF) testing using automated static perimetry[35]

i. Measures visual function

ii. VF testing is most precise method for quantifying progression
- Measures sensitivity of hill of vision using standardized threshold testing algorithms
- Every point in the VF has a visual threshold
- Testing looks for the weakest stimulus just visible compared to age-matched norms

iii. Normal boundaries
- 60° superior, 70° inferior, 90° temporal, 60° nasal
- Point of fixation in center of hill has highest sensitivity
  - Dim stimulus visible = low threshold
- decreases rapidly in the 10 degrees around fixation
  - Peripheral regions have low sensitivity
- Most retinal ganglion cells located within 30° of fixation
  - So, as you go out from fixation, need a bright stimulus = high threshold
- Height of hill affected by age, ambient light, stimulus size, and duration
- Measuring light intensity in units
  - 10,000 apotilbs (asb) is brightest illumination the Humphrey VF analyzer projects
  - Decibels (db) is a logmar relationship with apostilbs
  - 1 db = 1/10 log attenuation of maximum stimulus (see Table 8.4)

iv. Types of automated perimetry
- Humphrey visual field (HVF) is the recommended perimeter for diagnosis and evaluation of glaucoma
  - Although other perimeters are useful, within the glaucoma community, the HVF remains the gold standard

v. HVF testing algorithms
- VF testing is either threshold or suprathreshold algorithms
- Threshold
  - The brightness of a stimulus at which it can be detected on 50% of the occasions it is presented
  - Staircase strategy that changes light in increments of 4 dB until light is not seen, then increases light by 2 dB until it is seen again
  - Goal is to measure differential light sensitivity at each location
- Suprathreshold
  - An intensity of pre-determined age-matched stimuli is tested at each point
  - Enables quicker testing, but detects only gross defects so used primarily in screening

vi. HVF threshold testing strategies
- Full threshold 30–2 (10 mins)
  - Gold standard but longest test (76 points in central 30° tested 6° apart)
  - Edge point often depressed
  - Use this test for suspected non-glaucomatous/neurology pathology such as stroke, multiple sclerosis, arteritic/non-arteritic ischemic optic neuropathy, and pituitary tumor
  - Approximately 18–20-min test time per eye in real life
  - If young and normal VF, then time reduced to 10 mins
- Full threshold 24–2 (3–7 min)
  - 54-point subset of those points in 30–2 with less testing time but may not pick up progression as quickly with fewer points tested

TABLE 8.4 Relationship of Apostilbs to Decibels in Automated Perimetry

Relationship of Decibels (dB) to Apostilbs (asb)		
0 dB =	10,000 asb	Brightest
10 dB =	1000 asb	
20 dB =	100 asb	↓
30 dB =	10 asb	
40 dB =	1 asb	Dimmest

vii. SITA standard Swedish interactive threshold algorithm
- Gathers same info as full threshold but faster because it tests closer to the expected threshold
- Uses knowledge of how different points influence the outcome of other points
- Due to quicker testing with good repeatability, SITA Standard 24–2 is the recommended testing strategy for glaucoma
  - Only veer from this testing strategy when necessary
- Sita Fast or Sita Faster not standard in glaucoma but can be utilized if Sita Standard unreliable due to patient fatigue
  - Many practitioners do routinely substitute Sita Fast in glaucoma management

viii. Stimulus
- Decibel value Humphrey perimeter (see Table 8.4)
  - 0 dB = maximum brightest perimeter produces (10,000 apostilbs)
  - 51 dB is dimmest (.08 apostilbs)
  - 40 dB is the dimmest most normal, young patients can see
  - When maximum intensity of light of 10,000 apostilbs is not perceived, it is labeled as 0 dB retinal sensitivity (absolute scotoma)
- HVF has I–V stimuli
  - Size III white stimulus (0.43°) with duration of 0.2 sec is standard and used in patients with good visual acuity
  - In cases of decreased visual acuity, a size V maximum stimulus is used
  - I, II, and IV rarely used

ix. Pupil size and refractive error in HVF testing
- Pupil size needs to be consistent when comparing across tests
- Pupils <2 mm and >6 mm may cause artifacts
- Stick with either all dilated or all non-dilated VFs but administer dilated if the pupil size is <3 mm
- Correct refractive error
  - Myopia, hyperopia, and presbyopia
  - Astigmatism over 2D, otherwise use spherical equivalent
- Watch trial frame rings
  - Place trial lens as close to eye as possible without touching lashes
  - Aphakes/high myopes should wear a contact lens instead of using trial lens to minimize trial frame ring

x. STATPAC analysis package
- Software statistical analysis package available in full threshold 24–2 or 30–2 test and SITA to help interpret data
- Database is average of second and third VFs for age-adjusted *normal* patients
- Features glaucoma hemifield and change probability indices
- STATPAC single field analysis (SFA)
  - Compares results of single threshold test with age-related normative data to show abnormalities (this is the printout at conclusion of testing)
- Guided progression analysis (GPA)
  - Compares the changes between the baseline and follow-up tests (also available printout at conclusion of testing)
  - Developed for use in Early Manifest Glaucoma Trial study
  - Uses VF test-taking data collected in 16 trial centers to establish a normal rate of test-to-test variability between VFs
  - Only SITA tests may be chosen initially for GPA analysis
  - You may mix any combination of SITA-Standard, SITA-Fast or SITA-Faster tests to create a GPA analysis
  - Newer Humphrey models will automatically choose the two oldest compatible tests to be the baseline
  - Tests displaying high false positives ≥15% are excluded by default from GPA analysis
  - Possible progression: if same three test points are abnormal compared to a normative database on two consecutive VFs
  - Probable/likely progression: if same three test points are abnormal on three consecutive examinations
  - GPA saves time by simplifying results
  - Use it as another tool in identification of progression: clinically correlate all findings
- Review your baseline exam choices and change when any of the following occur
  - Significant change in course of therapy
  - Ocular surgery or significant trauma to the eye
  - Learning curve effects suspected or retrospectively identified

xi. Proper administration of test for optimum reliability
- Provide positive and clear standardized step-by-step instructions
- Position patient so comfortable and aligned with forehead against rest
- Test right eye first but consider altering which eye is tested first on subsequent tests in cases of poor second eye reliability due to fatigue/exhaustion
- Tell patient they can pause the test should they need to rest by pressing and holding the button on the clicker

- Operator should watch for
  - Fixation and proper plotting of blind spot
  - Patient backing away from forehead rest
  - Droopy upper eyelid blocking superior VF: tape lids up

xii. Tips and pearls
- Should not mix a 24–2 and 30–2
  - Higher sensitivities are found with the shorter test and you can't compare them
  - Keep testing strategy and type the same to ensure reproducibility
- Shorter test may look better and there may be a 1–2 dB change
- Standard 24–2 is not useful for monitoring visual field near fixation
- Remember for GPA to be effective re-baseline a patient when *any* new or change in treatment has been initiated
- VF testing is subjective
  - Dependent on the co-operation and responses of the patient as well as the skill of the test giver
  - Poor reliability is common due to patient's poor comprehension of test or poor response reflex
  - Dry eye can negatively affect performance: manage the ocular surface aggressively, especially if on numerous topical glaucoma medications

1. Advanced imaging instruments

i. Background
- Detects structural loss of RNFL
  - Typically occurs prior to the development of functional loss of VF[36]
  - In advanced disease, VF functional changes are more obvious
- High-speed Fourier-domain ocular coherence tomography (OCT) has higher diagnostic accuracy and reproducibility than other quantitative imaging technologies[37]
- Artifacts, anatomical factors, operator error, poor image capture can affect reliability of RNFL thickness measurements in all instruments
- Advanced imaging is most useful in detecting and monitoring RNFL loss in early to moderate disease

ii. Ocular coherence tomography (OCT)
- Provides thickness measurements of retinal nerve fiber layer (RNFL) and detail of retinal layers using low-coherence interferometry to obtain cross-sectional images
  - Imaging can aid in earlier detection before enough axons are damaged enough to be seen on perimetry (i.e., functional vision loss)
  - Used also to evaluate for disease progression
  - 5 μm resolution
  - Commonly used devices: Cirrus HD-OCT (Carl Zeiss Meditec; Dublin, CA), Spectralis (Heidelberg Engineering; Heidelberg, Germany), and RTVue-100 (Optovue; Fremont, CA)
- Each tomographer has different glaucoma scan patterns, software algorithms, and print outs interpretations comparing to a normative database
  - Cannot compare scans from different tomographers to each other: not interchangeable
- Useful in differentiating glaucoma suspects from physiologic cupping or other normal glaucoma mimickers
- RNFL thickness measured in a 3.5 mm-diameter, circular, cross-section centered at the ONH
  - Creates a TSNIT map (displays patient's RNFL measurement in clock hours along the calculation circle centered on ONH compared to normative data: temporal, superior, nasal, inferior, temporal)
- Tips and pearls
  - Make sure scan is high quality with good reliability parameters such as patient fixation, image clarity and that your patient's age is within the normative database
  - Scan both the RNFL and macula for glaucoma
  - Take multiple scans at a time to get the most reliable
  - You can take two of these scans and use as a baseline to trigger guided progression analysis (GPA) at follow-up testing
  - Remember RNFL thins with aging at a slower rate than thinning due to glaucoma

iii. Older testing technology
- Confocal scanning laser ophthalmoscopy (HRT)
  - Evaluates changes in the topography of the ON and surrounding RNFL
- Scanning laser polarimetry (GDx)
  - Evaluates RNFL using confocal scanning laser ophthalmoscope measuring the change in polarization of light as it doubly passes through the birefringent RNFL

2. Useful additional testing

a. 10–2 HVF full threshold

i. 24–2 test grid may miss damage to central VF due to the 6° separation between test points and only 12 points tested in central 10°
- 50% or more of total RGCs are contained within 16° of the foveal center represent 7.3% of the total retina[38]
- 10–2 tests 68 points in central 10° with points 2° apart

ii. Macular involvement may occur earlier than previously thought in glaucoma
- Comma-shaped defects can appear in the macular region—in early POAG not seen on 24–2

iii. Clinicians now incorporating both 24–2 and 10–2 in glaucoma VF testing

iv. Preferred test for end-stage glaucoma to monitor central vision

v. 10–2 under-used in *all* stages of glaucoma

b. HVF short-wavelength-automated perimetry (SWAP)

i. Uses size V blue stimulus on yellow background
- Background reduces sensitivities of the green and red cones

- Isolates the short-wavelength-sensitive blue cones
  - Tests koniocellular ganglion cells
  - By testing fewer cells less overlap in tested ganglion cell-receptive fields which reveals defects earlier
  - Defects found with SWAP often appear larger and deeper than with standard automated perimetry (SAP)
  - SWAP may identify VF defects 5 years earlier than SAP[39]
- Test can take 12–14 minutes per eye
- Difficult if cataracts—filter out blue light
- Higher inter-test variability than SAP

c. Corneal hysteresis (CH) (see Section I. B. b. iii.)
   i. Ocular response analyzer
   - Accounts for corneal biomechanics
   - Bi-directional non-contact applanation pneumotonometry
   - Normal CH value is around 10 mm Hg[40]
   - Combination of a low CH and a high IOP is predictive of VF loss
   - Repeat CH after any change in glaucoma therapy

d. OCT angiography
   i. Tracks movement in vasculature to indirectly evaluate blood flow of ONH and retina
   ii. Glaucoma findings
   - Decreased vessel density and flow in the peripapillary and macular area
   - Loss of choriocapillaris with PPA

e. Stereo disc photos
   i. Useful tool to monitor progression from baseline
   ii. Gives more dimensional detail for real time comparison purposes

f. Anterior segment OCT
   i. Uses longer wavelength light to obtain images of the anterior segment
   ii. Evaluates angle structure with no pressure on globe
   - Precisely measures angle opening distance, angle recess area, and the trabecula-iris space
   - Also used to evaluate results of iridotomy and trabeculectomy

g. Electrophysiology
   i. May be able to detect changes 8 years earlier than RNFL and VF loss[41]
   ii. Independent of patient response (totally objective) and compared to normative database
   iii. Can be used as a tiebreaker when other tests are borderline and inconclusive
   iv. Does not differentiate glaucoma from other ON/retinal diseases
   v. Visual evoked potential (VEP)
   - Amplitude of signals that measure function of visual pathway from the cornea to the visual cortex
     - Measure of "how much" information is getting to visual cortex: strength and speed of signal
     - Normal amplitude is above 6 μV
     - Normal speed is between 95 ms and 117 ms
   vi. Pattern electroretinogram (ERG)
   - Test's function (strength and speed) specifically of retinal ganglion cells

B. Analysis and Abnormalities (See Table 8.5)

1. IOP
   a. Elevated IOP >22 mm Hg is risk factor for POAG (see Section I. B. b. i.)
   b. Important to understand that many with ocular hypertension (OHTN) do not develop glaucoma and some with IOPs <22 mm Hg get glaucoma
2. Pachymetry (see Section I. B. b. iv.)
3. Gonioscopy
   a. Will have normal angle in most glaucoma patients
   b. Must differentiate between "open" and "narrow" angles (see Figure 8.7)
      i. Occludable angle: refer for laser iridotomy
      - If Schwalbe's line seen in two quadrants
      - If the angle width is less than 20°
      - If trabecular meshwork seen in all quadrants, monitor every 6–12 months

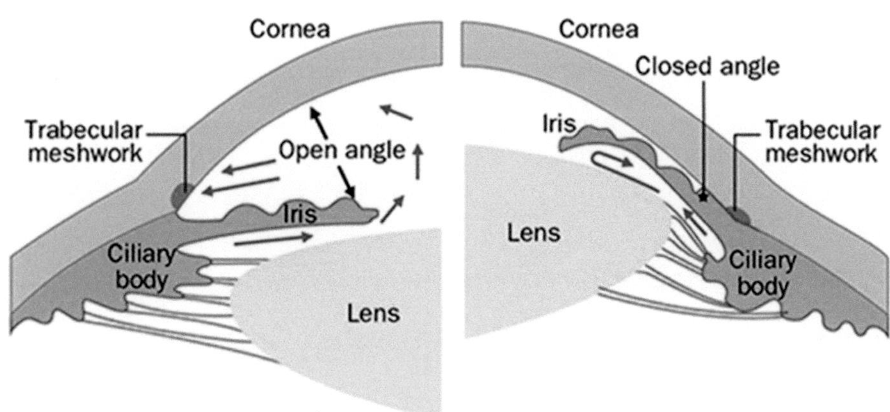

FIGURE 8.7 Schematic diagram of the ocular anterior segment in open-angle and closed-angle glaucoma. (*Source*: Janey L. Wiggs, Louis R. Pasquale, Genetics of glaucoma, Human Molecular Genetics, Volume 26, Issue R1, 01 August 2017, Pages R21–R27 by permission of Oxford University Press.)

c. Dense pigmentation
   i. Suggestive of pigment dispersion or pseudoexfoliation but consider trauma, melanoma, and hyphema
   ii. Non-uniform pigmentation seen especially superior angle
   iii. Sampolesi line
      - Highly pigmented Schwalbe's line
d. Angle recession
   i. Widening of the ciliary body
e. Peripheral anterior synechiae (PAS)
   i. Iris adhesion into TM (tent-like projection of iris to cornea)
   ii. Suggestive of past angle occlusion especially if superior
   iii. Can also suggest inflammatory glaucoma especially if inferior
   iv. Laser trabeculoplasty can also yield focal PAS
f. Neovascularization
   i. Abnormal blood vessel growth due to ischemia
      - Vessels cross scleral spur into TM instead of appearing radial
g. Peripheral roll or iris double hump
   i. Suggestive of plateau iris

4. Anterior segment (see Section II. A. 1. h.)
   a. Cornea: vertical pigment line on endothelium (Krukenberg's spindle), pseudoexfoliation (PXF) material on endothelium, posterior embryotoxon, edema
   b. Iris: PXF material on pupil border, transillumination defects, iris tears (iridodialysis), heterochromia, iris strands/hypoplasia, neovascularization
   c. Lens: PXF material on anterior capsule, pigment on lens zonules (Scheie's line), mature cataract, lens dislocation
5. Disc appearance—critical evaluation of disc (see Figure 8.8)
   a. Cup to disc ratio
      i. Size of optic disc and the size of cup are interrelated
         - Normal, large disc will have a large cup
         - Normal, small disc will have a small cup
      ii. Some large cups within big-sized discs tend to be mistaken as abnormal
      iii. Likewise, small cups in small discs may be wrongly considered normal
         - Large cup in a large disc can be normal but an average cup in a small nerve suggests glaucoma
      iv. Clinicians tend to under-diagnose glaucoma in patients with small discs and over-diagnose patients with large discs
      v. In my clinical experience:
         - C/D ratio <0.45 usually normal unless the patient has small optic disc (which then requires further testing)
         - C/D ratio between 0.5 and 0.8 can be normal (physiologic cupping if large disc), a glaucoma suspect or early to moderate glaucoma
         - C/D ratio ≥0.8 glaucomatous unless proven normal with testing
      vi. Cupping normally symmetrical between eyes
         - C/D ratio difference of 1.5–2.0 cup sizes between eyes should be considered a risk factor unless the overall disc size is also asymmetric (e.g., OD 0.4 C/D ratio and OS 0.6 C/D ratio with same size overall discs)
      vii. Framingham eye study glaucoma benchmarks[42]
         - CD >.6 cup only occurs in 3% normal population
         - Asymmetry >2 cup sizes only occurs in 6% normal population
   b. Rim
      i. *ISNT* rule in glaucomatous atrophy[43]
         - Thickest portion of rim is *I*nferior followed by *S*uperior, *N*asal, and *T*emporal quadrants in normal nerve
         - Deviation from this is an alert to glaucoma
         - Eventually, rim is lost in all sectors of optic disc
         - Independent of optic disc size
         - This rim loss is what gives the appearance of vertical elongation of cup
      ii. Notching (area of focalized thinning of rim)
         - Tends to be inferior temporal or superior temporal
         - May be associated with peri-papillary atrophy

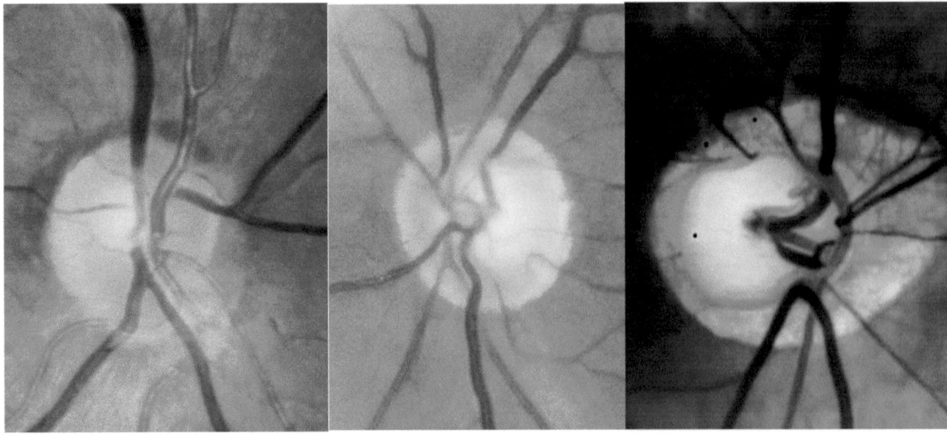

FIGURE 8.8 Normal and glaucomatous optic nerves.

- Becomes full-thickness notch with complete absence of rim
- Progression will cause this area to enlarge
- Notches will usually correspond to specific visual field defects and defects in RNFL

iii. Bayonetting of blood vessels
- Bend in vessel where vessels shift from a vertical orientation along the cup wall to a horizontal orientation on the retinal surface
- Change in the position of that bend is an indicator of disc change

iv. Nasalization of blood vessels
- Normal nerve vessels pass through cup center and travel initially down the central portion of the optic nerve
- Glaucoma damage causes cup enlargement: vessels, pushed aside and follow the receding nasal wall of the cup

v. Disc hemorrhage[44,45] (see Figure 8.9)
- Usually flame or splinter shaped located at edge of disc (Drance heme)
  - Shape due to axon orientation of the axons in RNFL
- Inferior location most common followed by superior
- Disappear in 6–10 weeks so may miss them occurring in time between exams
  - Important to always look at disc at every visit for glaucoma suspects or diagnosed patients whether dilated or not
- Current OCT technology can't image disc hemorrhage
- Independent predictive factor for the development of POAG in OHTN and NTG
- Rule out other sources for disc heme: posterior vitreous detachment, hypertension or diabetic retinopathy, retinal vascular disease, and non-arteritic anterior ischemic optic neuropathy (NAION)
- Maybe due to biomechanical forces on the lamina cribrosa as well as vascular component
- Occurs more in NTG than OHTN, prevalence
  - 0% to 0.4% in normal eyes
  - 0.4% to 10% in OHTN
  - 4.2% to 17.6% in eyes high IOPs
  - 20.5% to 33.3% in NTG
- Tend to occur earlier in glaucoma than later and may precede RNFL thinning
- Risk factor for glaucomatous progression in already established glaucoma
- Presence of disc heme is a risk factor but not indicative of glaucoma
  - May tip the scale if occurs in a suspect with other risks factors

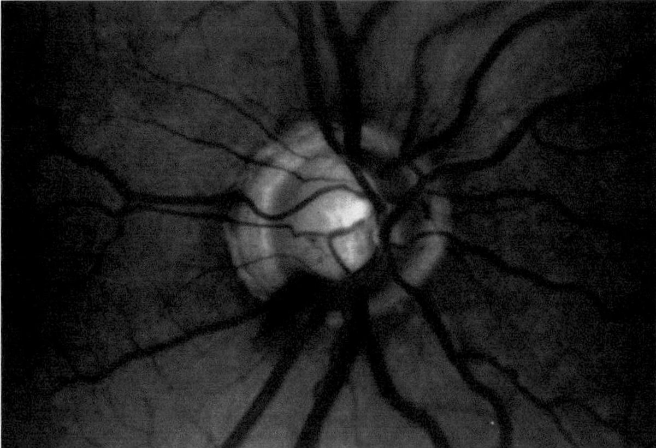

FIGURE 8.9 Drance hemorrhage with bayonetting of blood vessels. (*Source*: Photo by courtesy Tom S. K. Chi, M.D.)

6. Peripapillary atrophy (PPA)
   a. PPA relates to insufficient or impaired choriocapillaris circulation to the ONH
   b. As RPE loses nourishment, it becomes atrophic
   c. Area where PPA is widest corresponds to area with thinnest neuroretinal rim
   d. Beta zone associated with thinning and progression (area adjacent to disc)
7. RNFL
   a. NFL defect is a sign of pathology but not specific for glaucoma
      i. Need to correlate it to other risk factors
   b. Commonly see wedge defect
   c. Look for bright striations which represent healthy RNFL
      i. If RNFL loss is present, the bright striations of the background disappear
   d. Dark areas represent RNFL dropout
8. Unique/anomalous discs
   a. Represent a challenge in identifying glaucomatous change and must differentiate
   b. **I have seen many of these disc anomalies misdiagnosed as glaucoma in my career…I also have seen many cases of undiagnosed glaucoma**
      i. High myopic disc
         - Optic nerve head is more oval than normal with long vertical axis
         - Extensive peripapillary atrophy and white scleral crescent
         - Large cup but respects ISNT rule
         - RPE appears to be thinned and choroid vessels seen
         - Can develop staphyloma
           - Ectatic thinning and bulging of the wall of the globe

      ii. Tilted nerves
         - ON exits sclera at oblique angle (not at typical 90°)
         - Usually bilateral
         - Oval-shaped nerve with raised superior/temporal side and flat inferior/nasal side
         - Usually thinning of RPE inferior nasal quadrant
           - Will show up as abnormal on OCT
         - Unchanging with possible VF defect—superior temporal corresponding to inferior nasal conus

      iii. Optic pit
         - Can be congenital or acquired
         - Round/oval grey or white depression in the optic disc
         - Most common temporal

- Associated with visual field loss and serous sensory detachment of the macula
- If acquired
  - Classic sign of glaucoma damage
  - Focal loss of neural tissue associated with pronounced excavation
  - Loss of normal architecture of lamina cribrosa that resembles a pit
  - Extreme pallor of the affected area, in contrast to other areas
  - More prevalent in normal tension glaucoma

iv. Disc drusen
- Scalloped appearance at disc margin with little cup
- Retained calcified hyaline bodies/axoplasmic waste
- Early in childhood may appear more elevated and crowded
  - As ages, drusen calcify, autofluorescence
- Vessels not obscured, no hyperemia (differentiate from edema)
- Drusen can compress nerve fibers and the vascular supply
  - Visual field defects—enlargement of blind spot and NFL bundle defects
  - Vascular occlusion (NAION, CRAO)
  - Choroidal neovascular net (CNV)
- Over time VF loss can occur
- No proven treatment to treat ONH drusen
- If progressive VF loss occurs, lower IOP
- May be difficult to distinguish optic nerve drusen from progressing glaucoma as the cause

v. Macro disc
- Enlarged disc with a large physiologic cup
  - May occur unilaterally or bilaterally (>2.5 mm^2)
- May appear pale due to larger disc diameter allowing axons to be more spread out
- Anomalous multiple retinal vessels branching

vi. Hypoplastic disc
- Abnormally small nerve due to low axons
- Surrounded by a PPA halo
- Associated with
  - Endocrine disorders
  - Gestational diabetes
  - Maternal drug use
  - Fetal alcohol syndrome
  - Rubella or syphilis

vii. Morning glory disc
- Congenital funnel-shaped excavated disc that resembles a morning glory flower
  - Central glial tissue w/PPA
- Vessels at disc abnormally straighten out
- Unilateral, female > male, unknown pathogenesis
  - Possible variant coloboma or mesenchymal abnormality

c. What about imaging unique discs
  i. HRT/OCT/GDx are complementary tools that help aid our clinical assessment
  ii. Diagnostic and management decisions should be made by considering all findings
  iii. Imaging may not be useful on unique nerves
  iv. Not reflected in normative database
  - **Unique nerves will always give you an abnormal OCT/HRT/GDx!**
  - Can use as a baseline
  - Only useful in looking for change over time

9. Interpretation of the VF
  a. VF defects are not limited to glaucoma and keep in mind the visual pathway (see section on "Visual Pathway Anatomy")
  b. 25–40% of retinal nerve fibers in a region need to be damaged before corresponding scotoma is detected[46]
  c. Non-glaucomatous VF findings
    i. Sign of damage anywhere in the visual system from retina to visual cortex
    ii. General overall depression suggests preretinal cause (cataracts)
    iii. Unilateral prechiasmal defects can resemble glaucoma but can be due to many other causes
    iv. Bitemporal VF defects suggest chiasmal lesion
    v. VF that respects the vertical midline are usually post-chiasmal
    - Homonymous hemianopia due to lesions in optic tract to the visual cortex
  d. Glaucomatous VF patterns (see Figure 8.10)
    i. Hallmark glaucomatous defect is a nerve fiber bundle defect due to corresponding damage at the optic nerve head
    - Follows distribution of retinal fibers (see "Review of Clinical Anatomy," 2. a. i. and Figure 8.1)
    - Superior and inferior optic nerve head most susceptible to glaucomatous damage
    ii. Rarely are glaucoma defects outside 30°
    iii. Typical glaucomatous VF defects
    - Nasal step
      - Most common early defect and easily missed
      - Progresses to arcuate defect in later stages
    - Bjerrum or arcuate defect
      - Most common pattern and occurs in the area 10–20° from fixation
      - Arches from the blind spot (optic disc) and ends at the nasal raphe
    - Paracentral scotoma
      - Located closer to fixation when they occur in the superior hemifield
    - Altitudinal defect
      - Severe VF defect that respects the horizontal meridian
      - Usually due to retina or ON
      - Glaucoma is a common cause but there are other conditions that cause similar VF patterns (excludes non-arteritic ischemic optic neuropathy, retinal detachment)
    - Temporal wedge
      - Damage to nerve fibers on the nasal side of the optic disc
      - Less common and often do not respect horizontal meridian

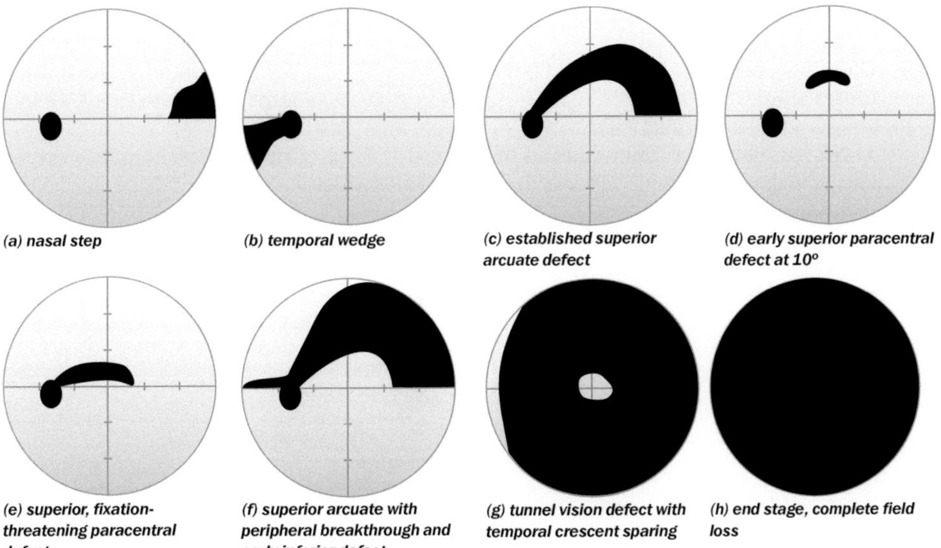

FIGURE 8.10 Common visual field patterns of glaucomatous optic neuropathy. (*Source*: Photo by courtesy David Broadway, M.D.)

e. Understanding the single field analysis (SFA) printout (see Figure 8.11)
   i. Proper review of VF analysis ensures accurate test
      - Assess reliability
      - Examine VF for glaucomatous defects
      - Evaluate global indices
   ii. Key reliability indices
      - Repeat VF test if poor reliability
         – Never change or initiate treatment based on an unreliable test
         – It can take a patient multiple test attempts to become reliable
         – Keep in mind cognitive decline and test anxiety affects performance
      - Fixation losses (FLs)
         – Fixation monitored by showing a stimulus in the blind spot
         – Excess FLs may be due to mis-plotted blind spot
         – May mask true defects
         – FL >20% is unreliable test
      - False negatives (FNs)
         – Occurs when patient does not respond to a stimulus that should be easily seen
         – No response to light 9 dB brighter than previously seen at same point
         – Common due to "falling asleep at the wheel" (inattention) but also found in advanced glaucoma VF loss
      - False positives (FP)
         – Occurs when patient responds when no stimulus displayed ("trigger happy")
         – Value of 40 dB or higher indicates that the patient may be trigger happy (normal around 30 dB)
         – FPs will make VF appear better than it actually is
         – FP rate of 15% or more indicates an unreliable test
   iii. Key probability values
      - Total deviation (TD) shows decibel deviations from norm
      - Pattern deviation (PD) similar to TD but filters out generalized depressions like media opacities
         – PD most important STATPAC analysis when glaucoma suspected
   iv. Greyscale
      - Shows values closer to 0 dB in black and those closer to 50 dB in white
      - Use as "first look" and as an excellent visual patient education tool
         – Remember that areas between test points are extrapolated
         – Data is not compared to normal ranges
      - Does present profound loss
   v. Glaucoma hemifield test (GHT)
      - Compares points in the upper field to corresponding points in the lower field below the horizontal midline to look for significant differences (mirror image)
      - Inferior and superior threshold response to stimuli should correspond symmetrically
      - If results outside normal limits
         – Indicates the upper and lower fields differ by an amount found in less than 1% of normals
      - If results borderline
         – This difference found in only 1–3% of normal
   vi. Important global indices
      - Gives a numerical quantification in decibels of the visual field loss and reduced sensitivity
      - Mean total deviation (MD)
         – The average difference from normal expected value from patient age-matched normative database
         – Normal value is above −2.0

- Moderate stage glaucomatous visual field loss (−6 dB to −12 dB)
- Does not take into account cataract progression
- Pattern standard deviation (PSD)
  - Measured deviation from normal for localized loss adjusting out loss from media opacities
  - May be the most useful STATPAC analysis because it highlights localized defects common in glaucoma

f. Standards for an abnormal VF in glaucoma in HVF testing[47]
   i. Criteria below must be present in a *repeatable* test
      - Cluster of three contiguous non-edge points on the same side of the horizontal meridian

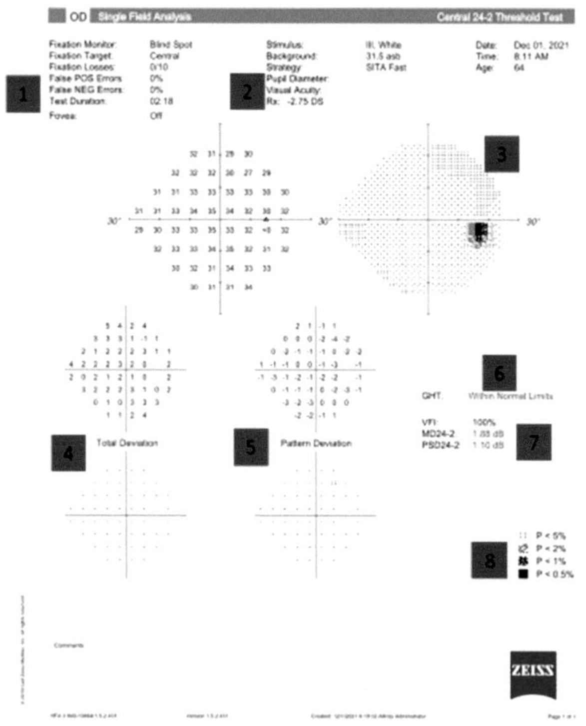

1= Reliability Indices
- False Positives (responding when no stimulus shown)
  - >15% is unreliable test
- False Negatives (no response when bright stimulus shown in previously established normal locations
- Fixation Losses (maintaining fixation straight ahead)
  - >20% FL is an unreliable test

2=Threshold Values
- Sensitivity at each point measured in decibels

3=Greyscale
- Translates raw decibel sensitivity but not compared to normal range
- Shows values closer to 0 dB in black and those closer to 50 dB in white
- Use as "first look"

4=Total Deviation Maps
- Show deviation in decibels from expected norm

5=Pattern Deviation Maps
- Shows localized loss after filtering out other factors affecting hill of vision like media opacities

6=Glaucoma Hemifield Test
- Compares points in the upper field to corresponding points in the lower field below the horizontal midline to look for significant differences (mirror image)

7=Indices
- Visual Field Index- Stages VF from 0-100 (100% in normal VFs, 0% blind VF)
- Mean Deviation- How much deviation from normative database (normal is above -2.0)
- Pattern Standard Deviation-Measured deviation from normal for localized loss adjusting out loss from media opacities

8=Probability Symbols
- Indicates statistically significant deviation that occurs in fewer than 5%, 2%, 1%, or 0.5% of normals

FIGURE 8.11 Interpretation guide to Humphrey VF printout.

TABLE 8.5 Key Glaucoma Testing Values

Test	Normal Values	Abnormal Values
Central Corneal Thickness (CCT)	535–565 μm (555 μm = avg.) Goldmann Applanation calibrated for 520 μm CCT	Very Thin <510 μm Thin <535 μm Thick >565 μm Very Thick >600 μm
Corneal Hysteresis	Average = 10 mm Hg	< 10 mm Hg
Ocular Perfusion Pressure OPP = 2/3 [diastolic BP + 1/3 (systolic BP—diastolic BP)] —IOP	>56 mm Hg	<56 mm Hg is associated with a 6 × 2 increased risk of glaucoma
HVF 242	• MD should be above 2.0 • Average stimulus brightness seen is 30 dB	• 3 contiguous nonedged points on same side of horizontal with P<5% with one point at P<1—GHT "outside normal limits" • PSD where P<5%
VF and OCT Progression	• Normal RNFL thinning due to age 0.48 μm/per year for Cirrus and 0.60 μm/year for Spectralis (so approximately <1 μm for both) • RNFL testing reproducibility is around 4 μm	VF: rapid <2 dB/yr RNFL: decrease of 8 μm in superior or inferior from previous scan and/or repeatable decreased of 4 overall RNFL average
RNFL	• RNFL thickness symmetry between eyes should not differ by more than 2 μm • Average thickness is 82 μm	<75 μm mild RNFL loss <64 μm moderate RNFL loss <56 μm advanced RNFL loss
Optic Nerve/Rim	• Small = 1.0 mn 1.3 mm w/mean C/D ratio 0.3 • Average = 1.4 mm 1.8 mm w/mean C/D ratio 0.45 • Large >1.8 mm w/mean C/D ratio 0.55	• C/D ratio difference of 2 cup sizes between eyes same overall disc size • 0.6 C/D ratio in average disc size • Deviations from ISNT rule in rim

with P <5% (10 dB lower) with one at P <1% (5 dB lower) in the pattern deviation plot
  - Abnormal clusters typical of glaucoma: nasal step, Bjerrum arcuate bundle and paracentral defects that respect the horizontal midline
  - An abnormal isolated point may not be clinically significant, but a cluster of abnormal points is most likely a real depression in the VF
- Glaucoma hemifield test (GHT) reads "outside normal limits"
  - If repeatable, this is a stand-alone criterion for diagnosing glaucoma
- Pattern standard deviation (PSD) where P <5%

g. Staging glaucomatous VF loss: guides for classifying glaucoma as mild, moderate, or advanced
   i. Hodapp, Parish, and Anderson staging chart[48]
   ii. The Advanced Glaucoma Intervention Study (AGIS) staging system[49]
   iii. Glaucoma staging, the American Glaucoma Society work group[50]
   - Mild = glaucomatous ON abnormalities with no VF defect on standard HVF but could have abnormal short wavelength automated perimetry test
   - Moderate = glaucomatous ON abnormalities with glaucomatous VF defect in one hemifield, and not within 5° of fixation
   - Severe/advanced/end-stage = glaucomatous ON abnormalities with glaucomatous VF defect in both hemifields, and/or loss within 5° of fixation in at least one hemifield

10. Interpretation in advanced imaging
   a. Axial length, disc size, gender, age, and neuro-ophthalmic and retinal diseases can affect RNFL thickness[51]
   b. Not useful in monitoring advanced disease but switching to macular scans can be helpful
      i. RNFL thinning maxes out around 50 μm and almost never below 40 μm (floor effect)[52]
   c. OCT
      i. Inferior RNFL quadrant generally undergoes the greatest amount of thinning correlating with ON tissue findings in glaucoma
      ii. Understanding important indices (software analysis, normative database, and printout vary from each manufacturer but all have similar key indices) (see Figure 8.12)
      - Errors in interpretation
        - Optimum scan quality signal strengths: Cirrus >6 (0–10), RTVue >45 (0–100), Spectralis >15 (0–40)[53]
        - Eye movement or excessive blinking – cause RNFL to appear thinner than it is
        - Super important to have a healthy ocular surface for optimum image capture: lubricate before scanning!
        - Misplaced segmentation lines
        - Decentration of the ONH
        - Scanning individuals outside the age normative database for each tomographer
        - Poor representation of high myopes and diverse ethnicities in database
      - ONH analysis
        - Outlines the disc, rim, and cup
        - Provides measurements of disc and rim area, average NFL thickness, cup-to-disc ratio and symmetry between eyes
      - TSNIT map
        - displays RNFL thickness measurements in clock hours
      - Macular thickness analysis
        - Macular thinning is early indicator for glaucoma and more reliable when advanced disease or high myopia
        - Important to scan both macula and RNFL to look for glaucomatous damage
      - Ganglion cell complex
        - Encompasses three retinal layers that are damaged in glaucoma: RNFL, ganglion cell layer, and the inner plexiform layer (IPL)
        - Earliest changes may be loss of dendrites in IPL
   d. Standards for abnormal imaging/structural changes from normal
      i. Color map–patient compared to normative database
      - White – upper 5% of normals
      - Green – middle 90% of normals
      - Yellow – lower 5% of normals
      - Red – lowest 1% of normals
      - Gray – not compared
        - Don't be fooled into just looking at the color map
        - Red areas could be thinning due to other diseases than glaucoma or false positives due to increase in axial length or small discs
        - Green areas that look normal could have evidence of glaucoma in early stage "green disease" (e.g., early glaucoma where RNFL thickness is labeled green, but there is asymmetry between eyes or focal areas of thinning, and/or progressively decreasing RNFL thickness on serial scans despite thickness falling within normal "green" classification)
      ii. RNFL thickness symmetry between eyes if normal should not differ by more than approximately 9 to 12 μm[54]
      iii. Average normal RNFL thickness = 82.1 ± 6.2 μm, with the superonasal sector being the thickest and the inferior sector the thinnest[55]
      iv. Glaucoma RNFL average thickness[56]
      - Early = 75.2 ± 6.8 μm
      - Moderate = 64.4 ± 8.4 μm
      - Advanced = 55.6 ± 7.6 μm

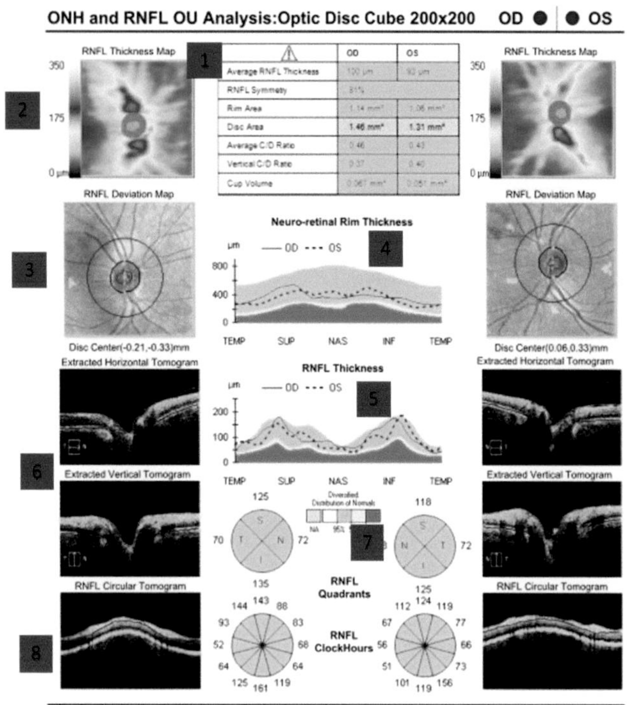

1= Key values compared to normative database

2= RNFL topographical thickness map

- Normal thickness will glow with red/yellow

3= RNFL Deviation Map

- Shows calculation circle and areas thinner than norm

4= Neuro-retinal rim thickness

- 90% of measurements fall into green area
- Thinnest 5% measurements fall into yellow area
- Thinnest 1% measurements fall into red area and considered outside normal limits

5= RNFL TSNIT Graph

- Shows RNFL measurement around calculation circle compared to normative database

6= Horizontal and Vertical B Scans from data cube through disc center

7= RNFL Quadrant and Clock Hour

- Average thickness compared to normative database

8=RNFL Calculation Circle

- Centered on disc with RNFL boundaries shown

FIGURE 8.12 Normal OCT with interpretation guide of report.

C. Clinical Correlation of Findings

1. Glaucoma risk factors, testing abnormalities, ON findings, VF loss, and advanced imaging should all "make sense" and correlate to point to a diagnosis of glaucoma, or not! (see Figure 8.13)
2. Challenges
   a. Differentiating between patients that are at risk of blindness and those that are not
   b. No single perfect reference standard for establishing the diagnosis of glaucoma
   c. Early diagnosis can be challenging, and multiple clinicians may disagree when presented with a case
   d. Many findings of glaucoma also occur in people without the condition
      i. Enormous variability of nerve appearance in healthy populations
      ii. Both elevated or normal IOP can occur in glaucoma
   e. OCT should complement, not replace the clinical exam of the ONH and RNFL
   f. Disagreement in the structure/function relationship can occur
      i. Due to non-linear relationship between changes in structure and function as well as numerous other confounding factors
      ii. Resolve the discrepancy
         - Look for other non-glaucomatous explanations
         - Repeat VF and OCT testing

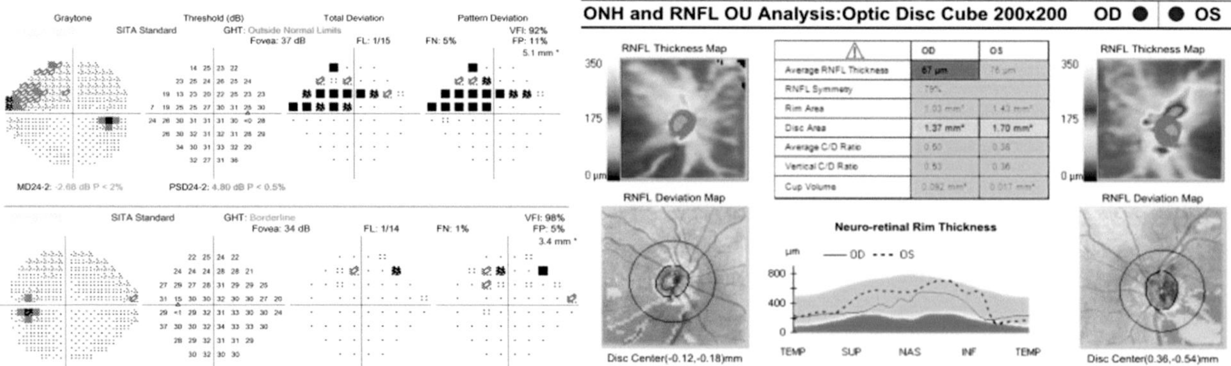

FIGURE 8.13 Patient example of correlation between OCT and VF testing.

- Re-evaluate macula and utilize disc photography
- Consider OCT-A to evaluate vasculature

iii. Keep in mind many patients show progressive functional VF loss in the absence of clear structural changes to the ONH[57]
- Imaging devices, despite their increasing use and erroneous replacement for ON photography, are not substitutes for VF testing
  - **VFs are still the single most critical tool for monitoring glaucomatous disease!**

3. Findings specific to glaucoma
   a. Focal pallor and thinning of the disc rim
   b. An acquired ON pit
   c. Asymmetry in cup to disc ratio between eyes
   d. RNFL loss associated with a correlating VF defect
   e. Change in ONH and VF over time
4. Each stage of glaucoma requires different strategies in testing for progression
   a. Early glaucoma
      i. RNFL and macula OCT important for patients with normal or unreliable VF
   b. Moderate glaucoma
      i. Correlating exam findings, OCT measurements and VF help confirm progression
      ii. Comparison of disc photos also beneficial
   c. Advanced glaucoma
      i. RNFL OCT not helpful due to floor effect
      ii. Use macular OCT and 10–2 visual field tests to detect progress

III. Glaucoma Conditions by SOAP Notation

A. Glaucoma Suspects

1. Ocular Hypertension (OHTN)/Primary Open Angle Glaucoma (POAG) Suspect

Subjective

- Asymptomatic
- Found on routine exam
- Normal appearance on gonioscopy
- IOP usually above 22 mm Hg and considered OHTN
- (see "Current Concepts in Glaucoma," A.–B.)

Objective

- Risk factors (see "Diagnosing Glaucoma," A.–C.)
- No glaucomatous neuropathy but has some risk factors and/or borderline abnormal tests that could convert to glaucoma over time

Assessment

- Rule out glaucoma, physiologic cupping, secondary open angle glaucoma suspects (pigment dispersion syndrome, pseudoexfoliation, steroid-response, normal tension suspect)

Plan

- Monitor every 6–12 months for conversion to glaucoma
- Initiate treatment if conversion (see "Treatment and Management" below and Table 8.8)

2. Normal/Low Tension Glaucoma (NTG/LTG) Suspect

Subjective

- Same findings as POAG suspect but IOP is under 22 mm Hg at all time points

Objective

- Risk Factors (see "Diagnosing Glaucoma," A.–C.)
- Decreased CCT (<520 μm)
- No glaucomatous neuropathy but has some risk factors and/or borderline abnormal tests that could convert to glaucoma over time

Assessment

- Rule out NTG, physiologic cupping, secondary open angle glaucoma suspects (pigment dispersion syndrome, pseudoexfoliation, and steroid-response)

Plan

- Monitor every 6–12 months for conversion to glaucoma
- Initiate treatment if conversion (see "Treatment and Management" below and Table 8.8)

3. Narrow Angle without Glaucoma (See Figure 8.14)

Subjective

- Asymptomatic
- Found with Van Herick on biomicroscopy, confirmed with gonioscopy

Objective

- Gonioscopy shows trabecular meshwork in all quadrants

Assessment

- Determine if angle at risk for closure (Schwalbe's line seen in two quadrants)

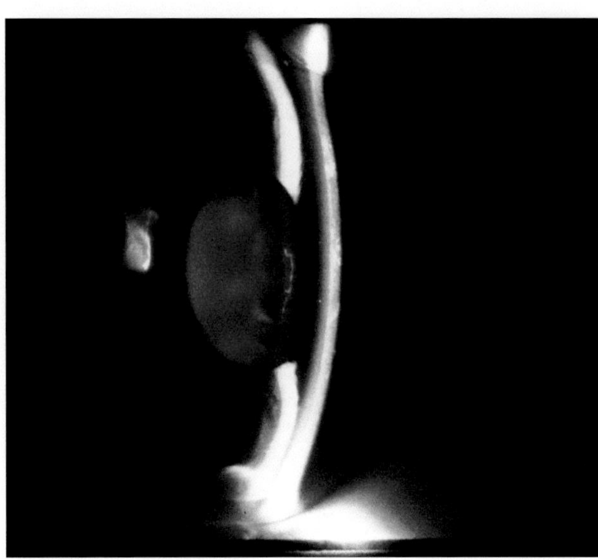

FIGURE 8.14 Decreased anterior chamber depth in a narrow angle. (*Source*: Photo by courtesy Tom S. K. Chi, M.D.)

Plan

- Monitor every 6–12 months if not yet occludable
- Refer for Laser Peripheral Iridotomy (LPI) if occludable (see Section I. B. 3. b.)
- If occludable consider 1% pilocarpine b.i.d. until LPI performed

4. Narrow Angle with Evidence of Closure (No Glaucomatous Damage)

Subjective

- Past episodes of blurred vision, halos around lights, pain

Objective

- Narrowed angle, peripheral anterior synechiae, elevated IOP
- Risk factors (see Section I. A.)
- No glaucomatous damage of the optic nerve

Assessment

- Rule out secondary causes of angle closure

Plan

- Refer for LPI (see Section I. B. 3. b.)
- If IOP elevated, initiate IOP lowering methods including 1% Pilocarpine b.i.d. until LPI performed
- Obtain baseline VF, OCT to ensure no evidence of glaucoma

5. Pigment Dispersion Syndrome

Subjective

- Asymptomatic, bilateral but asymmetric
- Often younger myopic males

Objective

- Midperipheral spoke-like iris transillumination defects (see Figure 8.15)
- Grade 4 pigmentation of the angle on gonio 360° especially inferior
- Sampaolesi's line—pigmented Schwalbe's line
- Vertical pigment band on cornea: Krukenberg spindle
- Pigment on posterior equatorial lens surface: Scheie's line
- Normal IOPs and no glaucomatous optic neuropathy

Assessment

- Rule out pigmentary glaucoma, pseudoexfoliation, uveitis, pigment liberation post-surgery, iris melanoma

Plan

- Monitor for conversion to glaucoma based on risk factors and testing (see Section II.)
- If IOP elevates and/or glaucoma is diagnosed, begin treatment (see "Treatment and Management" below and Table 8.8)

6. Pseudoexfoliation Syndrome (PXF)

Subjective

- Asymptomatic in early stages
- Can be unilateral or bilateral (but often asymmetric)

Objective

- White flaky "dandruff-like" material located on iris pupillary margin and sometimes on corneal endothelium
- Moth eaten appearance of peri-pupillary margin of iris with transillumination defects
- Same material located on peripheral anterior surface of lens and zonules (see Figure 8.16)
- Grade 4 pigmentation of the angle on gonio 360° especially inferior
- Sampaolesi's line: pigmented Schwalbe's line
- Poor response to dilation
- Normal IOPs and no glaucomatous atrophy
- Weak zonules: pseudophacodonesis/phacodonesis (tremulousness or vibration of crystalline lens during eye movement)

Assessment

- Rule out pseudoexfoliation glaucoma, pigment dispersion syndrome, uveitis, true exfoliation, amyloidosis

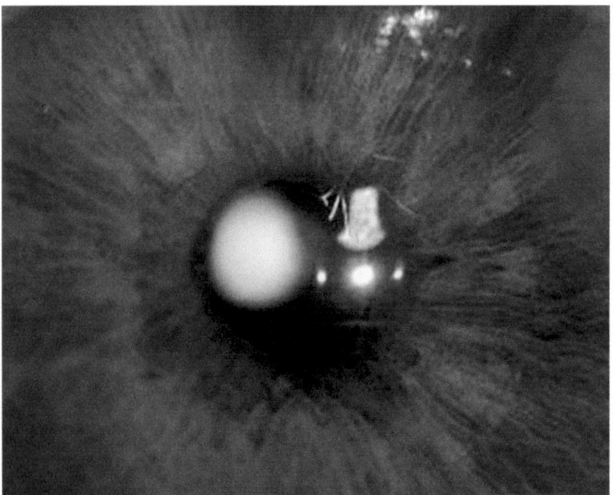

FIGURE 8.15 Iris transillumination defects in pigmentary dispersion syndrome.

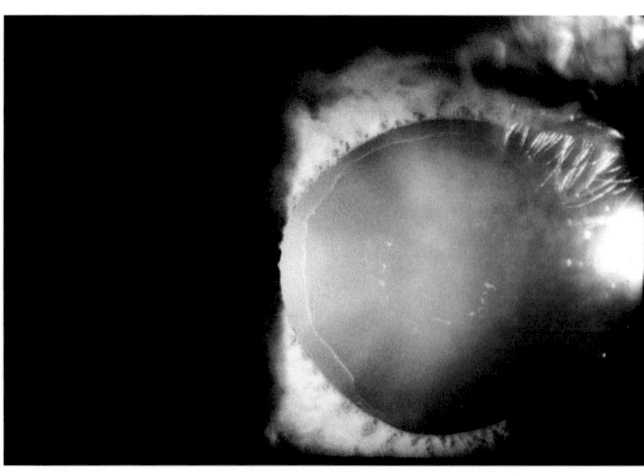

FIGURE 8.16 Pseudoexfoliaton on the anterior lens. (*Source*: Photo by courtesy Tom S. K. Chi, M.D.)

Plan

- Monitor for conversion to glaucoma based on risk factors and testing (see Section II.)
- If IOP elevates and/or glaucoma is diagnosed, begin treatment (see "Treatment and Management" below and Table 8.8)
- IOP is often volatile so monitor every 6 months for conversion

7. Angle Recession

Subjective

- Asymptomatic, unilateral
- History of blunt force trauma to eye
- Can take 10–20 years after injury to convert to glaucoma

Objective

- Torn iris/iridodialysis (see Figure 8.17)
- Widening of ciliary body and whitening of scleral spur on gonioscopy (see Figure 8.18)
- Normal IOPs and no glaucomatous atrophy

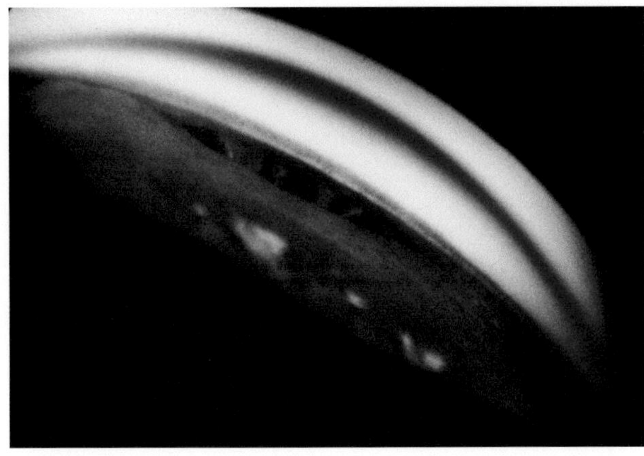

FIGURE 8.17 Gonioscopic view of iridodialysis. (*Source*: Photo by courtesy Tom S. K. Chi, M.D.)

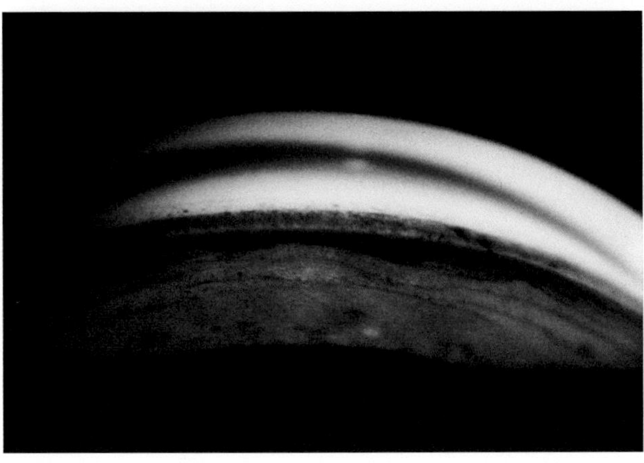

FIGURE 8.18 Gonioscopic view of angle recession. (*Source*: Photo by courtesy Tom S. K. Chi, M.D.)

Assessment

- Rule out open angle glaucoma suspect

Plan

- Monitor for conversion to glaucoma based on risk factors and testing (see Section II.)
- If IOP elevates and/or glaucoma is diagnosed, begin treatment (see "Treatment and Management" below and Table 8.8)

B. Open Angle Glaucoma

1. Primary Open Angle Glaucoma (POAG)

Subjective

- Same findings as in POAG suspect (see Section III. A. 1. above)

Objective

- Same findings as in POAG suspect (see Section III. A. 1. above) accompanied by glaucomatous findings on testing (see Section II. A.–C.)
- Pressure is elevated over 22 mm Hg

Assessment

- Rule out OHTN, physiologic cupping, NTG, secondary open angle glaucoma (pigment dispersion syndrome, pseudoexfoliation, steroid-response), optic atrophy, previous glaucoma damage where the trigger is removed and is now static, congenital ON defects, VF defects from non-glaucomatous conditions

Plan

- Initiate treatment and IOP lowering (see "Treatment and Management" below and Table 8.8)

2. Normal (Low) Tension Glaucoma (NTG/LTG)

Subjective

- Same findings as in normal tension suspect (see Section III. A. 2. above)

Objective

- Same findings as in normal tension suspect (see Section III. A. 2. above) accompanied by glaucomatous findings on testing (see Section II. A.–C.)
- Higher incidence of disc hemorrhages

Assessment

- Rule out physiologic cupping, OHTN, POAG, secondary open angle glaucoma (pigment dispersion syndrome, pseudoexfoliation, steroid-response), optic atrophy, previous glaucoma damage where the trigger is removed and is now static, congenital ON defects, VF defects from non-glaucomatous conditions, previous episode of systemic hypotension (acute blood loss/h/o cardiac bypass)

Plan

- Initiate treatment and IOP lowering (see "Treatment and Management" below and Table 8.8)

C. Primary Angle Closure Glaucoma (ACG)/Pupillary Block

1. Acute

Subjective

- Sudden onset eye pain, halos around lights, decreased vision
- Nausea, vomiting, severe headache (HA)
- Typically unilateral
- Risk factors: older age, female, hyperopia >3D, Asian, family history, recent mydriasis

Objective

- Closed angle on gonioscopy
- Elevated or asymmetric IOP
- Microcystic corneal edema
- Mid-dilated pupil, shallow AC peripherally
- Glaucomatous neuropathy
- Possibly occludable or narrow angle in other eye

Assessment

- Rule out IOP spike due to secondary causes—herpetic infection, inflammation, neovascularization, post-surgical, trauma

Plan

- Break attack immediately and lower IOP so surgeon can perform laser peripheral iridoplasty
- Goal is to get IOPs in low 30s before patient leaves office (see Table 8.6)
  1. Give oral acetazolamide two 250-mg tablets in office unless contraindicated
  2. Start rotation of topical glaucoma meds from every drug class (beta-blocker, alpha-agonist, CAI, prostaglandin, rho kinase inhibitor, parasympathomimetic agonists) every 5–10 minutes and repeat one time if IOP not responding in 60 minutes
  3. Instill topical prednisolone to decrease corneal edema and inflammation (repeat every 15 minutes up to 1 hour)
  4. Try compressive gonioscopy to manually open angle and break attack
  5. Check IOP and VA every 30–60 minutes until you reach IOP in low 30s
     a. If IOP not responding with two rounds of topical meds and 500 mg of oral acetazolamide, hyperosmotic (oral glycerol or isosorbide) can be considered but direct referral for immediate surgical intervention is now indicated
  6. Send patient home with all topical glaucoma meds including 1% pilocarpine q.i.d., topical prednisolone q.i.d. and oral acetazolamide 500 mg b.i.d. until LPI performed
  7. **Don't forget the other eye!** If occludable, initiate 1% pilocarpine b.i.d.

TABLE 8.6 Angle Closure Emergency Kit

30 count 250 mg Acetazolamide
2% Pilocarpine 5 mL
1% Prednisolone Acetate 5 mL
0.5% Timolol 5 mL
0.1% Alphagan P™ or generic equivalent 5 mL or 0.5% Apraclonidine
1% Brinzolomide or 2% Dorzolamide 5 mL
Prostaglandin analog 2.5 mL
Oral Glycerol 50% 1 g/kg (contraindicated in diabetics) or Oral isosorbide 1.5–2.0 g/kg

2. Chronic

Subjective

- Usually asymptomatic but may have past history of HA, halos around lights
- If advanced, decreased VA or loss of VF on confrontations or automated perimetry

Objective

- Areas of multiple peripheral anterior synechiae, usually in three quadrants
- Elevated IOP
- Glaucomatous nerve with NFL thinning on OCT and possible VF loss

Assessment

- Rule out acute angle closure glaucoma, and other secondary closure from uveitis or neovascular glaucoma caused by diabetic proliferative disease/retinal vein occlusions
- Perform glaucoma workup testing to evaluate stage

Plan

- If angle closure glaucoma is due to pupillary block, initiate 1% pilocarpine and if IOP elevated, topical therapy with beta-blocker, alpha-agonist, and CAI
- Refer for LPI (see Section I. B. 3. b.) but if unsuccessful, may need argon laser iridoplasty if plateau iris or goniosynechialysis with clear lens extraction

3. Plateau Iris

Subjective

- Typically asymptomatic unless in acute angle closure glaucoma

Objective

- Flat iris plane with normal anterior chamber depth
- Convex peripheral iris with anterior insertion into the ciliary body
- Large ciliary body or pars plicata
- Often not detected until post LPI when angle may not open up

Assessment

- Rule out pupillary block (which shows decreased anterior chamber depth and entire iris convex), aqueous misdirection (which is shallow anterior chamber occurring post-surgery)
- Typically identified post LPI if angle does not open or IOP rises post dilation despite patent peripheral iridotomy

Plan

- Consider argon laser iridoplasty or clear lens extraction

D. Secondary Glaucoma

1. Pseudoexfoliation Glaucoma

Subjective

- All findings with pseudoexfoliation syndrome, but if advanced, decreased vision or VF loss

Objective

- All findings with pseudoexfoliation syndrome plus glaucomatous optic nerve and VF findings

Assessment

- Rule out pigmentary dispersion and pigmentary glaucoma, uveitis, amyloidosis, true lens exfoliation

Plan

- Initiate treatment and IOP lowering (see "Treatment and Management" below and Table 8.8)

2. Pigmentary Glaucoma

Subjective

- All findings with pigmentary dispersion syndrome but if advanced, decreased vision or VF loss

Objective

- All findings with pigmentary dispersion syndrome plus glaucomatous optic nerve and VF findings

Assessment

- Rule out pigmentary dispersion syndrome, pigment liberation post-surgery, pseudoexfoliation glaucoma, uveitis

Plan

- Initiate treatment and IOP lowering (see "Treatment and Management" below and Table 8.8)

3. Aphakic Glaucoma

Subjective

- May be asymptomatic until advanced, particularly in children
- History of lens extraction (especially at young age)
- Pre-op history of dense cataract, complicated cataract surgery, high myopia, trauma
- Common cause of pediatric glaucoma when aphakic: possible due to cataract surgery affecting development of TM or possible low grade chronic trabeculitis post-op

Objective

- Aphakia
- Elevated IOP, corneal clouding, glaucomatous optic nerve changes, VF loss, peripheral anterior synechiae

Assessment

- Rule out retained lens fragment glaucoma, pupillary block due to vitreous herniation, shallowing of anterior chamber over time, uveitis, aqueous misdirection

Plan

- Initiate Treatment and IOP lowering (see "Treatment and Management" below and Table 8.8)
- May be difficult to treat medically or surgically

4. Drug-Induced Glaucoma

a. Corticosteroid

Subjective

- Asymptomatic unless advanced with vision or VF loss

Objective

- Elevated IOP with use of corticosteroids
- Most common 2–4 weeks after initiating corticosteroids, especially in those already with glaucoma risk factors
- Seen most commonly with topical or intravitreal but can occur with nasal, oral, intramuscular, or intravenous
- Potency of steroid can contribute to IOP elevation—dexamethasone (highest) ⇒ difluprednate ⇒ prednisolone ⇒ loteprednol or fluorometholone (weakest)
- IOP can return to normal when discontinued but affected by amount of IOP elevation and length of steroid use
- Due to resistance in outflow of trabecular meshwork from reacted glucocorticoid receptors that alter extracellular matrix and decrease phagocytosis

Assessment

- Rule out uveitis as cause of elevated IOP: many patients being treated for uveitis are also on steroids
- Perform gonioscopy and rule out all other forms of glaucoma

Plan

- Discontinue steroid use or switch to weaker steroid or topical NSAID
- If IOP not responding, then initiate treatment and IOP lowering (see "Treatment and Management" below and Table 8.8)

b. Topiramate (Topamax)

Subjective

- Bilateral blurry vision and headache
- Loss of uncorrected distance acuity with better uncorrected near vision
- Halos around lights
- New topiramate use 10–14 days prior or recent increased dose

Objective

- Sudden myopic shift
- Bilateral signs of angle closure (see above)
- Due to choroidal effusion causing anterior rotation of ciliary body and forward displacement of iris-lens diaphragm: seen on anterior segment OCT
- Topiramate causes increase permeability of the ciliochoroidal vasculature ⇒ choroidal effusion
- Optic nerve changes/VF loss if IOP spike is high without early intervention

Assessment

- Rule out other forms of angle closure glaucoma and inflammatory glaucoma

Plan

- Patient to stop topiramate use
- Initiate 1% cyclopentolate b.i.d.: relaxes the ciliary body and tightens zonules, keeping the iris-lens diaphragm in check
- Break attack initiating treatment as outlined in acute angle closure glaucoma except for using oral carbonic anhydrase inhibitors as this can increase effusion
- Send patient home with topical meds, steroid, and cycloplegic agent
- Recheck IOP in 1–2 days and taper off topical treatment over 1–2-week period as improvement noted
- Myopic shift should resolve within 1–2 weeks

c. Glaucoma Due to Intravitreal/Retinal Injections

Subjective

- Usually asymptomatic and often detected by retinal specialist first

Objective

- IOP increasing over time after series of multiple retinal injections—(AntiVEGF or Corticosteroid)
- Glaucomatous nerve changes and VF loss if high spike or undetected

Assessment

- Rule out other forms of OHTN/POAG

Plan

- Initiate treatment and IOP lowering (see "Treatment and Management" below and Table 8.8)

E. Traumatic Glaucoma

1. Angle Recession Glaucoma (See Also Chapter 6)

Subjective

- See angle recession subjective
- Occurs 10–20 years after initial trauma

Objective

- Same as angle recession with glaucomatous nerve changes and VF loss

Assessment

- Rule out other forms of POAG

Plan

- Initiate treatment and IOP lowering (see "Treatment and Management" below and Table 8.8)

2. Acute Glaucoma Due to Hyphema

Subjective

- Recent history of blunt force trauma, pain, decreased vision
- In absence of trauma, ask about use of blood thinners, clotting disorder such as sickle cell or easy bruising, past ocular surgery

Objective

- Red blood cells in anterior chamber: can be circulating or starting to layer (see Figure 8.19)
    1. Evaluate amount of hyphema in anterior chamber 0–100%
- Elevated IOP
- If trauma, may have additional injuries to orbit, anterior and posterior segments—important to dilate and evaluate

Assessment

- If trauma, rule out ruptured globe and other injuries avoiding gonioscopy
- If spontaneous consider uveitis/glaucoma/hyphema (UGH) syndrome, blood clotting disorders, anticoagulant use

Plan

- Prescribe cycloplegic (homatropine or atropine b.i.d.), topical steroid q2h, IOP lowering agents
- Topical beta-blocker, alpha-agonist, CAI if no sickle cell
- Limit activity with head elevation 30°, eye shield always
- Stop anticoagulants
- Recheck IOP in 1 day
- If IOP non-responsive, oral CAI unless sickle cell or otherwise contraindicated
- If IOP still not responsive (>60 mm Hg for 48 hrs), corneal blood staining, or >50% hyphema at day 8, then surgical evacuation
- Special considerations if Black or Mediterranean
- Suspect sickle cell and order laboratory screening test whether hyphema traumatic or spontaneous
- Order: sickle cell prep blood test: screener for sickle cell
    1. If prep positive, order hemoglobin electrophoresis: diagnostic in determining sickle cell trait or disease
    2. May take time to get results so proceed keeping possibility in mind
    3. Approximately 10% carry the HbS gene

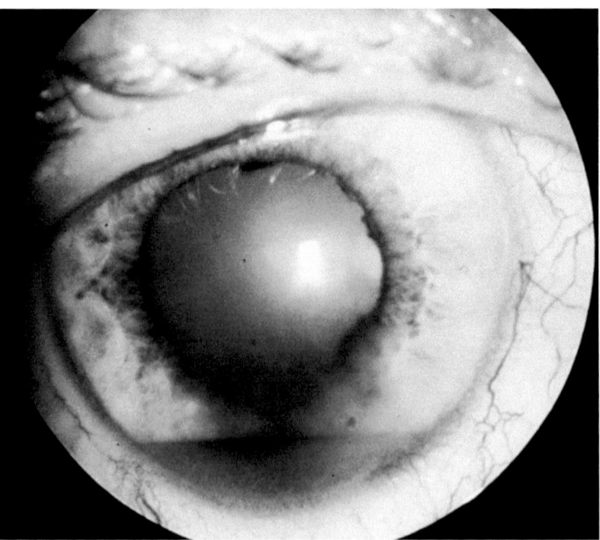

FIGURE 8.19 Layered hyphema. (*Source*: Photo by courtesy Tom S. K. Chi, M.D.)

- Red blood cells can sickle in anterior chamber ⇒ clog trabecular meshwork
    1. As IOP rises, further hypoxia occurs increasing sickling
- Central retinal artery under stress at lower IOPs (24 mm Hg) increased risk of CRAO and AION at IOPs that most would tolerate otherwise
- Occurs with all phenotypes: sickle trait < sickle disease < sickle anemia
- Avoid oral or topical CAIs as this increases pH promoting sickling
- May need paracentesis or surgical evacuation sooner if IOP spikes >30 mm Hg or >24 mm Hg more than a few days[58]

F. Inflammatory Glaucoma

1. Uveitis (Can Be Open or Closed Angle or Steroid-Induced)

Subjective

- Boring pain, photophobia, decreased vision, unilateral

Objective

- Cells/flare in anterior chamber
- Cornea: possible keratic precipitates, Descemet's folds/edema, dendrite if due to herpetic infection
- Conjunctival injection
- Possible posterior synechiae with possible irregular pupil
- Possible pigment on lens capsule
- Initially open angle on gonioscopy but may have some degree of peripheral anterior synechiae that can lead to pupillary block/secondary angle closure glaucoma
- Elevated IOP: can be acute or chronic due to obstruction from inflammatory cell
- Glaucomatous optic neuropathy and VF loss if chronic or late stage

Assessment

- Rule out Fuchs's heterochromia iridocyclitis, neovascular and pigmentary glaucoma

Plan

- Workup for underlying systemic etiology (see Chapter 6, Sections II. and III.)
- Treat underlying inflammation (see Chapter 6, Sections II. and III.)
- Initiate treatment and IOP lowering (see "Treatment and Management" below and Table 8.8)
    1. Prostaglandins and miotics can increase inflammation and are not recommended as first-line IOP lowering agents
- As inflammation subsides, meds can be discontinued
- May need long-term steroid management which can lead to steroid-induced glaucoma
- Consider oral immunosuppressive systemic agents if underlying autoimmune etiology and referral to rheumatology

2. Neovascular

Subjective

- May be asymptomatic if early
- Pain, conjunctival injection, decreased vision, photophobia
- History of diabetes, cardiovascular disease, or ischemia

Objective

- Neovascularization of iris and angle (see Figure 8.20)
    1. Lacy, non-radial, blood vessels along pupillary margin
    2. Various degrees of angle closure/peripheral anterior synechiae due to fibrovascular sheath over trabecular meshwork
- Elevated IOP
- Possible cells and flare in AC, corneal edema, hyphema
- Glaucomatous optic neuropathy and VF loss if later stages
- Underlying ischemic retinal condition: severe diabetic retinopathy, vascular occlusion, carotid occlusive disease
    1. Rarely: ocular tumor, trauma

Assessment

- Rule out uveitic inflammatory glaucoma and primary angle closure glaucoma
- Determine underlying cause

Plan

- Manage inflammation—topical steroid q2h, cycloplegic b.i.d.
- Initiate treatment and IOP lowering (see "Treatment and Management" below and Table 8.8)
    1. Prostaglandins can increase inflammation and not recommended in acute phase but may help lower IOP once inflammation controlled
    2. Miotics are contraindicated due to increase in inflammation and synechiae
- Refer for antiVEGF treatment and/or pan retinal photocoagulation (PRP)
- If IOP not responding to topical and oral therapy once vessel regression seen, filtration tube-shunt surgery indicated and/or cyclodestructive procedure if refractory
- If visual recovery limited, goal is comfort care and preserve vision in other eye
    1. Enucleation may be necessary if eye is painful and risk of sympathetic ophthalmia
- Refer for systemic re-evaluation of diabetes, cardiovascular, and carotid disease

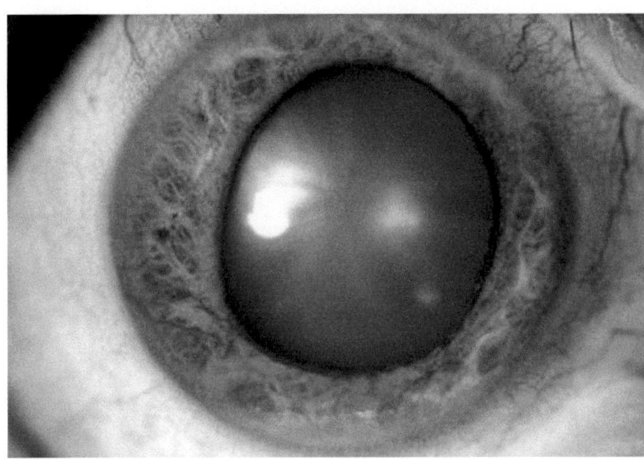

FIGURE 8.20 Neovascularization of the iris.

G. Post-Surgical OHTN/Glaucoma

1. Cataract Surgery

Subjective

- Acute: pain, nausea, vomiting 1–2 hours post-surgery
- Within first week: asymptomatic

Objective

- Acute
  1. IOP spike >40 mm Hg
- Within first week
  1. Elevated IOP <30 mm Hg

Assessment

- Acute
  1. Typically due to retained viscoelastic
  2. Rule out hyphema, significant inflammation, surgical pigment dispersion, pupillary block
- Within first week
  1. Can be due to slow filtration on viscoelastic or low-grade inflammation
  2. Rule out retained lens fragment, hyphema, steroid response (usually 2–4 weeks post-op but can occur as early as 1 week), UGH syndrome
  3. If later onset, evaluate for steroid response or rebound iritis

Plan

- Acute
  1. Give 500 mg oral acetazolamide unless contraindicated
  2. Initiate IOP lowering with topical beta-blocker, alpha-agonist, CAI, steroid
  3. If not responding and patient still vomiting, consider paracentesis
  4. Patient to continue topical and oral therapy for 24 hours and recheck IOP in 1 day
  5. When IOP responding, reduce or discontinue therapy starting with oral agent first
- Within first week
  1. To treat or monitor? If patient ON not already compromised, can consider monitoring if IOP in 20s
  2. Initiate IOP lowering with beta-blocker, alpha-agonist, CAI, or combo med for 1–2 weeks post-operatively if IOP over 28–30 mm Hg and/or ON compromised
  3. If IOP climbing over 4 weeks, consider steroid response (see "Steroid-Induced Glaucoma" above) and rule out rebound inflammation

2. Aqueous Misdirection (Malignant Glaucoma)

Subjective

- Pain, conjunctival injection, photophobia *occurring immediately after surgery* in patients with history of risk factors for angle closure or past ACG
  1. Occurs more commonly after glaucoma surgery

Objective

- Shallowing of AC *both* centrally and peripherally with elevated IOP persisting despite having had an iridotomy/iridectomy
  1. Central AC shallowing is critical sign and helps differentiate from regular pupillary block
- Lens/iris diaphragm shifted forward

Assessment

- Diagnosis of exclusion and rare
  1. Rule out all forms pupillary block (iris bombe, acute angle closure/angle closure glaucoma suprachoroidal hemorrhage, choroidal effusion/detachment)—IOP usually low
  2. If laser iridotomy does not reduce IOP and deepen anterior chamber, most likely misdirection
- Unknown etiology but aqueous not able to percolate through vitreous and lens/iris diaphragm forwardly displaced

Plan

- Initiate treatment using oral and topical IOP lowering agents
  1. Mannitol or glycerol may help dehydrate vitreous
- Cycloplegic (atropine) b.i.d. to prevent ciliary muscle contraction which posteriorly moves lens
- Usually improves in 4–7 days: taper off meds gradually with cycloplegic agent last
- If no improvement, surgical vitrectomy/iridectomy and lens extraction if phakic

3. Uveitis/Glaucoma/Hyphema (UGH) Syndrome

Subjective

- Sudden change in vision, blurry vision, photophobia, injection

Objective

- Cells/flare and/or hyphema in anterior chamber
- Pseudophakia
- Vitreous in anterior chamber
- IOL haptics out of capsule/malpositioned IOL
- Elevated IOP
- Pigment dispersion with transillumination defects
- CME with chronic inflammation
- With prolonged elevated IOP, glaucomatous nerve and VF changes

Assessment

- Rule out pigment dispersion/pigmentary glaucoma, spontaneous, or traumatic hyphema, inflammatory glaucoma (NVG/uveitic)
- Due to mechanical rubbing of IOL against anterior chamber structures

Plan

- Refer for IOL repositioning or exchange
- Treat underlying inflammation and lower IOP (see hyphema) until surgery performed
- Avoid miotics as they can increase IOL chafing

H. Pediatric Glaucoma

1. Congenital

Subjective

- May be asymptomatic
- Photophobia, epiphora, blepharospasm
- Onset
  1. Newborn—present at birth
  2. Infantile glaucoma: 12–24 months

Objective

- Corneal diameter >12 mm before 1 year
- Enlarged globe (buphthalmos)

- Haab striae, corneal edema
- Elevated IOP (usually 30–40 mm Hg), glaucomatous disc changes

Assessment

- Rule out congenital corneal anomalies—megalocornea, trauma at birth, endothelial dystrophies,
- Often associated with other systemic or anterior segment structural disorders (see "Secondary Juvenile" below)

Plan

- Refer to pediatric specialist for management and surgical intervention

2. Juvenile

Subjective

- Onset after 3 years of age
- Same symptoms as in congenital glaucoma
- Parents may note abnormal appearance of the eyes: cloudiness or a blue tint to sclera, large globe, chronic eye rubbing, or avoiding bright light

Objective

- Corneal diameter >13 mm
- All other similar findings as in congenital glaucoma

Assessment

- See "Congenital" above

Plan

- See "Congenital" above

3. Secondary Juvenile

Subjective

- Due to associated congenital or acquired systemic or anterior segment structural anomalies
- Sturge–Weber, neurofibromatosis
- Aniridia, Axenfeld/Reiger/Peters anomalies, posterior polymorphous, and ICE dystrophy (see Figure 8.21)
- Post-congenital cataract surgery
- Same symptoms as above

Objective

- Same findings as in congenital glaucoma with additional anterior chamber structural or systemic anomalies associated with underlying disease (see Chapter 5 and Table 5.6)

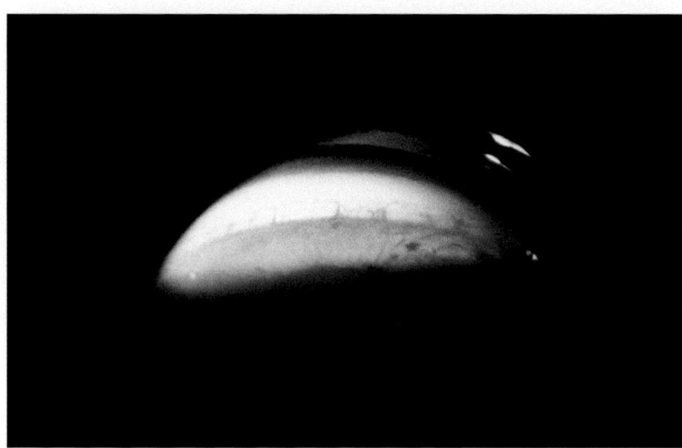

FIGURE 8.21 Gonioscopic view of iris processes in Axenfelds anomaly. (*Source*: Photo by courtesy Tom S. K. Chi, M.D.)

Assessment

- Rule out primary causes of pediatric glaucoma

Plan

- See "Congenital" above

Section 2: Treatment and Management

I. Treating Glaucoma: IOP Lowering

A. Lowering IOP Is Only Proven Method to Treat Glaucoma

1. Goal is to slow disease progression and preserve quality of life
   a. Set IOP target where you believe rate of progression will be slowed enough to prevent functional loss
      i. Aim for a 20% to 50% reduction from baseline[59]
      ii. Should progression occur despite maintaining initial target IOP, lower target IOP once again
2. Important considerations in setting IOP goal
   a. Life expectancy (how aggressive should treatment be to prevent functional vision loss if patient lives to 100 years of age)
   b. Baseline IOP at time of diagnosis
   c. Disease severity at time of diagnosis
      i. If severe, need aggressive IOP lowering and goal
   d. Risk of future prognosis/aggressiveness of disease
   e. Risk factors: (see Section I. A. 3. above)
3. Relevant landmark clinical studies key points
   a. Importance of applying evidence-based medicine in glaucoma management
   b. Advanced Glaucoma Intervention Study (AGIS)[60]
      i. Those with unstable glaucoma were randomized to ALT or trabeculectomy
      ii. Eyes in which 100% of visits over a 6-year period had an IOP <18 mm Hg showed little VF progression
      iii. Those with IOPs 15 mm Hg showed half the progression of those with 18 mm Hg, and those with 13 mm Hg showed half the progression of 15 mm Hg
         - With unstable or advanced glaucoma, set IOP goal <13 mm Hg
      iv. Race should be factored when designing a surgical treatment
   c. Early Manifest Glaucoma Trial (EMGT)[61]
      i. Does treatment slow progression?
      ii. Glaucoma progressed slower in the treated group but is variable
      iii. Every 1 mm Hg matters
         - For every 1 mm Hg reduction in IOP, risk of progression decreases by 10%.
      iv. Follow progression closely and reset target IOP when progression confirmed
      v. Pseudoexfoliation glaucoma doubled risk of VF loss
   d. Collaborative Initiative Glaucoma Treatment Study (CIGTS)[62]
      i. Do newly diagnosed patients benefit more from initial treatment with topical therapy (35% IOP reduction) or trabeculectomy (48% IOP reduction)?
         - Quality of life outcome was similar between two groups

- Prescribe individualized treatment and no surgery until it is indicated
- Those with advanced VF loss at baseline (−10 dB), of older age, of African descent or have diabetes are more at risk for VF progression and benefit from earlier filtering surgery

e. Collaborative Normal Tension Glaucoma Study (CNTGS)[63]
 i. Is IOP a factor in normal-tension glaucoma?
  - Found IOP reduction important for normotensives
  - 30% IOP lowering slows progression
   - 35% of untreated eyes progressed with VF loss compared to only 12% of eyes that received treatment
 ii. Those at risk of aggressive progression include women, migraine sufferers, and patients with disc hemorrhages

f. Ocular Hypertensive Treatment Study (OHTS)[64]
 i. Does treating OHTN prevent POAG and what risk factors in OHTN develop into glaucoma?
  - Risk of POAG in OHTN patients is reduced by almost 50% at 5 years with treatment (treatment delays onset)
  - Risk factors for developing POAG: older age, elevated IOP, larger vertical C/D ratio, and thinner central corneal thickness
  - High-risk patients may benefit from early treatment
  - In the control group (no treatment), 9.5% of those with OHTN developed glaucoma compared to 4.4% in the treated group
   - Consider observation in low risk OHTN patients

B. Treatment Options

1. Pharmacologic agents (see Table 8.7)
 a. Reach target IOP with fewest medications to preserve ocular surface and minimize side effects
 b. Two methods to lower IOP
  i. Reduce aqueous production from ciliary body (beta-blockers, carbonic anhydrase inhibitors, alpha-agonists)
   - Rate dependent on blood flow to ciliary body (CB)
   - Dependent on rate of secretion from cells
  ii. Increase outflow via
   - Trabecular meshwork (cholinergic, nitric oxide donors, rho kinase inhibitors)
   - Uveoscleral pathway (prostaglandins)
  iii. Topical agents can be used as monotherapy, adjunctive therapy, or replacement therapy
 c. Beta-blockers
  i. Non-selectively antagonizes beta-1 and beta-2 adrenergic receptors
  ii. Lowers IOP by inhibiting cyclic adenosine monophosphate (cAMP) production in ciliary epithelium
  iii. Reduces aqueous humor secretion 20–50% with a corresponding IOP reduction of 20–30%[65]
   - Effect occurs within 1hr of instillation
  iv. Standard starting dose b.i.d. but commonly used 1× daily in AM
  v. Potential systemic adverse effects:
   - Bronchospasm (especially in asthmatics)
   - Bradycardia, lowered blood pressure
   - Lethargy, mood changes, depression,
   - Light-headedness, syncope, visual disturbance
   - Reduced glucose tolerance in diabetics
    - Hypoglycemic signs and symptoms can be masked
   - Studies indicate topical beta-blockers are not associated with increased risks of cardiovascular and respiratory diseases but still use with caution[66]
  vi. Commercially available
   - Levobunolol 0.25%, 0.5% (Betagan)
   - Timolol hemihydrate 0.25%, 0.5% (Betimol)
   - Timolol maleate 0.5% (Istalol)
   - Timolol maleate 0.25%, 0.5% (Timoptic, Timolol Ocudose preservative free)
   - Timolol maleate gel 0.25%, 0.5% (Timoptic XE, Timolol GFS)
   - Betaxolol 0.25% (Betoptic–S)
    - Beta-1 selective and is a safer choice to use in those with pulmonary issues, but IOP lowering effect may be less
 d. Prostaglandins (PG)
  i. Increases uveoscleral outflow[67]
   - Stimulation of PG receptors in the ciliary body and iris which activate metalloproteinase
   - This stimulates collagenase which breaks down the collagen of the extracellular matrix in CB
   - Results in widening and decompressing the connective tissue-filled spaces among the ciliary muscle bundles
   - Allows freer movement of aqueous into the vasculature of the iris and ciliary body face
  ii. Potent 22–39% reduction in IOP (6–8 mm Hg) and dosed q.d. h.s.[68]
  iii. Bimatoprost most efficacious of prostaglandin analogues[69]
  iv. Common side effects
   - Conjunctival hyperemia
   - Hyperpigmentation of eyelashes
   - Darkening of iris and skin discoloration
   - Hair/lash growth
  v. Less common side effects
   - Uveitis
   - Worsening herpetic keratitis
   - Cystoid macular edema (CME)
  vi. Commercially available
   - Latanoprost 0.005% (Xalatan)
    - Only prostaglandin that needs refrigerated prior to opening
   - Latanoprost emulsion 0.005% (Xelpros)
    - Benzalkonium chloride (BAK) free has polysorbate as preservative
    - Drug delivered with LIPIXELLE: micelle microemulsion formulation (nanomedicine)
    - Helps improve latanoprost solubility which typically requires BAK to stay in solution and makes it stable at room temperature

- Travoprost 0.004% (Travatan Z)
  - IOP lowering at all times of day/flattening diurnal curve[70]
  - Brand does not contain BAK
- Bimatoprost 0.01%, 0.03% (0.1% Lumigan)
  - Prostamide, not prodrug (activated after instillation) because it remains mostly unchanged when in the eye
  - 0.01% Lumigan has 4× the amount of BAK than 0.03%
- Tafluprost 0.0015% (Zioptan)
  - Preservative free (vials)
  - 5–8 mm Hg reduction from baseline[71]
- Latanoprostene bunod 0.024% (Vyzulta)
  - First nitric oxide (NO_2) donating prostaglandin F2α analog
  - Molecule splits into prostaglandin agonist (latanoprost acid) and NO_2
  - Proposed dual mechanism of action—increases outflow in both uveoscleral (prostaglandin) and trabecular meshwork (TM) (NO_2) pathways [72]
  - NO_2 is mediator of smooth muscle relaxation and vasodilation which relaxes TM increasing outflow

e. Selective alpha agonists[73]
  i. Lower IOP through alpha-2 agonist-mediated aqueous suppression and a secondary mechanism that increases uveoscleral outflow
  ii. Used either as monotherapy, as second-line therapy, or in fixed combination with beta-blockers
  iii. Dosed t.i.d. but many practitioners off-label initially dose b.i.d. for compliance purposes
  iv. Side effects
    - Ocular
      - Follicular conjunctivitis
      - Dry eye
      - Allergy—delayed hypersensitivity with highest in apraclonidine >0.2% brimonidine >0.15% >0.1%
    - Systemic
      - Headache, dry mouth
      - Fatigue, bradycardia, hypotension
      - Contraindicated in patients receiving monoamine oxidase (MAO) inhibitor antidepressants, which have been replaced with safer antidepressants
  v. Commercially available
    - Apraclonidine 0.5% (Iopidine)
      - Not commonly prescribed for daily use due to high allergy
      - Used mostly in surgery to prevent IOP spike
    - Brimonidine 0.2%, 0.15%, 0.1% (0.1% Alphagan P)
      - IOP lowering 20% as monotherapy
      - Reduces IOP within 1 hour, peak IOP effect 2–3 hours after dosing
      - More effective than dorzolamide when used as adjunctive therapy with beta-blocker
      - Less effective than dorzolamide when used as adjunctive therapy with latanoprost
      - Possible neuroprotective effect for RGCs
      - 0.1% and 0.15% branded brimonidine preserved with purite, not BAK, and an improved pH of 7.7

f. Carbonic anhydrase inhibitors
  i. Lowers IOP by decreasing aqueous production
    - Direct antagonist activity on the ciliary epithelial carbonic anhydrase
  ii. Available both orally and topically
  iii. Oral indicated for glaucoma as well as pseudotumor cerebri
  iv. Systemic side effects (common with oral, rarer in topical administration)
    - Transient myopia
    - Metallic taste
    - Paresthesia of the fingers, toes
    - Urinary frequency
    - Metabolic acidosis
    - Malaise, fatigue
    - Potassium depletion
    - Renal calculi formation
  v. Ocular side effects
    - Burning/stinging
    - Higher risk of allergy
      - With topical
      - If also a history of sulfonamide allergy because of increased immune sensitivity, but less risk that may be expected from a cross-reactivity mechanism[74]
  vi. Commercially available oral CAIs
    - Acetazolamide (Diamox) 125 mg, 250 mg, 500 mg ER
      - Dose 125–250 mg b.i.d.–q.i.d. p.o., or 500 mg ER b.i.d.
    - Methazolamide (Neptazane) 25 mg, 50 mg
      - Dose 50–100 mg b.i.d.–t.i.d. p.o.
    - 40% IOP lowering with oral agent, but side effects are high[75]
  vii. Commercially available topical CAIs
    - Can be used first line but better as adjunct agent
    - Improves prostaglandin efficacy
    - Identified as good option as second adjunct therapy to prostaglandin[76]
    - Dosed t.i.d. but used b.i.d. off-label
    - Dorzolamide 2% (Trusopt)[77]
      - IOP lowering 4 to 6 mm Hg at peak (2 hours post-dose)
      - 3 to 4.5 mm Hg at trough (8 hours post-dose)
    - Brinzolamide 1% (Azopt)[78]
      - Reduced IOP by 18%
    - Dorzolamide 5.6 pH while brinzolamide 7.5 pH
    - More stinging and ocular surface disruption with dorzolamide
    - Brinzolamide is available as a suspension

g. Parasympathomimetic agonists
  i. Lower IOP by increasing outflow through miosis
    - Causes contraction of longitudinal ciliary muscle
      - Pulls scleral spur to tighten trabecular meshwork, increasing outflow of aqueous humor

- ii. Topical side effects
    - Brow ache
    - Induced myopia
    - Miosis (leading to decreased vision), shallowing of the anterior chamber
    - Retinal detachment
- iii. Commercially available
    - Pilocarpine HCL 1%, 2%, 4%, 6% (Isopto Carpine in 1%, 2%, and 4%)
        - Dosed q.i.d.
    - 20% reduction in IOP[79]
- iv. Uses today
    - Last line option when on max meds prior to filter surgery
    - Used in angle closure glaucoma or prevention of closure while awaiting iridotomy
    - Used post-goniotomy surgery to prevent angle from scarring

h. Rho kinase inhibitors[80]

- i. Prevents the phosphorylation of myosin light chains in smooth muscle cells
- ii. Inhibiting this helps trabecular meshwork cells stay relaxed which increases outflow
- iii. Side effects
    - Most common is hyperemia (53%)
        - Mild in 83%
    - No systemic side effects
    - Corneal verticillata (9%) → whorl keratopathy
    - Deposits onset ranged from 6 to 13 weeks after therapy initiation
        - Resolved by 13 weeks after discontinuation
    - Conjunctival hemorrhage (15%)
- iv. Commercially available
    - Netarsudil 0.02% (Rhopressa)
    - Lowers IOP through three effects on aqueous humor dynamics
        - Increases trabecular outflow facility
        - Decreases production of aqueous humor
        - Decreases episcleral venous pressure
    - Dosed topically q.d. h.s.
    - Up to 5 mm Hg lowering at peak
        - 4 mm Hg lowering of diurnal curve at 90 days irrelevant of baseline IOP
    - May be effective for normal tension glaucoma (NTG)
    - May not get patient to IOP goal of 18 mm if >27 mm Hg at baseline

i. Combination medications

- i. Can be first-line or adjunct therapy
- ii. Advantages[81]
    - Enhanced convenience with less drop confusion
    - Improved compliance and adherence
    - Reduced exposure to preservatives by decreasing total drops on ocular surface
    - Potential cost savings
    - Combination agents reduce IOP more effectively than their component medications when used separately as monotherapy
- iii. Commercially available
    - 2% dorzolamide/0.5% timolol (Cosopt)
        - IOP reduction of up to 40%[82]
        - Generic has common complaint of stinging due to lower pH
        - Lower pH can be toxic to ocular surface
        - Available in preservative free vials (Cosopt PF)
    - 0.2% brimonidine/0.5% timolol (Combigan)
        - IOP reduction 33% (7.6 mm Hg) from baseline and 40% were consistently below 18 mm Hg[83]
        - Combigan prescribed as adjunct to a prostaglandin further lowers IOP another 25 to 35%[84]
        - 50% lower incidence in ocular allergy with Combigan compared with 0.2% brimonidine monotherapy[85]
    - 0.2% brimonidine/1% brinzolamide (Simbrinza)
        - Beta-blocker free
        - Dosed t.i.d. but used off label as b.i.d.
        - Reduced IOP 8.5 mm Hg in clinical trials with 28.6 to 37.6% reduction when dosed b.i.d.[86]
        - Up to 7.1 mm Hg additional IOP lowering effect when added to prostaglandin[87]
        - Approved as an initial, first-line therapy
        - Serve as a complete replacement for patients who failed PGA use
        - Suspension formula: needs shaken
    - 0.02% netarsudil/0.005% latanoprost (Rocklatan)
        - 34% IOP reduction from baseline with 2 mm Hg more than latanoprost alone[88]
        - Similar side effects of individual components
- iv. Available outside the United States
    - 0.005% latanoprost/0.5% timolol (Xalcom)[89]
        - IOP lowering 9.4 mm Hg
        - Dosed once daily
        - IOP lowering less than with timolol twice daily and latanoprost once daily
        - Contains BAK
    - 0.3 bimatoprost/0.5% timolol (Ganfort)[90]
        - Dosed once daily in AM
        - IOP lowering of 9.6 mm Hg compared with a maximum 8.8 mm Hg in the bimatoprost monotherapy group
        - BAK preserved
    - 0.004% travoprost/0.5% timolol (DuoTrav)[91]
        - Dosed once daily in AM or PM
        - Preserved with polyquad
        - 8–10 mm Hg IOP lowering with AM dose
    - 1.0% brinzolomide/0.5% timolol (Azarga)[92]
        - Efficacy similar to Cosopt
        - Dosed twice daily
        - BAK preservative

j. Medical marijuana (tetrahydrocannabinol)

- i. Shown to lower IOP but too short acting to be effective with risks
    - 2–3-hour duration
    - Would need to smoke around the clock with resultant cognitive impairment
    - Risk of lung carcinoma
    - Other routes of administration not effective in IOP lowering
    - Not recommended at this time as a treatment since other pharmacologic therapy longer acting with fewer side effects

k. Understanding role of preservatives[93]
   i. Extends shelf-life of medications by decreasing microbial contamination
   ii. Often toxic to ocular surface and disrupts cell–cell junctions in epithelium and decreases tear stability
      - Corneal surface break-down allows for greater drug penetration into the aqueous
   iii. Benzalkonium chloride (BAK)
      - Found in 70% of glaucoma medications
      - Most toxic preservative
      - Mechanism of action is to destroy cell membranes to kill pathogens (quaternary ammonium detergent)
      - Does not discriminate between bacterial cell membranes and human cell membranes
      - 0.01% BAK cellular apoptosis occurs
      - 0.05 to 0.1% BAK cell necrosis occurs
   iv. Polyquad
      - Less toxic
         – Detergent quaternary ammonium similar to BAK but larger molecule
         – Not internalized by epithelial cells on the eye
         – Found in DuoTrav (outside United States)
   v. Purite
      - Less toxic
         – Preservative that breaks down upon contact with the air
         – Oxidizes microbial cellular components
      - No significant effect on human ocular tissues
      - Found in 0.1% Alphagan P
   vi. SofZia
      - Least toxic
         – Becomes inactive when in contact with potassium and sodium ions in the eye
         – Oxidative damage and subsequent death in bacteria that lack the enzymes cytochrome oxidase or catalase
         – Human cells possess these enzymes and are thus not similarly harmed
         – Found in Travatan Z
   vii. Potassium Sorbate
      - Synthetic salt that inhibits bacteria and fungi
      - Found in Xelpros

l. Considerations in selecting medication
   i. Patient's other systemic diseases and medications
      - Critical to evaluate to reduce drug interactions
   ii. Ability to comply and adhere to dosing and schedule (see Section II. C.)
   iii. Adverse effects
   iv. Cost
      - Generics versus branded

TABLE 8.7 Medications for Glaucoma (United States)

Category	Generic Name	Brand Name™	pH	Preserved
Beta-Blocker	Betaxolol 0.25%	Betoptic-S	7.6	0.01% BAK
	Levobunolol 0.25%, 0.5%	Betagan	5.5–7.5	0.004% BAK
	Timolol Maleate 0.25%, 0.5%	Generic, Timoptic, Istalol (0.5% only)	6.5–7.5	0.01% BAK
	Timolol Maleate 0.25%, 0.5%	Timolol Ocudose	7.0	None
	Timolol Hemihydrate 0.25%, 0.5%	Betimol	6.5–7.5	0.01% BAK
	Timolol Maleate Gel 0.25%, 0.5%	Timoptic XE, Timolol GFS	7.0	0.012% Benzododecinium bromide
Prostaglandin Analogue	Bimatoprost 0.03%	Generic	6.8–7.8	0.005% BAK
	Bimatoprost 0.01%	Lumigan	6.8–7.8	0.02% BAK
	Latanoprost 0.005%	Generic, Xalatan	6.7	0.02% BAK
	Latanoprost ophthalmic emulsion 0.005%	Xelpros	7.0	0.47% Potassium Sorbate
	Latanoprostene bunod 0.024%	Vyzulta	5.5	0.02% BAK
	Travoprost 0.004%	Generic, Travatan Z	5.7	Ionic Buffered Solution SofZia
	Tafluprost 0.0015%	Zioptan	5.5–6.7	None
Alpha-Agonist	0.5% Apraclonidlne	lopidine	4.4–7.8	0.01% BAK
	Brimonidne 0.02%	Generic	5.6–6.6	0.005% BAK
	Brimonidine 0.15%	Generic	6.9–7.4	0.001% Polyquad
	Brimonidine 0.1%	Alphagan P	7.4–8.0	0.005% Purite
Carbonic Anhydrase Inhibitor	Brinzolamide 1%	Generic, Azopt	7.5	0.01% BAK
	Dorzolomide 2%	Generic, Trusopt	5.6	0.0075% AK
	Acetazolomide 125 mg, 250 mg, 500 mg ER oral	Diamox	N/A	N/A
	Methazolamide 25 mg, 50 mg oral	Neptazane	N/A	N/A
Para-sympathomimetic Agonist	Pilocarpine HCL 1%, 2%, 4%, 6%	Generic, Isopto Carplne (1%, 2%, 4% only)	3.5–5.5	0.01% BAK
Rho-Kinase Inhibitor	Netarsudil 0.02%	Rhopressa	5.0	0.015% BAK
Combination	0.2% brimonidine/1% brinzolamide	Simbrinza	6.5	0.003% BAK
Agents	0,2% brimonidine/0.5% timolol	Combigan	6.5–7.3	0.005% BAK
	2% dorzolomide/0.5% timolol	Generic	5.65	0.0075% BAK
	2% dorzolomide/0.5% timolol	CosoptPF	5.65	None
	0.02% netarsudil/0.005% latanoprost	Rocklatan	5.0	0.02% BAK

- Combination meds versus separate generic components
- Preservative free versus preserved

v. Ocular surface integrity
- Important to reduce amount of corneal surface disease due to topical medications and their preservatives
- May take 8–12 weeks to reverse corneal staining and increase TBUT from preservative toxicity
- Preservative free is best, followed by disappearing preservatives, followed by oxidative preservatives, and worst with detergent preservatives (e.g., BAK)

vi. Efficacy monotherapy treatments
- Prostaglandin analogs generally provide the greatest IOP-lowering efficacy, followed by beta-blockers, α_2-adrenergic agonist, and CAI[94]

2. Intracameral implant
   a. Bimatoprost 10 mcg (Durysta)[95]
      i. Time released biodegradable pellet of bimatoprost injected into the anterior chamber
      ii. Increase outflow of aqueous humor through both the trabecular meshwork (conventional) and the uveoscleral routes (unconventional)
      iii. Continuous drug delivery for several months
      iv. Advise trying topical bimatoprost first prior to implantation to ensure tolerability
      v. Side effects
         - Conjunctival hyperemia, foreign-body sensation, eye pain, photophobia, conjunctival hemorrhage, dry eye, eye irritation, iritis
      vi. Reduced IOP by approximately 30% from baseline at 3 months primary efficacy period
3. Surgical
   a. Selective laser trabeculoplasty (SLT)
      i. Indications
         - First-line therapy
         - Primary open-angle glaucoma or mixed mechanism glaucoma (certain cases)
         - Maximum medical therapy
         - Intolerance of medical therapy
         - On multiple drops
         - Reduce a medication when using multiple
         - Medication too costly
         - Non-compliant patients
         - Non-believers
         - Dementia/Alzheimer's memory issues
      ii. Mechanism of action
         - 532 nm frequency-doubled Q-switched Nd:YAG laser with a 3 ns pulse and 400 μm beam selectively targets non-pigmented TM cells
         - Spares adjacent cells from thermal heat transfer and damage
         - Activated cells release cytokines that trigger targeted macrophage response
           - Phagocytize matter in the TM, increasing outflow
         - IOP reduction[96]
           - Approximately 20–25% IOP lowering from baseline
           - IOP lowering effect decreases over time with 50% failing (IOP not at 20% below baseline) at 2 years post-SLT
           - Higher IOP baseline is associated with better SLT success
           - 66–75% response rate (IOP lowering >20%)
         - Can be used in NTG, PXF, pigmentary, and steroid-induced glaucoma
           - Watch for IOP spike immediately post-op in pigmentary glaucoma
           - Set energy lower if pigmentary glaucoma
      iii. Procedure protocol
         - Topical alpha-agonist before and after to prevent an IOP spike
         - TM treated 360° for best results
           - Treatment of 180° can also be done
         - Topical steroid to prevent inflammation for 3 days
         - Check for an IOP spike 1 hour immediately after surgery
      iv. Post-op
         - Adjust the medications at 4–6 weeks or once lowering effect demonstrated
         - Based on IOP goal
         - Many surgeons will not perform SLT on the second eye until response seen in first eye
         - Once response seen, set up second eye
         - If no response, then glaucoma medications or other procedures will be needed
         - SLT can lose its effectiveness over time and IOP may rise
           - Can repeat yielding resultant IOP reduction[97]
           - The number of times SLT can be repeated has not been established, but one study suggests it can be repeated two times (total of three procedures) with another study underway looking at repeating SLT annually[98,99]
      v. Adverse effects
         - Redness, pain, photophobia
         - IOP spike which usually resolves in 24 hours and reduced using pre/post op alpha agonist
         - Rare—hyphema, cystoid macular edema (CME)
   b. Laser peripheral iridotomy (LPI)
      i. Indications
         - Definitive treatment for pupillary block
         - Angle-closure glaucoma (primary and secondary), angle closure, angle closure suspects
         - Can be considered in pigmentary glaucoma to reduce iris concavity by equalizing pressure in anterior (AC)/posterior chamber (PC)
      ii. Mechanism of action
         - LPI establishes alternative route for aqueous flow between the AC and PC by creating a hole in the iris
         - Q-switched Nd:YAG laser or Argon Nd:YAG-KTP 532 nm
      iii. Procedure protocols
         - 1% pilocarpine with brimonidine or apraclonidine instilled 10 minutes prior to the LPI
           - Prevent postoperative IOP spike
         - Iridotomies now placed temporal to reduce linear dysphotopsias from light reflecting off upper/lower lid tear prisms
         - Recheck IOP 1 hr after procedure to check for spike

- Schedule return in 2 weeks pending no complications

iv. Post-op
- Topical steroid for 4–5 days
- Ensure patency of iridotomies (see Figure 8.22)
  - Use retroillumination
  - If non-patent, repeat LPI
  - Late closure can also occur up to 6 weeks postoperatively
- Perform gonioscopy and evaluate for openness

v. Adverse effects
- Transient, acute IOP spike
- Focal corneal endothelial damage
- Iris bleeding/hyphema
- Focal lens opacity
- Persistent iritis
- Glare
- Need for repeat LPI due to closure

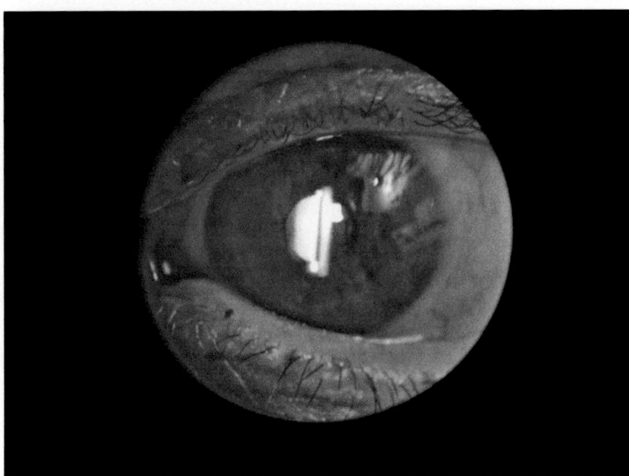

FIGURE 8.22 Retroillumination of patent peripheral iridotomy at 3:00. (*Source*: Photo by courtesy Tom S. K. Chi, M.D.)

c. Ciliary body (CB) procedures

i. Mechanism Of Action
- Reduce IOP by CB destruction or thermal shrinking
- Reducing aqueous production or increasing outflow by pulling it away from trabecular meshwork (TM)
- Old methods reserved for advanced and refractory glaucoma
- Can be repeated

ii. Continuous wave transscleral photocoagulation
- Older-diathermy, cryotherapy
- Newer-iridex G probe
  - Probe at limbus through sclera aimed at CB, retrobulbar anesthesia
  - Complications: pain, inflammation, hyphema, loss BCVA, hypotony, IOP spikes, macular edema
  - 30–50% IOP reduction[100]

iii. Endoscopic cyclophotocoagulation (ECP)
- Ciliary processes ablation in conjunction with cataract surgery
- Indicated for mild to moderate COAG
- Light, diode laser, and camera in probe to visualize ciliary epithelium
- 4 mm Hg IOP reduction with one less medication[101]

iv. Micropulse transscleral diode laser CPC (MP3)
- Series of short (microsecond), repetitive bursts of low energy pulses that effectively confines the thermal effect to the absorbing tissue in CB
  - Thermal effect but no tissue destruction
- Indicated for those on maximum therapy but can be done prior to a filter
- Approximately 5 mm Hg IOP lowering[102]

v. Post-op considerations of ciliary body procedures
- Control inflammation
  - 4–6 weeks taper of steroids
  - Use topical NSAID
- Oral acetazolamide 250 mg b.i.d. for first 2 days
- Manage glaucoma meds based on post-op pressures, IOP goal, and severity of disease
- Watch for CME and rebound iritis

d. Micro-invasive glaucoma surgery (MIGS)

i. Background
- Indicated for mild/moderate glaucoma
- Angle-based surgery
  - Angle must be open
- Criteria for classification of MIGS procedure:
  - Incision w/o conjunctival dissection (ab interno)
  - Minimal trauma
  - Efficacious in IOP lowering
  - Positive safety profile
  - Rapid recovery
- Usually performed with cataract surgery

ii. IOP lowering
- MIGS resultant IOP lowering effect is directly related to where you target the device and enhance outflow
- Schlemm's canal
  - Target TM and increase outflow through collector channels
  - Resultant IOP usually in mid-teens
- Supraciliary space
  - Device vaults TM into this space
  - Space has larger surface area and is very absorptive
  - Produces substantially lower IOP by avoiding episcleral venous resistance
- Subconjunctival space
  - Shunting aqueous into subconjunctival space to bypass TM
  - Procedures that target this area are bleb-forming
  - Have largest IOP lowering effect
  - However, increased risk of hypotony

iii. iStent inject[103] (see Figure 8.23)
- Mushroom-shaped titanium stent device that is injected through TM into Schlemm's (two preloaded stents are inserted) canal
- Shown to lower IOP more than cataract surgery alone
  - 7 mm Hg IOP lowering from baseline
  - Reduction in medication
  - Comparable safety profile to standalone cataract surgery

- Post-op considerations
  - Same corneal edema, risk of capsular haze, risk of post-op IOP elevation
  - Sometimes implantation not possible so iStent aborted
  - Mild initial bleeding at insertion site
  - On gonio, stent should be parallel not at angle
  - Same postoperative drop schedule as cataract surgery (antibiotic/steroid)
  - Keep on all pre-op glaucoma meds
  - Doesn't work immediately: can take at least 6 weeks (if not longer) to see effect
  - Adjust current glaucoma meds when you see the pressure drop anytime: can be as early as 1 week
  - Gonio every 6–12 months to ensure stent still patent and not extruded

iv. Hydrus microstent[104] (see Figure 8.24)
- Easy to implant, flexible, nitinol open-back stent
- Scaffolds and dilates TM inferonasal quadrant 3 clock hours
- 66% of mild POAG medication free at 5 years and 77% achieved IOP lowering >20%
- Reduced need for future invasive surgery

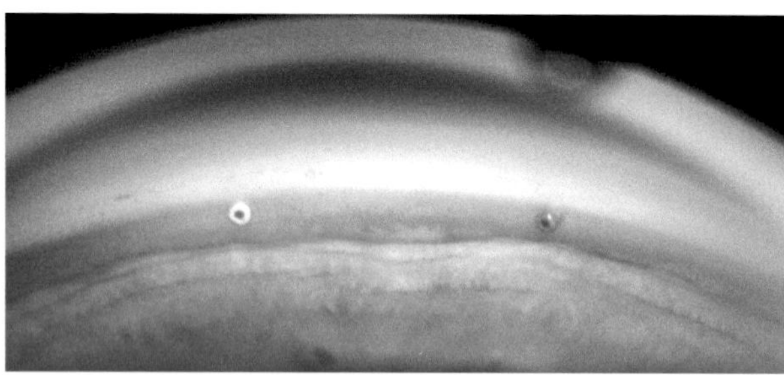

FIGURE 8.23 Gonioscopic view of placement of Istent Inject two clock hours apart. (*Source*: Photo by courtesy Tom S. K. Chi, M.D.)

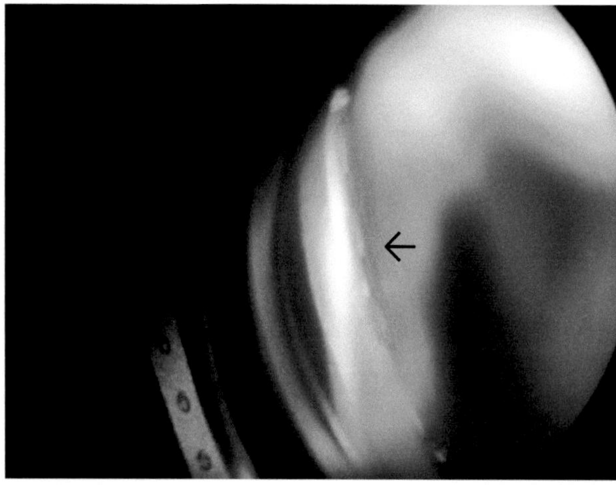

FIGURE 8.24 Gonioscopic view of placement of hydrus microstent in angle. (*Source*: Photo by courtesy Tom S. K. Chi, M.D.)

- Post-op
  - Device obstruction, higher inflammation, hyphema, PAS, rebound iritis
  - Same postoperative drop schedule as cataract surgery (antibiotic/steroid)
  - Taper off glaucoma agents when IOP starts decreasing—can be as early as 1 week

v. Goniotomy/trabeculotomy
- Removes strip of TM with Kahook dual blade or electrocautery (Trabectome) to expose collector channels
- Post-op
  - 1% pilocarpine b.i.d. for 1 month to prevent peripheral anterior synechiae
  - Topical antibiotic q.i.d. for 1 week
  - Topical steroid q.i.d. × then taper over 6 weeks according to inflammation
  - This procedure causes a high degree of postoperative inflammation and may need steroid longer
- Resume glaucoma medications and adjust as IOP decreased

vi. Xen Gel Stent[105]
- Collagen-derived porcine gelatin tube cross-linked with glutaraldehyde that hydrates on implantation
- Shunts fluid from the anterior chamber (AC) to subconjunctival space through a scleral tunnel which yields lower resultant IOPs than other stents
- Device dependent on bleb formation and limitation of fibrosis
- Patients will be on a longer course of prednisolone postoperatively (3 months) to prevent scarring of bleb which causes failure

vii. Omni canaloplasty[106]
- Microcatheterization and transluminal viscodilation of Schlemm's canal combined with trabeculotomy
- 27% reduction in IOP from baseline
- Post-op
  - Inflammation (13%), IOP spikes (6%), hyphema, corneal edema, and BCVA loss 4%
  - Steroid 4–6× daily (week 1) and taper over 4–6 weeks
  - Antibiotic q.i.d. for 1 week
  - Adjust glaucoma meds when done with steroid

e. Filtering surgery: trabeculectomy and aqueous drainage devices

i. Indications
- Disease progression despite all other efforts exhausted
  - IOP not at goal despite maximum meds, past laser intervention and/or previous MIGS intervention
- IOP same as episclerous venous pressure but worsening VF or cupping
- Poor compliance/intolerance to drops
- Will the patient go blind in their lifetime if surgery not performed?
- Choose between trabeculectomy (trab) or aqueous drainage device (tube)

- Some surgeons prefer tubes over trabeculectomy and vice versa
- Higher rate of complications and loss of BCVA so important to exhaust all other measures of IOP lowering

C. Evaluating for Progression

1. Once glaucoma diagnosis is made, clinician now shifts toward monitoring progression as well as estimating approximate rate of progression
2. Functional VF loss negatively affects quality of life (mobility, reading, and driving) and goal as clinician is to reduce or avoid this devasting outcome
   a. Rate of progression is individual and may take years to establish or could be rapid
   b. Helpful to know if parent or sibling lost vision during their disease course: is this genetically aggressive or slower?
   c. Important to test VFs and OCTs frequently in early diagnosis to establish reliable baseline and rule out rapid progression
   d. Rates of MD change in most glaucoma patients vary from 0 to −2.5 dB/year, depending on the severity of disease, treatment, and population samples[107] (see Figure 8.25)
      i. Rapid visual field progression is approximately ≤−2 dB/year[108]
   e. With intervention, most do not progress at a rate that would lead to functional impairment, but 3–17% of patients will continue to lose vision despite

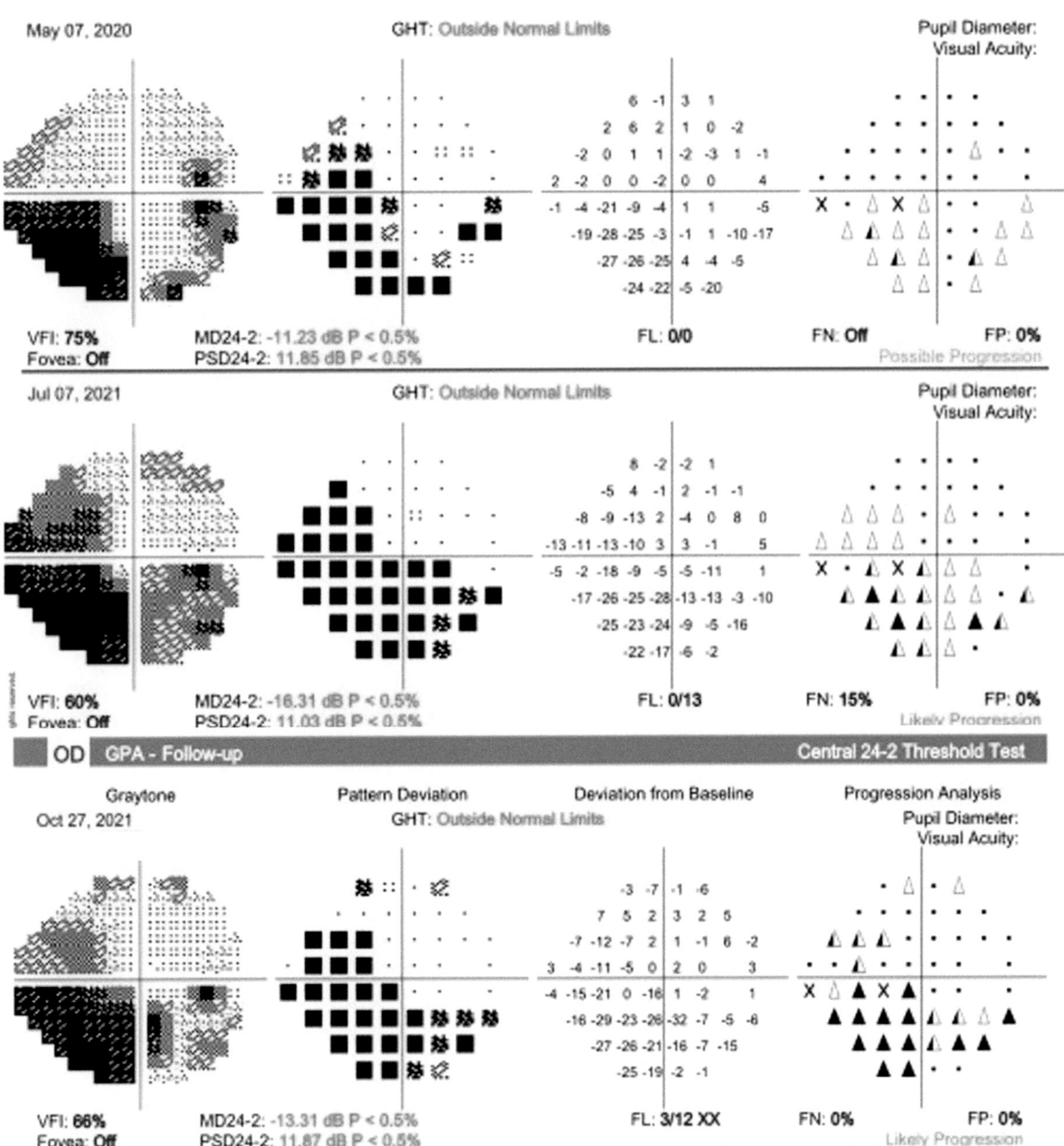

FIGURE 8.25 Confirmed progression in repeat visual field testing.

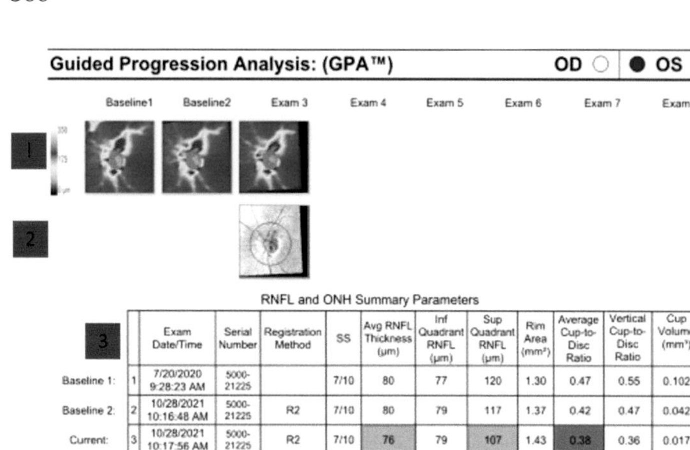

		Exam Date/Time	Serial Number	Registration Method	SS	Avg RNFL Thickness (µm)	Inf Quadrant RNFL (µm)	Sup Quadrant RNFL (µm)	Rim Area (mm²)	Average Cup-to-Disc Ratio	Vertical Cup-to-Disc Ratio	Cup Volume (mm³)
Baseline 1:	1	7/20/2020 9:28:23 AM	5000-21225		7/10	80	77	120	1.30	0.47	0.55	0.102
Baseline 2:	2	10/28/2021 10:16:48 AM	5000-21225	R2	7/10	80	79	117	1.37	0.42	0.47	0.042
Current:	3	10/28/2021 10:17:56 AM	5000-21225	R2	7/10	76	79	107	1.43	0.38	0.36	0.017

1= RNFL Thickness Map

- Shows RNFL thickness baseline and subsequent scans

2= RNFL Thickness Change Map

- Shows change in RNFL thickness

3= Summary of Parameters

- Shows a spreadsheet of relevant data from all scans for comparison purposes
- Overall RNFL thickness as well as Inferior and Superior are compared for change and highlighted if possible or likely progression

- 4=Definitions of Summary Parameters

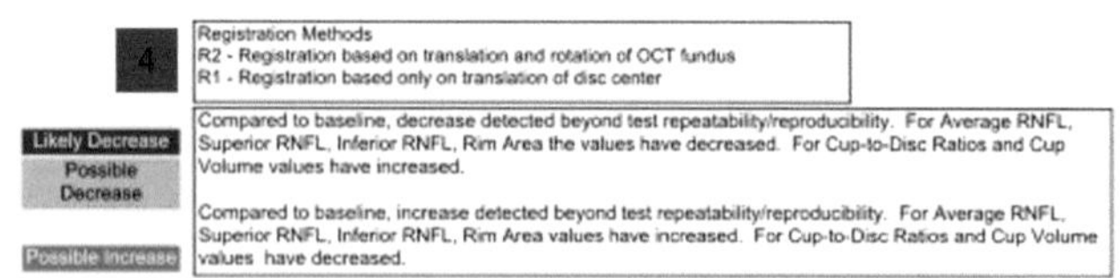

FIGURE 8.26 Cirrus OCT interpretation guide for guided progression analysis report.

optimum IOP lowering and progress to blindness within 20 years[109]

3. Structural changes using advanced imaging
   a. OCT[110]
      i. Can be event or trend based similar to VF analysis
      ii. Suggestive of progression
         - Difference of ≥7 µm thinning in superior and inferior quadrants between scans
         - Difference of ≥4–5 µm thinning for average RNFL difference between scans
      iii. Glaucoma progression analysis (see Figure 8.26)
         - Compares baseline and subsequent RNFL thickness of individual clusters of A-scans (pixels) to estimated test/retest variability
         - Pixels exceeding such test–re-test variability are coded in yellow at the first event, and in red if the same changes are seen on three consecutive images
         - Two baseline scans with three follow-up scans are needed to get a trend plot
         - Linear regression line in um/yr, represents rate of change
         - Reset baseline when change in treatment
      iv. Typical RNFL progression patterns[111]
         - Widening of existing RNFL defect
         - Deepening of current RNFL defect
         - Development of a new RNFL defect
           – Inferior temporal location most common site of progression
      v. Evaluating progression in advanced glaucoma is best using serial VFs since retinal thinning bottoms out (floor effect)
         - Once thinning hits floor, progression can still occur but OCT can't detect it
           – Use macular OCT and HVF 10–2 to monitor progression in advanced glaucoma
      vi. Correlate OCT findings to VF changes and exam findings to help confirm progression
4. Monitoring for change over time can be challenging to identify
   a. Progression software is event (tells us if progression occurred) or trend based (tells us rate of progression)
   b. Event-based compares current test with past baseline
   c. Trend-based quantifies rate of change using linear regression of a given metric with time
   d. Only trend-based analyses can be used to evaluate rates of change
5. If individuals fall outside normative databases or have unique ONHs, they still have a baseline, even if deemed abnormal by imaging or perimetry
   a. Changes from initial baseline assessment in ONH, RNFL thickness, and perimetry outside of normal aging should raise a red flag for progression

D. Author's Recommended Minimum Guidelines for Monitoring

1. Glaucoma suspects
   a. Should be followed every 6–12 months depending on low to high risk
   b. Baseline 24–2 VF, OCT, and disc photo and establish diurnal curve and maximum IOP (T_{max})
      i. Is there a T_{max} that you would treat regardless of CCT with normal ONH, VFs, and OCT testing? What is that threshold number for you? My threshold for treatment is 27 mm Hg no matter the CCT
      ii. Repeat testing every 6 months or annually depending on risk factors

iii. Consider 10–2 baseline additionally for macular defects
c. Gonioscopy
i. Baseline, then every 1–3 years
d. Perform diagnostic testing mentioned in Section II. A., if available
e. Clinically correlate findings and watch for change over time
f. Initiate treatment when abnormal testing is clinically correlated indicating progression from normal baseline to a glaucoma diagnosis

2. Glaucoma diagnosis: mild to moderate
a. Clinical assessment of IOPs and ONH every 4–6 months depending on mild or moderate
b. Establish target IOP (see "Treatment and Management," Section I. A.) and initiate treatment
c. Stagger AM and PM IOP readings at follow-up
i. Ensure flattening of diurnal curve
ii. Ensure IOP at target goal
d. 24–2 VFs to evaluate progression
i. European Glaucoma Society guidelines: VF testing three times per year in the first 2 years after initial glaucoma diagnosis[112]
ii. Need to obtain enough VFs initially to get reliability and repeatability
iii. Minimum every 12 months if reliable and rate of progression deemed slower
- More frequent if high risk or progression identified
iv. Perform 10–2 from time to time to look for macular defects not seen on 24–2
e. Imaging
i. Repeat every 6–12 months depending on if mild to moderate
ii. Evaluate both macular and ON tomography
iii. ON imaging may not be beneficial for advanced disease due to "floor effect" (see Section II. C. 2. c. i.)
f. Gonioscopy
i. Initially at baseline then every 1–2 years
ii. Anytime you suspect narrowing of angle on Van Herick
iii. If BRVO or CRVO monthly for the first 3 months then every 3 months the first year
iv. Post-MIGS surgery: annually and if the IOP starts to elevate post-MIGS at any time postoperatively
v. Annually in stable angle closure glaucoma
g. Disc photos—repeat every 1–3 years depending on progression of disease
i. Modify treatment based on IOP at target goal and/or signs of progression
ii. Further lower IOP goal with adjunct therapy
iii. Reassess IOP in 4–6 weeks to ensure IOP at new target when change in treatment
iv. If using HVF GPA, reselect latest VF as new baseline when treatment initiated or modified

3. Glaucoma diagnosis advanced
a. Clinical assessment of IOPs and ONH every 3–4 months
b. VF testing every 3–6 months depending on functional loss and rate of progression
i. 24–2 and 10–2 testing with macular imaging (e.g., OCT)
c. Gonioscopy
i. Initially at baseline then every 1–3 years
ii. Anytime you suspect narrowing of angle on Van Herick
d. Strict IOP goal and filtering surgical intervention if progressing on max meds/previous less invasive procedures

4. What is realistic?
a. The above guidelines are evidence-based but often may not be practical for clinicians and patients
i. Frequency may be burdensome to healthcare and affect compliance
ii. Compromise of two reliable baseline standard automated perimetry VFs followed by annual or biannual VF testing
- Modify based on risk: more frequent if moderate/advanced VF damage or younger age; or less frequent if OHTN/suspect[113]
iii. One must also keep in mind cost and healthcare plan coverage and work within system while providing optimal care

5. No "cookbook" for managing glaucoma
a. Every patient must be treated as an individual
b. This requires YOU to use your clinical skills

6. Author's algorithm in treatment and management (see Table 8.8)

II. Patient Education

A. Glaucoma Key Patient Educational Points

1. Important to be honest but not scare patient!
a. Anxiety over blindness can cause patient to never return
b. Follow every potentially scary statement with a statement of hope

2. Always show patients (and explain) VFs and OCTs
a. Helps them understand why you are testing as well as demonstrate any loss that may be asymptomatic or perceived
b. Creates buy-in and makes them part of the care team
i. Improves compliance
ii. Gives them feeling of control/power over disease

3. Be concerned, empathetic, but confident in delivering test results and treatment options/changes

4. Initial explanation/talking oints
a. Disease where fluid inside of eye builds up and puts pressure on the optic nerve and damages it
b. Nerve damage is unrepairable and results in loss of vision but fortunately there is treatment
c. Silent disease caught often on routine exam
i. By the time you notice vision changes, the disease stage is moderate
ii. You may not have symptoms now which means we caught this early
d. Regardless of presenting IOP, lowering IOP reduces risk of progression
e. Glaucoma is not cured, and treatment is lifelong
f. Treatment options include medicated eyedrops, non-invasive laser, and even surgery
g. Without treatment, vision loss and blindness can occur
h. Treatment is highly effective at preventing and reducing vision loss but sometimes despite best efforts, progression may occur

TABLE 8.8 Muckley's Treatment Algorithm and Management Plan after POAG Diagnosis

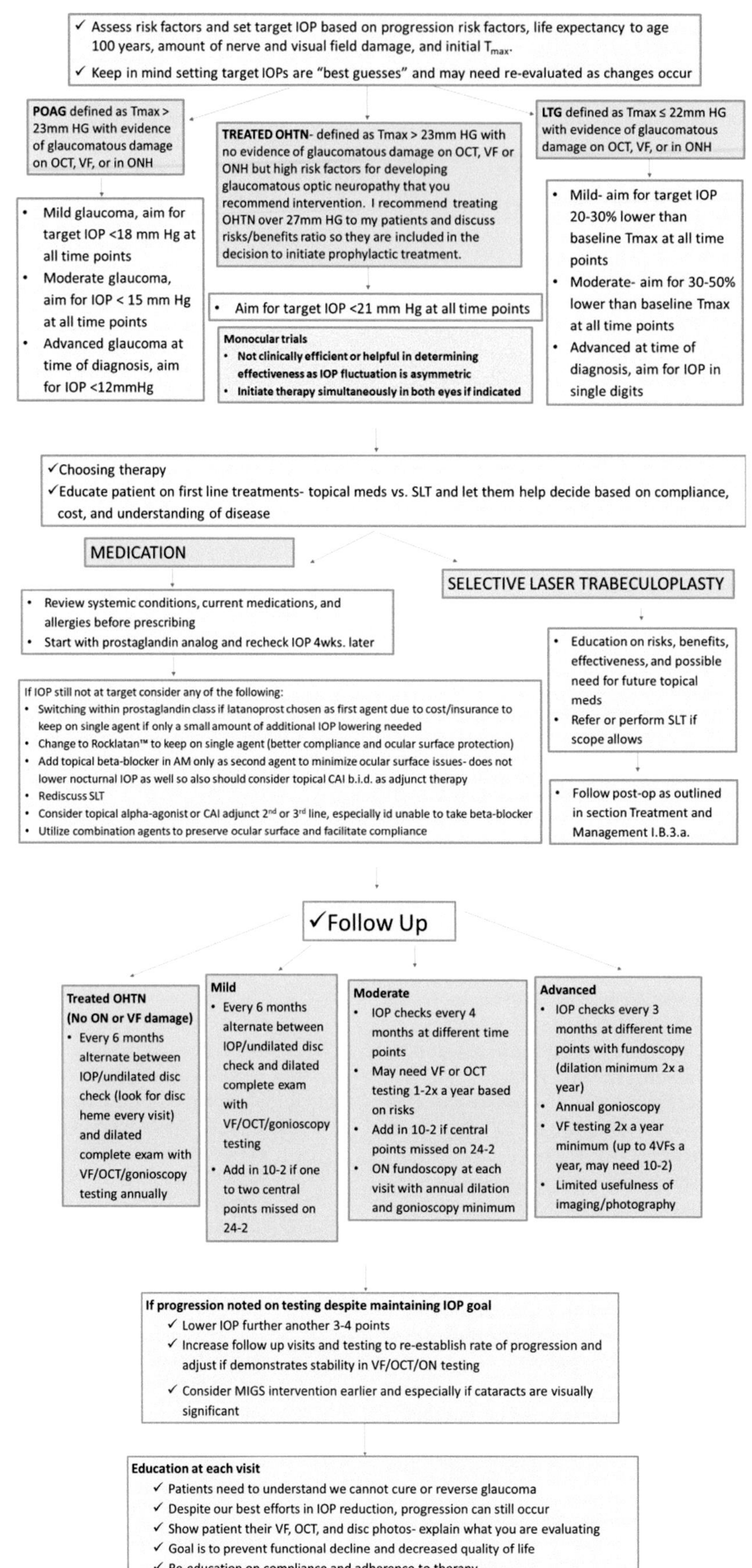

i. You need to do your part by adhering to my treatment and follow-up recommendations

5. Outside-the-box analogies of explaining glaucoma if unable to understand
   a. ON is like a cable that connects the eye to brain, just like a satellite dish cord connects to a TV. If you step on the cable over and over, you crush the cord causing the signal not to reach the TV to get a clear picture. The pressure in the eye is the same. If it builds up, it can crush the optic nerve and cause you to lose your picture signal just like the TV and satellite dish cable
   b. Eye is like a sink that connects to a drain. Over time the sink drainpipe becomes partially obstructed and cannot totally drain fluid in the basin from the running faucet. Eventually the sink is under pressure and can crack or break. This is what happens in the eye as fluid builds up in the back of the eye and causes nerve damage
6. Talking points if damage at time of presentation
   a. Unfortunately, your glaucoma has already caused some blind spots in your vision. However, we can start treatment today to aggressively lower the IOP and reduce the risk of further loss

B. Risk of Progression over Lifetime

1. Important to remind patients that even with IOP lowered, progression can occur despite best efforts
2. Progression explanations to patient
   a. Once a retinal nerve cell starts dying, it sends a message to the surrounding healthy cells that the environment is toxic, which causes them to die despite appearance of controlled IOP
   b. Think of ON like a tightrope that initially could hold a 200-lb person. Over time, a few individual threads snap and eventually the rope can no longer hold 200 lbs and you must lower the weight to 100 lbs
      i. So, if we see nerve damage despite your pressure being at original goal, we will need to adjust your target goal lower

C. Considerations in Compliance and Adherence

1. Compliance = level to which one follows medical advice
   a. Significant challenge in management
      i. Is my patient progressing because of the disease or because they are non-compliant?
   b. Non-compliance is one of main reasons for progression
      i. 50% of patients stopped glaucoma meds within first 6 months. of treatment[114]
         - Intentional factors: dissatisfaction, denial of disease, cost associated with medication
         - Unintentional factors: memory, confusion, difficulty with instilling drops, life interruptions
      ii. Other stats[115]
         - 20% do not follow up in the 18 months after diagnosis
         - Rates of non-adherence with glaucoma medications are 16 to 30%
      iii. Most common compliance barriers
         - Failing to have an Rx filled
         - Taking an incomplete dose
         - Taking the medication at the wrong time
         - Forgetting to take one or more meds
         - Stopping the medication
      iv. Categories of non-compliance
         - Regimen factors
           – Difficulty squeezing bottle, poor aim, side effects, obtaining refills (filling out mail forms, getting to pharmacy)
         - Patient factors
           – Cognitive disorders, motivation, acceptance of disease, fear, personal belief regarding medications, depression, male gender
         - Provider factors
           – Poor patient/doctor communication
           – Dissatisfaction with provider/healthcare system
           – Concealing noncompliance to be perceived as a "good patient"
         - Environmental factors
           – Lack of support
           – Major life event interrupters: health crisis, death of spouse, travel, change in insurance or formulary
         - The five big personality traits
           – Neuroticism: measures degree of emotional stability
           – Extraversion: describes degree of interpersonal interactions
           – Openness to experiences: estimates willingness to accept novel ideas
           – Agreeableness: estimates the quality of interpersonal orientation
           – Conscientiousness: estimates motivation in goal behavior motivation (best trait for adherence but influenced by extraversion and neuroticism)
2. Detecting non-compliance
   a. Ask open ended questions about treatment habits
      i. Tell/describe how you use your drops
   b. Look for signs of eyedrop use
      i. Long lashes with prostaglandin
      ii. Hyperemia
   c. Are pressures good but patient still progressing?
   d. Ask the patient to explain their understanding of glaucoma
   e. When in doubt, call the pharmacy to verify refills
3. Overcoming barriers
   a. Regimen factors
      i. Drop holders/auto droppers/bottle squeezer
      ii. Dosing schedule (once per day meds, AM versus PM)
      iii. Single agent, combination meds
      iv. Demonstrate/teach instillation
      v. Cost
         - Choosing from formulary
         - 90-day supply
         - Use generics
         - Drug company coupons or patient assistance programs
         - Recommend SLT, drug delivery devices, or MIGS procedures
      vi. Minimize tolerability/side effects (see "Treatment and Management," Section I. B. j.)
   b. Patient factors
      i. Memory cues
         - Written instructions

- Placing the drop with an item/activity done every day (toothbrush, saltshaker)
- Smartphone glaucoma apps
- Set phone alarm daily
- Online support from pharmaceutical companies for refill reminders
- Involve family member to help/social support

ii. Acceptance of disease

- Patient education (see Section II. A. and B.)

c. Environmental factors

i. Travel

- Give patient extra copy of Rx with 1 refill
- Have patient take sample size in carry on

ii. Major life events

- Enlist support of family and friends
- Help patient create new habits

iii. Provider factors

- Provider barrier is the one factor the optometrist can improve and control!!!
- Clinician–patient communication is foundation for adherence
- Communication issues
  - Education of disease and treatment options
  - Explanation of how to use meds and side effects
  - Give clear recommendation for follow-up visits
  - Listen to patient and let them help in decision making
  - Do not demean and scold patient
- Engage patient
  - Involve them in treatment decisions
  - Use eye contact, mindful body language, and active listening skills
- Expect patients to be non-compliant with drops
- Understand the categories of non-compliance and their barriers
- Recognize your patient's personality
- Consider non-compliance as a reason for progression
- Carefully document chart of non-compliant patients

III. Co-Management

A. Referral Relationship

1. Between glaucoma surgeon and optometrist for shared responsibility in patient's care
   a. Transfer of care
   b. Shared communication between providers

B. Optometrist Responsibility

1. Establish a relationship with local glaucoma specialist
2. Define roles of who is managing what
3. Observe specialist in clinic and surgery
   a. Know their surgical techniques and management preferences
4. Build mutual trust when co-managing patients
5. If you and surgeon are not in sync with regards to post-surgical treatment and management, increased risk of litigation

C. When to Refer

1. When you or the patient want a second opinion
2. When case is beyond scope of practice or risk of functional vision loss is increasing
3. When IOP is not at target despite modifications you made and surgery is best option
4. When on multiple medications and may need third-consider surgical evaluation for MIGS earlier than later
5. Non-compliance

IV. Reducing Liability

A. Follow Standard of Care and Preferred Practice Patterns

1. Don't be an outlier!
2. Keep up on latest technology

B. Get Second Opinion

1. Don't be afraid to collaborate if diagnosis not straightforward
2. Always follow through on an abnormal finding and order proper testing
3. If unclear, refer for second opinion

C. Refer for Surgical Intervention

1. If progression despite maximum medical therapy
2. Don't wait until vision loss advanced! Too late!

D. Detailed Chart Documentation for Risk Management

1. Non-compliance with recommendations
   a. Treatment
   b. Follow up visits
      i. Send certified letter if no-show or canceled and did not reschedule
   c. Testing
      i. If unable to perform or declines any testing, document reason
2. If patient declines your recommendations and you discuss risk of vision loss

E. Initial Documentation of Diagnosis

1. Glaucoma education and discussion with patient over importance of treatment, risks, loss of vision despite best efforts, and lifetime disease

F. Communication Excellence

1. Develop a trusting doctor–patient relationship
2. Be available to answer questions/concerns
3. Do not abandon
4. Communicate all findings and *listen*!

G. Financial Constraints

1. Consider cost as barrier to compliance
   a. Payment plans for office visits
   b. Set up medication assistance with drug company
      i. Provide samples of medications if available
   c. Refer for laser/MIGS if unable to afford meds
   d. Seek out free clinics and teaching institutions if no insurance
   e. If patient is a U.S. veteran, may qualify for VA benefits

H. Co-Management

1. Office staff should make an appointment before the patient leaves
2. Patient should be given the information about specialist
3. Provide information on patient's glaucoma status, medical records, and testing at every encounter promptly
4. Read consultation reports and act on recommendations of specialist

I. Reducing Medication Errors

1. In office
   a. Review and document all systemic and topical medications including dose with patient
      i. Over-the-counter medications
      ii. Nutritional supplements
      iii. Herbal drugs
   b. Confirm all drug allergies, past side effects, and intolerances
2. The prescription
   a. If written, ensure legible
   b. Specify correct medicine with correct dosage, site, frequency, and duration
   c. 90-day supply, large bottles, 1 year refill to increase compliance
   d. Document "Dispense As Written" (DAW) if no substitution wanted
   e. Review systemic meds and allergies before prescribing
3. Patient comprehension of regimen
   a. Provide written instructions (large font if sight challenged), include color coding of bottle caps
   b. Ask patient how and when they are using their drops—open ended questions
   c. Demonstrate proper drop instillation techniques
   d. Enlist help of family members
   e. Utilize artificial intelligence/smart technology to set reminders

J. Reasons Patients Go Blind from Glaucoma

1. Failure to diagnosis and/or advanced disease at time of initial diagnosis
2. Failure to lower IOP sufficiently and consistently at all time points
3. Inability to establish rate of progression
4. Poor patient compliance

It is our job as optometrists to use our diagnostic skills and all tools available to detect and treat glaucoma effectively in order to preserve functional vision and quality of life for the patients that have entrusted us!

References

1. Allingham RR, Damji KF, Freedman S, Moroi SE and Shafranov G. *Shields' Textbook of Glaucoma*. Philadelphia: Lippincott Williams Wilkins, 2005.
2. Gupta M, Bordoni B. Neuroanatomy, visual pathway. [Updated 2021 Feb 9]. In: *StatPearls* [Internet]. Treasure Island: StatPearls Publishing; 2021 Jan-. Available from: https://www.ncbi.nlm.nih.gov/books/NBK553189/
3. Tham YC, Li X, Wong TY, Quigley HA, Aung T, Cheng CY. Global prevalence of glaucoma and projections of glaucoma burden through 2040: a systematic review and meta-analysis. *Ophthalmology.* 2014;121(11):2081–2090. doi:10.1016/j.ophtha.2014.05.013
4. Friedman DS, Wolfs RC, O'Colmain BJ, et al. Prevalence of open-angle glaucoma among adults in the United States [published correction appears in Arch Ophthalmol. 2011 Sep;129(9):1224]. *Arch Ophthalmol.* 2004;122(4):532–538. doi:10.1001/archopht.122.4.532
5. U.S. Department of Health and Human Services, National Institutes of Health, National Eye Institute. 2010. https://www.nei.nih.gov/learn-about-eye-health/outreach-campaigns-and-resources/eye-health-data-and-statistics/glaucoma-data-and-statistics
6. Allison K, Patel D, Alabi O. Epidemiology of glaucoma: the past, present, and predictions for the future. *Cureus.* 2020;12(11):e11686. Published 2020 Nov 24. doi:10.7759/cureus.11686
7. McMonnies CW. Glaucoma history and risk factors. *J Optom.* 2017;10(2):71–78. doi:10.1016/j.optom.2016.02.003
8. Ritch R, Steinberger D, Liebmann JM. Prevalence of pigment dispersion syndrome in a population undergoing glaucoma screening. *Am J Ophthalmol.* 1993;115(6):707–710.
9. Fan BJ, Pasquale LR, Rhee D, et al. LOXL1 promoter haplotypes are associated with exfoliation syndrome in a U.S. Caucasian population. *Invest Ophthalmol Vis Sci M.* 2011;52(5):2372–2378.
10. Alward WL, Kwon YH, Khanna CL, et al. Variations in the myocilin gene in patients with open-angle glaucoma. *Arch Ophthalmol M.* 2002;120(9):1189–1197.
11. Lim SH, Tran-Viet KN, Yanovitch TL, et al. CYP1B1, MYOC, and LTBP2 mutations in primary congenital glaucoma patients in the United States. *Am J Ophthalmol M.* 2013;155(3):508–517.
12. World Health Organization. 2021. https://www.who.int/news-room/fact-sheets/detail/blindness-and-visual-impairment
13. Susanna R Jr, De Moraes CG, Cioffi GA, Ritch R. Why do people (still) go blind from glaucoma?. *Transl Vis Sci Technol.* 2015;4(2):1. Published 2015 Mar 9. doi:10.1167/tvst.4.2.1
14. Burgoyne CF, Downs JC, Bellezza AJ, Suh JK, Hart RT. The optic nerve head as a biomechanical structure: a new paradigm for understanding the role of IOP-related stress and strain in the pathophysiology of glaucomatous optic nerve head damage. *Prog Retin Eye Res.* 2005;24(1):39–73. doi:10.1016/j.preteyeres.2004.06.001
15. Weinreb RN, Aung T, Medeiros FA. The pathophysiology and treatment of glaucoma: a review. *JAMA.* 2014;311(18):1901–1911. doi:10.1001/jama.2014.3192
16. Barnett EM, Fantin A, Wilson BS, Kass MA, Gordon MO; Ocular Hypertension Treatment Study Group. The incidence of retinal vein occlusion in the ocular hypertension treatment study. *Ophthalmology.* 2010;117(3):484–488. doi:10.1016/j.ophtha.2009.08.022
17. Berdahl JP, Allingham RR, Johnson DH. Cerebrospinal fluid pressure is decreased in primary open-angle glaucoma. *Ophthalmology.* 2008;115(5):763–768. doi:10.1016/j.ophtha.2008.01.013
18. Kiuchi T, Motoyama Y, Oshika T. Postural response of intraocular pressure and visual field damage in patients with untreated normal-tension glaucoma. *J Glaucoma.* 2010;19(3):191–193. doi:10.1097/IJG.0b013e3181a98f30
19. Kim KN, Jeoung JW, Park KH, Kim DM, Ritch R. Relationship between preferred sleeping position and asymmetric visual field loss in open-angle glaucoma patients. *Am J Ophthalmol.* 2014;157(3):739–745. doi:10.1016/j.ajo.2013.12.016
20. Zimprich L, Diedrich J, Bleeker A, Schweitzer JA. Corneal hysteresis as a biomarker of glaucoma: Current insights. *Clin Ophthalmol.* 2020;14:2255–2264. Published 2020 Aug 10. doi:10.2147/OPTH.S236114
21. Gordon MO, Beiser JA, Brandt JD, et al. The ocular hypertension treatment study: baseline factors that predict the onset of primary open-angle glaucoma. *Arch Ophthalmol.* 2002;120(6):714–830. doi:10.1001/archopht.120.6.714
22. Shimmyo M, Ross AJ, Moy A, Mostafavi R. Intraocular pressure, Goldmann applanation tension, corneal thickness, and corneal curvature in Caucasians, Asians, Hispanics, and

African Americans. *Am J Ophthalmol.* 2003;136(4):603–613. doi:10.1016/s0002-9394(03)00424-0

23. Tezel G. TNF-alpha signaling in glaucomatous neurodegeneration. *Prog Brain Res.* 2008;173:409–421. doi:10.1016/S0079-6123(08)01128-X
24. Chen H, Cho KS, Vu THK, et al. Commensal microflora-induced T cell responses mediate progressive neurodegeneration in glaucoma [published correction appears in Nat Commun. 2018 Sep 20;9(1):3914]. *Nat Commun.* 2018;9(1):3209. Published 2018 Aug 10. doi:10.1038/s41467-018-05681-9
25. Flammer J, Orgül S, Costa VP, et al. The impact of ocular blood flow in glaucoma. *Prog Retin Eye Res.* 2002;21(4):359–393. doi:10.1016/s1350-9462(02)00008-3
26. Quaid P, Simpson T, Freddo T. Relationship between diastolic perfusion pressure and progressive optic neuropathy as determined by Heidelberg retinal tomography topographic change analysis. *Invest Ophthalmol Vis Sci.* 2013;54(1):789–798. Published 2013 Jan 28. doi:10.1167/iovs.12-11177
27. Kwon J, Jo YH, Jeong D, Shon K, Kook MS. Baseline systolic versus diastolic blood pressure dip and subsequent visual field progression in normal-tension glaucoma. *Ophthalmology.* 2019;126(7):967–979. doi:10.1016/j.ophtha.2019.03.001
28. Zheng W, Dryja TP, Wei Z, et al. Systemic medication associations with presumed advanced or uncontrolled primary open-angle glaucoma. *Ophthalmology.* 2018;125(7):984–993. doi:10.1016/j.ophtha.2018.01.007
29. Tamm ER, Braunger BM, Fuchshofer R. Intraocular pressure and the mechanisms involved in resistance of the aqueous humor flow in the trabecular meshwork outflow pathways. *Prog Mol Biol Transl Sci.* 2015;134:301–314. doi:10.1016/bs.pmbts.2015.06.007
30. Cavet ME, Vittitow JL, Impagnatiello F, Ongini E, Bastia E. Nitric oxide (NO): an emerging target for the treatment of glaucoma. *Invest Ophthalmol Vis Sci.* 2014;55(8):5005–5015. Published 2014 Aug 14. doi:10.1167/iovs.14-14515
31. Greenfield DS. Glaucomatous versus nonglaucomatous optic disc cupping: clinical differentiation. *Semin Ophthalmol.* 1999;14(2):95–108. doi:10.3109/08820539909056069
32. Wong B, Parikh D, Rosen L, Gorski M, Angelilli A, Shih C. Comparison of disposable goldmann applanation tonometer, ICare ic100, and tonopen XL to standards of care goldmann nondisposable applanation tonometer for measuring intraocular pressure. *J Glaucoma.* 2018;27(12):1119–1124. doi:10.1097/IJG.0000000000001059
33. Goldmann H, Schmidt T. Uber Applanationstonometrie [Applanation tonometry]. *Ophthalmologica.* 1957;134(4):221–242. doi:10.1159/000303213
34. Lichter PR. Iris processes in 340 eyes. *Am J Ophthalmol.* 1969;68(5):872–878. doi:10.1016/0002-9394(69)94583-8
35. Hejl A, Patella V, *Bengtsson B. The Field Analyzer Primer: Effective Perimetry.* Carl Zeiss Meditec Incorporated, 2012.
36. Quigley HA, Dunkelberger GR, Green WR. Retinal ganglion cell atrophy correlated with automated perimetry in human eyes with glaucoma. *Am J Ophthalmol.* 1989;107(5):453–64.
37. Le PV, Zhang X, Francis BA, et al. Advanced imaging for glaucoma study: design, baseline characteristics, and intersite comparison. *Am J Ophthalmol.* 2015;159(2):393-403.e2. doi:10.1016/j.ajo.2014.11.010
38. Rolle T, Dallorto L. Bonetti B. Retinal and macular ganglion cell count estimated with optical coherence tomography RTVUE-100 as a candidate biomarker for glaucoma. *Invest Ophthalmol Vis Sci.* 2016;57(13):5772–5779. doi:10.1167/iovs.15-18882
39. Johnson CA, Adams AJ, Casson EJ, Brandt JD. Blue-on-yellow perimetry can predict the development of glaucomatous visual field loss. *Arch Ophthalmol.* 1993;111(5):645–650. doi:10.1001/archopht.1993.01090050079034
40. Zimprich L, Diedrich J, Bleeker A, Schweitzer JA. Corneal hysteresis as a biomarker of glaucoma: current insights. *Clin Ophthalmol.* 2020;14:2255–2264. Published 2020 Aug 10. doi:10.2147/OPTH.S236114
41. Banitt MR, Ventura LM, Feuer WJ, et al. Progressive loss of retinal ganglion cell function precedes structural loss by several years in glaucoma suspects. *Invest Ophthalmol Vis Sci.* 2013;54(3):2346–2352. Published 2013 Mar 28. doi:10.1167/iovs.12-11026
42. Kahn HA, Leibowitz HM, Ganley JP, et al. The framingham eye study. I. Outline and major prevalence findings. *Am J Epidemiol.* 1977;106(1):17–32. doi:10.1093/oxfordjournals.aje.a112428
43. Harizman N, Oliveira C, Chiang A, et al. The ISNT rule and differentiation of normal from glaucomatous eyes. *Arch Ophthalmol.* 2006;124(11):1579–1583. doi:10.1001/archopht.124.11.1579
44. Drance SM, Begg IS. Sector haemorrhage: a probable acute ischaemic disc change in chronic simple glaucoma. *Can J Ophthalmol.* 1970;5(2):137–141.
45. Budenz DL, Huecker JB, Gedde SJ, Gordon M, Kass M; Ocular Hypertension Treatment Study Group. Thirteen-year follow-up of optic disc hemorrhages in the ocular hypertension treatment study. *Am J Ophthalmol.* 2017;174:126–133. doi:10.1016/j.ajo.2016.10.023
46. Quigley HA, Addicks EM, Green WR. Optic nerve damage in human glaucoma. III. Quantitative correlation of nerve fiber loss and visual field defect in glaucoma, ischemic neuropathy, papilledema, and toxic neuropathy. *Arch Ophthalmol* 1982 Jan;100(1):135–146.
47. Keltner JL, Johnson CA, Cello KE, et al. Classification of visual field abnormalities in the ocular hypertension treatment study [published correction appears in Arch Ophthalmol. 2008 Apr;126(4):561]. *Arch Ophthalmol.* 2003;121(5):643–650. doi:10.1001/archopht.121.5.643
48. Hodapp E, Parrish RK II, Anderson DR. *Clinical decisions in glaucoma.* St Louis: The CV Mosby Co; 1993. pp. 52–61.
49. Advanced Glaucoma Intervention Study. 2Visual field test scoring and reliability. *Ophthalmology.* 1994;101(8):1445–1455.
50. Ronald L, Fellman OCS, Mattox CG. Know the new glaucoma staging codes. *Eyenet.* Published Oct 2011. file:///C:/Users/dredm/Downloads/Know-the-New-Glaucoma-Staging-Codes-PDF%20(1).pdf
51. Budenz DL, Anderson DR, Varma R, et al. Determinants of normal retinal nerve fiber layer thickness measured by Stratus OCT. *Ophthalmology.* 2007;114(6):1046–1052.
52. Hood D, Kardon R. A framework for comparing structural and functional measurements of glaucomatous damage. *Prog Retin Eye Res* 2007;26:688–710.
53. Lim HB, Kim YW, Nam KY, et al. Signal strength as an important factor in the analysis of peripapillary microvascular density using optical coherence tomography angiography. *Sci Rep* 2019;9:16299. https://doi.org/10.1038/s41598-019-52818-x
54. Budenz DL. Symmetry between the right and left eyes of the normal retinal nerve fiber layer measured with optical coherence tomography (an AOS thesis). *Trans Am Ophthalmol Soc.* 2008;106: 252–275.
55. Mwanza JC, Durbin MK, Budenz DL, et al. Profile and predictors of normal ganglion cell-inner plexiform layer thickness measured with frequency-domain optical coherence tomography. *Investig Ophthalmol Vis Sci* 2011;52:11:7872–7879.
56. Xu X, Xiao H, Guo X, et al. Diagnostic ability of macular ganglion cell-inner plexiform layer thickness in glaucoma suspects. *Med.* 2017;96:51:e9182.
57. Anderson AJ. Significant glaucomatous visual field progression in the first two years: what does it mean? [published correction appears in Transl Vis Sci Technol. 2017 Feb 10;6(1):10]. *Transl Vis Sci Technol.* 2016;5(6):1. Published 2016 Nov 1. doi:10.1167/tvst.5.6.1
58. Deutsch TA, Weinreb RN, Goldberg MF. Indications for surgical management of hyphema in patients with sickle cell trait. *Arch Ophthalmol.* 1984;102(4):566–569. doi:10.1001/archopht.1984.01040030444022
59. American Academy of Ophthalmology Preferred Practice Patterns Committee GP. *Ophthalmology.* Chicago: American Academy of Ophtalmology; 2010. Preferred practice pattern: primary open-angle glaucoma

60. The Advanced Glaucoma Intervention Study (AGIS): 4. Comparison of treatment outcomes within race. Seven-year results. *Ophthalmology.* 1998;105(7):1146–1164. doi:10.1016/s0161-6420(98)97013-0
61. Heijl A, Leske MC, Bengtsson B, et al. Reduction of intraocular pressure and glaucoma progression: results from the early manifest glaucoma trial. *Arch Ophthalmol.* 2002;120(10):1268–1279. doi:10.1001/archopht.120.10.1268
62. Musch DC, Lichter PR, Guire KE, Standardi CL. The collaborative initial glaucoma treatment study: study design, methods, and baseline characteristics of enrolled patients. *Ophthalmology.* 1999;106(4):653–662. doi:10.1016/s0161-6420(99)90147-1
63. Comparison of glaucomatous progression between untreated patients with normal-tension glaucoma and patients with therapeutically reduced intraocular pressures. Collaborative Normal-Tension Glaucoma Study Group [published correction appears in Am J Ophthalmol 1999 Jan;127(1):120]. *Am J Ophthalmol.* 1998;126(4):487–497. doi:10.1016/s0002-9394(98)00223-2
64. Kass MA, Heuer DK, Higginbotham EJ, et al. The ocular hypertension treatment study: a randomized trial determines that topical ocular hypotensive medication delays or prevents the onset of primary open-angle glaucoma. *Arch Ophthalmol.* 2002;120(6):701–830. doi:10.1001/archopht.120.6.701
65. Sambhara D, Aref AA. Glaucoma management: relative value and place in therapy of available drug treatments. *Ther Adv Chronic Dis.* 2014;5(1):30–43. doi:10.1177/2040622313511286
66. Chen HY, Huang WC, Lin CL, Kao CH. Association between topical beta-blockers and risks of cardiovascular and respiratory disease in patients with glaucoma: a retrospective cohort study. *BMJ Open.* 2020;10(7):e034361. Published 2020 Jul 22. doi:10.1136/bmjopen-2019-034361
67. Toris CB, Gabelt BT, Kaufman PL. Update on the mechanism of action of topical prostaglandins for intraocular pressure reduction. *Surv Ophthalmol.* 2008;53(SUPPL1):S107–S120. doi:10.1016/j.survophthal.2008.08.010
68. Perry CM, McGavin JK, Culy CR, Ibbotson T. Latanoprost: an update of its use in glaucoma and ocular hypertension. *Drugs Aging.* 2003;20(8):597–630. doi:10.2165/00002512-200320080-00005
69. Tang W, Zhang F, Liu K, Duan X. Efficacy and safety of prostaglandin analogues in primary open-angle glaucoma or ocular hypertension patients: A meta-analysis. *Medicine.* 2019;98(30):e16597. doi:10.1097/MD.0000000000016597
70. García-Feijoo J, Martínez-de-la-Casa JM, Castillo A, Méndez C, Fernández-Vidal A, García-Sánchez J. Circadian IOP-lowering efficacy of travoprost 0.004% ophthalmic solution compared to latanoprost 0.005%. *Curr Med Res Opin.* 2006;22(9):1689–1697. doi:10.1185/030079906X120959
71. Chabi A, Varma R, Tsai JC, et al. Randomized clinical trial of the efficacy and safety of preservative-free tafluprost and timolol in patients with open-angle glaucoma or ocular hypertension. *Am J Ophthalmol.* 2012;153(6):1187–1196. doi:10.1016/j.ajo.2011.11.008
72. Weinreb RN, Ong T, Scassellati Sforzolini B, et al. A randomised, controlled comparison of latanoprostene bunod and latanoprost 0.005% in the treatment of ocular hypertension and open angle glaucoma: the VOYAGER study. *Br J Ophthalmol.* 2015;99(6):738–745. doi:10.1136/bjophthalmol-2014-305908
73. Cantor LB. Brimonidine in the treatment of glaucoma and ocular hypertension. *Ther Clin Risk Manag.* 2006;2(4):337–346. doi:10.2147/tcrm.2006.2.4.337
74. Strom BL, Schinnar R, Apter AJ, et al. Absence of cross-reactivity between sulfonamide antibiotics and sulfonamide nonantibiotics. *N Engl J Med.* 2003;349(17):1628–1635. doi:10.1056/NEJMoa022963
75. Gábor Holló. *Glaucoma* (Second Edition) Volume 1, pages 559–565, 2015. Elsevier.
76. Tanna AP, Rademaker AW, Stewart WC, Feldman RM. Meta-analysis of the efficacy and safety of alpha2-adrenergic agonists, beta-adrenergic antagonists, and topical carbonic anhydrase inhibitors with prostaglandin analogs. *Arch Ophthalmol.* 2010;128(7):825–833. doi:10.1001/archophthalmol.2010.131
77. Balfour JA, Wilde MI. Dorzolamide. *Drugs & Aging* 1997;10:384–403.
78. Lester M. Brinzolamide ophthalmic suspension: a review of its pharmacology and use in the treatment of open angle glaucoma and ocular hypertension. *Clin Ophthalmol.* 2008;2(3):517–523. doi:10.2147/opth.s3182
79. Drance SM, Nash PA. The dose response of human intraocular pressure to pilocarpine. *Can J Ophthalmol.* 1971;6(1):9–13.
80. Serle JB, Katz LJ, McLaurin E, et al. Two phase 3 clinical trials comparing the safety and efficacy of netarsudil to timolol in patients with elevated intraocular pressure: rho kinase elevated IOP treatment trial 1 and 2 (ROCKET-1 and ROCKET-2). *Am J Ophthalmol.* 2018;186:116–127. doi:10.1016/j.ajo.2017.11.019
81. Higginbotham EJ. Considerations in glaucoma therapy: fixed combinations versus their component medications. *Clin Ophthalmol.* 2010;4:1–9. Published 2010 Feb 2.
82. Henderer JD, Wilson RP, Moster MR, et al. Timolol/dorzolamide combination therapy as initial treatment for intraocular pressure over 30 mm Hg. *J Glaucoma.* 2005;14(4):267–270. doi:10.1097/01.ijg.0000169389.09804.33
83. Sherwood MB, Craven ER, Chou C, et al. Twice-daily 0.2% brimonidine-0.5% timolol fixed-combination therapy vs monotherapy with timolol or brimonidine in patients with glaucoma or ocular hypertension: a 12-month randomized trial. *Arch Ophthalmol.* 2006;124(9):1230–1238. doi:10.1001/archopht.124.9.1230
84. Fechtner RD, Harasymowycz P, Nixon DR, et al. Twelve-week, randomized, multicenter study comparing a fixed combination of brimonidine-timolol with timolol as therapy adjunctive to latanoprost. *Clin Ophthalmol.* 2011;5:945–953. doi:10.2147/OPTH.S19999
85. Motolko MA. Comparison of allergy rates in glaucoma patients receiving brimonidine 0.2% monotherapy versus fixed-combination brimonidine 0.2%-timolol 0.5% therapy. *Curr Med Res Opin.* 2008;24(9):2663–2667. doi:10.1185/03007990802333167
86. Gandolfi SA, Lim J, Sanseau AC, Parra Restrepo JC, Hamacher T. Randomized trial of brinzolamide/brimonidine versus brinzolamide plus brimonidine for open-angle glaucoma or ocular hypertension. *Adv Ther.* 2014;31(12):1213–1227. doi:10.1007/s12325-014-0168-y
87. Fechtner RD, Myers JS, Hubatsch DA, Budenz DL, DuBiner HB. Ocular hypotensive effect of fixed-combination brinzolamide/brimonidine adjunctive to a prostaglandin analog: a randomized clinical trial. *Eye.* 2016;30(10):1343–1350. doi:10.1038/eye.2016.126
88. Asrani S, Bacharach J, Holland E, et al. Fixed-dose combination of netarsudil and latanoprost in ocular hypertension and open-angle glaucoma: pooled efficacy/safety analysis of phase 3 MERCURY-1 and -2. *Adv Ther.* 2020;37(4):1620–1631. doi:10.1007/s12325-020-01277-2
89. https://www.pfizer.ca/sites/default/files/202005/XALACOM_PM_E_237590_2020.05.07.pdf
90. https://allergan-web-cdn-prod.azureedge.net/allerganaustralia/allerganaustralia/media/allergan-australia/products/pdfs/pi/ganfort-0-3-5-piv4-cds3-02oct19.pdf
91. https://www.novartis.com.sg/sites/www.novartis.com.sg/files/product-info/Duotrav-Jun2020.SIN-App110920-pdf.pdf
92. Călugăru M, Călugăru D. Azargao nouă şi utilă combinatie medicaméntoasă fixă în tratamentul glaucomului [Azarga, a new and useful fixed combination in glaucoma treatment]. *Oftalmologia.* 2011;55(3):38–46.
93. Goldstein MH, Silva FQ, Blender N, et al. Ocular benzalkonium chloride exposure: problems and solutions. *Eye.* 2022;36:361–368.
94. van der Valk R, Webers CA, Schouten JS, Zeegers MP, Hendrikse F, Prins MH. Intraocular pressure-lowering effects of all commonly used glaucoma drugs: a meta-analysis of randomized clinical trials. *Ophthalmology.* 2005;112(7):1177–1185. doi:10.1016/j.ophtha.2005.01.042
95. Medeiros FA, Walters TR, Kolko M, et al. Phase 3, randomized, 20-month study of bimatoprost implant in open-angle glaucoma and ocular hypertension (ARTEMIS 1). *Ophthalmology.* 2020;127(12):1627–1641. doi:10.1016/j.ophtha.2020.06.018

96. Leahy KE, White AJ. Selective laser trabeculoplasty: current perspectives. *Clin Ophthalmol.* 2015;9:833–841. Published 2015 May 11. doi:10.2147/OPTH.S53490
97. Garg A, Vickerstaff V, Nathwani N, et al. Efficacy of repeat selective laser trabeculoplasty in medication-naive open-angle glaucoma and ocular hypertension during the LiGHT trial. *Ophthalmology.* 2020;127(4):467–476. doi:10.1016/j.ophtha.2019.10.023
98. Bournias TE, Lai J. *AAO Paper.* Las Vegas; 2006.
99. Realini. Clarifying the optimal application of SLT therapy trial (COAST). *ClinicalTrials.gov* Identifier: NCT04967989. https://clinicaltrials.gov/ct2/show/NCT04967989
100. Aquino MC, Barton K, Tan AM, et al. Micropulse versus continuous wave transscleral diode cyclophotocoagulation in refractory glaucoma: a randomized exploratory study. *Clin Exp Ophthalmol.* 2015;43(1):40–46. doi:10.1111/ceo.12360
101. Francis BA, Berke SJ, Dustin L, Noecker R. Endoscopic cyclophotocoagulation combined with phacoemulsification versus phacoemulsification alone in medically controlled glaucoma. *J Cataract Refract Surg.* 2014;40(8):1313–1321. doi:10.1016/j.jcrs.2014.06.021
102. Tong W, Shen TYT, Wong HC, Aquino MC, Chew P, Lim D. One-year outcomes of micropulse cyclophototherapy for primary open-angle glaucoma. *J Glaucoma.* 2021;30(10):911–920. doi:10.1097/IJG.0000000000001925
103. Samuelson TW, Sarkisian SR Jr, Lubeck DM, et al. Prospective, randomized, controlled pivotal trial of an ab interno implanted trabecular micro-bypass in primary open-angle glaucoma and cataract: two-year results. *Ophthalmology.* 2019;126(6):811–821. doi:10.1016/j.ophtha.2019.03.006
104. Ahmed IIK, Rhee DJ, Jones J, et al. Three-year findings of the HORIZON trial: A schlemm canal microstent for pressure reduction in primary open-angle glaucoma and cataract. *Ophthalmology.* 2021;128(6):857–865. doi:10.1016/j.ophtha.2020.11.004
105. Lewis RA. Ab interno approach to the subconjunctival space using a collagen glaucoma stent. *J Cataract Refract Surg.* 2014;40(8):1301–1306. doi:10.1016/j.jcrs.2014.01.032
106. Vold SD, Williamson BK, Hirsch L, et al. Canaloplasty and trabeculotomy with the OMNI system in pseudophakic patients with open-angle glaucoma: The ROMEO study. *Ophthalmol Glaucoma.* 2021;4(2):173–181. doi:10.1016/j.ogla.2020.10.001
107. Chauhan BC, Garway-Heath DF, Goñi FJ, et al. Practical recommendations for measuring rates of visual field change in glaucoma. *Br J Ophthalmol.* 2008;92(4):569–573. doi:10.1136/bjo.2007.135012
108. Kirwan JF, Hustler A, Bobat H, Toms L, Crabb DP, McNaught AI. Portsmouth visual field database: an audit of glaucoma progression. *Eye.* 2014;28(8): 974–979. doi:10.1038/eye.2013.294
109. Saunders LJ, Medeiros FA, Weinreb RN, Zangwill LM. What rates of glaucoma progression are clinically significant?. *Expert Rev Ophthalmol.* 2016;11(3):227–234. doi:10.1080/17469899.2016.1180246
110. Mwanza JC, Chang RT, Budenz DL, et al. Reproducibility of peripapillary retinal nerve fiber layer thickness and optic nerve head parameters measured with Cirrus HD-OCT in glaucomatous eyes. *Invest Ophthalmol Vis Sci.* 2010;51(11):5724–5730.
111. Leung CK, Yu M, Weinreb RN, et al. Retinal nerve fiber layer imaging with spectral-domain optical coherence tomography: patterns of retinal nerve fiber layer progression. *Ophthalmology.* 2012;119:1858–1866.
112. Crabb DP, Russell RA, Malik R, et al. *Frequency of visual field testing when monitoring patients newly diagnosed with glaucoma: mixed methods and modelling.* Southampton: NIHR Journals Library; 2014 Aug.
113. Wu Z, Saunders LJ, Daga FB, Diniz-Filho A, Medeiros FA. Frequency of testing to detect visual field progression derived using a longitudinal cohort of glaucoma patients. *Ophthalmology.* 2017;124(6):786–792. doi:10.1016/j.ophtha.2017.01.027
114. Nordstrom BL, Friedman DS, Mozaffari E, Quigley HA, Walker AM. Persistence and adherence with topical glaucoma therapy. *Am J Ophthalmol.* 2005;140(4):598–606. doi:10.1016/j.ajo.2005.04.051
115. Robin AL, Muir KW. Medication adherence in patients with ocular hypertension or glaucoma, *Expert Rev Ophthalmol.* 14:4–5, 199–210. doi:10.1080/17469899.2019.1635456

Chapter 9
SYSTEMIC CONSIDERATIONS IN ANTERIOR SEGMENT CARE
Diagnostic Entities by Medical Specialties and Classification

Chapter Outline

DOI: 10.1201/9781003255598-9

I. Medical Specialties

A. Cardiology

1. Marfan's Syndrome (MFS)[1–3]

a. Etiology and pathogenesis
   i. 75% autosomal-dominant with variable expression
   ii. Defective formation of collagen and elastic fibers
   iii. May occur sporadically as mutation
b. Physical findings
   i. Skeletal
      - Slender, tall stature
      - Long arms, legs, fingers
      - Flat-footed and long and narrow feet
      - High arched palate
      - Hyperextensible joints
   ii. Cardiac
      - Mitral valve prolapse (floppy heart valves)
      - Aneurysmal dilation
      - Dissecting aneurysm
   iii. Ocular
      - Crystalline lens displaced superior, and temporal (ectopic lentis superotemporally) (diagnostic for MFS) causes mild to moderate visual impairment
      - Segmental hypoplasia of iris
      - Early and severe myopia due to increased axial length
      - Strabismus
      - Flat cornea
      - Early cataract
      - Retinal detachment
      - Fetal anterior chamber angle
      - Zonular lysis
c. Laboratory test
   i. Urinary excretion of hydroxyproline
   ii. Differentiate from homocystinuria
d. Clinical course
   i. May survive to 70 years old
   ii. Average death 30 to 40 years old, attributable to aortic rupture

2. Subacute Bacterial Endocarditis[4,5]

a. Epidemiology
   i. Occurs on damaged heart valves, as in rheumatic heart disease or congenital heart disease
   ii. Artificial valves
   iii. Intravenous (IV) drug abusers
b. Etiology and pathogenesis
   i. *Streptococcus viridens* infection of a previously damaged heart valve in presence of turbulent blood flow
c. Symptomatology
   i. Fever, night sweats, malaise, fatigue, backache, myalgia, arthralgia
   ii. Symptoms for weeks or months
   iii. Often responsible for fevers of unknown origin (FUO)
d. Physical findings
   i. Ocular manifestations of embolic disease
      - Roth spot hemorrhage of retina or conjunctiva
      - Retinal hemorrhage
      - Infectious vitritis
   ii. Osler's nodes: raised, purple-pink, tender lesions on pads of fingers and toes
   iii. Janeway lesions: irregular, non-tender, hemorrhagic lesions of palms or soles
   iv. New or changing cardiac murmur
   v. Pale skin, splenomegaly
e. Diagnostic tests
   i. Blood cultures, echocardiogram
   ii. Increased erythrocyte sedimentation rate (ESR), leukocytosis, anemia
   iii. Cardiac ultrasound
f. Treatment
   i. Antibiotics: prolonged IV therapy 4 to 6 weeks
   ii. Prophylaxis: patients with acquired valve disorder or artificial valves should take antibiotics prior to any surgical manipulation (e.g., dental work)
g. Clinical course
   i. Untreated, it is usually fatal
   ii. Usual cause of death in treated cases is congestive heart failure
   iii. Cardiac valve destruction
   iv. Renal damage
   v. Hemiplegia or other embolic phenomena 25%

B. Dermatology

1. Acne Rosacea[6] *(See Chapter 5, III. D. 1.)*

a. Epidemiology (Figure 9.1)
   i. Equal gender distribution, 30 to 60 years old
   ii. More common with alcoholics, high carbohydrate intake, and hyperchlorhydria
   iii. Approximately 20% of patients have ocular findings
   iv. Approximately 4% keratitis

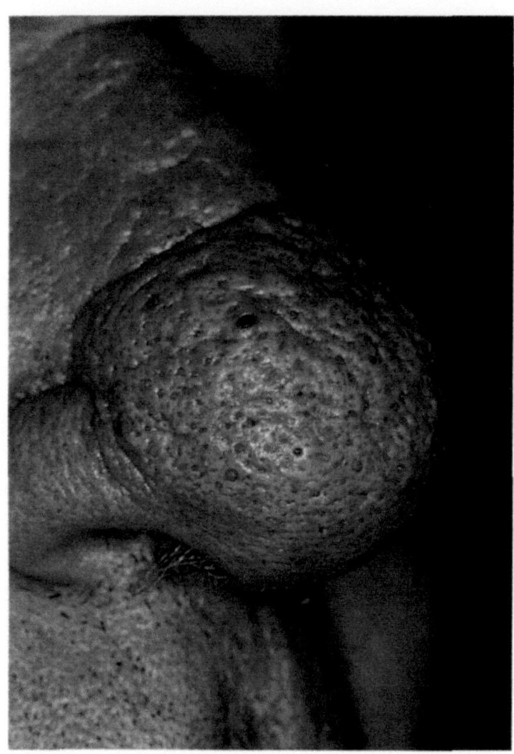

FIGURE 9.1 Acne rosacea (rhinophyma) is a dermatological disorder with a high frequency (greater than 50%) of associated ocular involvement ranging from blepharitis and recurrent chalazia to complicated blepharokeratoconjunctivitis. This figure shows rhinophyma (the "W.C. Fields' look"), which is a common dermatological sign in rosacea.

b. Symptomatology
  i. Transient attacks of flushing of the nose and cheeks occur initially
  ii. Variable ocular (lids and eye) involvement
c. Physical findings
  i. Mid-face: chronic congestion of capillaries, telangiectasis, sebaceous gland hypertrophy, rhinophyma of nose
  ii. Red areas of malar region with blepharitis, keratitis, conjunctivitis
d. Treatment
  i. Topical treatments
    - Metronidazole 0.75% gel
    - Finacea (azelaic acid) foam
    - Mirvaso (brimonidine) gel
    - Ivermectin cream 1%
  ii. Doxycycline orally to decrease propionibacteria and free fatty acids (FFA)
  iii. Balanced nutrition
  iv. Cleansing and drying preparations
  v. Penetrating keratoplasty if severe keratitis
e. Clinical course
  i. Approximately 25% recur soon after doxy stopped
  ii. Approximately 50% recur within 6 months of stopping doxy
  iii. Approximately 20% long-term remission
f. Anterior segment manifestations
  i. Blepharoconjunctivitis: thickened vascularized lids
  ii. Keratitis: marginal vascular infiltration followed by subepithelial-infiltrates that ulcerate and progress centrally
  iii. Recurrent chalazia secondary to superimposed staphylococcal infection

2. *Allergic Contact Dermatitis*[7]

a. Etiology
  i. T cell-mediated local allergic reaction to a usually innocuous agent (allergen)
  ii. Frequent lid involvement secondary to makeup or rubbing the eyes with contaminated fingers
b. Physical findings: classic signs of inflammation (redness, swelling, oozing, warmth) and symptoms (itch)
c. Diagnosis
  i. Inspection
  ii. History
  iii. Patch test to identify allergen
d. Treatment
  i. Removal of caustic agent
  ii. Protective arrangement with proper clothes
  iii. Topical steroid
  iv. Topical calcineurin-inhibitors (e.g., tacrolimus) for chronic treatment
  v. Benadryl for itching
e. Anterior segment manifestation
  i. Atopic blepharoconjunctivitis

3. *Basal Cell Epithelioma (See Chapter 3, II. A.)*

a. Epidemiology
  i. Most common malignancy of eyelid, 20 to 40 times more common than squamous cell
  ii. Sun-exposed skin
  iii. Lower lid more frequently than upper
  iv. Light-skinned patients most often affected
  v. Usually over 40 years of age
b. Etiology and pathogenesis
  i. Excessive exposure to ultraviolet (UV) irradiation from sunlight
  ii. Cumulative throughout life
c. Physical findings
  i. Painless, indurated, firm, pearly nodule, with heaped-up telangiectatic border
  ii. Ulceration may or may not be present
  iii. Less than 2 cm in diameter
  iv. Multiple sites
  v. Individual lesions may vary greatly from classic lesions
d. Diagnostic tests
  i. Inspection
  ii. Excisional biopsy, confirmation by microscopy
e. Treatment
  i. Excision most frequently
  ii. Chemosurgery and lasers
  iii. Topical fluorouracil
f. Clinical course
  i. Incapable of metastasis but recurs if incompletely excised
  ii. Morpheoform, rare but aggressive

4. *Herpes Zoster (Varicella Virus)*[8,9]

a. Etiology
  i. Herpesvirus
  ii. Usually a benign self-limited disease
  iii. However may be debilitating, even fatal
b. Underlying causes
  i. Immunosuppression secondary to steroids, chemotherapy
  ii. Patient with a malignancy (e.g., lymphoma)
c. Physical findings
  i. Rash of vesicles on an erythematous base in a dermatomic distribution
  ii. Thoracic: 70%
  iii. Trigeminal: 25%
  iv. Rash is characteristic, but hallmark is pain
d. Clinical course
  i. Ocular (globe) involvement >50% or variable when tip of nose involved (Hutchinson's sign)
  ii. Postherpetic neuralgia (PHN): subsides in 6 months but may last years
    - Painful
    - Has caused patients to commit suicide
  iii. Vesicles, conjunctivitis, keratitis, uveitis, secondary glaucoma, anything!
e. Treatment
  i. Isolation from immunosuppressed patients
  ii. Prednisone: 60 mg/day PO, for 1 week, 30 mg/day for 1 week, 15 mg/day for 1 week
  iii. Acyclovir: 800 mg 5×/day for 10 days or valacyclovir 1000 mg tid for 10 days
  iv. PHN can be treated with oral NSAIDs or narcotic analgesics

5. *Molluscum Contagiosum*

a. Etiology
  i. Viral infection that causes a skin growth

ii. Sometimes confused with basal cell carcinoma or papilloma
iii. Can lead to chronic unilateral conjunctivitis
b. Diagnosis
i. Inspection
ii. Biopsy
c. Treatment
i. Surgical removal
ii. Curette out central core during active phase

6. *Nevus of Ota*[10]

a. Epidemiology
i. Common in Asians, no risk of malignancy
ii. Rare in Caucasians; malignancy reported only with whites: uveal melanoma
iii. Melanosis oculi: when only the eye is involved
b. Etiology/pathogenesis
i. Hyperpigmentation
ii. A type of blue nevus
c. Symptomatology
i. Asymptomatic
ii. Cosmetic concern
d. Physical findings
i. Usually unilateral
ii. Blue hyperpigmentation of sclera, conjunctiva, and skin in the distribution of the ophthalmic and maxillary divisions of the trigeminal nerve
iii. 10% risk of glaucoma
e. Course: benign

7. *Psoriasis*[11–13]

a. Epidemiology
i. 2% of adult white population, uncommon in Black population
ii. Hereditary in 30% of cases
iii. Bimodal onset peaks but can develop at any age; 16–35 and 50–60 years of age
iv. Multisystem inflammatory disease mostly affecting skin and joints due to production of pro-inflammatory cytokines
b. Symptomatology
i. 20% of patients symptomatic
ii. Painful at times, itchy, but some lesions asymptomatic
iii. Monoarticular and polyarticular pain, tenderness, and morning stiffness
iv. Emotional and psychosocial effects due to visible skin lesions
c. Physical findings
i. Sharply demarcated red plaques covered with silvery scales
ii. Location: scalp, elbows, knees, back, buttocks
iii. Removal of scales; multiple punctate bleeding points: Auspitz sign
iv. Pitting of nail surface
v. Ocular psoriatic blepharitis produces yellowish-red plaques on conjunctiva with neovascularized marginal keratitis
vi. Psoriatic arthritis occurs in about 30% of psoriatic patients and follows the skin diagnosis by about 10 years
d. Diagnostic tests
i. Clinical appearance
ii. Biopsy of confusing cases
iii. Increased erythrocyte sedimentation rate
iv. Hyperuricemia, positive rheumatoid factor (RF)
e. Treatment
i. Topical
- Steroids, coal tar, salicylic acid combined with steroids
- Calcipotriol (vitamin D3 analog)
- Combination steroid and calcipotriol, more effective with fewer steroid side effects
ii. Methotrexate, in severest forms
iii. Phototherapy
- PUVA (psoralen plus UVA)
- Broadband UVB
- Narrowband UVB (NB-UVB)
- Dermatologist may refer for eye consultation prior to treatment for baseline lens evaluation
- Periodic monitoring during treatment course (months) also advisable
iv. Systemic biologics (e.g., infliximab, certolizumab pegol, risankizumab-rzaa) to control systemic inflammation
f. Clinical course
i. Exacerbation and remissions
ii. Can be disabling (with arthritis)
iii. Koebner reaction: lesions appear in areas of epidermal injury, beltline typical
g. Anterior segment manifestations
i. Conjunctivitis
ii. Blepharitis
iii. Uveitis
iv. Punctate keratitis

8. *Stevens–Johnson Syndrome*[14–17]

a. Epidemiology
i. Can occur at any age
ii. Very rare but can be fatal due to multisystem organ failure (sepsis, kidney, liver)
iii. 50% or greater have ocular involvement
b. Etiology and pathogenesis
i. A severe cutaneous allergic reaction
ii. Reaction to drugs (most common), infections, visceral malignancy
- Most common drugs involved in reaction
  - Antibiotics (most frequent are sulfonamides such as trimethoprim/sulfamethoxazole, β-lactam antibiotics, etc.)
  - Allopurinol (for gout and kidney stones)
  - Anticonvulsants (carbamazepine, phenytoin, phenobarbital)
  - NSAIDs
c. Symptomatology
i. Prodromal symptoms: fever, malaise, headache, upper respiratory infection (URI) symptoms, difficulty swallowing, ocular itch
ii. Bullous eruptions of skin and mucous membranes
d. Physical findings
i. Target lesion: red with clear center: characteristic lesion
ii. Macules, papules, vesicles, and bullae on extremities
iii. Mucous membrane lesions: oral, pharynx, larynx, esophagus, trachea, bronchi, genitals
iv. Ocular

- Conjunctivitis: pseudo- or membranous
- Corneal ulceration
- Symblepharon
- Entropion
- Destruction of goblet cells and lacrimal punctae
- Keratitis sicca syndrome
- Necrosis and purulent inflammatory reactions
- Corneal scarring, neovascularization, and perforation

e. Diagnostic tests
   i. Clinical appearance
   ii. Keratitis sicca testing

f. Treatment
   i. Immediate discontinuation of offending agent (however, tissue damage does not regress)
   ii. Supportive
   - Manage airway and renal function
   - Wound care options: skin debridement, whirlpool baths, petrolatum-impregnated gauze, and non-adherent nanocrystalline gauze containing silver

   iii. Systemic: no treatment has been overly effective
   - Steroids mixed results
   - Antibiotics for cutaneous infections and to avoid sepsis
   - Intravenous immunoglobin
   - Oral cyclosporin

   iv. Correction of electrolyte imbalances due to body fluid loss from skin disruption
   v. Ocular treatment to minimize keratopathy and complication of corneal scarring, neovascularization, and perforation that negatively impacts vision
   - Topical antibiotics and steroids to prevent ulcers and symblepharon
   - Amniotic membrane therapy early in disease process
   - Lid-margin mucous membrane grafting (MMG)
   - Fluid-filled scleral lenses

g. Clinical course
   i. Mortality is 15–20%
   ii. Erythema multiforme is minor form, only involving skin

C. Endocrinology

1. Diabetes Mellitus[18–21]

a. Epidemiology
   i. Metabolic disorder characterized by hyperglycemia
   ii. Chronic hyperglycemia damages organs such as blood vessels, eyes, kidneys, heart, and nerves
   iii. When diabetes is combined with hypertension and dyslipidemia, it is called metabolic syndrome
   iv. Global prevalence (2013) of 382 million and expected to increase to 592 million by 2035
   - Globally (2010) 800,000 blind and 3.7 million visually impaired due to diabetic retinopathy

   v. Appears at any age
   vi. Prevalence increases with each decade; 10% of population by age 70

b. Etiology and pathogenesis
   i. Disease of insufficient insulin action secondary to either not enough insulin or peripheral resistance to insulin or both
   ii. Genetics
   - Type 1: insulin-dependent diabetes mellitus (IDDM), or juvenile-onset diabetes
     - Immune-mediated destruction of pancreatic β-cells
     - Viral infections (e.g., enterovirus, rotavirus, herpes virus, cytomegalovirus, etc.) possible causative agent
     - Maybe idiopathic in nature
     - Typically diagnosed in children and adolescents but can happen at any age
     - Prone to other autoimmune conditions (e.g., Addison's disease, Graves' disease, myasthenia gravis, pernicious anemia)
     - Not hereditary but genetic factors involved
     - Persons have their disease much longer before development of diabetic retinopathy but, when it comes, it is severe
   - Type 2: non-insulin-dependent diabetes mellitus (NIDDM), or adult-onset diabetes
     - Resistance to insulin action
     - 90–95% of diabetes
     - Obesity or abnormal amount of abdominal fat common
     - With childhood obesity on the rise, Type 2 diabetes in children and adolescents has risen
     - Has more hereditary pattern
     - Persons have their disease a shorter time period before development of retinopathy, usually not as severe
   - Other types
     - Diseases of exocrine process (e.g., pancreatic tumor, pancreatitis, trauma, etc.)
     - Drugs (systemic steroids)
     - Endocrine disease with hormone excess (glucocorticoids, glucagon, epinephrine, human growth hormone)
   - Gestational
     - Previously undiagnosed Type 1 or 2 that manifests during pregnancy

c. Symptomatology
   i. Polyuria, polydipsia, polyphagia
   ii. Blurred vision, weight loss, fatigue
   iii. Can be asymptomatic early in Type 2 which delays treatment
   iv. Slow healing
   v. Women: monilia vaginitis
   vi. Refractive fluctuation
   - Increased minus
   - Decreased plus

   vii. Uncontrolled diabetes can cause confusion and stupor and cause death if not treated from ketoacidosis (Type 1)

d. Physical findings
   i. Affects all organs and systems, secondary to metabolic or vascular involvement
   ii. Basement membrane thickening
   iii. Microangiopathy

e. Diagnostic tests
   i. Elevated serum glucose (hyperglycemia)
   - Fasting blood sugar (FBS) >126 mg/dL
   - Hemoglobin A1c (HbA1c) >6.5
     - A chronic marker of hyperglycemia average over a 3-month period

ii. Glycosuria
iii. Glucose tolerance test (GTT), 2-hour postprandial

f. Treatment
   i. Diet control, weight reduction
   ii. Type 1
      - Insulin
         - Rapid (e.g., Novolog), short, (e.g., Humalog), intermediate (NPH), long-term acting (e.g., Lantas) injections
         - Premixed (e.g., Humalog 25) are a combination of short and intermediate action
   iii. Type 2
      - Oral medications
         - Biguanides (e.g., Metformin)
         - Sulfonylureas (e.g., Glipizide, Glimepiride)
         - Long-acting insulin may be added to metformin regimen

g. Clinical course
   i. Increased incidence of atherosclerosis, cardiovascular, peripheral vasculature, and cerebrovascular disease: 50% of adult onset die from coronary disease
   ii. Renal failure: leading cause of death in juvenile diabetes
   iii. Peripheral neuropathy
      - Most common
      - Bilateral symmetric sensory impairment in lower extremities
      - Foot ulcers and chance of amputation
   iv. Autonomic neuropathy
      - Gastrointestinal
      - Genitourinary
      - Cardiovascular
      - Sexual dysfunction
   v. Retinopathy, at same time as glomerulonephrosis of kidneys
   vi. Oculomotor palsy
   vii. Cerebrovascular accident (CVA), myocardial ischemia (MI)
   viii. Gangrene resulting in amputations
   ix. Ketoacidosis (always a threat)
   x. Shortens life expectancy by 8 to 10 years

2. *Hyperparathyroidism*[22,23]

a. Etiology and pathogenesis
   i. Excessive production of parathyroid hormone (PHT)
      - Primary: produced by >1 parathyroid glands (most common is adenoma)
      - Secondary: organic cause (e.g., kidney, bowel, or liver disease)
      - Tertiary: persistent parathyroid stimulation
   ii. PHT responsible for calcium (causes hypercalcemia) and potassium levels

b. Symptomatology
   i. Most do not present with symptoms
   ii. Non-specific due to hypercalcemia
      - Malaise
      - Fatigue
      - Headache
      - Anxiety and depression
      - Diffuse aches and pains
   iii. Polyuria, polydipsia, GI symptoms such as constipation and obstructive uropathy from nephrolithiasis (kidney stone)
   iv. Nausea, anorexia, vomiting

c. Diagnostic tests
   i. Elevated blood levels of calcium, uric acid, and parathyroid hormone
   ii. Decreased serum phosphate
   iii. Increased urine calcium and phosphate
   iv. Radiographic findings of bone cortex reabsorption

d. Treatment
   i. Surgical exploration
   ii. Removal of parathyroid adenoma (only definitive treatment)
   iii. Vitamin D and calcium supplement
   iv. Thiazide diuretics to reduce urinary calcium and kidney stone formation

e. Clinical course
   i. The disease of "bones, stones, abdominal groans, and psychic moans"
      - Risk of bone fractures, anxiety/depression, cardiovascular disease
   ii. Peptic ulcer disease, gout, hypertension, osteitis fibrosa cystica, renal stones

f. Anterior segment manifestations
   i. Band keratopathy of Bowman's layer
   ii. Limited to intrapalpebral area

3. *Hyperthyroidism (Graves' Disease Most Common Form)*[24–27]

a. Epidemiology (Figure 9.2)
   i. Female to male ratio: 7:1
   ii. Young to middle age
   iii. Marked familial pattern
   iv. Approximately 50% of Graves' patients have ophthalmic signs
   v. Approximately 10% have infiltrative ocular signs
   vi. Approximately 20% with infiltrative ophthalmopathy are euthyroid

b. Etiology/pathogenesis
   i. Autoimmune disease
      - Thyroid-stimulating antibodies in the blood activate thyroid-stimulating hormone (TSH) receptors, triggering thyroid hormone synthesis
   ii. Exophthalmos-producing substance

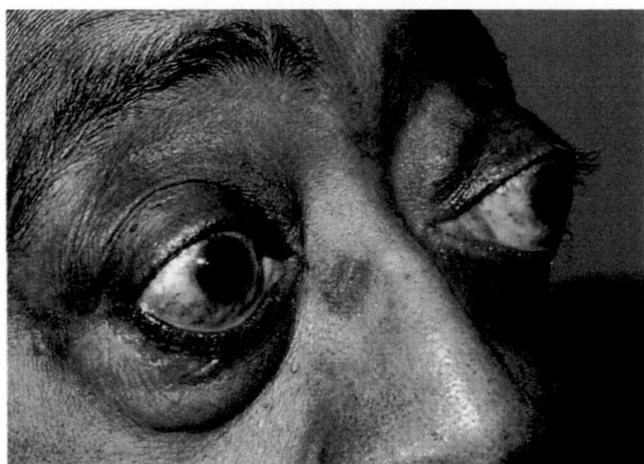

FIGURE 9.2 Hyperthyroidism (Graves' disease) producing bilateral exophthalmos along with numerous other abnormal signs associated with the eyelids, extraocular muscles, and pupils.

c. Symptomatology
 i. Nervousness, anxiety, restless overactivity, tremor, palpitation
 ii. Sensitivity to heat, sweating, weight loss,
 iii. Occasionally, altered mental status, depression, anxiety, nausea, hyperdefecation, diarrhea

d. Physical findings
 i. Diffuse goiter
 ii. Infiltrative ophthalmopathy
 iii. Infiltrative dermopathy (pretibial myxedema, reddish nodules on anterior surface of lower legs)
 iv. Flushing of the face, erythema of the palms, and hyperhidrosis (excessive sweating) of the palms and soles
 v. Thyroid acropachy (a form of clubbing of the digits)
 vi. Smooth skin, tachycardia

e. Diagnostic tests
 i. Radioimmunoassay (RIA) tests
  - Triiodothyronine (T3), thyroxine (T4), free T3, free T4, thyroid-stimulating hormone (TSH)
  - Usually T3 and T4 increased, TSH decreased
 ii. A radioactive iodine uptake test and thyroid scan
 iii. 90% of euthyroid Graves' patients positive to T3-suppression test

f. Treatments
 i. Hyperthyroidism (Graves' disease)
  - Thyroidectomy
  - Radioactive iodine ablation most common treatment of Graves' disease in the United States
  - Antithyroid drug therapy: propylthiouracil (high risk of liver cancer with use), methimazole is preferred except in first trimester of pregnancy
 ii. Beta-blockers control adrenergic symptoms (e.g., palpitations, tremors, tachycardia, anxiety, jitters, etc.)
 iii. Ocular complications, treated as warranted

g. Clinical course
 i. Highly variable
 ii. Continuously present
 iii. Intermittent flareups or even spontaneous hypothyroidism
 iv. Ocular proptosis not affected by thyroid treatment
  - New infusion drug to treat thyroid eye disease (e.g., proptosis and diplopia)
   – Teprotumumab (Tepezza)
   – Monoclonal antibody inhibitor of tyrosine kinase receptor
 v. Heart failure may develop

h. Anterior segment manifestations
 i. Most common cause of unilateral and bilateral proptosis
 ii. Thickened extraocular muscles
 iii. Conjunctival chemosis and congestion
 iv. Superior limbic keratoconjunctivitis
 v. Lid retraction and lag
 vi. Exposure keratitis due to incomplete eye closure
 vii. Diplopia

4. *Hypoparathyroidism*[28–30]

a. Etiology and pathogenesis
 i. Iatrogenic (most common): when parathyroids are removed during neck (e.g., thyroid) surgery
 ii. Autoimmune
 iii. Genetic: DiGeorge's syndrome (most common genetic cause)
 iv. Caused by infiltration by iron (hemochromatosis), copper (Wilson's disease), and certain metastases
 v. Caused by severe magnesium deficiency
 vi. Idiopathic

b. Symptomatology
 i. Relates to hypocalcemia: tingling in lips, fingers
 ii. Cramps, spasm, tonic contraction of any muscle
 iii. Psychiatric, neurological, and cardiovascular

c. Physical findings
 i. Chovstek's signs: tap facial nerve at zygomatic arch; watch involuntary contractions of orbicularis oris muscle (ipsilateral upturn twitch of the facial muscles)
 ii. Trousseau's signs: tetany (muscle spasms) of hand following 2 minutes of upper arm constriction with sphygmomanometer (above systolic pressure)
 iii. Higher bone density due to reduced bone turnover rate

d. Diagnostic tests
 i. Serum tests: low Ca, high PHT, hyperphosphatemia, low vitamin D
 ii. Urine: high calcium levels
 iii. Radiographs show increased bone density

e. Treatment
 i. Synthetic parathyroid hormone injections
 ii. Supplemental calcium salts
 iii. Vitamin D analogs: 50,000 to 150,000 IU/day

f. Anterior segment manifestations
 i. Cataracts: cortical (idiopathic type), posterior and peripheral location in adults

5. *Hypothyroidism*[31–33]

a. Epidemiology
 i. Most common cause worldwide: environmental iodine insufficiency
 ii. Hashimoto's thyroiditis is most common, in women aged 20 to 50 years

b. Etiology/pathogenesis
 i. 95% primary hypothyroidism: the thyroid gland does not produce enough T3 or T4 hormones
  - Iodine insufficiency: most common cause worldwide
  - Autoimmune damage (e.g., Hashimoto's thyroiditis) to thyroid gland
 ii. Other causes
  - Thyroid gland damage (surgical, radioactive iodine therapy for Graves' disease, radiotherapy for head and neck cancer, etc.)
  - Insufficient delivery of TSH by pituitary disease

c. Symptomatology
 i. Gradual onset of lethargy, intolerance to cold, decreased sweating, weight gain, constipation, menstrual irregularities
 ii. Mental confusion, slowing of mentation, forgetfulness
 iii. Voice changes: deep, harsh, thick tongue
 iv. Bizarre sense of humor, frank psychosis often inappropriately committed to mental institutions

d. Physical findings
 i. Skin: cool, coarse, dry, yellow-orange (carotene), puffy face
 ii. Hair: brittle, alopecia

iii. Deep tendon reflexes, relaxation phase delayed
iv. Bradycardia, hypothermia
v. Myxedema, non-pitting edema

e. Diagnostic tests
i. Same tests as for hyperthyroidism
ii. TSH increased; T4 decreased, T3 resin uptake decreased
iii. Serum Na depressed, elevated creatine phosphokinase (CPK), elevated cerebrospinal fluid (CSF), and protein

f. Treatment
i. Oral levothyroxine (a synthetic T4)
ii. Titrated until TSH levels normalized
iii. Lifelong replacement of levothyroxine (L-T4)

g. Clinical course
i. Ability to handle stress is diminished
ii. Mild illnesses may cause coma
iii. Drug metabolism is decreased
iv. Associated risks
- Anemia 20%
- Increased risk for arteriosclerotic heart disease

h. Anterior segment manifestations
i. Ptosis, edema, cataract, keratoconjunctivitis sicca (KCS), extraocular muscle myotonia
ii. Thyroid eye disease (TED) is rare but can happen (systemic hypothyroidism is diagnosed prior to TED)
- Less severe than Graves' disease

D. Gastroenterology

1. *Crohn's Disease (Regional Enteritis)*

(Refer to Chapter 6 for a complete discussion.)

2. *Ulcerative Colitis*

(Refer to Chapter 6 for a complete discussion.)

3. *Wilson's Disease (WD) (Hepaticolenticular Disease)*[34,35]

a. Epidemiology
i. Autosomal recessive
- Two pathologic genetic mutations in 98% of WD patients

ii. Under 30 years of age, can present as chronic active hepatitis without mental or corneal changes

b. Etiology and pathogenesis
i. Unknown metabolic defect
ii. Copper deposits
- Brain
- Kidney
- Liver
- Cornea

c. Symptomatology
i. Neurological
- Irregular, jerky, dystonic tremor
- Parkinsonian syndrome-like movements (e.g., loss of coordination, etc.)
- Difficulty speaking, swallowing, and excessive salivation
- Various types of seizures (e.g., grand mal, focal)

ii. Psychiatric
- Most common are increased irritability or disinhibition, personality changes, anxiety, and depression
- Behavioral disturbances characterized by impulsivity
- Dementia and psychosis

iii. Acute and chronic liver disease

d. Physical findings
i. All patients with neuropsychiatric signs have Kayser–Fleischer ring
ii. Tremors
iii. Dystonia of facial and mandible muscles leads to "Wilson's face" (masked facies)
- Open mouth
- Dull look
- Mindless smile
- Hypersalivation

e. Diagnostic tests
i. Low serum ceruloplasmin level
ii. Low serum copper
iii. Elevated hepatic transaminase levels
iv. Aminoaciduria
v. Hemolytic anemia
vi. Urine copper level increased
vii. MRI abnormalities

f. Treatment
i. Cooper chelators
- Penicillamine
- Trientine
- Tetrathiomolybdate

ii. Zinc salts (drug of choice for lifetime treatment)
iii. One of few treatable causes of dementia and liver disease

g. Clinical course
i. Can be reversible with treatment
ii. Cirrhosis of liver begins by 6 years of age, often fatal
iii. Cavitations develop in lenticular nucleus in the brain

h. Anterior segment manifestations
i. Copper deposits in peripheral Descemet's membrane (Kayser–Fleischer ring) (Figure 9.3) are a greenish-brown color

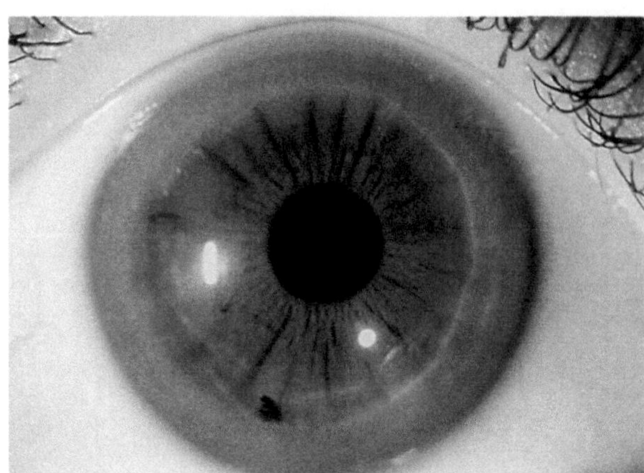

FIGURE 9.3 Kayser–Fleisher ring (Wilson's hepaticolenticular disease) is a definitive ocular finding in this infrequently-presenting gastroenterologic disease. Eye care practitioners are often asked by neurologists for a slit-lamp biomicroscopic evaluation to rule out this posterior corneal brownish-orange copper ring in the anterior chamber angle.

ii. Sunflower cataract (copper under anterior lens capsule)
iii. Both disappear with chelation therapy

E. Hematology

1. *Anemias*[36–38]

a. Etiology and pathogenesis
  i. Deficiency in hemoglobin to transport oxygen to the lungs and carbon dioxide from the lungs
    - Excessive blood loss
    - Deficient red blood cell (RBC) production (nutritional, suppression)
    - Excessive RBC destruction (hemolytic)
    - Disorders with both deficient RBC production and excessive RBC destruction (hemoglobinopathies, infection, thalassemia)

b. Symptomatology
  i. Weakness, vertigo, headache, tinnitus, spots before eyes, fatigue, intolerance to exercise
  ii. Drowsiness, irritability, euphoria, psychotic behavior
  iii. Amenorrhea, loss of libido, gastrointestinal (GI) complaints, jaundice

c. Physical findings: Pale skin and mucous membranes

d. Diagnostic tests
  i. Hemoglobin and hematocrit are decreased
  ii. Reticulocyte count, increased, decreased, or normal, depending on type of anemia
  iii. RBC indices (cell morphology): normocytic, microcytic (and hypochromic), or macrocytic

e. Treatment
  i. Symptomatic: rest
  ii. Diet: high protein from animal (cow, poultry, fish, fowl) or plant (legumes and non-leafy vegetables) sources
  iii. Supplements (e.g., iron, vitamin B12, folate)
  iv. Erythropoiesis-stimulating agents (e.g., epoetin alfa [Procrit], darbepoetin alfa [Aranesp]) to stimulate bone marrow to produce RBCs
  v. Transfusion when necessary: packed red blood cells (PRBC)

f. Anterior segment manifestations
  i. Ischemia (pallor)
  ii. Subconjunctival hemorrhage

2. *Polycythemia*[39–43]

a. Etiology and pathogenesis
  i. Preleukemic (myeloproliferative neoplasm) disorder of bone marrow causing an excess of circulating RBC
  ii. Increase in blood viscosity increases risks of microvascular and thrombotic complications
  iii. Can be secondary to chronic lung disease

b. Symptomatology
  i. Headache, tinnitus, pruritis (itching), dyspnea, weakness, GI complaints, atypical chest pain
  ii. Amaurosis fugax, hemianopia, blurring (secondary to impaired cerebral circulation)

c. Physical findings
  i. Hepatosplenomegaly, hypertension

d. Diagnostic tests
  i. Increased hematocrit, hemoglobin, and decreased serum EPO
  ii. Bone marrow biopsy hyperplasia
  iii. Complete blood count (CBC) shows leukocytosis with neutrophils

e. Treatment
  i. Phlebotomy (to reduce RBC mass)
  ii. Low dose aspirin and other platelet aggregation inhibiting drugs
  iii. Cytoreductive drugs (e.g., hydroxyurea, busulfan)
  iv. Ruxolitinib

f. Clinical course
  i. Variable, depending on occurrence of serous cerebrovascular hemorrhage (CVA) and thrombosis, from which 30% of patients die
  ii. Survival 15 years
  iii. 15% of patients will develop leukemia

g. Ocular manifestations
  i. Vascular congestion of conjunctiva
  ii. Vascular engorgement of iris
  iii. Fundus appears like impending central retinal vein occlusion, retinal hemorrhages, Roth spots

3. *Sickle Cell Anemia*[44–48]

a. Epidemiology
  i. 1:600 Black patients in the United States
  ii. 80% Black patients heterozygous for HbS (trait)

b. Etiology and pathogenesis
  i. Genetic: substitution of a valine for a glutamine in the sixth position of the b-hemoglobin (Hb) chain
  ii. Inherited from parents
  iii. The altered hemoglobin forms crystalline aggregates, leading to sickled shape of RBC
  iv. Multisystem disorder

c. Symptomatology
  i. Acute (sickle cell crisis)
    - Vaso-occlusive events (e.g., acute chest syndrome which is like pneumonia)
    - Pain in extremities, abdomen, back, or chest
    - Episodes of arthralgia, fever, other symptoms of anemia (crisis)
  ii. Chronic
    - Large vessel vasculopathy (e.g., cerebrovascular disease, pulmonary disease, and retinopathy)
    - Progressive ischemic organ damage (hyposplenism, renal failure, bone disease, liver damage, cerebral infarcts)
    - Deep bone pain secondary to microvascular necrosis

d. Physical findings
  i. "Sun-ray" findings on radiographs of the skull
  ii. Recurrent leg ulcers
  iii. Poorly developed, short trunk with long extremities, tower skull

e. Diagnostic tests: electrophoresis demonstrating HbS

f. Treatment
  i. Symptomatic
    - Regular blood transfusions
    - Pain relief (narcotics)
  ii. Penicillin prophylaxis in children
  iii. Stroke prevention
  iv. Hydroxyurea (FDA-approved drug) inhibits the HbS polymerization that causes sickling
  v. Hematopoietic stem cell transplantation from HLA-matched siblings is curative

g. Clinical course
   i. Disease apparent by 2 to 3 years of age
   ii. Chronic course of exacerbations of the anemia accompanied by pain in abdomen or skeleton secondary to microvascular occlusions
   iii. Median life expectancy 42 years old for men and 48 years old for women because of intercurrent infection, pulmonary emboli, or thrombosis
h. Anterior segment manifestations
   i. Comma-shaped capillary segments on bulbar conjunctiva
i. Other ocular manifestations
   i. Retinopathy
      - Non-proliferative
         - Salmon-patch retinal findings
         - Angioid streaks
         - Venous tortuosity
      - Proliferative
         - Vascular occlusion and ischemia
         - Seafan neovascular tuft
         - Vitreal hemorrhage and retinal detachments

F. Infectious Disease

1. Acquired Immune Deficiency Syndrome (AIDS)[49–53]

a. Epidemiology
   i. High-risk categories
      - Intravenous drug users (reusing or sharing needles)
      - Homosexual males
      - Female sex workers
      - 10× greater in Black population compared to white population
      - Heterosexuals with unsafe sexual habits (25% of HIV/AIDS are women)
   ii. Epidemic spread among high-risk categories
   iii. Prevalence of human immunodeficiency virus (HIV) infection (diagnosed or undiagnosed) is estimated to be slightly greater than 100,000
   iv. Incubation period from infection to disease estimated at approximately 5 years
b. Etiology and pathogenesis
   i. Acquired through transmission of bodily fluids (blood, semen, breast milk, vaginal and anal secretions)
      - Found in tears and ocular tissues but no evidence of transmission
   ii. HIV attacks and destroys CD4 T lymphocytes (T_H cell-mediated immunity) as well as other immune cells (e.g., macrophages, immature dendritic cells) which are key regulators of the immune system
   iii. Patient becomes vulnerable to opportunistic infection
c. Symptomatology
   i. May be asymptomatic with HIV infector until secondary infection or complication present
   ii. Symptomatology usually consistent with type and degree of complications
d. Physical findings
   i. Cytomegalovirus retinitis very common
   ii. High incidence of *Pneumocystis carinii* infection and esophageal candidiasis
   iii. Disseminated opportunistic infectors common
      - Herpes simplex virus
      - Herpes zoster virus
      - Syphilis
      - Tuberculosis
      - Toxoplasmosis
   iv. Increased frequency of neoplasia
      - Kaposi's sarcoma
      - Lymphoma
e. Diagnostic tests
   i. Careful history for risk factors and risk categories associated with unresponsive, complicated infectious disease
   ii. <200 CD4 cells/cubic mm blood
   iii. Blood test for HIV viral antibodies
f. Treatment
   i. Six classes of antiretroviral therapy (ART) affect HIV life cycle at different stages
   ii. Current treatment is highly active antiretroviral therapy (HAART)
      - Three drugs from two classes
      - Drug classes
         - Nucleoside reverse transcriptase inhibitors (NRTIs)
         - Non-nucleoside reverse transcriptase inhibitors (NNRTIs)
         - Protease inhibitors (PIs)
         - Integrase inhibitors
         - CCR5 antagonists
         - Fusion inhibitors
      - Successful drug treatment has made this a chronic but manageable disease
   iii. Specific treatment for secondary infector
g. Clinical course
   i. Initial HIV infection to clinical disease (opportunistic infection and complications) variable
   ii. Virus can mutate and has caused resistance at times to ART medications
   iii. Kaposi's sarcoma (red plaque-like neoplasia on lid or conjunctiva) frequent late complication of disease
   iv. Mortality rate is 100% without treatment

2. Cat-Scratch Disease[54,55]

a. Etiology and pathogenesis
   i. *Bartonella henselae* (gram-negative bacteria) responsible microorganism
   ii. Cat scratch or bite 1 to 2 weeks prior to symptoms
   iii. Granulomatous abscess formation
b. Symptomatology
   i. Fever
   ii. Headache
   iii. Malaise
c. Physical findings
   i. Unilateral regional lymphadenitis with enlargement, tenderness, and occasional suppuration in 50% of patients
   ii. Inflamed scratch or papular lesion with central necrosis
   iii. Unilateral conjunctivitis and adenitis of preauricular, submandibular, or cervical lymph nodes
   iv. Neuroretinitis
d. Diagnostic tests
   i. Serology

- Indirect fluorescent assay
- Enzyme-linked immunosorbent assay

e. Treatment
  i. Supportive
    - Most patients have self-limited lymphadenopathy lasting 2 to 8 weeks
    - Antibiotics (e.g., azithromycin) can be used for moderate cases

f. Clinical course
  i. Relatively benign disease
  ii. Spontaneous remissions in weeks to months

3. *Lyme Disease*[56–58]

a. Epidemiology (Figure 9.4)
  i. Infectious agent is the *Borrelia burgdorferi* spirochete in the United States and *B. burgdorferi*, *B. afzelii*, and *B. garinii* in Eurasia
  ii. Worldwide prevalence with high-concentration endemic areas including the northeast United States (particularly Lyme, Connecticut), north central states, and the West Coast

b. Etiology and pathogenesis
  i. Life cycle of the spirochete includes the Ixodes deer tick
  ii. Transmission to humans is by tick bite
  iii. Pathology is mainly due to host inflammatory response

c. Symptomatology
  i. Non-specific malaise, fatigue, fever, and muscular aches and pains
  ii. Symptomatology causes difficulty in differential diagnosis if risk factors and/or physical findings are not obvious
  iii. Increasing "over" diagnosis of disease due to prevalence

d. Physical findings
  i. Red rash (erythema chronicum migrans) (bull's eye appearance) appears approximately 1 to 3 weeks after bite in 70% of patients and may spontaneously resolve
  ii. The associated annular lesion (achrodermatitis chronicum atrophicans) persists for years and is highly diagnostic
  iii. Multiorgan and systems disease occurring in 3 stages

  Stage 1: Early, localizing stage (1–28 days after initial infection) with dermatologic (rash) (70% of cases), flu-like symptoms

  Stage 2: Disseminated stage (3–12 weeks after initial infection) with flu-like symptoms, dizziness, headaches, facial (VII) nerve palsy, ophthalmic conditions, meningitis, cardiac disease

  Stage 3: Late stage (months or years after initial infection) with arthritis (knee frequent joint) and neurological signs (meningitis, Bell's palsy, cognitive deficits)
  iv. Anterior segment findings found in all stages

  Stage 1: Conjunctivitis

  Stage 2 and Stage 3: Keratitis, uveitis, vitritis, multifocal choroiditis, and panophthalmitis

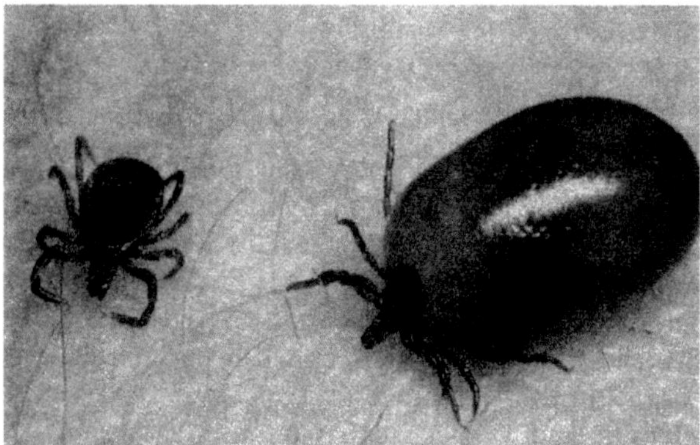

FIGURE 9.4 Ixodes deer ticks responsible for Lyme disease in humans through the transmission of the spirochete *Borrelia burgdorferi*. The small deer tick, only a few millimeters in size (left organism), "snacks" and engorges itself (right organism) on spirochetes from rodent droppings and then translocates itself from a deer to foliage to a passing, "rubbing," human.

e. Diagnostic tests
  i. ELISA (enzyme-linked immunoabsorption assay*)*
  ii. Western blot
  iii. Use specific blood tests to rule out other possible infectious diseases (e.g., fluorescent treponemal antibody-absorption test [FTA-ABS] for syphilis)

f. Treatment
  i. Oral antibiotics
    - Doxycycline for 10 days
    - Amoxicillin is drug of choice for children
  ii. Treat until Lyme titer negative

g. Clinical course
  i. Without treatment infection can linger sub clinically for years
  ii. Appropriate antibiotics are usually neutral titer within 1 month, but treatment may be required in some cases for longer periods

4. *Severe Acute Respiratory Syndrome Coronavirus 2 (SARS-CoV-2) (COVID-19)*[59–67]

a. Epidemiology
  i. All populations are susceptible
    - Risk factors are age, immunocompromised, hypertension, cancer, diabetes, obesity, cardiovascular disease, chronic lung disease
  ii. Caused worldwide pandemic (2020–to be determined)

b. Etiology and pathogenesis
  i. SARS-CoV-2 is the causative virus
    - Single-stranded RNA enclosed in a capsid with protein spikes
  ii. Believed to have originated in a bat (Wuhan, China) and transmitted to humans
  iii. Belongs to a family of coronaviruses that have caused common colds, upper respiratory infection, and acute respiratory distress
  iv. Transmission is through infectious respiratory droplets from mucous membranes
  v. Various droplet (aerosols) sizes can be expelled by sneezing, coughing, and even talking
  vi. Asymptomatic people may spread disease
  vii. Virus has mutated and variants (e.g., Alpha, Beta, Gamma, Delta, Omicron) have been produced

c. Symptomatology
  i. Can be asymptomatic
  ii. Viral-like symptoms such as fever, fatigue, muscle pain, cough, nasal congestion, and runny nose

- iii. Loss of smell and taste
- iv. Chest tightness and dyspnea (labored breathing)
- v. Symptoms increase with more severe disease

d. Physical findings
- i. Low blood oxygen (hypoxemia)
- ii. Lung lesions
- iii. Lymphopenia and elevated C-reactive protein

e. Diagnostic tests
- i. Polymerase chain reaction (PCR) (gold standard): laboratory direct testing for virus RNA (3–4 days)
- ii. Rapid diagnostic tests (results in minutes)
  - Point of care nucleic acid amplification test (NAAT): test for virus RNA
  - Antigen test: tests for virus antigens
  - Less sensitive than PCR
- iii. Chest x-ray as disease progresses (pneumonia)
- iv. Serological testing can detect viral antibodies and antigens

f. Treatment
- i. Standard of care is disease prevention
  - Mitigation procedures
    - Avoid crowds especially indoors and poorly ventilated spaces
    - Social distance, at least 6 ft and minimize duration time (avoid symptomatic people)
    - Wear a mask over nose and mouth especially indoors
    - Wash hands frequently
  - Vaccines
    - mRNA: provides instructions to our cells to manufacture the "spiked protein" of the COVID-19 virus to cause an immunological response (production of antibodies against the virus)
      - o Moderna and Pfizer-BioNTech vaccines were approximately 94% effective
    - Vector vaccines: a modified virus (usually a harmless adenovirus) with the COVID-19 virus instructions placed inside which provides instructions to our cells to manufacture the "spiked protein" of the COVID-19 virus to cause an immunological response (production of antibodies against the virus)
      - o Johnson & Johnsen Janssen was 66% effective at preventing disease
- ii. Supplemental oxygen
  - Nasal canula (mild disease)
  - Positive airway pressure (PAP) and mechanical ventilation for moderate to severe disease
- iii. Remdesivir
  - Intravenous therapy
  - Inhibits viral replication
- iv. Monoclonal antibodies (e.g., Regeneron and Eli Lilly produced)
  - Not effective against all variants
- v. Convalescent plasma (CCP)
  - Plasma from recovered patients has antibodies for the virus
  - High titer CCP used early in hospitalization period
- vi. Oral antiviral treatments
  - For mild to moderate disease
  - Initiate treatment within 5 days of symptom onset
  - FDA issued Emergency Use Authorization in December 2021
  - Paxlovid (Pfizer)
    - Hospitalization/deaths 0.8% versus 6.3% for placebo
  - Lagevrio (Merck)
    - Hospitalization/deaths 6.8% versus 9.7% for placebo

g. Clinical course
- i. Pneumonia and acute respiratory distress syndrome
- ii. Can cause neurological, liver, heart, and kidney damage
- iii. Tissue injury causes severe inflammatory response ("cytokine storm")
- iv. Microthrombi of the lungs, heart, liver, and kidneys can lead to severe organ damage
- v. Death (mortality rate approximately 3%)
- vi. Post-COVID syndrome (Long haul disease): symptoms after COVID-19 acute infection has resolved (most were not hospitalized)
  - Fatigue
  - Respiratory complaints
  - Cognitive impairment
  - Sleep disturbance
  - Mental health issues

h. Anterior segment manifestations
- i. Ocular symptoms: foreign-body sensation, dry eye, redness, tearing, eye pain
  - May be present a few hours to 2 days prior to systemic symptoms
- ii. Conjunctivitis very common
- iii. Lid margin hyperemia

5. *Sexually Transmitted Diseases (STDs)*[68,69]

a. Epidemiology
- i. Most common infectious diseases
- ii. Rising incidence because of availability of multiple sexual partners, asymptomatic infection, increasing affluence, leisure time, and mobility of patients
- iii. Syphilis and gonorrhea have increased since introduction of HAART therapy for HIV

b. Etiology and pathogenesis
- i. Chlamydia, gonorrhea, pediculosis, human papilloma virus (HPV) genital warts, genital herpes, trichomoniasis (protozoan parasite), syphilis, and AIDS
- ii. Acquired through sexual contact with infected partner

c. Symptomatology
- i. Male heterosexuals: infections of pharynx, urethra, anorectal region
  - Discharge ("the drip") and pain while urinating (men)
- ii. Male homosexuals: urethral, pharyngeal less common
- iii. Female heterosexuals: pharyngeal, vaginal, cervical, anorectal infection
- iv. Female homosexuals: very monogamous, hence rare infection
- v. Can be asymptomatic

d. Physical findings
- i. Urethral discharge, epididymitis, vaginal discharge, genital sore, rash, scabies, proctitis, salpingitis

(inflammation of fallopian tubes), prostatitis, genital ulcer
   ii. Skin lesion: condylomata (anogenital warts)
   iii. Mucosal sore
   iv. Corneal infiltrates in chlamydia
e. Diagnostic tests
   i. Cultures of infected areas
   ii. FTA-ABS, Venereal Disease Research Laboratory (VDRL) test for syphilis
   iii. HIV test for AIDS
f. Treatment
   i. Antibiotics (for bacterial causes) to infected patients and sexual contacts
   ii. Oral antivirals for herpes
   iii. Topical therapy for genital warts
   iv. HPV vaccine for prevention
   v. Education: to prevent infection
g. Clinical course
   i. Homosexual male: leads to intestinal pathology because of fecal–oral contact, hepatitis, Kaposi's sarcoma, AIDS
   ii. AIDS: suppression of cell-mediated immunity with life-threatening opportunistic infections
   iii. Risk group: homosexual males, intravenous drug abusers
   iv. Kaposi's sarcoma: red plaque-like growth on lid or conjunctiva
      - Up to 5-year incubation period
      - 100% mortality
   v. HPV can cause anogenital carcinoma

6. Sinusitis (Suppurative)[70,71]

a. Predisposing conditions
   i. Ciliary (hairlike structures line nasal mucosa) injury secondary to dryness, chemical irritants, inhalation of dust, exposure, or change in temperature
   ii. Most common in children
b. Etiology and pathogenesis
   i. Inflammation obstructing the drainage orifices leads to secondary infection in the nasal sinuses
   ii. Viral (e.g., rhinovirus, adenovirus, influenza, coronavirus) most common
   iii. Bacterial (*Streptococcus pneumonia*, *Staphylococcus aureus*, *Haemophilus influenzae*, *Moraxella catarrhalis*, group A Streptococcus)
c. Symptomatology
   i. Fever, chills, cloudy or colored nasal discharge, headache with changes in intensity with position
   ii. Dull aching around eyes, facial pressure, nasal blockage
   iii. Acute sinusitis
      - Symptoms lasting less than 10 days and not changing in severity usually viral
      - Symptoms that worsen within first 10 days or continue longer than 10 days usually bacterial
d. Physical findings
   i. Pain over infected sinuses
   ii. Erythema or edema of turbinates
   iii. Visualization of mucopus in the nose or nasopharynx
e. Diagnostic tests
   i. Not typically performed in primary care setting
   ii. Endoscopically directed middle meatal culture and CT scan can be done in otorhinolaryngological setting
f. Treatment
   i. Medical: appropriate antibiotics for bacterial sinusitis
      - Amoxicillin
      - Augmentin
   ii. Medical: decongestants, saline irrigation, intranasal steroid (e.g., fluticasone propionate)
   iii. Surgical for chronic sinusitis: functional endoscopic sinus surgery (FESS)
g. Clinical course
   i. May lead to orbital cellulitis and osteomyelitis
   ii. Orbital abscess
   iii. Meningitis: death
   iv. Cavernous sinus thrombosis with clinical hallmarks
      - Proptosis
      - Chemosis
      - Ophthalmoplegia
      - Blindness in contralateral eye
      - Can be fatal, even with antibiotics

G. Nephrology

1. Cystinosis[72,73]

a. Epidemiology
   i. Rare
   ii. Autosomal-recessive trait
   iii. Infantile (diagnosed up to 2 years old)
   iv. Juvenile (diagnosed later childhood/adolescence)
   v. Non-nephropathic adult form
b. Etiology and pathogenesis
   i. Autosomal recessive inherited lysosomal storage disease due to genetic mutations
   ii. Cystine crystal deposits accumulate in multiple organs resulting in a multisystem disorder, initially in the kidneys and eyes later in thyroid, testes, pancreas, muscles, and brain
c. The adult form has no renal abnormalities
d. Symptomatology: as disease progresses photophobia, headache, burning, stinging, foreign-body sensation, blepharospasm
e. Physical findings
   i. Hexagonal cystine crystals in the anterior stroma starting peripherally and spreading centrally
   ii. Clusters around vessels in conjunctiva
   iii. Cystine crystals can accumulate in all ocular tissues
f. Diagnostic tests: quantified determination of cystine in blood leukocytes (approximately 30 times normal)
g. Treatment
   i. Adult form benign, no treatment necessary
   ii. Cystadrops (EU approved): topical cysteamine to reduce corneal cystine crystals in adults and children
   iii. Differential is multiple myeloma, similar corneal crystals
   iv. Oral cysteamine (Cystagon) reduces cystine crystals in all organs except the eye
g. Clinical course
   i. Infantile type: Franconi syndrome (a proximal kidney tubule disorder) results in substances which are normally absorbed into the bloodstream by the kidneys are released into the urine instead) and renal insufficiency during first decade of life
   ii. Juvenile type: renal disease during second decade of life
   iii. Adult type: benign with no renal disease

2. *Nephrotic Syndrome*[74]

a. Definition: the clinical expression of any glomerular disease that produces massive proteinuria
b. Etiology and pathogenesis: the decreased plasma oncotic pressure results in consequent edema and serosal effusion
c. Causative renal pathology
   i. Primary glomerulonephritis
   ii. Secondary glomerulonephritis
      - Diabetes
      - Systemic lupus erythematosus
      - Infectious disease (e.g., HIV, CMV, etc.)
      - Renal vessel thrombosis
      - Neoplasms
      - Drug effects (e.g., NSAIDs)
d. Physical findings
   i. Weight gain
   ii. Fatigue
   iii. Generalized edema
   iv. Edema of eyelids
   v. Increased melanin "allergic shiner" in recurrent periorbital edema
e. Diagnostic tests
   i. Urine protein loss exceeding 3 to 4 g/day (hallmark finding)
   ii. Albuminuria, hypoalbuminemia, hyperlipidemia
f. Treatment
   i. Treat underlying cause
   ii. Diet high in protein, low in sodium and fluid uptake
   iii. Gradual reduction of edema (e.g., oral furosemide)
   iv. Treat complications (venous thrombosis, infection, dyslipidemia, etc.) when appropriate

3. *Post-Transplant*[75–77]

a. Definition: organ or stem cell replacement
b. Etiology
   i. Organ transplant: primary treatment for end-stage organ failure
      - Heart, lung, kidney, liver, and small bowel
   ii. Stem cell replacement: replace unhealthy bone marrow and immune cells following cancer treatment (chemotherapy or radiotherapy) with healthy bone marrow and immune cells
      - Used to treat multiple myeloma, lymphoma, leukemias, myeloproliferative neoplasms
c. Clinical course: complications common
   i. Organ transplant
      - Obesity, diabetes, hypertension, heart failure, malignancies
      - Caused by immunosuppressive medications, damage caused by end-stage organ failure, lifestyle, genetic susceptibility
      - Long-term graft failure major reason for mortality and morbidity
   ii. Stem cell transplant
      - Neutropenia (low neutrophil or white blood cell count) and resulting infections
      - Gastrointestinal toxicities and organ dysfunction
      - Graft versus Host disease (allogenic transplantation only)
         – Chronic disease will affect skin, lungs, liver, gastrointestinal tract, salivary, and lacrimal glands (sicca syndrome)
      - Relapse of disease major cause of mortality
d. Ocular complications
   i. Posterior subcapsular cataracts very common due to systemic, topical, intravitreal, and inhaled steroid use
   ii. Secondary to immunosuppressive antirejection treatment
      - Opportunist infections (herpes simplex, herpes zoster, CMV retinitis, rhino-orbital fungus)
      - Conjunctival and eyelid squamous cell carcinoma
      - Central vein occlusion

4. *Uremia*[78]

a. Widespread systemic disorder associated with chronic renal failure
b. Pathogenesis: unknown, but accumulation of metabolic by-products may be the cause
c. Symptoms: pruritis, polydipsia, nausea, vomiting, weight loss, mental confusion
d. Physical findings
   i. Wasting, sallow complexion, mouth ulcers, hypertension
   ii. Band keratopathy, pericarditis, neuropathies, pleural effusions
e. Laboratory findings
   i. Elevated blood urea nitrogen (BUN) and creatinine, anemia
   ii. Urine specific gravity 1.010, isothenuria, proteinuria, tubular casts
f. Treatment
   i. Conflicting evidence on protein restriction
   ii. Potassium, phosphate, and sodium intake should be approximately 2 g/day
   iii. Dialysis
   iv. Kidney transplantation

5. *Wilms' Tumor*[79]

a. Kidney tumor
   i. 95% found in children
b. Third most common organ cancer in children under 10 years of age
c. Mesodermal in origin, hence association with aniridia
d. Symptoms caused by tumor's large size, abdominal
e. Abdominal ultrasound is initial imaging of choice
f. Treatment: chemotherapy, radiotherapy, nephrectomy
g. 5-year survival rate exceeds 90%

H. Neurology

1. *Myasthenia Gravis*[80–83]

a. Epidemiology
   i. Any age
   ii. Prevalence one in 5000 patients
   iii. Thymoma: 10%
   iv. Divided into early onset (<45 years old) (female to male 3:1) and late onset (>45 years old) (male to female 5:1)
b. Etiology and pathogenesis
   i. Defective neuromuscular transmission across motor end plates of skeletal muscles
   ii. Autoimmune reaction against acetylcholine receptors (AChR)
c. Symptomatology

i. Ocular complaint: ptosis and diplopia found in about 85% of initial complaints
   - Can be transient, fluctuating, and progressive throughout the day

ii. 5% have thyrotoxicosis

d. Physical findings
   i. Weakness without other signs of neurological deficit
   ii. Variability of muscle function within minutes, hours, or weeks
   iii. Predilection for extraocular, facial, and oropharyngeal muscles
   iv. Approximately 20% of MG patients will only have ocular issues

e. Diagnostic tests
   i. Tensilon test 10 mg (IV effects immediate)
   ii. Single fiber electromyography
   iii. Specific lab test for autoantibodies
   iv. Chest radiographs to rule out thymoma
   v. Must be considered in any extraocular muscle problem

f. Treatment
   i. The domain of the neurologist
   ii. Neostigmine, pyridostigmine PO
   iii. Systemic immunosuppressants
      a. Steroids
      b. Azathioprine
   iv. Plasmapheresis, immunoadsorption, and the intravenous administration of immunoglobulins are used for crisis intervention
   v. Thymectomy: beneficial in more than 50% of patients

g. Clinical course
   i. Long, chronic course with periods of remission
   ii. Highly variable and not predictable in any one patient
   iii. Can be fatal if respiratory muscles in volved
   iv. Remission achieved in 25% of patients
   v. One-third remain ocular after 3 years duration
   vi. If only ocular after 2 years, low chance of progression

2. *Temporal Arteritis (Cranial or Giant-Cell Arteritis)*[84–86]

a. Epidemiology
   i. Rare under 60 years of age (80% are over 70 years of age)
   ii. Female incidence greater than males (3:1)
   iii. Ophthalmic artery involved in more than 50% of cases
   iv. Rare among Black patients

b. Etiology and pathogenesis
   i. Autoimmune reaction to elastin fibers
   ii. An inflammatory disorder affecting medium-size arteries
   iii. Considered an ophthalmic emergency since can lead to significant irreversible vision loss

c. Symptomatology
   i. Headache, scalp tenderness, intermittent jaw claudication, fever, weight loss, fatigue
   ii. Polymyalgia rheumatica (50% of GCA patients): stiffness, aching, and pain in the muscles of the neck, shoulders, lower back, hips, and thighs
   iii. Loss of vision due to Arteritis Anterior Ischemic Optic Neuropathy (AAION)
   iv. Pain on combing hair

d. Physical findings
   i. Palpable nodular enlargement of temporal artery
   ii. Overlying skin: edematous, erythematous
   iii. Skip lesions: long segments of involved arteries unaffected
   iv. Clinical signs and symptoms can vary
      - Silent variant: systemic conditions prominent and cranial features absent
      - Occult variant: systemic signs and symptoms are absent

e. Diagnostic tests
   i. CRP and ESR (≥50 mm/h) elevated
   ii. Imaging: non-invasive techniques
      - Ultrasound: "halo" sign of temporal arteries
      - CTA/MRA/PET scans
   iii. Biopsy of temporal artery with mononuclear-cell infiltration or granulomatous inflammation, loss of internal elastic lamina
   iv. Anemia, thrombocytosis, leukocytosis

f. Treatment
   i. New onset cases: intravenous steroids for 3 days
   ii. Oral corticosteroids to reduce ESR (1 mg/kg body weight/day)
      - Continued for several months and eventually slowly tapered
   iii. Secondary immunosuppressive agents include infliximab, methotrexate, cyclophosphamide
   iv. Pain relief with aspirin, indomethacin (Indocin)

g. Clinical course
   i. Once blindness occurs, return of vision rare
   ii. Chronic course, eventually leading to remission
   iii. Blindness in other eye 25% if untreated
   iv. Aorta often involved with aneurysm, dissection
   v. Mesenteric arteritis, MI, claudication of legs (if iliacs involved)

I. Oncology

1. *Breast Cancer*[87,88]

a. Currently the most common form of cancer in women in the United States

b. Mortality rates are decreasing for breast cancer but increasing for lung cancer in females

c. 1:7 to 1:12 in women

d. Prognosis depends on type of tumor, lymph node involvement, age, and size of tumor
   i. Best prognosis: <2 cm tumor
   ii. Less chance of recurrence with HR positive and HER2 negative cancers
   iii. Highest chance of recurrence with hormone receptor (HR) negative and HER2 negative cancers ("triple negative")

e. Treatment
   i. Lumpectomy (breast conservation therapy)
      - Radiation is adjuvant therapy to eliminate residual microscopic disease
   ii. Chemotherapy
      - Neoadjuvant: makes inoperable breast cancer resectable
      - Systemic chemotherapy for high-risk patients (e.g., 5-fluorouracil, methotrexate)
   iii. Endocrine treatment for HR positive disease

- Selective estrogen receptor modulators (tamoxifen)
- Aromatase inhibitors (AI) (anastrozole, letrozole, and exemestane)

iv. Biologics for HER2 positive
- Paclitaxel, docetaxel, trastuzumab, pertuzumab

v. Surgery (mastectomy)
- Total mastectomy
- Skin-sparing mastectomy
- Nipple areolar-sparing mastectomy
- Postmastectomy radiation

vi. Anterior segment manifestations
- Treatment side effects
  - Ocular surface disease may be induced by treatment or just associated with postmenopausal women who are more likely suffer from breast cancer
  - Docetaxel and 5-fluorouracil induce epiphora (canicular stenosis)
  - Tamoxifen: corneal deposits and posterior subcapsular cataracts
  - AI induced bone loss and subsequent bisphosphonates Rx and potential uveitis and scleritis

2. *Bronchogenic (Lung) Cancer*[89,90]

a. Symptoms
  i. 25% asymptomatic, found incidentally on chest radiography
  ii. 75% symptomatic cough, fatigue, weight loss, chest pain, dyspnea (difficulty breathing), hemoptysis (coughing up blood)
  iii. Risk factors include history of smoking, exposure to secondhand smoke, workplace exposure (e.g., asbestos), radon, and air pollution

b. May present with ipsilateral Horner's syndrome (ptosis, miosis, anhidrosis), and ulnar nerve pain
  i. Pancoast tumor (pulmonary apex location)
  ii. In apical field, it impinges on cervical sympathetic plexus

c. Two classes of cancer
  i. Small cell lung carcinoma (SCLC)
  ii. Non-small cell lung carcinoma (NSCLC) more common (85%)
  - Adenocarcinoma represents 85% of NSCLC

d. Most common cause of mortality among all cancers (18%)

e. Overall 5-year survival, 10%

3. *Metastatic Neoplasm*[91,92]

a. General
  i. Malignant neoplasms disseminate by one of three pathways
  - Direct seeding within body cavity (e.g., basal cell rare)
  - Lymphatic spread (e.g., breast cancer)
  - Hematogenous (via the bloodstream) spread (e.g., colon cancer)

b. Ocular involvement
  i. No predilection for right or left eye
  ii. Bilateral 20%
  iii. Commonly carcinomas, not melanoma or sarcoma
  iv. 25% of patients with ocular involvement will have no cancer history
  v. Choroid most common site for ocular metastases
  vi. Women: breast cancer, history of breast cancer of 2 years duration
  vii. Men: lung cancer, ocular metastasis before primary is found, also typical of kidney cancer
  viii. 40% of metastatic tumors to anterior segments have iridocyclitis

c. Rare for primary ocular malignancy to metastasize

4. *Multiple Myeloma*[93–96]

a. Epidemiology
  i. 3:100,000
  ii. 50 to 70 years of age

b. Etiology and pathogenesis: proliferation of abnormal plasma cells in the bone marrow that produce monoclonal immunoglobulin (M band)

c. Symptomatology
  i. Severe bone pain, initial symptom in two-thirds of patients
  ii. Symptoms of anemia: fatigue, malaise, anorexia

d. Physical findings
  i. Pathological fractures
  ii. Recurrent infections

e. Diagnostic tests
  i. Test for serum protein electrophoresis (SPEP), characteristic Monoclonal (usually IgA or IgG) spike
  ii. Osteolytic bone lesions on radiographs
  iii. Bone marrow biopsy: plasma cells (>10%)
  iv. Complete blood count reveals anemia

f. Treatment
  i. Chemotherapy (alkylating agents, anthracyclines, and steroids)
  ii. Proteasome inhibitors
  iii. Immunomodulatory drugs
  iv. Monoclonal antibodies
  v. Autologous stem cell transplantation
  vi. Allogenic stem cell transplantation

g. Clinical course
  i. Infection (pneumonia is common) is most common cause of death, secondary to patients' depressed immunological defenses (bone marrow failure)
  ii. Bone pain can be exceptionally disabling!
  iii. Five-year survival rate low
  iv. Uremia (sign of kidney failure) and hypercalcemia are worst prognostic signs

h. Anterior segment manifestations
  i. Crystals in cornea and conjunctiva
  ii. Microcystic-like epithelial changes secondary to treatment with antibody-drug conjugates (monoclonal antibody and chemotherapy)
  iii. Band keratopathy from hypercalcemia
  iv. Recurrent subconjunctival hemorrhages
  v. Ciliary body cysts
  vi. Lid edema if kidneys are damaged

5. *Primary Neoplasm*

a. Hodgkin's disease[97]
  i. 10% of systemic lymphomas
  ii. Symptoms and signs
  - Fever, night sweats, and weight loss
  - Painless lymphadenopathy

iii. Diagnosis: biopsy reveals microscopic presence of Reed–Sternberg cells
iv. Prognosis: depends on staging
v. Ocular: extremely rare involvement

b. Non-Hodgkin's lymphoma[98–101]
i. Majority of systemic lymphomas
ii. Heterogenous group of lymphoproliferative malignancies
iii. Majority of lymphomas affecting ocular adnexa (greater spread to extranodal locations)
iv. Symptom: lymphadenopathy (cervical is most common of head and neck presentations)
v. Diagnosis: biopsy
vi. Prognosis: nodular better than diffuse
vii. Most common: nodular, poorly differentiated, lymphocytic tumors
- Conjunctival lymphoid tumors
  - 50 to 60 years of age
  - 90% not associated with systemic disease
  - Predilection for the fornix
  - Biopsy is the only *way* to tell benign from malignant
  - 80% of lymphoid tumors represent reactive hyperplasia
- Orbital lymphoid tumors
  - Orbital pseudotumor: explosive onset, pain, proptosis, extraocular movement disturbance
  - Orbital lymphoid tumors: insidious onset, painless, usually anterior superior location; proptosis, ptosis, chemosis, and ocular motility (painful or restrictive); 50% have systemic disease; diagnosis based on biopsy, computed tomography (CT) and MRI scans; treatment: excision, radiation, chemotherapy

c. Malignant melanoma[102–105]
i. Skin cancer (cutaneous melanoma)
- Any age, peak incidence 50 to 60 years
- UV protection most modifiable risk factor, sun protection options when outside
  - Sunscreen (>15 SPF)
  - Wearing protective clothes (wide brim hats, long sleeve shirts, and long pants)
  - Staying in the shade
- Most arise from preexisting nevi or moles and more likely in fair skin, red or blond hair, and light-colored eyes
- 30% of population have nevi, 1:25,000 have melanoma
  - Nevi: rounded, regular, distinct borders, tan to brown
  - Melanomas: irregular margins, brown to black background with foci
- Metastasis based on depth of skin penetration
- Death by visceral involvement

ii. Malignant melanoma of iris
- Usually asymptomatic
- Patients are usually young (<20 years of age)
- Arise from previously noted iris nevi or a new pigment spot
- 6% of all uveal melanoma (least common of uveal melanomas)
- Presents as mass, heterochromia, glaucoma, uveitis, distorted pupil, hyphema
- Rarely metastasize
- Mortality rate 4%

iii. Malignant melanoma of conjunctiva
- Arise from nevi, primary acquired melanosis (approximately 60%), and de novo
- Rare from congenital ocular melanocytosis
- Typically found on bulbar conjunctiva and patients are over 60 years of age
- Exceedingly rare in Black patients
- Mortality
  - 5-year and 10-year survival rate is approximately 80% and 70% respectively
  - Nevi: approximately 5% in those acquired from nevi
  - De novo: approximately 40% in those that are de novo

J. Pediatrics

1. *Chickenpox*[106]

a. Varicella virus
i. Chickenpox in non-immune host (usually child)
ii. Shingles (zoster) in the immune host (*always* adult)

b. Droplet infection (from nasopharynx) communicable from 1 day prior to 6 days after appearance of physical findings

c. Discrete erythematous macules and papules about 10–21 days after infection over thorax, scalp, and mucous membranes
i. Crust forms in 2 to 4 days
ii. Duration of 2 to 3 weeks

d. Pruritis: most annoying feature

e. Complications are rare in healthy children but can happen in immunosuppressed children, teenagers, and adults

f. Treatment symptomatic

g. Vaccine for prevention

2. *Galactosemia*[107,108]

a. Epidemiology
i. Autosomal-recessive trait resulting in impaired galactose metabolism
ii. 1% of population is heterozygous for galactosemia gene
iii. Incidence 1:50,000

b. Etiology and pathogenesis
i. Deficiency of galactose-1-phosphate uridyltransferase
- Cataract
- Cirrhosis (neonatal jaundice)
- Long-term complications
  - Cognitive impairment
  - Speech and language impairment
  - Motor disturbance
  - Primary ovary deficiency

ii. Deficiency of galactokinase cataract formation

c. Symptomatology
i. Days to weeks after birth, failure to thrive
ii. Reluctant to ingest breast milk or formula
iii. Poor weight gain, vomiting, diarrhea

d. Physical findings
i. Oil droplet cataracts develop over weeks to months secondary to galacticol
ii. Jaundice, hepatomegaly, liver disease

e. Diagnostic tests
  i. High galactose in blood
  ii. Definitive: demonstrating the enzyme deficiency in RBC
  iii. Measure urine galactitol
  iv. Can be diagnosed by amniocentesis
f. Treatment
  i. Galactose-free diet usually leads to dramatic improvement but does not prevent long-term complications
  ii. All clinical features (except long-term complications) may improve
  iii. Lenses clear or regress if treated early

3. *Kawasaki's Disease*[109,110]

a. Autoimmune disease with inflammation in blood vessels throughout the body
  i. Cardiac vessels: aneurysms and myocardial infarctions
b. Patients are usually <5 years old, Asian countries especially Japan
c. Physical findings
  i. Fever >5 days
  ii. Bilateral injection of conjunctiva
  iii. Fissured lips, strawberry tongue, reddening of oral and pharyngeal mucosa
  iv. Polymorphous rash of trunk
  v. Peripheral edema, peripheral erythema (reddening of palms, soles)
  vi. Acute non-suppurative swelling of cervical nodes
d. 1% to 2% die from coronary artery thrombosis, aneurysm, myocarditis, or pericarditis
e. Treatment: high dose aspirin and intravenous immunoglobulin

4. *Mumps*[111,112]

a. Paramyxovirus
b. Humans: only natural host for mumps
c. Peak ages 6 to 10 years old but can affect adults
d. Incidence has declined due to vaccine acceptance
e. Physical signs
  i. Headache, muscle pain, low-grade fever, and malaise
  ii. Sudden onset of parotitis
f. Anterior segment manifestations
  i. Conjunctivitis
  ii. Episcleritis
  iii. Keratitis
  iv. Anterior uveitis
  v. Dacryoadenitis
  vi. Sixth nerve palsy
g. Mild disease in children
h. Complication in adults
  i. Orchitis in 30% of postpubertal males
  ii. Meningitis
i. Supportive treatment
j. Live attenuated vaccine for prevention

K. Rheumatology

1. *Ankylosing Spondylitis*

(Refer to Chapter 6 for a complete discussion.)

2. *Gout*[113,114]

a. Epidemiology
  i. Disease of middle-aged or elderly men (85 to 90% of patients)
  ii. Associated with overeating, alcohol, and periods of stress
  iii. 10% preceded by nephrolithiasis
b. Etiology
  i. Release of microcrystals of monosodium urate monohydrate into joint cavities
  ii. Disorder of purine metabolism
c. Symptomatology
  i. Acute monoarticular pain often of nocturnal onset
  ii. Symptoms of acute inflammation: erythema, heat, swelling, pain
d. Physical findings
  i. Initial presentation: first metatarsophalangeal joint (big toe)
  ii. Recurrent attacks may also involve ankles, knees, fingers, wrist, olecranon (elbow) bursa
e. Diagnostic tests
  i. Elevated serum uric acid level
  ii. Synovial fluid analysis: urate crystals
f. Treatment
  i. Non-pharmacological
    - Increase physical activity and weight loss
    - Dietary restrictions (no meat, crustaceans, yeast, sugar-containing drinks) and alcohol reduction
  ii. Pharmacological
    - Acute: nonsteroidal agents, steroids, colchicine, and canakinumab (monoclonal antibody)
    - Chronic: allopurinol, probenecid, lesinurad
g. Clinical course
  i. Can lead to bone erosion, joint deformity, and renal insufficiency
  ii. Variable beginning; many months to years between attacks; later attacks are more frequent and more severe and affect more and more joints
h. Anterior segment manifestations
  i. Cornea: scintillating crystals scattered in epithelium, Bowman's membrane, and stroma
  ii. Crystals deposited in conjunctiva, iris, and sclera
  iii. Chronic conjunctivitis with congested and tortuous vessels and subconjunctival hemorrhages (SCH) (spot and patchy)
  iv. Uveitis, scleritis, episcleritis

3. *Reactive Arthritis (Reiter's Syndrome)*

(Refer to Chapter 6 for a complete discussion.)

4. *Rheumatoid Arthritis (RA)*[115–117]

a. Epidemiology
  i. Affects 4% of women and 1.5% of men
  ii. Onset: 35 to 60 years old
  iii. All races and ethnic groups
  iv. Typical case: women 30 to 50 years of age
b. Etiology and pathogenesis
  i. Chronic, symmetrical, inflammatory autoimmune disease
  ii. Non-suppurative, proliferative synovitis affecting small joints first and then larger joints

iii. Anti-IgG antibodies

c. Symptomatology
   i. Joint pain, stiffness, limited motion, morning stiffness greater than 30 minutes
   ii. Constitutional symptoms precede arthritis: fatigue, fever, neurasthenia

d. Physical findings
   i. Ulnar deviation of wrist
   ii. Swan neck deformity of fingers
   iii. Rheumatoid nodules: asymptomatic, subcutaneous, 25% of patients
   iv. Carpal tunnel syndrome

e. Diagnostic tests
   i. Rheumatoid factor (RF) and anticitrullinated protein antibodies (ACPAs) in serum
   ii. Synovial fluid analysis: polymorphonuclear cells (PMNs) and decreased complement level
   iii. MRI of joints

f. Treatment
   i. First-line treatment: nonsteroidal anti-inflammatory drugs (NSAIDs)
      - ASA 3 to 6 g/day
         - Ibuprofen
         - Naproxen
   ii. Steroids short term for flare ups
   iii. Second-line treatment: disease-modifying antirheumatic drugs (DMARDs)
      - Methotrexate
      - Hydroxychloroquine
   iv. Biologics
      - Tumor necrosis factor (TNF) inhibitors: etanercept (Enbrel), infliximab (Remicade), adalimumab (Humira)
   v. Physical therapy and exercise
   vi. Arthritis surgery: end-stage disease

g. Clinical course
   i. Leads to destruction of articular cartilage and progressive disabling arthritis in 10% of patients after 20 years duration
   ii. Extra-articular involvement of skin, heart vessels (cardiovascular disease is leading cause of death for RA patients), muscles, lungs (amyloidosis in 5 to 10%)
   iii. After 10 years, disease stabilizes in 50% of patients
   iv. Not predictable, but men do slightly better than women

h. Anterior segment manifestations
   i. K sicca associated with secondary Sjögren's syndrome
   ii. Episcleritis
   iii. Scleritis (less frequent and associated with more severe disease)
   iv. Peripheral ulcerative keratitis and corneal melt: requires systemic treatment of underlying RA disease

5. *Sarcoidosis*

(Refer to Chapter 6 for a complete discussion.)

6. *Sjögren's Syndrome*[118,119]

a. Epidemiology
   i. 90% are women
   ii. Average age 50 years old
   iii. All races involved

b. Etiology and pathogenesis
   i. Immunological attack (T cells) on exocrine organs including lymphocyte infiltration of lacrimal and salivary glands, lungs, liver, and kidneys
   ii. B cell hyperactivity which releases autoantibodies

c. Symptomatology
   i. Dry eye
   ii. Difficulty chewing, swallowing, phonation
   iii. Morning stiffness and joint pain mimicking RA
   iv. Fatigue

d. Physical findings
   i. Filamentary keratitis
   ii. Fissures and ulcers of tongue, buccal mucosa, and lips
   iii. Rampant dental caries
   iv. 50% have parotid or submandibular gland enlargement
   v. Arthralgias and arthritis
   vi. Cutaneous lesions

e. Diagnostic tests
   i. Diagnosis: no single diagnostic test available, use the following as a guide
      - Lymphocytic infiltrate in salivary gland (biopsy)
      - Blood antinuclear autoantibodies (Ro/SSA and anti-La/SSB)
      - Definite KCS (ocular surface staining and reduced Schirmer's test)
      - Hyposalivation
      - Any connective tissue or lymphoproliferative disorder presenting rheumatoid arthritis, systemic lupus erythematosus, systemic sclerosis, polymyositis
   ii. Difficult to recognize and patients may go 10 years with symptoms but no diagnosis
   iii. Differential: local glandular disorder, depression, parasympathomimetic drugs

f. Treatment
   i. Symptomatic
      - Ocular: see KCS (Chapter 5, Section I. D.)
      - Oral: limit sugar and acid in diet, excellent oral hygiene, sugar-free lozenges/gum, and pharmacological stimulation (e.g., pilocarpine and cevimeline)
   ii. Corticosteroids and immunosuppressive drugs for
      - Severe functional disability
      - Life-threatening complications
      - A balanced risk/benefit ratio has not been established

g. Clinical course
   i. One-third only have KCS and xerostomia (dry mouth)
   ii. Raynaud's in 20%
   iii. One-third have interstitial nephritis

- iv. Lymphomas occur more frequently than in general population
- v. Esophageal webs may develop

h. Anterior segment manifestations

- i. Ocular complications: corneal ulceration, vascularization, opacification, and rarely perforation
- ii. All secondary to dry eye or keratitis sicca problems
- iii. Uveitis and scleritis have been reported

L. Trauma

1. Head Injury

a. General

- i. Leading cause of death under 40 years of age
- ii. Severity of head injury may not become manifest for days to weeks

b. Special entity

- i. Carotid cavernous fistulas[120]
  - Traumatic three times more common than spontaneous type
  - Usually in men 20 to 30 years of age, following severe head trauma
  - Symptoms: bothersome orbital bruit, red eye, foreign-body sensation, diplopia
  - Signs: pulsating exophthalmos, chemosis, conjunctival and episcleral vessel dilation, ocular motor palsy (VI nerve common), exposure keratitis, Goldmann tonometry will show more movement of the mires on the side of the ocular signs
  - Diagnosis: cerebral angiography (computer tomographic angiography or magnetic resonance angiography)
  - Treatment
    - Low flow: observe since may close spontaneously
    - High flow: endovascular treatment (transarterially or transvenously)
- ii. Epidural hematoma[121]
  - 1% to 3% of major head injuries
  - Male to female, 4:1
  - Auto accidents common, also with trivial falls and sports injuries
  - Fracture of temporal skull in 80% of cases
  - Clinical picture: "talk and die picture"
    - Unconscious, then regains relatively normal function
    - As hematoma enlarges, it causes herniation of the uncus compressing cranial nerve III with ipsilateral pupil dilation or ptosis
    - Contralateral hemiparesis develops
  - Computed tomography (CT) is gold standard for diagnosis
- iii. Basal skull fracture[122]
  - If anterior basilar fracture is present, damaging the anterior venous sinuses, blood leaks into periorbital tissue producing raccoon or panda sign (dark discoloration of lids with no subconjunctival involvement)

2. Orbital/Periorbital Trauma

(See Chapter 3, "Orbital Irritations and Injuries.")

II. "Top 100" Systemic Diagnoses Related to Anterior Segment Care

A. "Top 100" Specific Diagnoses

See Table 9.1.

B. "Top 100" Diagnoses by Pathological Classification

See Table 9.2.

C. "Top 100" Diagnoses by Ocular Anatomical Classification

See Table 9.3.

TABLE 9.1 "Top 100" Specific Diagnoses

Systemic Disorder	Pathological Classification	Anterior Segment Manifestation	Primary Eyecare Management	Co-Management or Referral
1. Acne rosacea[123]	Dermatological	Blepharitis, meibomian gland dysfunction Conjunctivitis, keratitis	Warm compresses, lid hygiene Steroids, oral doxycycline	Dermatologist
2. AIDS	Infectious	Kaposi's sarcoma	Monitor and counsel	Primary physician
3. Addison's disease[124]	Endocrine	Lid pigmentation Conjunctiva pigmentation	Counsel	Internist
4. Albinism	Metabolic	Depigmentation	Palliative	Vision rehabilitation
5. Alcoholism	Nutritional	Meibomianitis Conjunctivitis	Antibiotics Steroids (limited)	Primary physician
6. Alkaptonuria	Metabolic	Pigmentation Pathognomonic "oil-drop" lesions of the limbus	Counsel	Internist
7. Allergies	Allergic	Lid and conjunctival edema Hyperemia	Cold compresses Antihistamine mast cell stabilizer Steroids (limited)	Primary physician Allergist
8. Alport's syndrome[125]	Renal	Anterior lenticonus Anterior polar cataract	Counsel	Internist
9. Amyloidosis[126]	Metabolic	Lid nodules Conjunctival masses Bruising around eyes Dry eye, lattice dystrophy	Counsel Palliative	Internist
10. Anemia(s)	Hematologic	Pallor Subconjuctival hemorrhage	Counsel	Primary physician
11. Ankylosing spondylitis	Collagen vascular	Anterior uveitis	Cycloplege and dilate Steroids	Rheumatologist
12. Asthma[127]	Pulmonary	Conjunctivitis	Antihistamine/Mast cell stabilizer Steroids (limited)	Internist
13. Behçet's disease[128]	Dermatological (?) Ophthalmologic (?)	Anterior uveitis Cataracts	Cycloplege and dilate Steroids	Gynecologist Primary physician
14. Breast cancer (carcinoma)	Neoplastic	Metastasis	Counsel	Surgeon, Oncologist Ophthalmologist
15. Cardiovascular disease	Cardiovascular	Arcus senilis Lipid keratopathy	Counsel	Cardiologist Primary physician
16. Cat-scratch fever	Infectious	Follicular conjunctivitis	Supportive	Primary physician
17. Chlamydial disease	Infectious	Conjunctivitis Keratitis	Oral azithromycin	Primary physician
18. Cogan's syndrome[129]	Collagen vascular	Interstitial keratitis Conjunctivitis, iritis	Steroids, counsel	Neurologist Cardiologist
19. Crohn's disease (regional enteritis)	Gastrointestinal	Anterior uveitis	Cycloplege and dilate Steroids	Gastroenterologist
20. Dermatitis	Dermatological	Blepharitis Conjunctivitis	Calcineurin-inhibitors, Steriods	Dermatologist
21. Dermatomyositis (polymyositis)[130]	Collagen vascular	Lid edema/ptosis Lid erythema, chemosis exophthalmous	Cold compresses	Dermatologist Internist
22. Diabetes mellitus	Endocrine	Recurrent erosion Rubeosis irides	Supportive	Internist
23. Down syndrome	Chromosomal	Epicanthal folds Keratoconus Brushfield's spots	Monitor closely	Pediatrician
24. Eczema[131]	Dermatological	Blepharoconjunctivitis Dry eye syndrome	Supportive	Dermatologist
25. Ehlers–Danlos syndrome[132]	Dermatological	Blue sclera Steeper/thinner cornea	Counsel	Primary physician

(Continued)

TABLE 9.1 (CONTINUED) "Top 100" Specific Diagnoses

Subjective Systemic Highlight	Objective Systemic Highlight	Standard Medical Management	Complications (Ocular and Systemic)	Prognosis (Ocular and Systemic)
Recurrent Middle age	Skin flush Papillae Telangiectasia	Oral doxycycline Topical metronidazole Intense pulse light	O: Scarring S: Recurring	O/S: 10–15-year course
Risk category	HIV positive	Antiretroviral drugs	O: CMV retinitis S: Infection	O: Good S:Good
Weakness Fatigue	Skin pigmentation in body creases	Steroids	O: Papilledema S: Diabetes	O/S: Good
Genetic	Depigmentation	Counsel	O: Numerous S: Sunlight	O: Guarded S: Good
Addiction	Gastrointestinal Dermatological	Rehabilitation	O: Neurological S: Liver disease	O: Good S: Guarded
Genetic, brown urine	Skin pigmentation	Nitisinone Vitamin C	O: Central vein occlusion, elevated IOP S: Arthritis, Numerous	O/S: Good
Long history Seasonal	Nasal congestion Asthmatic	Antihistamines Decongestants Steroids	O: Recurrent S: Steroids	O: Guarded S:Good
Genetic	Nerve deafness Hypertension	Antihypertensive	O: Posterior pole S: Renal, Cardiovascular	O/S: Guarded
Genetic	Serum protein Amyloid deposits	Surgery	O: Posterior pole, vitreous opacites, glaucoma S: Numerous	O: Guarded S: Poor
General weakness	Laboratory blood Workup	Vitamins/ Minerals, EPO stimulating	O: Posterior Pole S: Numerous	O: Good S: Guarded
Lower back pain	HLA-B27+	Steroids Biologics	S: Rheumatoid arthritis, Steroids	O: Good S: Guarded
Family history	Breathing problems	Beta-2 adrenergic agonists, steroids	O: Steroids S: Steroids	O: Good S: Guarded
Greater in Orientals	Mouth ulcers Genital lesions Systemic vasculitis	Steroids Cytostatic agents	O: Hyphema S: Vascular	O: Poor S: Guarded
Cancer history	Biopsy+	Surgery	O: Posterior pole S: Metastasis	O/S: Poor
Risk factors	Angina Arterosclerosis	Reduce risk factors Pharmacotherapy Invasive procedures	O: Posterior pole S: Renal	O: Guarded S: Poor
Cat history	Lymphadenopathy Fever	Palliative Azithromycin ?	O: Retinitis	O/S: Good
Venereal	Genitourinary	Oral azithromycin Counsel	O: Adult scarring S: Genitourinary	O/S: Good
Tinnitus Vertigo	Vestibular deafness	Immunosuppressants Rehabilitation	O: Photophobia S: Cardiovascular Neurological	O/S: Guarded
Recurrent cramping	Bloody diarrhea	Steroids Biologics Surgery	S: Metabolic disturbance	O: Good S: Guarded
Atopic history	Skin rash	Steroids	O: Keratitis	O: Good
Contact History	Erythema Dermatological Systemic	Steroids Immunosuppressants	S: Steroids O: Posterior pole S: Steroids	S: Guarded O: Good S: Guarded
Polyuria	Hyperglycemia	Oral meds, Insulin	O: Posterior pole S: Numerous	O/S: Guarded
Congenital Trisomy 21	Stigmata of syndrome "Funny-looking kid" (FLK)	Counsel	O: Cataracts numerous S: Cardiac	O: Good S: Guarded
Atopia	Excoriated, nodular, red lesions	Steroids (limited) Topical calcineurin inhibitors, systemic immunosuppression	O: Cataracts S: Asthma	O: Good S: Guarded
Skin fragility	Hyperelasticity	Counsel	O: Retinal detachment S: Hematomas	O: Guarded S: Good

(*Continued*)

TABLE 9.1 (CONTINUED) **"Top 100" Specific Diagnoses**

Systemic Disorder	Pathological Classification	Anterior Segment Manifestation	Primary Eyecare Management	Co-Management or Referral
26. Fabry's disease[133,134]	Metabolic	Conjunctival vessel tortuosity	Monitor closely	Pediatrician
		Corneal "whirl like" opacities		Internist
27. Facial deformity syndromes	Musculoskeletal	Lower lid colobomas	Counsel	Pediatrician
		Epibulbar dermoids		
28. Galactosemia[135]	Metabolic	Cataract	Counsel	Pediatrician
29. Gaucher's disease[136]	Metabolic	Conjunctival infiltrates	Counsel	Pediatrician
		Corneal opacity		Corneal surgeon
30. Gonorrhea	Infectious	Hyperacute purulent conjunctivitis	Topical antibiotic	Primary physician
31. Gout[113,137]	Metabolic	Corneal crystals Tortuous conjunctival vessels	Steroids	Internist
		Anterior uveitis		
32. Hay fever	Allergic	Conjunctivitis	Antihistamine/mast cell stabilizers	Primary physician
			Steroids (limited)	Allergist
33. Hemophilia[138–140]	Hematological	Ecchymosis	Cold compresses	Hematologist
		Subconjunctival hemorrhage	Monitor closely	Primary physician
34. Herpes simplex	Infectious	Blepharitis Dendritic keratitis	Trifluridine, Ganciclovir, Oral antivirals	Primary physician
35. Herpes zoster	Infectious	Dermatoblepharitis	Oral antivirals	Dermatologist
		Keratitis	Steroids (limited)	
		Anterior uveitis		
36. Histiocytosis[141]	Metabolic	Unilateral exophthalmos	Monitor exophthalmometry	Internist
37. Histoplasmosis[142]	Infectious	Conjunctival nodule	Palliative	Primary physician
38. Hives (urticaria)	Allergic	Lid edema Lid erythema	Cold compresses	Allergist
39. Homocystinuria[143]	Metabolic	Dislocated lens	Monitor closely	Pediatrician
40. Hyperparathyroidism	Endocrine	Band keratopathy	Monitor closely	Endocrinologist
41. Hyperthyroidism[144] (Graves' disease)	Endocrine	Lid signs Exophthalmos	Monitor closely	Internist
		Exposure keratitis		
		SLK		
42. Hypervitaminosis[145]	Nutritional	Band keratopathy	Monitor closely	Primary physician
43. Hypoparathyroidism[30,146,147]	Endocrine	Cataract	Monitor closely	Endocrinologist
44. Hypothyroidism	Endocrine	Lid edema, K sicca	Monitor closely	Primary physician
45. Impetigo[148]	Infectious	Lid pustules	Antibiotics	Pediatrician
46. Influenza[149,150]	Infectious	Conjunctivits	Palliative	Primary physician
47. Kaposi's sarcoma[151]	Neoplastic	Lid tumor	Counsel	Oncologist
48. Leukemia(s)[152]	Neoplastic	Proptosis Subconjunctival	Counsel	Oncoclogist
		hemorrhages		
49. Lipidoses	Metabolic	Arcus senilis	Monitor closely	Internist
50. Liver disease[153]	Nutritional	Icteric sclera	Monitor closely	Internist

(*Continued*)

TABLE 9.1 (CONTINUED) "Top 100" Specific Diagnoses

Subjective Systemic Highlight	Objective Systemic Highlight	Standard Medical Management	Complications (Ocular and Systemic)	Prognosis (Ocular and Systemic)
Red-purple maculopapular skin lesions	Genetic deficiency of a lysosomal enzyme	Counsel Enzyme replacement therapy	O: Posterior pole S: Cardiovascular, Renal	O/S: Guarded
"Funny-looking kid" (FLK) syndromes	Goldenhar Hallerman–Streiff	Counsel	O: Numerous S: Retardation	O: Guarded S: Good
Congenital	Galactose intolerance	Discontinue galactose	O: Amblyopia, Posterior pole	O/S: Good
Congenital	Genetic deficiency of a lysosomal enzyme	Supportive	S: Retardation O: Posterior S: Numerous	O: Guarded S: Poor
Venereal	Genitourinary	Ceftriaxone I/M	O: Corneal ulcer S: Reproductive	O: Guarded S: Good
Pain	Arthritis	NSAIDs, Steroids	O: Glaucoma S: Renal disease, cardiovascular	O/S: Guarded
Seasonal	Rhinitis	Antihistamine decongestants Steroids	S: Steroids	O/S: Guarded
Genetic, bruise easy	Hemorrhaging	Hemostatic agents, clotting factor concentrates Precaution	O: Posterior pole S: Blood loss	O: Good S: Guarded
Venereal	Genitourinary	Oral antiviral	O: Scarring S: Recurrence	O/S: Guarded
Severe pain	Dermatitis (shingles)	Oral antiviral, pain medications Steroids	O: Numerous S: Scarring	O: Guarded S: Poor
Childhood	Granulomas	Steroids Bone biopsy	O: Granuloma S: Musculoskeletal	O/S: Guarded
Regional	Laboratory workup	Amphrotericin B, itraconazole, steroids	O: Posterior pole S: Respiratory	O: Guarded S: Good
Atopic history Allergen	Dermatitis Edema	Remove allergen Steroids (limited)	S: Anaphylaxis	O: Good S: Guarded
Congenital	Fair complexion Urinanalysis	Diet and vitamins Counsel	O: Cataract S: Vascular disease, skeletal	O/S: Guarded
Pain	Hypercalcemia	Anticalcemic Surgery	O: Conjunctival S: Renal, skeletal	O/S: Guarded
Aggitation	Laboratory workup Enlarged thyroid	Euthyroid	O: Neurological S: Numerous	O: Good S: Guarded
GI upset, headache	Intracranial pressure	Dietary	O: Cataract	O/S: Good
Psychiatric symptoms	Tetany	Calcium and vitamin D	O: Papilledema S: Numerous	O/S: Good
Lethargy, Mental confusion	Dry skin, hair	Thyroxin substitute	O: Cataract S: Myxedema	O: Good S: Guarded
Hygiene problems	Maculopapule rash	Antibiotics Hygiene	O/S: Secondary infection (e.g., cellulitis, sepsis)	O/S: Good
General malaise, chills, sore throat, cough	Myalgia, fever	Palliative	O: Posterior pole S: Pulmonary, Rare neurological	O/S: Good
Predominant male	AIDS victim, transplant recipients	Radiation, cryotherapy, highly active antiretroviral therapy	S: Metastasis	O: Guarded S: Poor
Weakness, weight loss, bruising	Hematologic	Chemotherapy, monoclonal antibodies, bone marrow transplantation	O: Posterior pole Anterior uveitis S: Cardiovascular	O/S: Guarded
Diet Risk factors	Laboratory workup	Diet control	S: Cardiovascular	O: Good S: Guarded
Malaise Weakness	Jaundice	Diet and vitamin supplementation	O: Night vision S: Hepatitis	O: Good S: Guarded

(Continued)

TABLE 9.1 (CONTINUED) **"Top 100" Specific Diagnoses**

Systemic Disorder	Pathological Classification	Anterior Segment Manifestation	Primary Eyecare Management	Co-Management or Referral
51. Louis–Barr syndrome[154]	Phakomatoses	Conjunctival telangiectasia	Monitor	Gynecologist (ataxiatelangiectasia) Neurologist
52. Lowe's syndrome[155]	Renal	Cataracts Corneal and conjunctival keloids	Monitor closely	Nephrologist
53. Lung cancer (carcinoma)	Neoplastic	Metastasis Ophthalmologist	Counsel	Surgeon
54. Lyme disease	Infectious	Conjunctivitis, keratitis Uveitis	Treat topically	Primary physician
55. Lymphoma(s)[156]	Neoplastic	Uveitis, conjunctival mass	Cycloplege and dilate	Internist
56. Malnutrition	Nutritional	Edema Keratopathy	Supportive	Primary physician
57. Marfan's syndrome	Metabolic	Subluxated lens	Monitor closely	Internist
58. Measles (rubeola)[157,158]	Infectious	Conjunctivitis, keratitis Koplik's spots	Supportive	Pediatrician
59. Melanoma (skin cancer)	Neoplastic	Conjunctival lid nevus	Monitor closely	Dermatologist
60. Mononucleosis	Infectious	Upper lid edema Conjunctivitis Uveitis	Palliative Steroids (limited)	Primary physician
61. Mucopolysaccharidosis[159,160]	Metabolic	Corneal opacities	Counsel	Pediatrician
62. Multiple myeloma	Hematological	Corneal crystals Iris cysts	Monitor closely	Internist
63. Multiple sclerosis[161]	Neurological	Pain with eye movements Ptosis	Counsel	Neurologist
64. Mumps[162,163]	Infectious	Keratoconjunctivitis	Warm compresses Steroids (limited)	Pediatrician
65. Muscular dystrophy[164]	Musculoskeletal	Ptosis	Counsel	Pediatrician
66. Myasthenia gravis[165]	Neurological	Ptosis, diplopia	Monitor	Neurologist
67. Occlusive arterial disease	Cardiovascular	Hypoxia Hemorrhages	Counsel	Primary physician Cardiologist
68. Occlusive venous disease	Cardiovascular	Edema Rubeosis iridis	Counsel Cold compresses	Primary physician Cardiologist
69. Osteogenesis imperfecta[166,167]	Musculoskeletal	Blue sclera	Monitor	Primary physician
70. Pemphigoid (benign, ocular)[168]	Dermatological	Conjunctivitis Keratitis sicca	Palliative steroids (limited)	Ophthalmologist Dermatologist
71. Periarteritis nodosa	Collagen vascular	Episcleritis Uveitis	Supportive Steroids	Internist
72. Pneumonia	Infectious	Hemorrhagic blepharoconjunctivitis	Antibiotics Supportive	Primary physician
73. Polycythemia vera	Hematological	Conjunctival hyperemia	Cold compresses Palliative	Internist
74. Psoriasis[169]	Dermatological	Conjunctivitis, blepharitis	Supportive	Dermatologist
75. Reactive arthritis (Reiter's syndrome)	Collagen vascular	Conjunctivitis Uveitis	Cycloplege and dilate Steroids	Internist
76. Rheumatoid arthritis (and JRA)	Collagen vascular	Uveitis, K sicca, episcleritis	Cycloplege and dilate Steroids	Rheumatologist
77. Rubella (German measles) congenital form	Infectious	Glaucoma, cataract	Monitor	Pediatrician

(*Continued*)

TABLE 9.1 (CONTINUED) **"Top 100" Specific Diagnoses**

Subjective Systemic Highlight	Objective Systemic Highlight	Standard Medical Management	Complications (Ocular and Systemic)	Prognosis (Ocular and Systemic)
Familial (rare)	Spasms	Counsel	O: Motility S: Cerebellar	O/S: Poor
Congenital Males	Conduct disturbances	Counsel	O: Glaucoma S: Renal disease, Conduct disturbances	O/S: Guarded
Cancer history	Biopsy+	Surgery Chemotherapy	O/S: High-risk metastasis	O/S: Poor
History of tick bite, flu-like symptoms	Annular rash	Oral antibiotics	O: Posterior pole S: Recurrence Arthritis, neurological	O: Good S: Guarded
Painless adenopathy, fever, unexplained weight loss	Biopsy Hematologic	Chemotherapy	O: Posterior pole S: Metastasis	O/S: Poor
History of weakness	Weight loss	Nutrition	O: Xerophthalmia Night blindness	O: Guarded S: Good
Tall, slender stature	Arachnodactylae (long fingers) Cardiovascular	Counsel Monitor	O: Myopia, lens dislocation Retinal detachment S: Cardiac	O: Guarded S: Good
Childhood	Koplik's spots, rash	Palliative	S: Respiratory, neurological	O/S: Good
Metastasis	Pigmented lesions	Surgery	O: Hyphema	O: Guarded S: Poor
Sore throat, swollen neck, malaise, fatigue	Laboratory workup	Rest	O: Posterior vitritis	O/S: Good
Congenital	"Funny-looking kids" Laboratory workup	Supportive Stem cell transplant, enzyme replacement	O: Glaucoma, pigmentary retinopathy S: Numerous	O/S: Guarded
Weakness, frequent infections	Laboratory workup	Stem cell transplant chemotherapy transfusion	O: Posterior S: Neurological	O: Guarded S: Poor
Uthoff's sign Lhermitte's sign	Neurological workup	Immunomodulatory	O: Optic neuritis S: Recurrences	O: Good S: Guarded
Malaise	Swollen glands	Isolation	O: Optic neuritis S: Meningitis, pelvic inflammation	O/S: Good
Congenital	Muscular	Supportive, physiotherapy	O: Ophthalmoplegia	O/S: Guarded
Weakness	Tensilon test	Pyridostigmine	O: Pupil defects	O/S: Good
Risk factors	Vascular disease	Anticoagulants	O: Posterior S: Ml or stroke	O: Good S: Guarded
Risk factors	Vascular disease	Specific to disease	O: Posterior S: Phlebitis	O: Good S: Guarded
Congenital	Fragile long bones	Supportive	O: Glaucoma S: Deafness	O: Good S: Guarded
Pain	Skin bullae	Dapsone	O: Scarring, symblepharon Corneal perforation	O/S: Guarded
Sick male	Fever High ESR	Steroids	O: Hemorrhages S: Vasculitis	O/S: Guarded
Malaise	Laboratory workup	Antibiotics Supportive	O: Corneal S: Vascular	O: Good S: Guarded
Weakness	Blood workup	Cytoreductive drugs Phlebotomy	O: Retinal S: Hemorrhage	O: Good S: Guarded
History	Skin scaling	Ultraviolet therapy Steroids, biologics	O: Uveitis	O: Good S: Guarded
Arthritic history	Urethritis (nongonococcal)	Oral antibiotics, NSAIDs	O: CME S: Vasculitis	O: Guarded S: Poor
Joint pain	High RF and ACPA	Anti-inflammatories (steroidal and nonsteroidal)	O: Peripheral ulcerative keratitis/corneal melt S: Musculoskeletal	O: Guarded S: Poor
Maternal history	Congenital findings	Supportive	O: Posterior S: Numerous	O/S: Guarded

(Continued)

TABLE 9.1 (CONTINUED) **"Top 100" Specific Diagnoses**

Systemic Disorder	Pathological Classification	Anterior Segment Manifestation	Primary Eyecare Management	Co-Management or Referral
78. Sarcoidosis	Collagen vascular	Uveitis	Cycloplege and dilate	Internist Steroids
79. Scleroderma[170]	Collagen vascular	Keratitis	Lubricants Supportive	Dermatologist
80. Septicemia (bacteremia)	Infectious	Subconjunctival hemorrhage Uveitis	Cycloplege and dilate Supportive	Internist
81. Sickle cell disease	Hematological	Comma-shaped conjunctival vessels	Counsel	Internist
82. Sjögren's syndrome	Collagen vascular	Keratitis sicca	Lubricants Anti-inflammatory	Internist
83. Stevens–Johnson disease	Dermatological	Conjunctivitis K sicca, symblepharon	Antibiotics/steroids Amniotic membrane	Dermatologist (erythema multiforme)
84. Sturge–Weber syndrome	Phakomatoses	Dilated episcleral veins Port wine stain, glaucoma	Counsel	Primary physician (encephalotrigeminal
85. Syphilis	Infectious	Interstitial keratitis Uveitis	Cycloplege and dilate Steroids	Internist
86. Systemic lupus erythematosus[171]	Collagen vascular	K sicca, rash on eyelid Episcleritis	Supportive	
87. Temporal (cranial) arteritis[172]	Collagen vascular	Uveitis	Cycloplege and dilate	Internist Steroids
88. Toxemia of pregnancy[173] (Pre-eclampsia)	Cardiovascular	Periorbital edema	Cold compresses Palliative	Obstetrician
89. Toxoplasmosis[174]	Infectious	Conjunctivitis Uveitis	Cycloplege and dilate Steroids	Internist
90. Trichinosis (trichinella)[175]	Infectious	Lid edema Chemosis	Cold compresses Palliative	Internist
91. Tuberculosis[176]	Infectious	Iritis Phlyctenular Keratoconjunctivitis	Steroids	Internist
92. Turner's syndrome[177]	Chromosomal	Epicanthal folds Oval corneas, ptosis	Counsel	Pediatrician
93. Ulcer (peptic)[178]	Gastrointestinal	Uveitis	Cycloplege and dilate Steroids (limited)	Primary physician
94. Ulcerative colitis	Gastrointestinal	Uveitis, episcleritis	Cycloplege and dilate Steroids	Internist
95. Varicella (chickenpox)[179]	Infectious	Lid vesicles Conjunctivitis, uveitis	Supportive, cycloplege and dilate, steroids	Pediatrician
96. Vitamin deficiencies	Nutritional	Xerosis	Lubricants	Nutritionist
97. Von Recklinghausen's (neurofibromatosis)[180]	Phakomatoses	Lid neurofibroma Lisch iris nodules Prominent corneal nerves	Counsel	Dermatologist Neurologist Internist
98. Wegener's granulomatosis[181,182]	Collagen vascular	Corneal margin ulceration Episcleritis	Steroids	Internist
99. Wilms' tumor (nephroblastoma)	Renal	Aniridia	Counsel	Nephrologist Pediatrician
100. Wilson's disease (hepaticolenticular)	Metabolic	Kayser–Fleischer ring (copper on posterior cornea)	Counsel	Neurologist

(*Continued*)

TABLE 9.1 (CONTINUED) **"Top 100" Specific Diagnoses**

Subjective Systemic Highlight	Objective Systemic Highlight	Standard Medical Management	Complications (Ocular and Systemic)	Prognosis (Ocular and Systemic)
Disseminated	Granulomas Chest radiograph	Steroids Biologics	O: Posterior S: Numerous	O: Guarded S: Good
Skin irritation	Leathery skin	Multiple drug therapy	O: Lid scarring S: SLE	O/S: Guarded
Gravely ill	Blood workup	Antibiotics	O: Endopthalmitis S: Multiorgan failure	O: Guarded S: Poor
Blacks	Hemoglobinopathy	Blood transfusions Hydroxyurea	O: Posterior S: Numerous	O: Guarded S: Poor
Fatigue Joint pain	Dry mouth Arthritis	Steroids Immunosuppressants	O: Corneal S: Polymyalgia Rheumatism	O: Good S: Guarded
History Sulfa drugs	Erythematous reactions	Steroids	O: Corneal scarring, perforation S: Multiorgan failure	O/S: Guarded
Congenital	Radiological (intracranial calcifications)	Counsel	O: Choroidal hemangiomas S: Brain angioma	O/S: Good
Acquired or congenital	FTA-ABS	Penicillin	O/S: "Anything"	O/S: Guarded
Females	Butterfly rash	Steroids, NSAIDs Antimalarial	O: Posterior pole S: Numerous	O: Good S: Guarded
Headache, jaw pain, amaurosis fugax	Prominent, tender temporal artery High erythrocyte sedimentation rate and C-reactive protein	Steroids	O: Posterior pole Ophthalmoplegia, Anterior ischemic optic neuropathy, blindness	O: Poor S: Guarded
Second to third trimester	Edema High blood pressure	Antihypertensives Diuretics	O: Posterior pole S: Renal	O: Good S: Guarded
Acquired Congenital	Laboratory workup	Sulphadiazine Pyrimethamine	O: Vitritis, chorioretinitis S: Neurological, pulmonary	O: Guarded S: Good
Diet history	Laboratory workup	Albendazole	O: Motility S: Hypersensitivity	O: Good S: Guarded
Hygienic history	Skin test Chest radiograph	Isoniazid	O: Posterior S: Pulmonary	O: Good S: Guarded
Congenital Females	"Funny-looking kid" (FLK) Dwarfism	Counsel Estrogens Human growth hormone	O: Cataracts Strabismus S: Cardiovascular	O: Guarded S: Guarded
GI pain Stressful males	Aggravated by diet, Endoscopy	Diet control Proton pump inhibitor	S: Numerous	O: Good S: Guarded
GI pain	Blood in stool	Antibiotics, Steroids Immunosuppressants	S: Carcinoma	O: Good S: Poor
Childhood	Vesicular patterns	Palliative	S: Adult shingles (herpes zoster)	O/S: Good
Diet	Serum levels	Dietary	O: Visual S: Numerous	O/S: Good
Disseminated findings	Neurofibromas Cafe-au-lait spots	Supportive	O: Glaucoma, Posterior hamartoma S: Numerous	O/S: Guarded
Purple rash	Upper airway, pulmonary	Steroids	O: Scleritis, Orbital S: Numerous	O: Guarded S: Poor
Childhood	Abdominal	Chemotherapy Surgery	O: Orbital mass S: Cardiovascular	O: Poor S: Guarded
Congenital Personality changes	Peripheral tremors	Penicillamine	O: Cataracts S: Neurologic Cirrhosis	O: Good S: Guarded

TABLE 9.2 **"Top 100" Diagnoses by Pathological Classification**

Pathological Classification	**Specific Systemic Disorder**	**No. on Top 100 Chart (Table 9.1)**	**Anterior Segment Manifestation**					
			Lids Adnexa	**Conjunctiva**	**Sclera Episclera**	**Cornea**	**Anterior Chamber**	**Lens**
Allergic	Allergies	7	X	X				
	Hay fever	32		X				
	Hives (urticaria)	38	X	X				
Cardiovascular	Arteriosclerosis	15				X		
	Occlusive arterial	67		X				
	Occlusive venous	68	X				X	
	Toxemia of pregnancy	88	X					
Chromosomal	Down syndrome	23	X			X	X	X
	Turner's syndrome	92	X			X		X
Collagen vascular	Ankylosing spondylitis	11					X	
	Dermatomyositis	21	X					
	Periarteritis nodosa	71			X		X	
	Reiter's syndrome	75		X			X	
	Rheumatoid arthritis	76			X	X	X	X
	Sarcoidosis	78					X	
	Scleroderma	79	X			X		X
	Sjögren's syndrome	82		X		X	X	
	Systemic lupus erythematosus	86	X	X	X	X	X	
	Temporal arteritis	87					X	
	Wegener's granulomatosis	98	X		X	X		
Dermatologic	Acne rosacea	1	X	X		X		
	Behçet's disease	13					X	X
	Dermatitis	20	X	X				
	Eczema	24	X	X		X		X
	Ehlers–Danlos syndrome	25			X	X		
	Pemphigoid	70		X		X		
	Psoriasis	74	X	X			X	
	Stevens–Johnson disease	83		X		X	X	
Endocrine	Addison's disease	3	X	X				
	Diabetes mellitus	22				X	X	
	Hyperparathyroidism	40		X		X		
	Hyperthyroidism	41	X			X		
	Hypoparathyroidism	43						X
	Hypothyroidism	44	X			X		X
Gastrointestinal	Crohn's disease	19					X	
	Ulcer (peptic)	93					X	
	Ulcerative colitis	94			X		X	
Hematologic	Anemia(s)	10		X				
	Hemophilia	33	X	X				
	Multiple myeloma	62				X	X	
	Polycythemia vera	73		X				
	Sickle cell disease	81		X				
	AIDS	2	X	X				
Infectious	Cat-scratch fever	16		X				
	Chlamydial disease	17		X		X		
	Gonorrhea	30		X		X		
	Herpes simplex	34	X	X		X	X	
	Herpes zoster	35	X	X		X	X	
	Histoplasmosis	37		x				
	Impetigo	45	X	X				
	Influenza	46		X		X		

(Continued)

TABLE 9.2 (CONTINUED) **"Top 100" Diagnoses by Pathological Classification**

Pathological Classification	Specific Systemic Disorder	No. on Top 100 Chart (Table 9.1)	Anterior Segment Manifestation					
			Lids Adnexa	Conjunctiva	Sclera Episclera	Cornea	Anterior Chamber	Lens
	Lyme disease	54	X	X	X	X	X	
	Measles	58		X		X		
	Mononucleosis	60	X	X			X	
	Mumps	64		X		X		
	Pneumonia	72	X	X		X		
	Rubella (congenital)	77						X
	Septicemia	80		X			X	
	Syphilis	85				X	X	
	Toxoplasmosis	89		X			X	
	Trichinosis	90	X	X				
	Tuberculosis	91		X		X	X	
	Varicella (chicken pox)	95	X	X			X	
Metabolic	Albinism	4	X			X		
	Alkaptonuria	6		X	X			
	Amyloidosis	9	X	X		X		
	Fabry's disease	26		X		X		
	Galactosemia	28						X
	Gaucher's disease	29		X		X		
	Gout	31		X		X		
	Histiocytosis	36	X					
	Homocystinuria	39						X
	Lipidoses	49	X			X		
	Marfan's syndrome	57						X
	Mucopolysaccharidosis	61				X		
	Wilson's disease	100				X		X
Musculoskeletal	Facial deformity syndrome	27	X					X
	Muscular dystrophy	65	X					
	Osteogenesis imperfecta	69			X			
Neoplastic	Breast cancer	14	X	X			X	
	Kaposi's sarcoma	47	X	X				
	Leukemia(s)	48	X	X				
	Lung cancer	53	X	X			X	
	Lymphoma(s)	55	X	X			X	
	Melanoma	59	X	X			X	
Neurological	Cogan's syndrome	18		X		X	X	
	Multiple sclerosis	63	X					
	Mysasthenia gravis	66	X				X	
Nutritional	Alcoholism	5	X	X				
	Hypervitaminosis	42		X		X		X

Note: Use Table 9.2 when patient presents symptoms in history (subjective) suggesting a specific pathological category or classification of systemic disease.

TABLE 9.3 "Top 100" Diagnoses by Ocular Anatomical Classification

Anterior Segment Manifestation	Specific Systemic Disorder(s)	Number on Top 100 Chart (Table 9.1)
Lids and Adnexa		
Blepharitis	Acne rosacea	1
	Dermatitis	20
	Eczema	24
	Eczema	24
	Herpes simplex	34
	Herpes zoster	35
	Impetigo	45
	Psoriasis	74
Blepharoptosis	Dermatomyositis	41
	Hypothyroidism	44
	Multiple sclerosis	63
	Muscular dystrophy	65
	Myasthenia gravis	66
Blepharospasm	Hypoparathyroidism	43
Changes eyebrows	Albinism	4
Colobomas	Facial deformity syndrome	26
Edema	Allergies	7
	Dermatomyositis	21
	Hives (urticaria)	38
	Hypothyroidism	44
	Malnutrition	56
	Mononucleosis	60
	Occlusive venous disease	68
	Toxemia of pregnancy	88
	Trichinosis	90
Epicanthal folds	Down syndrome	23
	Turner's syndrome	92
Erythema	Dermatomyositis	21
	Hives (urticaria)	38
	Lyme disease	54
Exophthalmos	Histiocytosis	36
	Hyperthyroidism	41
	Leukemia(s)	48
	Lymphoma	55
Hemorrhage	Hemophilia	33
	Pneumonia	72
Lumps and bumps	Acne rosacea	1
	AIDS	2
	Amyloidosis	9
	Facial deformity syndrome	27
	Kaposi's sarcoma	47
	Melanoma	59
	Neurofibromatosis	97
Pigmentary changes	Addison's disease	3
	Albinism	4
	Alkaptonuria	6
	Melanoma	59
	Sturge–Weber syndrome	84
	Systemic lupus erythematous	
Vesicles	Herpes simplex	34
	Herpes zoster	35
	Impetigo	45
	Varicella (chickenpox)	95

(Continued)

TABLE 9.3 (CONTINUED) "Top 100" Diagnoses by Ocular Anatomical Classification

Anterior Segment Manifestation	Specific Systemic Disorder(s)	Number on Top 100 Chart (Table 9.1)
Xanthalasma	Lipidoses	49
Conjunctiva		
Chemosis (edema)	Allergies	7
	Asthma	12
	Hives (urticaria)	38
	Occlusive venous disease	68
	Trichinosis	90
Conjunctivitis	Acne Rosacea	1
	Alcoholism	5
	Asthma	12
	Cat-scratch fever	16
	Chlamydial disease	17
	Cogan's syndrome	18
	Dermatitis	20
	Eczema	24
	Gonorrhea	30
	Hay fever	32
	Herpes zoster	35
	Hives (urticaria)	38
	Impetigo	45
	Influenza	46
	Lyme disease	54
	Measles (rubeola)	58
	Mononucleosis	60
	Mumps	64
	Pemphigoid	70
	Pneumonia	72
	Psoriasis	74
	Reactive arthritis	75
	Stevens–Johnson disease	83
	Toxoplasmosis	89
	Tuberculosis	91
	Varicella (chickenpox)	95
Hemorrhage	AIDS	2
	Anemia(s)	10
	Hemophilia	33
	Leukemia(s)	48
	Occlusive arterial disease	67
	Periarteritis nodosa	71
	Pneumonia	72
	Septicemia	80
Hyperemia	Allergies	7
	Fabry's disease	26
	Gout	31
	Louis–Barr syndrome	51
	Polycythemia vera	73
	Sickle cell disease	81
	Systemic lupus erythematosus	86
Hypoxia (pallor)	Anemia(s)	10
	Occlusive arterial disease	67
Lumps and bumps	AIDS	2
	Amyloidosis	9
	Histoplasmosis	37
	Kaposi's sarcoma	47
	Lowe's syndrome	52
	Lung cancer	53

(Continued)

TABLE 9.3 (CONTINUED) "Top 100" Diagnoses by Ocular Anatomical Classification

Anterior Segment Manifestation	Specific Systemic Disorder(s)	Number on Top 100 Chart (Table 9.1)
Lumps and bumps	Lymphoma	55
	Melanoma	59
Pigmentary changes	Addison's disease	3
	Alkaptonuria	6
	Melanoma	59
Xerosis	Malnutrition	56
	Vitamin deficiencies	96
Sciera and Episclera		
Episcleritis	Periarteritis nodosa	71
	Rheumatoid arthritis	76
	Systemic lupus erythematosus	86
	Ulcerative colitis	94
	Wegener's granulomatosis	96
Pigmentary changes	Ehlers–Danlos syndrome	25
	Liver disease	50
Sclerouveitis	Gout	31
Cornea		
Arcus	Cardiovascular disease	15
	Lipidoses	49
Clouding	Gaucher's disease	29
	Lowe's syndrome	52
	Mucopolysaccharidosis	61
	Rubella (congenital)	77
Changes in size/shape	Ehlers–Danlos syndrome	25
	Facial deformity syndrome	27
	Turner's syndrome	92
Deposits	Amyloidosis	9
	Fabry's disease	26
	Gout	31
	Multiple myeloma	61
Erosion	Diabetes mellitus	22
Infiltrates	Chlamydial disease	17
	Cogan's syndrome	18
	Syphilis	85
Keratitis	Acne rosacea	1
	Chlamydial disease	17
	Herpes simplex	34
	Herpes zoster	35
	Hyperthyroidism	41
	Hypothyroidism	44
	Influenza	46
	Liver disease	50
	Lyme	54
	Measles	58
	Mumps	64
	Pemphigoid	70
	Rheumatoid arthritis	76
	Scleroderma	79
	Sjögren's syndrome	82
	Stevens–Johnson disease	83
	Systemic lupus erythematosus	86
	Tuberculosis	91

(Continued)

TABLE 9.3 (CONTINUED) **"Top 100" Diagnoses by Ocular Anatomical Classification**

Anterior Segment Manifestation	Specific Systemic Disorder(s)	Number on Top 100 Chart (Table 9.1)
Keratoconus	Down syndrome	23
Keratopathy	Cardiovascular disease	15
	Hyperparathyroidism	40
	Hypervitaminosis	42
	Malnutrition	56
	Rheumatoid arthritis	76
Pigmentary changes	Alkaptonuria	6
	Wilson's disease	100
Prominent nerves	Neurofibromatosis	97
Ulceration	Gonorrhea	30
	Herpes simplex	34
	Herpes zoster	35
	Pneumonia	72
	Rheumatoid arthritis	76
	Sjögren's syndrome	82
	Wegener's granulomatosis	98
Anterior Chamber		
Brushfield's spots	Down syndrome	23
Glaucoma	(All steroid therapy)	
	Amyloidosis	9
	Osteogenesis imperfecta	69
	Neurofibromatosis	97
Hyphema	Behçet's disease	13
	Herpes simplex	34
	Melanoma	59
Iris abnormalities	Multiple myeloma	62
	Wilms' tumor	99
Pupil abnormalities	Marfan's syndrome	57
	Myasthenia gravis	66
Rubeosis iridis	Diabetes mellitus	22
	Occlusive venous disease	68
Uveitis	Ankylosing spondylitis	11
	Behçet's disease	13
	Cogan's syndrome	18
	Crohn's disease	19
	Gout	31
	Herpes zoster	35
	Leukemia(s)	48
	Lyme	54
	Lymphoma(s)	55
	Mononucleosis	60
	Periarteritis nodosa	71
	Reactive arthritis	75
	Rheumatoid arthritis (and JRA)	76
	Sarcoidosis	78
	Septicemia	80
	Syphilis	85
	Temporal arteritis	87
	Toxoplasmosis	89
	Tuberculosis	91
	Ulcer (peptic)	93
	Ulcerative colitis	94
	Varicella	95

(Continued)

TABLE 9.3 (CONTINUED) "Top 100" Diagnoses by Ocular Anatomical Classification

Anterior Segment Manifestation	Specific Systemic Disorder(s)	Number on Top 100 Chart (Table 9.1)
Lens		
Cataract	Alport's syndrome	8
	Behçet's disease	13
	Down syndrome	23
	Eczema	24
	Galactosemia	28
	Homocystinuria	39
	Hypervitaminosis	42
	Hypoparathyroidism	43
	Hypothyroidism	44
	Lowe's syndrome	52
	Rubella (congenital)	77
	Turner's syndrome	92
	Wilson's disease	100
Dislocation	Homocystinuria	39
	Marian's syndrome	57
Lenticonus	Alport's syndrome	8

Note: Use Table 9.3 when your objective examination of the anterior segment reveals physical signs suggestive of systemic origin.

References

1. Salik I, Rawla P. Marfan syndrome. In: *StatPearls*. Treasure Island: StatPearls Publishing; June 26, 2021.
2. Coelho SG, Almeida AG. Marfan syndrome revisited: From genetics to the clinic. Síndrome de Marfan revisitada – da genética à clínica. *Rev Port Cardiol.* 2020;39(4):215–226. doi:10.1016/j.repc.2019.09.008
3. Suwal R, Khadka S, Joshi P. Ocular manifestations and biometrics in Marfan's syndrome from Eastern Nepal. *Clin Ophthalmol.* 2020;14:2463–2472. Published 2020 Aug 25. doi:10.2147/OPTH.S269364
4. Strauss DS, Baharestani S, Nemiroff J, Amesur K, Howard D. Cecocentral scotoma as the initial manifestation of subacute bacterial endocarditis. *Clin Ophthalmol.* 2011;5:287–290. doi:10.2147/OPTH.S16237
5. Parashar K, Daveluy S. Osler node and janeway lesions. In: *StatPearls*. Treasure Island: StatPearls Publishing; July 30, 2021.
6. van Zuren EJ. Rosacea. *New England J Med.* 2017;377(18):1754–1764.
7. Kostner L, Anzengruber F, Guillod C, Recher M, Schmid-Grendelmeier P, Navarini AA. Allergic contact dermatitis. *Immunol Allergy Clin North Am.* 2017;37(1):141–152. doi:10.1016/j.iac.2016.08.014
8. Gross GE, Eisert L, Doerr HW, Fickenscher H, Knuf M, Maier P, ... Nast A. S2k guidelines for the diagnosis and treatment of herpes zoster and postherpetic neuralgia. *JDDG: J Dtsch Dermatol Ges.* 2020;18(1):55–78.
9. Whitley RJ, Weiss H, Gnann JW Jr, et al. Acyclovir with and without prednisone for the treatment of herpes zoster. A randomized, placebo-controlled trial. The National Institute of Allergy and Infectious Diseases Collaborative Antiviral Study Group. *Ann Intern Med.* 1996;125(5):376–383. doi:10.7326/0003-4819-125-5-199609010-00004
10. Agarwal P, Patel BC. Nevus of ota and ito. In: *StatPearls*. Treasure Island: StatPearls Publishing; July 25, 2021.
11. Korman NJ. Management of psoriasis as a systemic disease: what is the evidence?. *Br J Dermatol.* 2020;182(4):840–848. doi:10.1111/bjd.18245
12. Kim WB, Jerome D, Yeung J. Diagnosis and management of psoriasis. *Can Fam Physician.* 2017;63(4):278–285.
13. Menter A. Psoriasis and psoriatic arthritis overview. *Am J Manag Care.* 2016;22(8 Suppl):s216–s224.
14. Vazirani J, Donthineni PR, Goel S, et al. Chronic cicatrizing conjunctivitis: A review of the differential diagnosis and an algorithmic approach to management. *Indian J Ophthalmol.* 2020;68(11):2349–2355. doi:10.4103/ijo.IJO_604_20
15. Zhang J, Lei Z, Xu C, Zhao J, Kang X. Current perspectives on severe drug eruption [published online ahead of print, 2021 Jul 17]. *Clin Rev Allergy Immunol.* 2021;61:1–17. doi:10.1007/s12016-021-08859-0
16. Micheletti RG, Chiesa-Fuxench Z, Noe MH, et al. Stevens–Johnson syndrome/toxic epidermal necrolysis: A multicenter retrospective study of 377 adult patients from the United States [published correction appears in J Invest Dermatol. 2019 Feb;139(2):495-496]. *J Invest Dermatol.* 2018;138(11):2315–2321. doi:10.1016/j.jid.2018.04.027
17. Schneider JA, Cohen PR. Stevens–Johnson syndrome and toxic epidermal necrolysis: A concise review with a comprehensive summary of therapeutic interventions emphasizing supportive measures. *Adv Ther.* 2017;34(6):1235–1244. doi:10.1007/s12325-017-0530-y
18. Alam U, Asghar O, Azmi S, Malik RA, Chapter 15: General aspects of diabetes mellitus. In: Zochodne DW, Malik RA, editors. *Handbook of Clinical Neurology.* Elsevier, Volume 126, 2014, Pages 211–222, ISSN 0072-9752, ISBN 9780444534804.
19. American Diabetes Association. Diagnosis and classification of diabetes mellitus. *Diabetes Care.* 2014;37(Suppl 1):S81–S90. doi:10.2337/dc14-S081
20. Kharroubi AT, Darwish HM. Diabetes mellitus: The epidemic of the century. *World J Diabetes.* 2015;6(6):850–867. doi:10.4239/wjd.v6.i6.850
21. Skyler JS, Bakris GL, Bonifacio E, et al. Differentiation of diabetes by pathophysiology, natural history, and prognosis. *Diabetes.* 2017;66(2):241–255. doi:10.2337/db16-0806
22. Jawaid I, Rajesh S. Hyperparathyroidism (primary) NICE guideline: diagnosis, assessment, and initial management. *Br J Gen Pract.* 2020;70(696):362–363. Published 2020 Jun 25. doi:10.3399/bjgp20X710717
23. Insogna KL. Primary hyperparathyroidism. *N Engl J Med.* 2018;379(11):1050–1059. doi:10.1056/NEJMcp1714213
24. Kravets I. Hyperthyroidism: Diagnosis and treatment. *Am Fam Physician.* 2016;93(5):363–370.
25. Devereaux D, Tewelde SZ. Hyperthyroidism and thyrotoxicosis. *Emerg Med Clin North Am.* 2014;32(2):277–292. doi:10.1016/j.emc.2013.12.001

26. Lause M, Kamboj A, Fernandez Faith E. Dermatologic manifestations of endocrine disorders. *Transl Pediatr.* 2017;6(4):300–312. doi:10.21037/tp.2017.09.08
27. Smith T, J: Teprotumumab treatment for thyroid-associated ophthalmopathy. *Eur Thyroid J* 2020;9(suppl 1):31–39. doi: 10.1159/000507992
28. Bilezikian JP. Hypoparathyroidism. *J Clin Endocrinol Metab.* 2020;105(6):1722–1736. doi:10.1210/clinem/dgaa113
29. Clarke BL, Brown EM, Collins MT, et al. Epidemiology and diagnosis of hypoparathyroidism. *J Clin Endocrinol Metab.* 2016;101(6):2284–2299. doi:10.1210/jc.2015-3908
30. Shoback DM, Bilezikian JP, Costa AG, Dempster D, Dralle H, Khan AA, Peacock Munro, Raffaelli Marco, Silva BC, Thakker RV, Vokes T, Bouillon R. Presentation of hypoparathyroidism: Etiologies and clinical features. *J Clin Endocrinol Metabol.* 1 June 2016;101(6):2300–2312. https://doi.org/10.1210/jc.2015-3909
31. Chiovato L, Magri F, Carlé A. Hypothyroidism in context: Where we've been and where we're going. *Adv Ther.* 2019;36(Suppl 2):47–58. doi:10.1007/s12325-019-01080-8
32. Dubbs SB, Spangler R. Hypothyroidism: Causes, killers, and lifesaving treatments. *Emerg Med Clin North Am.* 2014;32(2):303–317. doi:10.1016/j.emc.2013.12.003
33. Kashkouli MB, Pakdel F, Kiavash V, Heidari I, Heirati A, Jam S. Hyperthyroid vs hypothyroid eye disease: the same severity and activity. *Eye.* 2011;25(11):1442–1446. doi:10.1038/eye.2011.186
34. Bandmann O, Weiss KH, Kaler SG. Wilson's disease and other neurological copper disorders. *Lancet Neurol.* 2015;14(1):103–113. doi:10.1016/S1474-4422(14)70190-5
35. Nagral A, Sarma MS, Matthai J, et al. Wilson's disease: Clinical practice guidelines of the Indian National Association for study of the liver, the Indian Society of Pediatric Gastroenterology, Hepatology and Nutrition, and the Movement Disorders Society of India [published correction appears in J Clin Exp Hepatol. 2020 Jan-Feb;10(1):99]. *J Clin Exp Hepatol.* 2019;9(1):74–98. doi:10.1016/j.jceh.2018.08.009
36. Schub T, Allen L, Pravikoff D. *Anemia: An Overview.* 2015. Clinical Information Systems, a division of EBSCO Information Services.
37. Aspuru K, Villa C, Bermejo F, Herrero P, López SG. Optimal management of iron deficiency anemia due to poor dietary intake. *Int J Gen Med.* 2011;4:741–750. doi:10.2147/IJGM.S17788
38. Sarma PR. Red cell indices. In: Walker HK, Hall WD, Hurst JW, editors. *Clinical Methods: The History, Physical, and Laboratory Examinations.* 3rd edition. Boston: Butterworths; 1990. Chapter 152. Available from: https://www.ncbi.nlm.nih.gov/books/NBK260/
39. Efferi A, Vannucchi AM, Barbui T. Polycythemia vera treatment algorithm 2018. *Blood Cancer J.* 2018;8:3. https://doi.org/10.1038/s41408-017-0042-7
40. Squizzato A, Romualdi E, Middeldorp S. Antiplatelet drugs for polycythaemia vera and essential thrombocythaemia. *Cochrane Database Syst Rev.* 2008;2:CD006503. Published 2008 Apr 16. doi:10.1002/14651858.CD006503.pub2
41. Benevolo G, Vassallo F, Urbino I, Giai V. Polycythemia vera (PV): update on emerging treatment options. *Ther Clin Risk Manag.* 2021;17:209–221. Published 2021 Mar 16. doi:10.2147/TCRM.S213020
42. Büyükaşik Y, Alİ R, Ar C, Turgut M, Yavuz S, Saydam G. Polycythemia vera: diagnosis, clinical course, and current management. *Turk J Med Sci.* 2018;48(4):698–710. Published 2018 Aug 16. doi:10.3906/sag-1806-43
43. Rao K, Shenoy SB, Kamath Y, Kapoor S. Central retinal artery occlusion as a presenting manifestation of polycythaemia vera. *BMJ Case Rep.* 2016;2016:bcr2016216417. Published 2016 Oct 20. doi:10.1136/bcr-2016-216417
44. Piel FB, Steinberg MH, Rees DC. Sickle cell disease. *N Engl J Med.* 2017;376(16):1561–1573. doi:10.1056/NEJMra1510865
45. Tisdale JF, Thein SL, Eaton WA. Treating sickle cell anemia. *Science.* 2020;367(6483):1198–1199. doi:10.1126/science.aba3827
46. Amissah-Arthur KN, Mensah E. The past, present and future management of sickle cell retinopathy within an African context. *Eye.* 2018;32(8):1304–1314. doi:10.1038/s41433-018-0162-8
47. El-Ghamrawy MK, El Behairy HF, El Menshawy A, Awad SA, Ismail A, Gabal MS. Ocular manifestations in egyptian children and young adults with sickle cell disease. *Indian J Hematol Blood Transfus.* 2014;30(4):275–280. doi:10.1007/s12288-014-0333-0
48. Williams TN, Thein SL. Sickle cell anemia and its phenotypes. *Annu Rev Genomics Hum Genet.* 2018;19:113–147. doi:10.1146/annurev-genom-083117-021320
49. Klimas N, Koneru AO, Fletcher MA. Overview of HIV. *Psychosom Med.* 2008;70(5):523–530. doi:10.1097/PSY.0b013e31817ae69f
50. Paranjape RS, Challacombe SJ. HIV/AIDS in India: an overview of the Indian epidemic. *Oral Dis.* 2016;22 Suppl 1:10–14. doi:10.1111/odi.12457
51. Centers for Disease Control and Prevention (CDC). HIV prevalence estimates: United States, 2006. *MMWR Morb Mortal Wkly Rep.* 2008;57(39):1073–1076.
52. Centers for Disease Control and Prevention. HIV transmission. 2020. https://www.cdc.gov/hiv/basics/transmission.html. Accessed 24 Mar 2020.
53. Bastiaans DE, Cressey TR, Vromans H, Burger DM. The role of formulation on the pharmacokinetics of antiretroviral drugs. *Expert Opin Drug Metabol Toxicol.* 2014;10(7):1019–1037.
54. Klotz SA, Ianas V, Elliott SP. Cat-scratch disease. *Am Fam Physician.* 2011;83(2):152–155.
55. Nelson CA, Saha S, Mead PS. Cat-scratch disease in the United States, 2005–2013. *Emerg Infect Dis.* 2016;22(10):1741–1746. doi:10.3201/eid2210.160115
56. Coburn J, Garcia B, Hu LT, et al. Lyme disease pathogenesis. *Curr Issues Mol Biol.* 2021;42:473–518. doi:10.21775/cimb.042.473
57. Skar GL, Simonsen KA. Lyme disease. In: *StatPearls.* Treasure Island: StatPearls Publishing; July 10, 2021.
58. Mikkilä HO, Seppälä IJ, Viljanen MK, Peltomaa MP, Karma A. The expanding clinical spectrum of ocular lyme borreliosis. *Ophthalmology.* 2000;107(3):581–587. doi:10.1016/s0161-6420(99)00128-1
59. Anka AU, Tahir MI, Abubakar SD, et al. Coronavirus disease 2019 (COVID-19): An overview of the immunopathology, serological diagnosis and management. *Scand J Immunol.* 2021;93(4):e12998. doi:10.1111/sji.12998
60. Salian VS, Wright JA, Vedell PT, et al. COVID-19 transmission, current treatment, and future therapeutic strategies. *Mol Pharm.* 2021;18(3):754–771. doi:10.1021/acs.molpharmaceut.0c00608
61. Nasiri N, Sharifi H, Bazrafshan A, Noori A, Karamouzian M, Sharifi A. Ocular manifestations of COVID-19: A systematic review and meta-analysis. *J Ophthalmic Vis Res.* 2021;16(1):103–112. Published 2021 Jan 20. doi:10.18502/jovr.v16i1.8256
62. Sen M, Honavar SG, Sharma N, Sachdev MS. COVID-19 and eye: a review of ophthalmic manifestations of COVID-19. *Indian J Ophthalmol.* 2021;69(3):488–509. doi:10.4103/ijo.IJO_297_21
63. Vanichkachorn G, Newcomb R, Cowl CT, et al. Post-COVID-19 syndrome (long haul syndrome): description of a multidisciplinary clinic at mayo clinic and characteristics of the initial patient cohort. *Mayo Clin Proc.* 2021;96(7):1782–1791. doi:10.1016/j.mayocp.2021.04.024
64. Younes N, Al-Sadeq DW, Al-Jighefee H, et al. Challenges in laboratory diagnosis of the novel coronavirus SARS-CoV-2. *Viruses.* 2020;12(6):582. Published 2020 May 26. doi:10.3390/v12060582
65. Cruz-Teran C, Tiruthani K, McSweeney M, Ma A, Pickles R, Lai SK. Challenges and opportunities for antiviral monoclonal antibodies as COVID-19 therapy. *Adv Drug Deliv Rev.* 2021;169:100–117. doi:10.1016/j.addr.2020.12.004
66. Emergency Use Authorization for Lagevrio. *Fact Sheet for Healthcare Providers.* Merck, December 2021.
67. Emergency Use Authorization for Paxlovid. *Fact Sheet for Healthcare Providers.* Pfizer, December 2021
68. Fuchs W, Brockmeyer NH. Sexually transmitted infections. *J Dtsch Dermatol Ges.* 2014;12(6):451–463. doi:10.1111/ddg.12310
69. Workowski KA, Bolan GA; Centers for Disease Control and Prevention. Sexually transmitted diseases treatment

guidelines, 2015 [published correction appears in MMWR Recomm Rep. 2015 Aug 28;64(33):924]. *MMWR Recomm Rep.* 2015;64(RR-03):1–137.

70. Al Thobaiti AD, Hamdi AM, Almalki MAO, Alghamdi WH, Albaz ME, Alshammari AM and et al. An overview of sinusitis diagnosis and management approach in PHC. *Arch Pharma Pract.* 2021;12(1):59–62.
71. Rosenfeld RM. Clinical practice. Acute sinusitis in adults. *N Engl J Med.* 2016;375(10):962–970. doi:10.1056/NEJMcp1601749
72. Kowalczyk M, Toro MD, Rejdak R, Załuska W, Gagliano C, Sikora P. Ophthalmic evaluation of diagnosed cases of eye cystinosis: A tertiary care center's experience. *Diagnostics.* 2020;10(11):911. Published 2020 Nov 7. doi:10.3390/diagnostics10110911
73. Wilmer MJ, Schoeber JP, van den Heuvel LP, Levtchenko EN. Cystinosis: practical tools for diagnosis and treatment. *Pediatr Nephrol.* 2011;26(2):205–215. doi:10.1007/s00467-010-1627-6
74. Graca A, Suszek D, Jeleniewicz R, Majdan M. Nephrotic syndrome in the course of type 1 diabetes mellitus and systemic lupus erythematosus with secondary antiphospholipid syndrome—diagnostic and therapeutic problems. *Reumatologia.* 2020;58(5):331–334. doi:10.5114/reum.2020.100105
75. Bazinet A, Popradi G. A general practitioner's guide to hematopoietic stem-cell transplantation. *Curr Oncol.* 2019;26(3):187–191. doi:10.3747/co.26.5033
76. Eisenga MF, Gomes-Neto AW, van Londen M, *et al.* Rationale and design of TransplantLines: a prospective cohort study and biobank of solid organ transplant recipients *BMJ Open.* 2018;8:e024502. doi: 10.1136/bmjopen-2018-024502
77. Dhal U, Raju S, Singh AD, Mehta AC. "For your eyes only": ophthalmic complications following lung transplantation. *J Thorac Dis.* 2018;10(11):6285–6297. doi:10.21037/jtd.2018.09.156
78. Cohen G, Vanholder R. Special issue: Immune dysfunction in uremia. *Toxins.* 2021;13(1):70. Published 2021 Jan 19. doi:10.3390/toxins13010070
79. Phelps HM, Kaviany S, Borinstein SC, Lovvorn HN 3rd. Biological drivers of Wilms tumor prognosis and treatment. *Children.* 2018;5(11):145. Published 2018 Oct 26. doi:10.3390/children5110145
80. Melzer N, Ruck T, Fuhr P, et al. Clinical features, pathogenesis, and treatment of myasthenia gravis: a supplement to the Guidelines of the German Neurological Society. *J Neurol.* 2016;263(8):1473–1494. doi:10.1007/s00415-016-8045-z
81. Sieb JP. Myasthenia gravis: an update for the clinician. *Clin Exp Immunol.* 2014;175(3):408–418. doi:10.1111/cei.12217
82. Jaber AL-Zwaini I, AL-Mayahi A. *Introductory Chapter: Myasthenia Gravis: An Overview.* https://doi.org/10.5772/intechopen.85761
83. Gilhus NEMD. Myasthenia gravis. *N Engl J Med.* 2016;375:2570–81. DOI: 10.1056/NEJMra1602678
84. Dejaco C, Ramiro S, Duftner C, et al. EULAR recommendations for the use of imaging in large vessel vasculitis in clinical practice. *Ann Rheum Dis.* 2018;77(5):636–643. doi:10.1136/annrheumdis-2017-212649
85. Weyand CM, Goronzy JJ. Clinical practice. Giant-cell arteritis and polymyalgia rheumatica. *N Engl J Med.* 2014;371(1):50–57. doi:10.1056/NEJMcp1214825
86. Dammacco R, Alessio G, Giancipoli E, et al. Giant cell arteritis: the experience of two collaborative referral centers and an overview of disease pathogenesis and therapeutic advancements. *Clin Ophthalmol.* 2020;14:775–793. Published 2020 Mar 11. doi:10.2147/OPTH.S243203
87. Moo TA, Sanford R, Dang C, Morrow M. Overview of breast cancer therapy. *PET Clin.* 2018;13(3):339–354. doi:10.1016/j.cpet.2018.02.006
88. Martín-Sánchez JC, Lunet N, González-Marrón A, et al. Projections in breast and lung cancer mortality among women: a bayesian analysis of 52 countries worldwide. *Cancer Res.* 2018;78(15):4436–4442. doi:10.1158/0008-5472.CAN-18-0187
89. Eisner A, Luoh SW. Breast cancer medications and vision: effects of treatments for early-stage disease. *Curr Eye Res.* 2011;36(10):867–885. doi:10.3109/02713683.2011.594202
90. Stapelfeld C, Dammann C, Maser E. Sex-specificity in lung cancer risk. *Int J Cancer.* 2020;146(9):2376–2382. doi:10.1002/ijc.32716
91. Collins LG, Haines C, Perkel R, Enck RE. Lung cancer: diagnosis and management. *Am Fam Physician.* 2007;75(1):56–63.
92. Augsburger JJ, GUTHOFF R. Chapter 148: *Metastatic Cancer to the Eye,* Posted by medtextfree on January 20, 2011 in Ophthalmology.
93. Lampaki S, Kioumis I, Pitsiou G, et al. Lung cancer and eye metastases. *Med Hypothesis Discov Innov Ophthalmol.* 2014;3(2):40–44.
94. Medical Masterclass Contributors. Firth J. haematology: multiple myeloma. *Clin Med.* 2019;19(1):58–60. doi:10.7861/clinmedicine.19-1-58
95. Bird SA, Boyd K. Multiple myeloma: an overview of management. *Palliat Care Soc Pract.* 2019;13:1178224219868235. Published 2019 Oct 9. doi:10.1177/1178224219868235
96. Farooq AV, Degli Esposti S, Popat R, et al. Corneal epithelial findings in patients with multiple myeloma treated with antibody-drug conjugate belantamab mafodotin in the pivotal, randomized, DREAMM-2 study [published correction appears in Ophthalmol Ther. 2020 Sep 12;:]. *Ophthalmol Ther.* 2020;9(4):889–911. doi:10.1007/s40123-020-00280-8
97. Sharma P, Madi HA, Bonshek R, Morgan SJ. Cloudy corneas as an initial presentation of multiple myeloma. *Clin Ophthalmol.* 2014;8:813–817. Published 2014 Apr 28. doi:10.2147/OPTH.S49283
98. Ansell SM. Hodgkin lymphoma: 2018 update on diagnosis, risk-stratification, and management. *Am J Hematol.* 2018;93(5):704–715. doi:10.1002/ajh.25071
99. Singh R, Shaik S, Negi BS, et al. Non-Hodgkin's lymphoma: a review. *J Family Med Prim Care.* 2020;9(4):1834–1840. Published 2020 Apr 30. doi:10.4103/jfmpc.jfmpc_1037_19
100. Jakobiec FA, Homer N, Zakka FR, Curtin HD, Fay A. Clinicopathologic and magnetic resonance imaging analysis of a multifocal orbital lymphoid tumor. *Ocul Oncol Pathol.* 2018;4(2):82–89. doi:10.1159/000478731
101. Eckardt AM, Lemound J, Rana M, Gellrich NC. Orbital lymphoma: diagnostic approach and treatment outcome. *World J Surg Oncol.* 2013;11:73. Published 2013 Mar 18. doi:10.1186/1477-7819-11-73
102. Shields CL, Shields JA. Tumors of the conjunctiva and cornea. *Indian J Ophthalmol.* 2019;67(12):1930–1948. doi:10.4103/ijo.IJO_2040_19
103. Jovanovic P, Mihajlovic M, Djordjevic-Jocic J, Vlajkovic S, Cekic S, Stefanovic V. Ocular melanoma: an overview of the current status. *Int J Clin Exp Pathol.* 2013;6(7):1230–1244. Published 2013 Jun 15.
104. Mahendraraj K, Shrestha S, Lau CS, Chamberlain RS. Ocular melanoma—when you have seen one, you have not seen them all: a clinical outcome study from the surveillance, epidemiology and end results (SEER) database (1973–2012). *Clin Ophthalmol.* 2017;11:153–160. Published 2017 Jan 5. doi:10.2147/OPTH.S120530
105. Watson M, Holman DM, Maguire-Eisen M. Ultraviolet radiation exposure and its impact on skin cancer risk. *Semin Oncol Nurs.* 2016;32(3):241–254. doi:10.1016/j.soncn.2016.05.005
106. Wong JR, Nanji AA, Galor A, Karp CL. Management of conjunctival malignant melanoma: a review and update. *Expert Rev Ophthalmol.* 2014;9(3):185–204. doi:10.1586/17469899.2014.921119
107. Freer G, Pistello M. Varicella-zoster virus infection: natural history, clinical manifestations, immunity and current and future vaccination strategies. *New Microbiol.* 2018;41(2):95–105.
108. Coelho AI, Rubio-Gozalbo ME, Vicente JB, Rivera I. Sweet and sour: an update on classic galactosemia. *J Inherit Metab Dis.* 2017;40(3):325–342. doi:10.1007/s10545-017-0029-3
109. Banford S, McCorvie TJ, Pey AL, Timson DJ. Galactosemia: towards pharmacological chaperones. *J Pers Med.* 2021;11(2):106. Published 2021 Feb 7. doi:10.3390/jpm11020106
110. Saneeymehri S, Baker K, So TY. Overview of pharmacological treatment options for pediatric patients with refractory

kawasaki disease. *J Pediatr Pharmacol Ther.* 2015;20(3):163–177. doi:10.5863/1551-6776-20.3.163

111. Pinna GS, Kafetzis DA, Tselkas OI, Skevaki CL. Kawasaki disease: an overview. *Curr Opin Infect Dis.* 2008;21(3):263–270. doi:10.1097/QCO.0b013e3282fbf9cd
112. Betáková T, Svetlíková D, Gocník M. Overview of measles and mumps vaccine: origin, present, and future of vaccine production. *Acta Virol.* 2013;57(2):91–96. doi:10.4149/av_2013_02_91
113. Khan B, Nasir S, Hanif S. Bilateral optic neuritis: A rare complication of mumps. *Cureus.* 2020;12(4):e7768. Published 2020 Apr 21. doi:10.7759/cureus.7768
114. Engel B, Just J, Bleckwenn M, Weckbecker K. Treatment options for gout. *Dtsch Arztebl Int.* 2017;114(13):215–222. doi:10.3238/arztebl.2017.0215
115. Ao J, Goldblatt F, Casson RJ. Review of the ophthalmic manifestations of gout and uric acid crystal deposition. *Clin Exp Ophthalmol.* 2017;45(1):73–80. doi:10.1111/ceo.12749
116. Bullock J, Rizvi SAA, Saleh AM, et al. Rheumatoid arthritis: a brief overview of the treatment. *Med Princ Pract.* 2018;27(6):501–507. doi:10.1159/000493390
117. Marcucci E, Bartoloni E, Alunno A, et al. Extra-articular rheumatoid arthritis. *Reumatismo.* 2018;70(4):212–224. Published 2018 Dec 20. doi:10.4081/reumatismo.2018.1106
118. Karampatakis V, Konidaris V, Michailidou M, Gerofotis A, Daniilidis M. Peripheral corneal ulceration associated with rheumatoid arthritis. *Am J Case Rep.* 2013;14:318–321. Published 2013 Aug 12. doi:10.12659/AJCR.883998
119. Argyropoulou OD, Tzioufas AG. Update on Sjögren's syndrome 2018. *Mediterr J Rheumatol.* 2018;29(4):193–198. Published 2018 Dec 18. doi:10.31138/mjr.29.4.193
120. Parisis D, Chivasso C, Perret J, Soyfoo MS, Delporte C. Current state of knowledge on primary Sjögren's syndrome, an autoimmune exocrinopathy. *J Clin Med.* 2020;9(7):2299. Published 2020 Jul 20. doi:10.3390/jcm9072299
121. Henderson AD, Miller NR. Carotid-cavernous fistula: current concepts in aetiology, investigation, and management. *Eye.* 2018;32(2):164–172. doi:10.1038/eye.2017.240
122. De Stefano F, Fiani B, Mayo T. A foundational "survival guide" overview of sports-related head injuries. *Cureus.* 2020;12(11):e11636. Published 2020 Nov 22. doi:10.7759/cureus.11636
123. Sivanandapanicker J, Nagar M, Kutty R, et al. Analysis and clinical importance of skull base fractures in adult patients with traumatic brain injury. *J Neurosci Rural Pract.* 2018;9(3):370–375. doi:10.4103/jnrp.jnrp_38_18
124. Picardo M, Eichenfield LF, Tan J. Acne and rosacea. *Dermatol Therapy.* 2017;7(1):43–52.
125. Ten S, New M, Maclaren N. Addison's disease 2001. *J Clin Endocrinol Metabol.* 1 July 2001;86(7):2909–2922.
126. Savige J, Sheth S, Leys A, Nicholson A, Mack HG, Colville D. Ocular features in Alport syndrome: pathogenesis and clinical significance. *Clin J Am Soc Nephrol.* 2015;10(4):703–709. doi:10.2215/CJN.10581014
127. Hashemian H, Jabbarvand M, Khodaparast M, Khalilipour E, Esfehani HR. Ocular presentations of amyloidosis. *Amyloidosis.* 2013;85.
128. Tesse R, Borrelli G, Mongelli G, Mastrorilli V, Cardinale F. Treating pediatric asthma according guidelines. *Front Pediatr.* 2018;6:234. Published 2018 Aug 23. doi:10.3389/fped.2018.00234
129. Paovic J, Paovic P, Sredovic V. Behçet's disease: systemic and ocular manifestations. *BioMed Res Int.* 2013;2013.
130. Iliescu DA, Timaru CM, Batras M, De Simone A, Stefan C. Cogan's syndrome. *Rom J Ophthalmol.* 2015;59(1):6–13.
131. Ophthalmic complications of dermatomyositis. In: *Dermatomyositis.* Berlin, Heidelberg: Springer, 2009. https://doi.org/10.1007/978-3-540-79313-7_13
132. Wollenberg A, Christen-Zäch S, Taieb A, Paul C, Thyssen JP, de Bruin-Weller M, ... European Task Force on Atopic Dermatitis/EADV Eczema Task Force. ETFAD/EADV Eczema task force 2020 position paper on diagnosis and treatment of atopic dermatitis in adults and children. *J Eur Acad Dermatol Venereol.* 2020;34(12):2717–2744.
133. Meester JAN, Verstraeten A, Schepers D, Alaerts M, Van Laer L, Loeys BL. Differences in manifestations of Marfan syndrome, Ehlers-Danlos syndrome, and Loeys-Dietz syndrome. *Ann Cardiothorac Surg.* 2017;6(6):582–594. doi:10.21037/acs.2017.11.03
134. Sodi A, Ioannidis A, Pitz S. Ophthalmological manifestations of Fabry disease. In: *Fabry Disease: Perspectives from 5 Years of FOS*, 2006. Oxford: Oxford PharmaGenesis.
135. Mahmud HM. Fabry's disease: A comprehensive review on pathogenesis, diagnosis and treatment. *J Pak Med Assoc.* 2014;64(2):189–194.
136. Bosch AM. Classical galactosaemia revisited. *Journal of Inherited Metabolic Disease: Official Journal of the Society for the Study of Inborn Errors of Metabolism*, 2006;29(4):516–525.
137. Stirnemann J, Belmatoug N, Camou F, et al. A review of gaucher disease pathophysiology, clinical presentation and treatments. *Int J Mol Sci.* 2017;18(2):441. Published 2017 Feb 17. doi:10.3390/ijms18020441
138. Lin J, Zhao GQ, Che CY, Yang SS, Wang Q, Li CG. Characteristics of ocular abnormalities in gout patients. *Int J Ophthalmol.* 2013;6(3):307–311. Published 2013 Jun 18. doi:10.3980/j.issn.2222-3959.2013.03.09
139. Aquino LM, Ranche FK. Hemophilia presenting as recurrent ocular hemorrhage. *GMS Ophthalmol Cases.* 2020;10:Doc15. Published 2020 Mar 18. doi:10.3205/oc000142
140. Srivastava A, Brewer AK, Mauser-Bunschoten EP, Key NS, Kitchen S, Llinas A, ... Treatment Guidelines Working Group the World Federation of Hemophilia. Guidelines for the management of hemophilia. *Haemophilia.* 2013;19(1):e1–e47.
141. Wang TY, Horng CT, Chen YC, Chang YH, Chien KH, Lu DW, ... Tsai ML. Management of ocular posterior segment hemorrhages in patients with hemophilia. *Asia Pacific J Oncol Hematol.* 2009;1(3):1.
142. Herwig MC, Wojno T, Zhang Q, Grossniklaus HE. Langerhans cell histiocytosis of the orbit: five clinicopathologic cases and review of the literature. *Surv Ophthalmol.* 2013;58(4):330–340. doi:10.1016/j.survophthal.2012.09.004
143. Pujari A, Rakheja V, Bajaj MS, Sen S, Yadav B. Isolated conjunctival histoplasmosis in an elderly patient: a rare but important scenario. *Canadian J Ophthalmol.* 2019;54(1), e15–e16.
144. Sacharow SJ, Picker JD, Levy HL. *Homocystinuria Caused by Cystathionine Beta-Synthase Deficiency.* PMID: 20301697
145. Chelala E, El Rami H, Dirani A, Fakhoury H, Fadlallah A. Extensive superior limbic keratoconjunctivitis in Graves' disease: case report and mini-review of the literature. *Clin Ophthalmol.* 2015;9:467–468. Published 2015 Mar 10. doi:10.2147/OPTH.S79561
146. Mathebula SD. Vitamin D in ocular and systemic health. *African Vis Eye Health.* 201574(1):5.
147. Rosa RG, Barros AJ, de Lima AR, et al. Mood disorder as a manifestation of primary hypoparathyroidism: a case report. *J Med Case Rep.* 2014;8:326. Published 2014 Oct 3. doi:10.1186/1752-1947-8-326
148. Liao X, Huang X, Lan C, Li J, Tan Q. Characteristic cataract associated with idiopathic hypoparathyroidism. *J Clin Exp Ophthalmol.* 2016;7(4):588.
149. Corredor-Osorio R, Corredor-Osorio M, Corredor-Osorio A. Eyelid nonbullous impetigo. *Our Dermatol Online.* 2016;7(3):291.
150. Belser JA, Lash RR, Garg S, Tumpey TM, Maines TR. The eyes have it: influenza virus infection beyond the respiratory tract. *Lancet Infect Dis.* 2018;18(7):e220–e227. doi:10.1016/S1473-3099(18)30102-6
151. Brydak-Godowska J, Turczyńska M, Przybyś M, Brydak LB, Kęcik D. Ocular complications in influenza virus infection. *Ocul Immunol Inflamm.* 2019;27(4):545–550. doi:10.1080/09273948.2017.1423335
152. Curtiss P, Strazzulla LC, Friedman-Kien AE. An update on Kaposi's sarcoma: epidemiology, pathogenesis and treatment. *Dermatol Ther.* 2016;6(4):465–470. doi:10.1007/s13555-016-0152-3
153. Davis A, Viera AJ, Mead MD. Leukemia: an overview for primary care. *Am Fam Physician.* 2014;89(9):731–738.

154. Lieber CS. Relationships between nutrition, alcohol use, and liver disease. *Alcohol Res Health.* 2003;27(3):220–231.
155. Rothblum-Oviatt C, Wright J, Lefton-Greif MA, McGrath-Morrow SA, Crawford TO, Lederman HM. Ataxia telangiectasia: a review. *Orphanet J Rare Dis.* 2016;11(1):159. Published 2016 Nov 25. doi:10.1186/s13023-016-0543-7
156. Loi M. Lowe syndrome. *Orphanet J Rare Dis.* 2006;1:16.
157. Lewis WD, Lilly S, Jones KL. Lymphoma: diagnosis and treatment. *Am Fam Physician.* 2020;101(1):34–41.
158. Ong APC, Watson A, Subbiah S. Rubeola keratitis emergence during a recent measles outbreak in New Zealand. *J Prim Health Care.* 2020;12(3):289–292. doi:10.1071/HC20013
159. Leung AK, Hon KL, Leong KF, Sergi CM. Measles: a disease often forgotten but not gone. *Hong Kong Med J.* 2018;24(5):512–520. doi:10.12809/hkmj187470
160. Del Longo A, Piozzi, E, Schweizer F. Ocular features in mucopolysaccharidosis: diagnosis and treatment. *Italian J Pediatr.* 2018;44:125.
161. Zhou J, Lin J, Leung WT, Wang L. A basic understanding of mucopolysaccharidosis: incidence, clinical features, diagnosis, and management. *Intractable Rare Dis Res.* 2020;9:1–9.
162. Graves J, Balcer LJ. Eye disorders in patients with multiple sclerosis: natural history and management. *Clin Ophthalmol.* 2010;4:1409–1422. Published 2010 Dec 6. doi:10.2147/OPTH.S6383
163. Choi KM. Reemergence of mumps. *Korean J Pediatr.* 2010;53(5):623–628. doi:10.3345/kjp.2010.53.5.623
164. Falsaperla R, Praticò AD, Ruggieri M, Parano E, Rizzo R, Corsello G, ... Pavone P. Congenital muscular dystrophy: from muscle to brain. *Italian J Pediatr.* 2016;42(1):1–11.
165. Nair AG, Patil-Chhablani P, Venkatramani DV, Gandhi RA. Ocular myasthenia gravis: a review. *Indian J Ophthalmol.* 2014;62(10):985–991. doi:10.4103/0301-4738.145987
166. Bregou Bourgeois A, Aubry-Rozier B, Bonafé L, Laurent-Applegate L, Pioletti DP, Zambelli PY. Osteogenesis imperfecta: from diagnosis and multidisciplinary treatment to future perspectives. *Swiss Med Wkly.* 2016;146:w14322. Published 2016 Jun 20. doi:10.4414/smw.2016.14322
167. Doolan E, O'Brien C. Abnormal corneal properties in osteogenesis imperfecta and glaucoma: a case series. *BMJ Open Ophthalmol.* 2021;6(1):e000684. Published 2021 Apr 15. doi:10.1136/bmjophth-2020-000684
168. Schonberg S, Stokkermans TJ. Ocular pemphigoid. In: *StatPearls.* Treasure Island: StatPearls Publishing; August 25, 2021.
169. Rajguru JP, Maya D, Kumar D, Suri P, Bhardwaj S, Patel ND. Update on psoriasis: A review. *J Family Med Prim Care.* 2020;9(1):20–24. Published 2020 Jan 28. doi:10.4103/jfmpc.jfmpc_689_19
170. Khanna D. Diagnosis and treatment of systemic and localized scleroderma. *Expert Rev Dermatol.* 2011;6(3):287–302.
171. Silpa-archa S, Lee JJ, Foster CS. Ocular manifestations in systemic lupus erythematosus. *British J Ophthalmol.* 2016;100(1):135–141.
172. Ness T, Bley TA, Schmidt WA, Lamprecht P. The diagnosis and treatment of giant cell arteritis. *Dtsch Arztebl Int.* 2013;110(21):376–386. doi:10.3238/arztebl.2013.0376
173. Al-Jameil N, Khan FA, Khan MF, Tabassum H. A brief overview of preeclampsia. *J Cli Med Res.* 2014;6(1):1.
174. Park YH, Nam HW. Clinical features and treatment of ocular toxoplasmosis. *Korean J Parasitol.* 2013;51(4):393–399. doi:10.3347/kjp.2013.51.4.393
175. Muflikhatun K, Nurdian Y. *Ocular System Involvement in Food-Borne Trichinellosis.* 2017. Researchgate.
176. Testi I, Agrawal R, Mehta S, et al. Ocular tuberculosis: Where are we today? *Indian J Ophthalmol.* 2020;68(9):1808–1817. doi:10.4103/ijo.IJO_1451_20
177. Sybert VP, McCauley E. Turner's syndrome. *New England J Med.* 2004;351(12):1227–1238.
178. Narayanan M, Reddy KM, Marsicano E. Peptic ulcer disease and *Helicobacter pylori* infection. *Mo Med.* 2018;115(3):219–224.
179. Gargouri S, Khochtali S, Zina S et al. Ocular involvement associated with varicella in adults. *J Ophthal Inflamm Infect.* 2016;6:47. https://doi.org/10.1186/s12348-016-0117-9
180. Abdolrahimzadeh B, Piraino DC, Albanese G, Cruciani F, Rahimi S. Neurofibromatosis: an update of ophthalmic characteristics and applications of optical coherence tomography. *Clin Ophthalmol.* 2016;10:851–860. Published 2016 May 13. doi:10.2147/OPTH.S102830
181. Rodrigues CEM, Callado MRM, Nobre CA, Moura FEA, Vieira RMRDA, Albuquerque LAFD, Vieira WP. Wegener's granulomatosis: Prevalence of the initial clinical manifestations-report of six cases and review of the literature. *Revista Brasileira de Reumatologia.* 2010;50:150–157.
182. Pakrou N, Selva D, Leibovitch I. Wegener's granulomatosis: ophthalmic manifestations and management. In *Seminars in Arthritis and Rheumatism* (Vol. 35, No. 5, pp. 284–292). WB Saunders, 2006, April.

APPENDIX 1: DIAGNOSTIC INDEX OF SUBJECTIVE SYMPTOMS

Subjective Symptoms Categories

A. Corneal irritation
B. Cosmetic concern (without pain)
C. Dull, aching ocular pain
D. Itching or burning irritation
E. Headache-type pain
F. Pain on palpation (or pressure) to eyelid or globe
G. Vision reduction (diminished visual acuity)
H. Visual loss (sudden or transient dimming or blindness)

A. Corneal Irritation

(Sandy, gritty, foreign-body sensation, or "something under my upper lid")

Eyelids and Adnexa

1. Chalazion (internal type), 84
2. Coloboma (large notch), 69
3. Ectropion, 70
4. Entropion, 70
5. Exophthalmos (exposure), 98
6. Foreign body on tarsus, 66
7. Lagophthalmos (band region), 72
8. Marginal blepharitis (infectious types), 81
9. Molluscum contagiosum (at margin), 73, 129
10. Subcutaneous cilia, 66
11. Trichiasis, 77
12. Verrucae (at margin), 78, 129

Conjunctiva, Sclera, and Episclera

1. Calcium concretions (severe on palpebral conjunctiva), 155
2. Conjunctivitis
   a. Bacterial (usually hyperacute forms), 118
   b. Viral, 129
   c. Toxic or irritative (chronic), 123
   d. Vernal, 118
3. Episcleritis (severe), 132
4. Giant papillary conjunctivitis, 117
5. Pinguecula (to pterygium), 111
6. Scleritis or sclerouveitis (advanced forms), 134

Cornea

1. Abrasion injuries, 140
2. Band keratopathy, 174
3. Bullous keratopathy, 174
4. Burns
   a. Chemical, 150
   b. Radiation, 104
   c. Thermal, 64
5. Chlamydial keratoconjunctivitis, 129
6. Cogan's microcystic degeneration, 175
7. Dendriform keratitis (HSV and infiltrative forms), 234
8. Dry eye or keratitis sicca syndromes (late day), 153
9. Dystrophies
   a. Epithelial layer, 179
   b. Bowman's layer, 179
   c. Posterior layer (Fuchs' endothelial), 181
10. Epithelial basement membrane disorders (EBMD) (AM syndrome), 179, 182
11. Epithelial edema (all forms), 37
12. Foreign-body injuries, 158
13. Infectious keratitis (all forms)
    a. Acanthamoeba, 219
    b. Bacterial, 220
    c. Fungal, 224
    d. Herpetic, 234
14. Microcysts (usually AM syndrome), 184
15. Mooren's ulcer, 245
16. Ocular rosacea, 241
17. Pellucid marginal degeneration, 190
18. Pterygium, 176
19. Recurrent corneal erosion (RCE) syndrome, 167
20. Salzmann's nodular degeneration, 177
21. Superficial keratitis (all forms), 208, 213, 240
22. Superior limbic keratoconjunctivitis (SLK), 246
23. Terrien's marginal degeneration (acute phase), 176, 181, 190, 247
24. Trachoma (acute phase), 247
25. Vernal keratoconjunctivitis, 118

Anterior Chamber, Iris, and Ciliary Body

1. Chronic uveitis (with posterior corneal decompensation), 275
2. Keratouveitis, 269
3. Sclerouveitis, 135

B. Cosmetic Concern (without Pain)

Eyelids and Adnexa

1. Blepharoptosis, 67
2. Blepharospasm, 68
3. Chloasma, 69
4. Coloboma, 69
5. Congenital anomalies, 69
6. Dermatochalasis, 69
7. Dermoid, 69
8. Epicanthus, 71
9. Exophthalmos, 98
10. Hemangioma, 71
11. Keratoses, 71
12. Madarosis, 72
13. Nevus, 71, 74
14. Papilloma, 74, 111
15. Poliosis, 75
16. Sebaceous cyst, 75
17. Sudoriferous cyst, 76
18. Verrucae, 78, 129
19. Xanthelasma, 79

Conjunctiva, Sclera, and Episclera

1. Acute bacterial conjunctivitis, 118
2. Blue sclera, 130, 171
3. Chronic (toxic) conjunctivitis, 123, 128
4. Dermolipoma, 106
5. Granuloma, 106
6. Hemangioma, 107

7. Hyaline plaques, 131
8. Icteric sclera, 109, 131
9. Inclusion (lymphatic) cyst, 108
10. Keratinization (xerosis), 108
11. Lithiasis (calcium concretions), 105
12. Lymphangiectasia, 108
13. Melanosis, 109, 110
14. Nevus, 110
15. Papilloma, 111
16. Pigmentations, 110, 111
17. Pinguecula, 111
18. Staphyloma, 132
19. Subacute viral conjunctivitis, 126

Cornea

1. Arcus senilis, 172
2. Megalocornea, 171
3. Microcornea, 171
4. Pigmentations, 190
5. Sclerocomea, 130, 171
6. White limbal girdle of Vogt, 177

Anterior Chamber, Iris, and Ciliary Body

1. Aniridia, 283
2. Atrophies, 283
3. Colobomas, 283
4. Persistent pupillary membrane(s) or remnant(s), 283, 284, 285
5. Pigmentation variations (of iris), 285

C. Dull, Aching Ocular Pain

Eyelids and Adnexa

1. Contusion (blunt) injuries, 65
2. Dacryoadenitis, 94
3. Dacryocystitis (acute form), 95
4. Herpes zoster blepharitis, 86
5. Hordeolum (internal type), 87
6. Insect bites or stings, 89
7. Orbital cellulitis, 98
8. Preseptal cellulitis, 98

Conjunctiva, Sclera, and Episclera

1. Episcleritis, 132
2. Hyperacute conjunctivitis, 123
3. Lacerating injuries, 105
4. Parinaud's oculoglandular fever, 129
5. Scleritis, 134

Cornea

1. Acanthamoeba keratitis, 219
2. Herpes simplex (stromal) keratitis, 238
3. Herpes zoster ophthalmicus, 238
4. Keratouveitis (all forms), 193

Anterior Chamber, Iris, and Ciliary Body

1. Acute anterior uveitis (all forms), 258
2. Chronic anterior uveitis (most forms), 272
3. Hyphema, 280
4. Pars planitis, 276
5. Trauma, 149

D. Itching or Burning Irritation

Eyelids and Adnexa

1. Allergic blepharitis, 80
2. Demodicosis, 84
3. Herpes simplex blepharitis, 85
4. Insect bites or stings, 89
5. Marginal (bacterial) blepharitis, 81
6. Molluscum contagiosum, 73, 129
7. Pediculosis, 91

Conjunctiva, Sclera, and Episclera

1. Allergic conjunctivitis, 113
2. Toxic or irritative (chronic) conjunctivitis, 123
3. Viral (and other follicular) conjunctivitis, 126

Cornea

1. Chlamydial (inclusion) keratoconjunctivitis, 128
2. Epidemic keratoconjunctivitis (EKC), 225
3. Herpes simplex keratitis, 234
4. Herpes zoster ophthalmicus, 238
5. Non-specific adenoviral keratoconjunctivitis, 126
6. Pharyngoconjunctival fever (PCF), 240
7. Vernal keratoconjunctivitis, 118

E. Headache-Type Pain

Eyelids and Adnexa

1. Blepharospasm, 68
2. Contusion (blunt) injuries, 97
3. Dacryoadenitis, 94
4. Dacryocystitis (acute or chronic form), 95
5. Herpes zoster blepharitis, 86
6. Insect bites or stings, 89
7. Orbital cellulitis, 98
8. Preseptal cellulitis, 98
9. Tumors, 74

Conjunctiva, Sclera, and Episclera

1. Episcleritis (nodular or advanced form), 134
2. Hyperacute conjunctivitis, 122
3. Parinaud's oculoglandular fever, 129
4. Scleritis, 134

Cornea

1. Blunt (concussion or contusion) injury, 149
2. Herpes zoster ophthalmicus, 238
3. Recurrent corneal erosion (RCE) syndrome, 167

Anterior Chamber, Iris, and Ciliary Body

1. Acute anterior uveitis (severe), 258, 285
2. Chronic anterior uveitis, 272
3. Hyphema, 280, 354
4. Iris bombe, 283, 284
5. Pars planitis, 276
6. Primary angle closure glaucoma, 352
7. Trauma, 149, 354

F. Pain on Palpation (or Pressure) to Eyelid or Globe

Eyelids and Adnexa

1. Blepharitis (acute forms), 80
2. Contusion (blunt) injuries, 65

3. Dacryoadenitis, 94
4. Dacryocystitis (acute and chronic), 95
5. Foreign bodies on tarsus, 66
6. Hordeolum, 87
7. Insect bites or stings, 89
8. Meibomianitis (acute form), 89
9. Neoplasias (sometimes), 73
10. Orbital cellulitis, 98
11. Preseptal cellulitis, 99

Conjunctiva, Sclera, and Episclera

1. Episcleritis, 132
2. Foreign bodies, 104
3. Hyperacute conjunctivitis, 122
4. Neoplasias (sometimes), 110
5. Parinaud's oculoglandular fever, 129
6. Scleritis, 134

Cornea

1. Blunt (concussion or contusion) injury, 149
2. Epidemic keratoconjunctivitis (EKC), 225
3. Filamentary keratitis, 208
4. Foreign bodies (embedded), 158
5. Herpes zoster ophthalmicus, 238
6. Superior limbic keratoconjunctivitis (SLK), 246
7. Vernal keratoconjunctivitis, 118

Anterior Chamber, Iris, and Ciliary Body

1. Acute anterior uveitis, 258, 285, 355
2. Chronic anterior uveitis (sometimes), 272, 355
3. Hyphema, 280, 354
4. Neoplasias (sometimes), 284
5. Trauma (especially blunt), 149, 354

G. Vision Reduction (Diminished Visual Acuity)

Eyelids and Adnexa

1. Chalazion (irregular astigmatism), 84
2. Entropion, 70
3. Lagophthalmos, 72
4. Orbital tumors (diplopia), 98
5. Subcutaneous cilia, 66
6. Trichiasis, 77

Conjunctiva, Sclera, and Episclera

1. Hyperacute conjunctivitis, 122
2. Scleritis (with photophobia), 134

Cornea (Visual Reduction Associated with Photophobia)

1. Abrasions, 140
2. Acne rosacea, 377
3. Band keratopathy, 174
4. Blunt (concussion or contusion) injuries, 149
5. Bullous keratopathy, 174
6. Burns, 64
7. Chlamydial (inclusion) keratoconjunctivitis, 129
8. Dry eye or keratitis sicca syndromes, 153
9. Dystrophies (most types), 180
10. Epithelial basement membrane disorders, 179, 182
11. Foreign bodies, 158
12. Infectious keratitis (all forms), 208, 216, 220
13. Keratoconus (irregular astigmatism), 188
14. Pellucid marginal degeneration, 190
15. Pterygium (irregular astigmatism), 176
16. Recurrent corneal erosion (RCE) syndrome, 167
17. Salzman's nodular degeneration, 177
18. Superior limbic keratoconjunctivitis (SLK), 246
19. Superficial keratitis (all forms), 208, 213, 239
20. Terrien's marginal degeneration, 176, 181, 190, 247
21. Trachoma, 125
22. Vernal keratoconjunctivitis, 118

Anterior Chamber, Iris, and Ciliary Body (Visual Reduction Associated with Photophobia)

1. Acute anterior uveitis, 258, 285, 355
2. Albinism, 285
3. Atrophies (iris), 283
4. Chronic anterior uveitis (insidious reduction), 272, 355
5. Hyphema, 280, 354
6. Pars planitis, 276
7. Trauma, 149, 354

H. Visual Loss (Sudden or Transient Dimming or Blindness)

Eyelids and Adnexa

1. Blepharoptosis, 67
2. Blepharospasm (essential type), 68
3. Dermatochalasis (insidious), 69
4. Insect bite or sting (with reaction), 89
5. Orbital tumor (compression types), 98
6. Trauma (head and ocular region), 97

Cornea

1. Blunt (concussion or contusion) injuries, 149
2. Burns (severe), 64
3. Herpes zoster ophthalmicus (severe), 86
4. Laceration (perforating), 142

Anterior Chamber, Iris, and Ciliary Body

1. Chronic anterior uveitis (insidious), 272, 355
2. Glaucoma (secondary and angle-closure types), 344, 352, 353
3. Hyphema, 280, 354
4. Trauma, 149, 354

APPENDIX 2: DIAGNOSTIC INDEX OF OBJECTIVE SIGNS

Eyelids and Adnexa

Conjunctiva, Sclera, and Episclera

c. Beal's (swimming pool) conjunctivitis, 240
d. Chlamydial (inclusion) conjunctivitis, 243
e. Folliculosis, 128
f. Hemorrhagic (acute) conjunctivitis, 128
g. Herpes virus (simplex and zoster), 129
h. Molluscum contagiosum, 73, 129
i. Newcastle's disease, 129
j. Parinaud's oculoglandular fever, 129
k. Toxic or irritative conjunctivitis, 123, 124
l. Trachoma, 125
m. Verrucae, 78, 129

4. **Hemorrhages**
   a. Acute bacterial conjunctivitis (especially Streptococcus), 119
   b. Granulomas, 106
   c. Hyperacute viral conjunctivitis, 126
   d. Neoplasias, 110
   e. Subconjunctival hemorrhage (spontaneous, idiopathic), 112
   f. Systemic diseases (especially blood dyscrasias), 407
   g. Telangiectasia ruptures, 113
   h. Trauma (lacerating, contusive, or foreign matter), 104–105

5. **Hyperemia**
   a. Acne rosacea (usually superficial circumcorneal), 377
   b. Anterior uveitis (deep circumcorneal), 258, 285
   c. Burns, 150
   d. Conjunctivitis (all forms), 122
   e. Corneal inflammation, 208
   f. Drug induced, 407
   g. Episcleritis (deep sector), 132
   h. Irritations (injuries to globe), 97
   i. Scleritis (deep diffuse), 134
   j. Systemic diseases, 407
   k. Toxic irritation (frequently angular), 123

6. **Lumps and bumps**
   a. Dermolipoma, 106, 111
   b. Granuloma, 106
   c. Hemangioma, 107
   d. Lithiasis (calcium concretions), 105
   e. Lymphangiectasia, 108
   f. Lymphatic (inclusion) cysts105, 108
   g. Neoplasias, 110
   h. Nevus, 106, 110
   i. Nodular episcleritis, 134
   j. Papilloma, 74, 111
   k. Phlyctenule, 124
   l. Pinguecula, 111
   m. Pterygium, 177
   n. Telangiectasia (in subconjunctival hemorrhage), 113

7. **Nodule**
   a. Nodular episcleritis, 134
   b. Phlyctenule, 124
   c. Pinguecula, 111

8. **Papillae**
   a. Allergic conjunctivitis, 113
   b. Bacterial conjunctivitis (acute and hyperacute), 122
   c. Corneal infection or inflammation (variable causes), 208
   d. Drug induced, 406
   e. Dry eye syndromes, 153
   f. Giant papillary conjunctivitis (GPC), 117
   g. Toxic or irritative conjunctivitis, 123, 128
   h. Trachoma, 125
   i. Vernal conjunctivitis and keratoconjunctivitis, 118

9. **Pigmentation changes**
   a. Argyrosis (silver), 111
   b. Axenfeld's loops, 130
   c. Blue sclera, 130, 131, 171
   d. Drug induced, 111
   e. Hemangioma, 107
   f. Hyaline plaques, 131
   g. Icteric sclera (jaundice), 109, 131
   h. Mascara staining, 111
   i. Melanosis, 109–111
   j. Nevus, 106, 110
   k. Ochronosis, 109–111
   l. Subconjunctival hemorrhage, 112
   m. Systemic diseases, 111
   n. Tattooing (usually by heavy metals), 111

10. **Pseudomembranes**
    a. Burns, 150
    b. Hyperacute conjunctivitis (most forms), 226

11. **Symblepharon**
    a. Burns, 150
    b. Chronic inflammation, 34

Cornea

1. **Arcus ring**
   a. Aging, 172, 175
   b. Central crystalline dystrophy, 180
   c. Familial, 173, 174
   d. Hyperlipidemias (e.g., hypercholesterolemia), 176

2. **Band keratopathy**
   a. Aging, 173–174
   b. Gout, 174
   c. Hypercalcemia (hyperparathyroidism), 174
   d. Juvenile rheumatoid arthritis (JRA; Still's disease), 174

3. **Bullous keratopathy**
   a. Aging, 174
   b. Fuchs' endothelial dystrophy, 175, 181
   c. Postoperative complication, 175
   d. Raised intraocular pressure, 175

4. **Breakup time (BUT) less than 10 seconds**
   a. Dry eye (keratitis sicca-type syndromes), 209
   b. Epithelial basement membrane disorders (instantaneous BUT), 179, 182–183

5. **Dellen**
   a. Contact lens edge, 176
   b. Postoperative complication, 176
   c. Raised conjunctival Lesion, 130, 175

6. **Dendrites**
   a. Atopic keratoconjunctivitis, 208, 214, 239–240
   b. Dry eye or keratitis sicca-type syndromes, 209

c. Herpes simplex keratitis (only ulcerative dendrites), 236
d. Herpes zoster keratitis, 238
e. Recurrent corneal erosion (RCE) syndrome, 167
f. SPK of Thygeson, 214
g. Superior limbic keratoconjunctivitis (SLK), 246
h. Vernal keratoconjunctivitis, 118

7. **Drying**
a. Band keratopathy, 174
b. Burns, 150
c. Degeneration (aging), 172, 175
d. Dellen, 175–176
e. Dry eye or keratitis sicca syndromes, 209
f. Epithelial basement membrane disorders, 179, 182–183
g. Eyelid disorders, 81, 89
h. Recurrent corneal erosion (RCE) syndromes, 167

8. **Edema**
a. Congenital, 169
b. Contusive injury, 149
c. Degeneration, 172, 175
d. Drug induced, 406
e. Dystrophy, 179–180
f. Endothelial dysfunction, 181
g. Hypersensitivity reactions, 191
h. Increased intraocular pressure (usually acute), 182
i. Inflammation (all types), 211, 216, 220
j. Injuries (foreign bodies, laceration, abrasion), 140

9. **Filaments**
a. Atopic keratoconjunctivitis, 208, 214, 239–240
b. Burns to cornea (radiation, thermal, chemical), 150
c. Dry eye-keratitis sicca syndromes, 209
d. Epidemic keratoconjunctivitis (EKC), 225
e. Herpes simplex keratitis, 85, 229–230
f. Herpes zoster ophthalmicus, 238
g. Mechanical (chronic) corneal irritation, 154
h. Postoperative response, 177
i. Prolonged pressure patching, 148
j. Recurrent corneal erosion (RCE), 167
k. Superior limbic keratoconjunctivitis (SLK), 246
l. Superficial punctate keratitis of Thygeson, 214
m. Vernal keratoconjunctivitis, 118

10. **Guttata**
a. Contact lens complications
b. Degeneration (aging), 172, 175
c. Fuchs' endothelial dystrophy (central), 181
d. Hassall–Henle warts (peripheral), 172, 176
e. Trauma (transient), 149
f. Uveitis (chronic, severe), 272

11. **Hypoasthesia (reduced corneal sensitivity)**
a. Contact lens wear
b. Diabetes, 397
c. Dystrophies (granular, lattice, macular), 179–180
d. Epidemic keratoconjunctivitis (EKC), 225
e. Herpes simplex keratitis, 236
f. Herpes zoster ophthalmicus, 238
g. Neurotrophic keratitis, 212
h. Postoperative

12. **Infiltrates**
a. Acanthamoeba (ring), 219
b. Acne rosacea(peripheral), 241
c. Burns (chemical), 150
d. Chlamydia, 243
e. Drug induced (topical or oral), 191
f. Dystrophies (stromal), 179–180
g. Infectious keratitis (bacterial, viral, fungal), 208, 216, 220
h. Interstitial keratitis, 235
i. Keratouveitis (chronic), 272
j. Marginal keratitis, 209
k. Staphylococcal keratitis, 209, 214, 241
l. Sterile keratitis, 214
m. SPK of Thygeson, 214
n. Superior limbic keratoconjunctivitis (SLK), 214
o. Syphilis (usually interstitial keratitis), 244
p. Systemic diseases, 378
q. Toxic keratitis, 209, 213, 240
r. Vernal keratoconjunctivitis, 118

13. **Limbal variations**
a. Band keratopathy (early at palpebral fissure zones), 174
b. Dellen, 175
c. Keratomelanocystosis, 189
d. Marginal furrow degeneration, 176, 190, 245, 247
e. Pellucid marginal degeneration, 176, 190, 245
f. Phlyctenular keratoconjunctivitis, 213
g. Posterior embryotoxon, 170
h. Pterygium, 176
i. Sclerocornea, 171
j. Superior limbic keratoconjunctivitis (SLK), 246, 247
k. Terrien's degeneration, 245, 247
l. Trachoma, 125
m. Vernal keratoconjunctivitis (superior Tranta's dots), 118
n. White limbal girdle of Vogt, 177

14. **Marginal (midperipheral) lesions**
a. Arcus, 172, 176
b. Central crystalline dystrophy, 180
c. Dellen, 175
d. Fungal ulceration (serpiginous), 224
e. Hassall–Henle bodies, 172, 176
f. Infiltrative keratitis (i.e., toxic, sterile, staphylococcal), 191, 214
g. Marginal furrow degeneration, 176, 190, 245, 247
h. Marginal keratitis, 209
i. Morren's ulcer (serpiginous), 225
j. Pellucid marginal degeneration, 176, 190, 245
k. Posterior embryotoxon, 170
l. Terrien's degeneration, 245, 247

15. **Microcysts**
a. Abrasions (during healing), 140
b. Cogan's microcystic degeneration, 175
c. Contact lens complications
d. Epithelial basement membrane disorders, 179, 182
e. Meesman's dystrophy
f. Postoperative, 252
g. Recurrent corneal erosion (RCE), 167

16. **Neovascularization and pannus**
    a. Acne rosacea, 241
    b. Burns (chemical), 150
    c. Chlamydia, 243
    d. Degenerations, 172, 175
    e. Dry eye or keratitis sicca syndromes, 209
    f. Dystrophies, 179
    g. Edema (chronic), 34
    h. Glaucoma, 286, 355
    i. Infectious keratitis, 208, 216, 220
    j. Keratouveitis, 268
    k. Neoplasia, 54
    l. Penetrating or perforating injury, 142
    m. Phlyctenular keratoconjunctivitis, 213
    n. Pterygium, 176
    o. Sterile keratitis (especially toxic, marginal types), 208, 214, 240
    p. Superior limbic keratoconjunctivitis (SLK), 247
    q. Uveitis (chronic), 274
    r. Vernal keratoconjunctivitis, 118

17. **Opacification**
    a. Burns (chemical, especially alkaline), 150
    b. Congenital, 169
    c. Degeneration (aging), 172, 175
    d. Drug induced, 402
    e. Dry eye-keratitis sicca syndromes, 209
    f. Dystrophies (usually stromal or posterior), 180
    g. Edema (stromal), 37
    h. Glaucoma, 172, 357
    i. Infectious keratitis, 208, 216, 220
    j. Keratouveitis, 268
    k. Systemic diseases, 375
    l. Vernal keratoconjunctivitis, 118

18. **Pigment variations**
    a. Argyrosis (silver), 190
    b. Blood staining (hemosiderosis), 190
    c. Chalcosis (copper)
    d. Chrysiasis (gold)
    e. Drug induced, 190
    f. Edema (brawny), 190
    g. Ferric ion lines, 190
    h. Melanosis (melanin)
    i. Posterior keratic precipitate (KP) patterns, 191
    j. Siderosis (iron)
    k. Tattooing, 191

19. **Raised lesions**
    a. Bullous keratopathy, 174
    b. Dermoids, 69
    c. Filaments, 208
    d. Phlyctenular keratoconjunctivitis, 213
    e. Pterygium, 176
    f. Salzmann's nodular degeneration, 177
    g. Tumors, 392

20. **Shagreen**
    a. Blunt (contusive) injury, 149
    b. Keratoconus, 188
    c. Post crocodile (degeneration), 172, 176
    d. Recurrent corneal erosion (RCE), 167
    e. Rubbing (habitual), 148

21. **Shape variations**
    a. Axenfeld–Reiger's (A–R) syndromes, 169
    b. Congenital, 171
    c. Keratoconus, 189
    d. Megalocornea, 171
    e. Microcornea, 171
    f. Rubella syndrome, 410
    g. Sclerocomea, 130, 171

22. **Striae**
    a. Buphthalmos (congenital glaucoma), 172
    b. Drug induced, 406
    c. Eyelid reactions (anterior), 64
    d. Infectious keratitis (deep), 235
    e. Inflammation, 34
    f. Intraocular pressure reduction or rise, 182
    g. Keratouveitis, 268
    h. Pressure patching, 148
    i. Systemic diseases, 375
    j. Trauma (especially at birth, vertical orientation), 172

23. **Superficial punctate keratitis (SPK)**
    a. Burns (radiation, thermal, chemical), 150
    b. Contusion, 149
    c. Dry eye or keratitis sicca syndromes, 209
    d. Edema (superficial or deep), 191
    e. Epithelial basement membrane disorders (EBMD), 182
    f. Epithelial dystrophies, 179
    g. Eyelid disorders, 64
    h. Foreign bodies (foreign-body tracking), 158
    i. Infectious keratitis (all forms), 208, 216, 220
    j. Inflammation, 206, 216, 220
    k. Recurrent corneal erosion (RCE) syndromes, 167–168
    l. Superficial keratitis (all types), 191, 214
    m. Toxins (e.g., from lids, conjunctiva, airborne, contact), 208, 214, 231
    n. Uveitis (chronic), 272

24. **Thinning**
    a. Congenital, 236
    b. Dellen, 175
    c. Inflammation (chronic), 235
    d. Interstitial keratitis, 236
    e. Keratoconus, 188
    f. Marginal furrow degeneration, 176, 190, 245, 247
    g. Pellucid marginal degeneration, 176, 190, 245
    h. Staphyloma, 132
    i. Terrien's degeneration, 189, 194, 245, 247
    j. Ulceration, 40

25. **Ulceration**
    a. Acanthamoeba, 219
    b. Bacterial, 220
    c. Dry eye or keratitis sicca syndromes, 210
    d. Fungal, 224
    e. Herpetic (simplex or zoster), 238
    f. Keratouveitis, 268
    g. Sterile causes, 214
    h. Systemic diseases, 375
    i. Toxic causes, 208, 214, 231

26. **Whorls**
    a. Amiodarone (arrhythmic systemic drug)
    b. Chloroquine toxicity
    c. Fabry's disease (systemic), 398
    d. Vortex dystrophy

Anterior Chamber, Iris, and Ciliary Body

1. **Aniridia**
    a. Congenital, 283
    b. Rieger's syndrome, 171, 357
    c. Traumatic, 280
    d. Wilms' tumor (Miller's syndrome), 389
2. **Aniscoria**
    a. Drug induced, 265
    b. Keratitis, 208, 216, 220
    c. Neurological, 264
    d. Physiological, 266
    e. Traumatic, 264
    f. Uveitis, 258
3. **Atrophy or hypoplasia (of iris)**
    a. Chandler's syndrome, 171
    b. Congenital, 283
    c. Degeneration (aging), 283
    d. Essential iris atrophy, 283
    e. Glaucoma, 265
    f. Inflammation, 283
    g. Iridoschisis, 283, 284
    h. Ischemia (multiple causes), 283
    i. Neurogenic (syphilitic), 409
    j. Rieger's syndrome, 169, 357
    k. Trauma, 264
4. **Cells and flare**
    a. Infection, 265
    b. Inflammation, 261
    c. Keratitis, 208, 216, 220
    d. Masquerade syndromes, 265
    e. Plasmoid aqueous, 264
    f. Systemic disease, 265
    g. Trauma, 264
    h. Unknown (idiopathic), 266
    i. Uveitis (anterior nongranulomatous, or granulomatous), 260
5. **Corectopia**
    a. Atrophy, 283, 284
    b. Coloboma, 283
    c. Congenital, 283
    d. Glaucoma, 265
    e. Iridodialysis, 284, 351, 354
    f. Posterior synechiae, 264
    g. Rieger's syndrome, 169
    h. Trauma, 268
    i. Tumors (iris), 94, 284
    j. Uveitis, 258
6. **Hyphema**
    a. Diabetes, 396
    b. Herpes simplex (acute uveitis), 282
    c. Neovascularization of angle or iris, 285, 355
    d. Trauma (blunt or contusive), 149, 354
    e. Tumors (iris), 94, 284
    f. Uveitis glaucoma hyphema (UGH) syndrome, 356
7. **Hypopyon**
    a. Drug induced, 265
    b. Endophthalmitis, 264
    c. Infectious keratitis, 216
    d. Uveitis (severe, acute anterior), 258
8. **Iridodonesis**
    a. Aphakia (and pseudophakia), 289
    b. Buphthalmos, 172
    c. Cataract (usually hypermature), 284
    d. Dislocated lens, 284
    e. Megalocornea, 171
9. **Iris processes**
    a. Axenfeld–Rieger's syndromes, 169, 337, 357
    b. Glaucoma (narrow angle types), 265, 350, 352
    c. Idiopathic (especially in dark eyes), 282, 337
    d. Inflammation (uveitis), 258
10. **Keratic precipitates (KPs), fine**
    a. Arlt's triangle, 262
    b. Degeneration (aging), 285
    c. Kruckenburg's spindle, 263, 342, 350, 353
    d. Pigment cells (normal melanin), 285
    e. Trauma, 149
    f. Uveitis (acute nongranulomatous), 258, 285
11. **Keratic precipitates (KPs), mutton fat**
    a. Endophthalmitis, 263
    b. Masquerade syndromes, 265
    c. Systemic disease, 375
    d. Uveitis (chronic granulomatous), 273
12. **Masses**
    a. Amyloidosis, 394
    b. Granulomas, 264
    c. Hemangiomas, 284
    d. Iris nevus (Cogan–Reese) syndrome, 283
    e. Juvenile xanthogranuloma (nevoxanthoendothelioma), 276
    f. Leiomyoma (neoplastic), 94, 284
    g. Leukemia (neoplastic), 267
    h. Lymphoma (neoplastic), 267
    i. Medulloepitheliomas, 94, 284
    j. Melanomas (neoplastic), 267
    k. Metastatic tumors (neoplastic), 94, 284
    l. Neurilemmomas, 284
    m. Neurofibromas, 284
    n. Nevi (iris freckles), 284
    o. Reactive lymphoid hyperplasia, 386
    p. Reticulum cell sarcoma (neoplastic), 94, 284
    q. Retinoblastoma (neoplastic), 267
13. **Miosis**
    a. Aging, 283, 284
    b. Drug induced, 396, 404, 406
    c. Keratitis, 208, 216, 220
    d. Migraine, 396, 404, 406
    e. Neurological, 403
    f. Parkinsonism, 383
    g. Physiological, 266
    h. Psychogenic, 266
    i. Uveitis, 258

14. **Mydriasis**
    a. Adie's tonic pupil, 55
    b. Drug induced, 265
    c. Idiopathic (especially in youth), 282
    d. Neurological, 403
    e. Physiological, 266
    f. Psychogenic, 266
    g. Trauma, 280
    h. Uveitis, 258

15. **Neovascularization of angle or iris (rubeosis iridis)**
    a. Diabetes, 286
    b. Glaucoma, 265, 355
    c. Inflammation, 285, 355
    d. Occlusive retinal vascular disease, 286
    e. Retinal diseases, 285
    f. Systemic vascular disease, 286
    g. Tumors (iris and other ocular tissue), 284

16. **Pigment variations**
    a. Aging, 285
    b. Congenital, 283
    c. Cysts (pigmented), 191
    d. Foreign body (intraocular siderosis), 285
    e. Fuchs' heterochromic iridocyclitis, 276
    f. Glaucoma (pigmentary), 191, 350, 353
    g. Hemangiomas (of iris), 107
    h. Hemosiderosis (from hyphema), 280
    i. Heterochromia (of iris), 285
    j. Melanoma, 284
    k. Nevi (of iris), 284

17. **Polycoria**
    a. Iris atrophy (or hypoplasia), 283
    b. Rieger's syndrome, 169
    c. Surgical, 284
    d. Traumatic, 284

18. **Synechiae**
    a. Axenfeld–Rieger's syndromes, 169, 357
    b. Glaucoma (especially angle closure and neovascular), 286, 350, 352, 355
    c. Iris atrophy, 283
    d. Iris bombe, 283
    e. Narrow (or closed) angles, 262, 336–337, 350, 352
    f. Trauma, 280
    g. Uveitis (usually chronic), 273

Other Objective Signs

1. **Bloody discharge**
    a. Granulomas, 106
    b. Hemangiomas, 107
    c. Lacerating injury (lids or conjunctiva), 66
    d. Lacrimal drainage tumors, 95
    e. Neoplasias, 284
    f. Telangiectasia, 113

2. **Dermatitis**
    a. Acne rosacea, 377
    b. Allergic reactions, 378
    c. Demodicosis, 84
    d. Drug induced, 377
    e. Herpes simplex, 86
    f. Herpes zoster, 86
    g. Molluscum contagiosum, 73, 129
    h. Systemic causes, 396, 404, 406
    i. Verrucae, 78, 129

3. **Intraocular pressure decrease**
    a. Congenital, 283
    b. Contusion (blunt) injury, 281
    c. Drug induced (topical or systemic), 396, 404, 406
    d. Idiopathic, 282
    e. Perforating wound, 142
    f. Retinal detachment, 267
    g. Systemic disease, 396, 404, 406
    h. Uveitis (anterior, usually early), 258

4. **Intraocular pressure increase**
    a. Aniridia, 283
    b. Aphakia, 353
    c. Axenfeld–Reiger's syndromes, 169, 357
    d. Cataract (usually mature or hypermature), 265
    e. Congenital or familial, 283, 356–357
    f. Dislocated lens, 407
    g. Drug induced (topical or systemic), 353, 396, 404, 406
    h. Essential iris atrophy, 283
    i. Glaucoma (all forms except "low-tension" glaucoma), 194 341, 349–357
    j. Hyphema, 280, 354
    k. Inflammation, 38, 355
    l. Megalocornea, 171
    m. Microcornea, 171
    n. Neovascularization of angle, 286, 355
    o. Plateau iris, 284, 342, 352
    p. Post-surgical (ocular), 293, 356, 441
    q. Sclerocornea, 170
    r. Shallow chamber (narrow angle), 341, 336–337, 352
    s. Steroid induced (topical or systemic), 9, 353–354
    t. Synechiae (anterior or posterior), 264, 336, 342
    u. Systemic disease, 396, 404, 406
    v. Trauma (usually unilateral), 280, 354
    w. Tumors (intraocular or retrobulbar), 284
    x. Uveitis, 258, 355

5. **Lissamine green staining**
    a. Filamentary keratitis, 219
    b. Keratitis sicca syndromes, 154, 157, 436
    c. Meibomian gland dysfunction, 89
    d. Superficial punctate keratitis, 191

6. **Lymphadenopathy or enlargement (preauricular)**
    a. Adenovirus, 128
    b. Chlamydial (inclusion) infection, 128
    c. Dacryoadenitis, 95
    d. Epidemic keratoconjunctivitis (EKC), 225
    e. Herpes simplex infection (primary and recurrent forms), 85, 229, 230
    f. Herpes zoster, 238
    g. Hyperacute conjunctivitis (bacterial or viral), 122
    h. Infectious keratitis (any advanced form), 208, 216, 220
    i. Newcastle's disease, 129
    j. Orbital cellulitis, 99
    k. Parinaud's oculoglandular ("cat-scratch") fever, 129
    l. Pharyngoconjunctival fever (PCF), 240
    m. Preseptal cellulitis, 99
    n. Trachoma, 125

7. **Mucoid discharge (nonpurulent)**
   a. Allergic blepharitis and conjunctivitis, 81, 114
   b. Burns (to any lid or ocular tissue), 104
   c. Conjunctival laceration, 104–105
   d. Dacryostenosis, 92
   e. Drug induced, 406
   f. Dry eye or keratitis sicca-type syndromes, 98
   g. Filamentary keratitis, 208
   h. Giant papillary conjunctivitis (GPC), 117
   i. Insect bites or stings, 89
   j. Pseudomembranous conjunctivitis (any cause), 224, 238
   k. Superior limbic keratoconjunctivitis (SLK), 246
   l. Toxic causes (chemical, environmental, irritants), 386
   m. Vernal keratoconjunctivitis, 118

8. **Purulent (or mucopurulent) discharge**
   a. Bacterial blepharitis (usually Streptococcus or gram-negative), 81
   b. Chlamydial infection, 128
   c. Dacryocystitis (acute or subacute), 95
   d. Fungal infection (any tissue), 225
   e. Hyperacute bacterial conjunctivitis (any type), 119
   f. Infectious keratitis (bacterial or fungal), 208, 216, 221

9. **Rose bengal staining**
   a. Chronic or toxic conjunctivitis, 123, 128
   b. Dendrites (infiltrative or ulcerative/herpetic), 208, 214, 240
   c. Dry eye or keratitis sicca-type syndromes, 209
   d. Filaments, 208
   e. Herpes simplex virus, 234
   f. Herpes zoster ophthalmicus, 238
   g. Necrotic-devitalized (dead or dying) epithelium, 154
   h. Recurrent corneal erosion (RCE) syndrome, 167

10. **Tearing (serous) discharge**
   a. Adenovirus, 128
   b. Chronic irritation (any cause), 92, 106, 140, 258
   c. Corneal abrasion, 140
   d. Dacryostenosis (obstruction), 92
   e. Drug induced, 396, 404, 406
   f. Dry eye or keratitis sicca-type syndromes, 153
   g. Entropion, 70
   h. Foreign bodies (on tarsus, conjunctiva, or cornea), 66, 104, 158
   i. Glaucoma (acute types), 194
   j. Herpes simplex keratitis, 85, 229, 230
   k. Herpes zoster ophthalmicus, 238
   l. Inflammation, 174, 214, 239
   m. Punctal anomalies, 93
   n. Recurrent corneal erosion (RCE) syndromes, 167
   o. Systemic causes, 396, 404, 406
   p. Trauma, 93
   q. Trichiasis, 77
   r. Uveitis (usually acute anterior), 258, 285

APPENDIX 3: INDEX OF DIFFERENTIAL DIAGNOSES (THINGS TO RULE OUT)

Eyelids and Adnexa

h. Nevus, 74, 110
i. Sebaceous cyst (subcutaneous), 75, 76
j. Verruca, 78, 129
k. Xanthelasma, 79

12. **Preseptal cellulitis**
 a. Abscess (lid), 99
 b. Allergic reaction, 80
 c. Blepharitis (acute), 81, 82
 d. Dacryocystitis, 95
 e. Hordeolum, 87
 f. Infectious causes, 99
 g. Orbital cellulitis, 99
 h. Systemic causes, 99

13. **Sebaceous cyst**
 a. Chalazion, 75, 76
 b. Cysts (other forms), 75, 76
 c. Dermoid, 69, 70
 d. Molluscum contagiosum, 73
 e. Neoplastic tumor, 73
 f. Papilloma, 74, 111
 g. Pustule (infectious), 76
 h. Subcutaneous type, 76
 i. Superficial type, 75, 76
 j. Xanthelasma, 79

14. **Sudoriferous cyst**
 a. Allergic or hypersensitivity, 80
 b. Drug induced, 75
 c. Milia (meibomianitis), 76
 d. Molluscum contagiosum, 73
 e. Papilloma (amclanotic), 74, 111
 f. Pustule (infectious), 76
 g. Sebaceous cyst (superficial), 75, 76

15. **Verrucae**
 a. Basal cell carcinoma, 78, 129
 b. Cysts (all forms), 75, 78
 c. Granuloma, 129
 d. Keratoses, 71
 e. Molluscum contagiosum, 73
 f. Neoplastic tumors, 73
 g. Nevus, 74, 110
 h. Papilloma, 74, 111
 i. Pustules (infectious), 80
 j. Xanthelasma, 79

16. **Vitiligo**
 a. Albinism, 79
 b. Burns, 64
 c. Drug induced, 80
 d. Familial, 79
 e. Hypopigmentation, 75, 78, 79
 f. Poliosis, 75, 79
 g. Syndromes, 79

17. **Xanthelasma**
 a. Familial, 79
 b. Hyperlipidemia (especially hypercholesterolemia), 79
 c. Neoplasia, 74
 d. Papilloma (amelanotic), 74, 111
 e. Sebaceous cyst(s) (superficial), 75, 76
 f. Systemic syndromes, 79

Conjunctiva, Sclera, and Episclera

1. **Allergic conjunctivitis**
 a. Adenovirus, 113, 126
 b. Bacterial (all forms), 118
 c. Blepharoconjunctivitis, 121
 d. Chlamydial, 128, 243
 e. Dermatologically related, 122
 f. Drug induced, 123
 g. Dry eye syndrome, 153, 156
 h. Epidemic keratoconjunctivitis, 127, 225
 i. Episcleritis, 132
 j. Follicular types, 126
 k. Foreign-body (or contact lens) reaction, 129
 l. Giant papillary conjunctivitis (GPC), 117, 118
 m. Glaucoma (acute-angle closure), 131
 n. Herpes simplex, 129, 229
 o. Herpes zoster, 129, 231
 p. Keratoconjunctivitis (all types), 128
 q. Pharyngoconjunctival fever, 126, 240
 r. Phlyctenular reaction, 124
 s. Pinguecula (inflamed), 112, 133
 t. Scleritis, 135
 u. Subconjunctival hemorrhage, 149
 v. Systemic related, 130
 w. Toxic or hypersensitivity, 123
 x. Uveitis (circumcorneal flush), 130
 y. Venereal causes, 123
 z. Vernal keratoconjunctivitis, 118

2. **Bacterial conjunctivitis**
 a. Adenovirus, 126
 b. Allergic, 119
 c. Blepharoconjunctivitis, 121
 d. Chlamydial, 128
 e. Dermatologically related, 122
 f. Drug induced, 123
 g. Dry eye syndrome, 124
 h. Epidemic keratoconjunctivitis, 127
 i. Episcleritis, 132
 j. Follicular types, 126
 k. Foreign-body (or contact lens) reaction, 130
 l. Giant papillary conjunctivitis (GPC), 118
 m. Glaucoma (acute-angle closure), 131
 n. Herpes simplex, 129
 o. Herpes zoster, 129
 p. Keratoconjunctivitis (all types), 118
 q. Pharyngoconjunctival fever, 126
 r. Phlyctenular reaction, 124
 s. Pinguecula (inflamed), 111
 t. Scleritis, 135
 u. Subconjunctival hemorrhage, 113
 v. Systemic related, 113
 w. Toxic or hypersensitivity, 123
 x. Uveitis (circumcorneal flush), 140
 y. Venereal causes, 123
 z. Vernal keratoconjunctivitis, 118

3. **Blue sclera**
 a. Acquired, 131
 b. Buphthalmos, 131
 c. Congenital, 131
 d. Congenital (or infantile) glaucoma, 131, 172
 e. Drug induced, 129

f. Ehler–Danlos syndrome, 130
g. Halleman–Strieff syndrome
h. Marfan's syndrome, 130
i. Melanoma, 131
j. Melanosis (conjunctival or scleral), 131
k. Nevus (hyperpigmentation), 131
l. Nevus of Ota (oculodermatomelanosis), 131
m. Ochronosis (alkaptonuria), 111
n. Osteogenesis imperfecta, 130
o. Paget's disease, 130
p. Staphyloma, 132
q. Turner's syndrome, 402

4. **Episcleritis**
   a. Conjunctivitis (any form), 132
   b. Drug induced, 132
   c. Dry eye syndrome, 124
   d. Foreign body, 131
   e. Lash (ingrown or in puncta), 67
   f. Phlyctenular reaction, 133
   g. Pinguecula (inflamed), 133
   h. Systemic related, 133
   i. Toxic or irritative, 133
   j. Traumatic, 150
   k. Uveitis (sector circumcorneal flush), 140

5. **Giant papillary conjunctivitis (GPC)**
   a. Contact lens complications (especially soft lens), 117
   b. Prosthetic eyes, shells, or retainers, 117
   c. Scleral buckles, implant, or explants, 129
   d. Superior limbic keratoconjunctivitis (SLK), 118
   e. Sutures (postoperative eruptions), 118
   f. Trachoma, 125
   g. Vernal keratoconjunctivitis, 118

6. **Granuloma**
   a. Allergic reaction, 113
   b. Bitot's spot (xerosis), 108
   c. Chalazion (palpebral conjunctiva), 84
   d. Concretions (calcium salts), 106
   e. Dermoid (dermolipoma), 98
   f. Foreign-body reaction, 104
   g. Neoplasia, 110
   h. Papilloma, 111
   i. Phlyctenule, 124
   j. Pterygium, 112

7. **Lymphangiectasia**
   a. Chemotic (allergic) patch, 114
   b. Concretion (calcium), 106
   c. Lymphatic (inclusion) cyst, 108
   d. Neoplasia, 110
   e. Phlyctenule, 124

8. **Melanosis**
   a. Acquired, 110, 131
   b. Blue sclera, 131
   c. Congenital, 131
   d. Conjunctival, 131
   e. Dermatological, 122
   f. Drug induced, 127
   g. Melanoma, 110
   h. Nevus, 110
   i. Pigmentation, 131
   j. Staphyloma, 132
   k. Systemic, 132

9. **Papilloma**
   a. Cyst, 74, 75
   b. Dermoid (dermolipoma), 106
   c. Granuloma, 106
   d. Neoplastic tumor, 110
   e. Nevus, 110

10. **Pinguecula**
    a. Angular conjunctivitis, 124
    b. Cyst, 111
    c. Dermoid, 98
    d. Episcleritis, 132
    e. Granuloma, 106
    f. Keratinization (Bitot's spot or xerosis), 108
    g. Neoplasia, 110
    h. Nodule, 110
    i. Papilloma, 111
    j. Phlyctenule, 124
    k. Pterygium, 112

11. **Scleritis**
    a. Conjunctivitis (any form), 134
    b. Drug induced, 134
    c. Endophthalmitis, 135
    d. Glaucoma (acute-angle closure), 134
    e. Keratitis (severe), 134
    f. Systemic related, 134
    g. Toxic or irritative, 134

12. **Subconjunctival hemorrhage**
    a. Blood dyscrasias (especially leukemia), 112
    b. Cardiovascular disease, 121
    c. Conjunctivitis (hemorrhagic), 112
    d. Diabetes, 113
    e. Febrile disease (acute), 112
    f. Hemangioma, 107
    g. Idiopathic, 112
    h. Menstruation, 112
    i. Postsurgical, 121
    j. Telangiectasia, 113
    k. Trauma, 112
    l. Valsalva-like maneuvers, 112

13. **Toxic or irritative (chronic) conjunctivitis**
    a. Adenovirus, 126
    b. Allergic, 113
    c. Bacterial (all forms), 118
    d. Blepharoconjunctivitis, 122
    e. Chlamydial, 128
    f. Dermatologically related, 122
    g. Drug induced, 129
    h. Dry eye syndrome, 124
    i. Epidemic keratoconjunctivitis, 127
    j. Episcleritis, 132
    k. Follicular types, 126
    l. Foreign-body (or contact lens) reaction, 130
    m. Giant papillary conjunctivitis (GPC), 118
    n. Glaucoma (acute-angle closure type), 135, 350, 352
    o. Herpes simplex, 129
    p. Herpes zoster, 129
    q. Keratoconjunctivitis (all types), 130
    r. Pharyngoconjunctival fever, 126
    s. Phlyctenular reaction, 124
    t. Pinguecula (inflamed), 133
    u. Scleritis, 134
    v. Subconjunctival hemorrhage, 112

w. Systemic related, 130
x. Uveitis (circumcorneal flush), 130
y. Venereal causes, 125
z. Vernal keratoconjunctivitis, 118

14. **Viral conjunctivitis**
a. Adenovirus, 126
b. Allergic, 133
c. Bacterial (all forms), 123
d. Blepharoconjunctivitis, 122
e. Chlamydial, 128
f. Dermatologically related, 122
g. Drug induced, 129
h. Dry eye syndrome, 124
i. Epidemic keratoconjunctivitis, 127
j. Episcleritis, 132
k. Follicular types, 124
l. Foreign-body (or contact lens) reaction, 129
m. Giant papillary conjunctivitis (GPC), 118
n. Glaucoma (acute-angle closure), 135, 350, 352
o. Herpes simplex, 129
p. Herpes zoster, 129
q. Keratoconjunctivitis (all types), 130
r. Pharyngoconjunctival fever, 126
s. Phlyctenular reaction, 124
t. Pinguecula (inflamed), 112
u. Scleritis, 134
v. Subconjunctival hemorrhage, 135
w. Systemic related, 130
x. Toxic or hypersensitivity, 123
y. Uveitis (circumcorneal flush), 135
z. Venereal causes, 126
aa. Vernal keratoconjunctivitis, 118

Cornea

1. **Anterior chamber cleavage syndromes**
a. Anterior synechiae, 169, 337, 342
b. Axenfeld's anomaly or syndrome, 170, 337, 357
c. Congenital glaucoma, 172, 356–357
d. Iridocorneal endothelial (ICE) syndromes, 171
e. Iris processes, 170, 337
f. Peter's anomaly, 170
g. Posterior embryotoxon, 170
h. Posterior polymorphous dystrophy, 171
i. Reiger's anomaly or syndrome, 170
j. Sclerocornea, 171

2. **Arcus**
a. Cardiovascular disease, 173
b. Degeneration, 172
c. Familial, 173
d. Hyperlipidemia (especially hypercholesteremia), 173
e. Marginal furrow degeneration, 176

3. **Band keratopathy**
a. Degeneration, 172
b. Glaucoma (absolute), 172
c. Gout, 133
d. Hypercalcemia (hyperparathyroidism), 174
e. Juvenile rheumatoid arthritis (Still's disease), 174
f. Postoperative, 175

4. **Bullous keratopathy**
a. Degeneration, 175
b. Fuchs' endothelial dystrophy, 176
c. Glaucoma (chronic), 172
d. Inflammation (chronic), 177
e. Postoperative, 175

5. **Chlamydial (inclusion) keratoconjunctivitis**
a. Adult (inclusion) type, 243
b. Bacterial keratoconjunctivitis, 243
c. Conjunctivitis (all forms), 240
d. Epidemic keratoconjunctivitis (EKC), 231
e. Episcleritis, 242
f. Inclusion bodies (on culture), 243
g. Maternal (inclusion blennorrhea) type, 243
h. Pharyngoconjunctival fever (PCF), 240
i. Reiter's syndrome, 257
j. Scleritis, 242
k. Superficial keratitis, 217
l. Trachoma, 243

6. **Dry eye or keratitis sicca syndrome**
a. Allergic response, 209
b. Blepharoconjunctivitis (especially Staphylococcus), 155
c. Burns (especially chemical), 150
d. Congenital alacrima, 169
e. Conjunctivitis (especially chronic), 155
f. Degeneration (aging), 168
g. Dermatologically related, 154
h. Drug induced, 155
i. Episcleritis, 135
j. Epithelial basement membrane disorders, 140, 143
k. Exposure keratitis, 147
l. Filamentary keratitis, 154
m. Follicular-type conjunctivitis, 133
n. Foreign-body (or contact lens) reaction, 140
o. Keratoconjunctivitis (all types), 154
p. Medicamentosa (topicals), 156
q. Neurotrophic keratitis, 212
r. Pemphigoid or ocular pemphigus, 212
s. Sarcoidosis, 133
t. Scleritis, 220
u. Seborrhea, 154
v. Sjögren's syndrome, 154
w. Staphylococcus, 157
x. Stevens–Johnson disease, 155
y. Systemic disease, 155
z. Vitamin A deficiency (xerosis), 155

7. **Epithelial basement membrane disorder**
a. Acquired (trauma or irritation), 188
b. Cogan's degeneration, 187
c. Degeneration (aging), 190
d. Diabetes, 184
e. Dry eye or keratitis sicca-type syndrome, 187
f. Dystrophic, 188
g. Fuchs' endothelial dystrophy, 182
h. Meesman's dystrophy
i. Recurrent corneal erosion (RCE) syndrome, 186
j. Superficial keratitis (any type), 191

8. **Infectious keratitis**
a. Acanthamoeba, 219
b. Bacterial (gram-positive or-negative), 220

c. Fungal, 224
d. Herpes simplex, 229
e. Herpes zoster, 233
f. Sarcoidosis, 277
g. Scleritis, 278
h. Syphilis, 277
i. Tuberculosis, 278

9. **Interstitial keratitis**
a. Burns (usually chemical), 150
b. Congenital (usually syphilis), 277
c. Herpes simplex (second most common cause), 274
d. Herpes zoster, 274
e. Sarcoidosis, 274
f. Syphilis (most common cause), 274
g. Toxic (especially chemical poisons), 268
h. Tuberculosis, 278

10. **Marginal furrow degeneration**
a. Acanthamoeba (ring ulcer), 219
b. Arcus senilis, 172, 174
c. Dellen, 175
d. Drug induced (especially steroids), 177
e. Fungal ulcer, 159
f. Marginal keratitis, 182
g. Mooren's ulcer, 176
h. Pellucid marginal degeneration, 190
i. Ring ulcers, 219
j. Systemic disorders (especially rheumatoid), 176
k. Terrien's marginal degeneration, 247
l. White limbal girdle of Vogt, 177

11. **Mooren's ulcer**
a. Acanthamoeba (ring ulcer), 219
b. Arcus senilis, 172, 174
c. Dellen, 175
d. Drug induced (especially steroids), 177
e. Fungal ulcer, 159, 224
f. Marginal furrow degeneration, 176
g. Marginal keratitis, 209, 211
h. Pellucid marginal degeneration, 190
i. Ring ulcers, 219
j. Systemic disorders (especially rheumatoid), 176, 247
k. Terrien's marginal degeneration, 247
l. White limbal girdle of Vogt, 177

12. **Ocular rosacea**
a. Atopic or allergic, 248
b. Blepharoconjunctivitis (especially staphylococcal), 241
c. Conjunctivitis (any type), 241
d. Dry eye or keratitis sicca syndrome, 221
e. Keratoconjunctivitis (all forms), 243
f. Marginal blepharitis, 241
g. Meibomian gland dysfunction, 241
h. Psoriasis, 258
i. Seborrhea, 241
j. Staphylococcus, 241
k. Systemic related, 241
l. Uveitis (anterior), 242

13. **Pterygium**
a. Allergic reaction, 112, 176
b. Dermoid, 178
c. Episcleritis, 177
d. Granuloma, 106
e. Marginal keratitis, 182
f. Neoplasia, 110
g. Pinguecula, 177
h. Phlyctenular keratoconjunctivitis, 213

14. **Recurrent corneal erosion (RCE) syndrome**
a. Degeneration (aging), 168
b. Dystrophies, 177
c. Epithelial basement membrane disorders, 182
d. Fuchs' endothelial dystrophy, 182
e. Trauma (tangential abrasion), 172

15. **Superior limbic keratoconjunctivitis (SLK)**
a. Atopic dermatokeratoconjunctivitis, 248
b. Contact lens (especially soft lens) related, 249
c. Giant papillary conjunctivitis (GPC), 246
d. Herpes simplex (with pseudodendrites), 246
e. Herpes zoster, 239
f. Hyperthyroidism, 246
g. Marginal keratitis, 214
h. Terrien's marginal degeneration, 247
i. Trachomatous, 247
j. Vernal keratoconjunctivitis, 247

16. **Trachoma**
a. Atopic keratoconjunctivitis, 154
b. Bacterial, 155
c. Chlamydial (inclusion) keratoconjunctivitis, 193
d. Cicatricial (scarring), 125
e. Giant papillary conjunctivitis (GPC), 118
f. Superior limbic keratoconjunctivitis (SLK), 246
g. Vernal keratoconjunctivitis, 247

17. **Vernal keratoconjunctivitis**
a. Atopic keratoconjunctivitis, 248
b. Chlamydial keratoconjunctivitis, 244
c. Giant papillary conjunctivitis, 247
d. Infectious keratitis (any form), 248
e. Superior limbic keratoconjunctivitis, 246
f. Trachoma, 247

18. **Viral keratoconjunctivitis**
a. Adenoviral, 127
b. Bacterial keratitis, 216
c. Chlamydial keratoconjunctivitis, 243
d. Dermatologically related, 242
e. Drug induced, 242
f. Dry eye or keratitis sicca-type syndromes, 221
g. Follicular types, 225
h. Herpes simplex keratitis, 229
i. Herpes zoster ophthalmicus, 231
j. Molluscum contagiosum, 73
k. Superficial punctate keratitis (SPK) of Thygeson, 227
l. Toxic or hypersensitivity, 240
m. Verrucae, 78

Anterior Chamber, Iris, and Ciliary Body

1. **Acute anterior uveitis**
a. Allergic or hypersensitivity, 258
b. Chronic anterior uveitis, 265

c. Conjunctivitis (severe forms), 261
d. Drug induced, 266
e. Episcleritis, 267
f. Foreign-body (or contact lens) reaction, 258
g. Glaucoma (acute-angle closure), 265, 350, 352
h. Keratouveitis, 268
i. Pars planitis, 276
j. Postoperative, 277
k. Scleritis, 267
l. Systemic related (recurrent forms), 260
m. Toxic (exogenous or endogenous), 268
n. Unknown etiology (most common), 277

2. **Chronic anterior uveitis**
   a. Acute anterior uveitis, 258
   b. Allergic or hypersensitivity, 268
   c. Conjunctivitis (especially chronic forms), 277
   d. Episcleritis, 267
   e. Foreign-body (or contact lens) reaction, 258
   f. Fuchs' heterochromic iridocyclitis, 264
   g. Glaucoma (chronic form), 265
   h. Keratouveitis, 268
   i. Lens induced, 268
   j. "Masquerade" syndromes, 267
   k. Pars planitis, 268
   l. Posterior involvement, 265
   m. Postoperative, 248
   n. Sclerouveitis, 268
   o. Systemic related (most common), 272
   p. Unknown etiology, 277

3. **Heterochromia (iris)**
   a. Congenital, 283
   b. Fuchs' heterochromic iridocyclitis, 285
   c. Melanoma, 285
   d. Nevus, 285
   e. Siderosis (intraocular foreign bodies), 285
   f. Syndromes (congenital or acquired), 282

4. **Persistent pupillary membrane**
   a. Anterior cleavage syndromes Axenfeld–Rieger, 169
   b. Congenital, 283
   c. Glaucoma (gonioscopy), 282
   d. Iris processes, 280, 337
   e. Postoperative, 282
   f. Syndromes (congenital or acquired), 282
   g. Synechiae (anterior and posterior), 283, 337, 342

5. **Rubeosis irides**
   a. Cranial (temporal) arteritis, 280
   b. Diabetes, 286
   c. Inflammation, 286
   d. Neoplastic tumors (intraocular), 284
   e. Neovascular glaucoma, 286, 355
   f. Retinal disease, 283
   g. Vascular disease (occlusive), 286

APPENDIX 4: COMMON CLINICAL DIAGNOSES BY DEGREE OF PRESENTATION

Lids/Adnexa			
Blepharitis, Allergic	**Mild**	**Moderate**	**Severe**
Etiology	Type I/IV/Atopic	Type I/IV/Atopic	Type I/IV/Atopic
Subjective	Itching	Itching	Itching/irritation
Objective	Edema	Edema/Erythema	Edema/Erythema Excoriation
Assessment	Rule out infectious	Rule out infectious	Rule out preseptal
Plan	Remove allergen Cold compresses	Remove allergen Cold compresses	Remove allergen Cold compresses
Drug	Antihistamine/Decongestant	Antihistamine/Decongestant Steroid cream (optional)	Antihistamine/Decongestant Steroid
Route	Orals Orals as directed	Orals Topical cream qid Orals as directed	Oral (both) Cream qid Orals as directed
RTC	PRN	48–72 hr	24–48 hr
Complications	No response	Slow response	Systemic response
Blepharitis, Marginal			
Etiology	Seborrhea/Staphylococcus	Staphylococcus	Staphylococcus/Streptococcus
Subjective	Chronic Cosmetic	Chronic Sticking shut	Acute presentation Irritation/Pain
Objective	"Granulated"	Tylosis/Rosettes/Redmadarosis/Poliosis/Trichiasis	Ulceration/Excoriation Edema/(unilateral)
Assessment	Rule out parasites	Rule out strep	Rule out preseptal
Plan	Staphylococcal prevention	Staphylococcal prevention	Heat
Drug	Bacitracin (optional)	Combination (optional)	Bacitracin/Keflex
Route	Topical ointment	Topical ointment	Topical/Oral
Dosage	hs	bid to tid	q4h/500 mg bid
RTC	2–4 wk	1–2 wk	48 hr
Complications	Chronicity	Acute reactions	Preseptal
Dacryocystitis, Adult			
Etiology	Blockage	Stenosis	Acute/Chronic
Subjective	Sudden onset	Chronic Painless	Pain (variable)
Objective	Tearing	Tearing	Inner canthal erythema Tearing
Assessment	Rule out infection	Rule out neoplasia	Rule out stenosis
Plan	Dilation and irrigation heat/Massage	Advise/refer (?)	Heat/Delay dilation and irrigation
Drug	Prophylactic (Polytrim)	Polytrim Keflex	Polytrim Keflex
Route	Topical drops	Topical and oral	Topical and oral
Dosage	tid × 1 wk	qid/500 mg bid	Topical qid, Oral 500 mg bid
RTC	pm	prn	48 h
Complications	Recurrent	Chronicity	Preseptal
Dacryocystitis, Congenital			
Etiology	Valve of Hasner	Streptococcus	Streptococcus/Fungi
Subjective	Congenital history	Congenital (or infantile)	Pain Nonresponsive
Objective	Tearing (unilateral)	Purulence (unilateral)	Unilateral or bilateral
Assessment	Rule out infectious	Rule out noncompliance	Rule out systemic foci
Plan	Heat/Massage	Heat/Massage/Irrigation	Advise/Refer
Drug		Polytrim	Augmentin

(Continued)

Dacryocystitis, Congenital (continued)	**Mild**	**Moderate**	**Severe**
Route		Topical drops	oral
Dosage		tid/qid	By weight
RTC	prn/6 wk	3–6 wk	1 wk/prn
Complications	Infection (systemic)	9–12 months old	Strictures
Ecchymosis			
Etiology	Mild contusion	Contusion	Crepitus
Subjective	Cosmesis	Concern Mild pain	Severe blow Palpable pain
Objective	Red blood Inferior lid	Black/Purple Superior/Inferior lid	Black/Purple Crackling sound
Assessment	Rule out eyeball	Rule out crepitus	Rule out blowout fracture
Plan	24 hr cold 3–5 days hot	24 hr cold 5–7 days hot	24 hr cold 7 days hot
Drug		Decongestant	Decongestant Antistaphylococcal agent
Route		Oral	Oral
Dosage		tid to qid	500 mg bid (e.g., Keflex)
RTC	5 days	3–5 days	24–48 hr
Complications	Slow resolution	Sneezing Organized hematoma	Blowout fracture Sneezing Orbital cellulitis
Hordeolum			
Etiology	Zeiss/Moll staphylococcal	Meibomian staphylococcal	Encapsulated
Subjective	Annoyance	Pain on palpation	Pain
Objective	External stye	Lump or edema	Abscess
Assessment	Rule out sebaceous cyst	Rule out chalazion	Rule out dacryocystitis (inferonasal)
Plan	Heat/Staphylococcal prevention	Heat/Staphylococcal	Heat/Drain ?
Drug	Ak-Poly-Bac	Ak-Poly-Bac or tobramycin	Tobramycin + oral antibiotic
Route	External lid ointment	External lid ointment	Topical/Oral (e.g., Keflex)
Dosage	bid to tid	qid	q4h/1g/day
RTC	3–5 days or PAN	48 hr	24–48 hr
Complications	Chalazion	Internal chalazion Preseptal cellulitis	Preseptal cellulitis
Lash Problems			
Etiology	Madarosis	Poliosis	Trichiasis
Subjective	Cosmesis	Cosmesis/Concern	Corneal pain
Objective	Sparse lashes Lashes "falling out"	White lashes	In-turning lashes Corneal foreign-body tracking
Assessment	Rule out alopecia	Rule out vitiligo	Rule out entropion
Plan	Staphylococcal prevention	Staphylococcal prevention	Epilation
Drug	Bacitracin/Hypochlorous acid 0.1%	Bacitracin/Hypochlorous acid 0.1%	Lubricant
Route	Ointment/Solution: Apply to lid margins	Ointment: Apply to lid margins	Topical eyedrops
Dosage	hs/bid	hs/bid	q4h × 24 hr
RTC	6 wk	6 wk	prn
Complications	Permanent	Permanent	Corneal infection
Sudoriferous Cyst			
Etiology	Zeiss/Moll gland	Zeiss/Moll gland	Zeiss/Moll gland
Subjective	General examination	Cosmesis/Concern	Concern
Objective	Small bubble in margin	Bigger bubble	"Balloon"
Assessment	Rule out milia	Rule out hordeolum	Rule out granuloma
Plan	Lance/Drain	Lance/Drain	Lance/Drain
Drug	Ak-Poly-Bac	Ak-Poly-Bac	Ak-Poly-Bac
Route	Topical ointment	Topical ointment	Topical ointment
Dosage	1 ×	1 ×	tid

(*Continued*)

Sudoriferous Cyst (continued)	Mild	Moderate	Severe
RTC	prn	prn	48 hr
Complications	Recurrence	Recurrence	Secondary infection

Conjunctiva/Episclera

Conjunctivitis, Allergic			
Etiology	Type I/IV	Type I/IV	Type I/IV
Subjective	Itching	Itching	Itching/Irritation
Objective	Patchy chemosis	Chemosis	"Watchglass" chemosis Hemorrhages
Assessment	Rule out infectious	Rule out infectious	Rule out infectious
Plan	Remove allergen	Remove allergen	Remove allergen
Cold	Cold	Cold	Cold
Drug	NSAID (optional) Antihistamine/Mast cell stabilizer	Antihistamine/Mast cell stabilizer Steroid (optional)	Antihistamine/Mast cell stabilizer Steroid Antihistamine
Route	Topical	Topical/Oral antihistamine	Topical/Oral
Dosage	qd/bid	qd/bid Oral, as directed	qd/bid; qid (steroid) Oral (antihistamine), as directed
RTC	prn	2–3 days	24–48 hr
Complications	No response	Slow response	Systemic reactions

Bacterial Conjunctivitis			
Etiology	Staphylococcus	Staphylococcus/Streptococcus	Streptococcus/Gram-negative
Subjective	Awareness	Spread	Concern/Irritation
Objective	Inferior hyperemia papillae	Meaty red/Pus	Hyperacute/Copious discharge
Assessment	Rule out viral	Rule out epithelial defect	Rule out ulcer
Plan	Staphylococcal prevention	Heat/Staphylococcal	Culture
Drug	Ak-Poly-Bac (optional)	Ciprofloxacin or tobramycin	Ak-Poly-Bac/Tobramycin or besifloxacin
Route	External lid ointment Drops	Drops	Ointment/Drops
Dosage	hs	qid (OU)	hs/q3–4h
RTC	1–2 wk or prn	2–3 days	24 hr
Complications	Chronicity/Superficial punctate keratitis	Pseudomembrane/Marginal keratitis	Ulcer/Scarring

Conjunctivitis, Chronic			
Etiology	Staphylococcal/Drying/UV	Staphylococcal/Drying/UV	Moraxella/Drying
Subjective	Chronic/Cosmesis	Chronic/Cosmesis	Dry irritation
Objective	Inferior injection Angular conjunctival hyperemia No discharge	Angular injection Papillary conjunctivitis No discharge	Papillary palpebral Angular conjunctivitis Xerosis
Assessment	Rule out cornea	Rule out infection	Rule out corneal/Infection
Plan	Lubrication/UV protection	Lubrications/UV tints	Lubrications/UV tints
Drug	Antistaphylococcal/Hypochlorous acid 0.1%	Antistaphylococcal/Hypochlorous acid 0.1%	Tobramycin
Route	Topical drops/Ointment	Topical drop/Ointments	Topical drops/Ointments
Dosage	bid to tid	tid	tid to qid
RTC	3–4 wk	2–3 wk	1–2 wk
Complications	No improvement	Increasing	Corneal involvement

Conjunctivitis, Viral			
Etiology	Non-specific	Pharyngoconjunctival fever/Epidemic keratoconjunctivitis	Epidemic keratoconjunctivitis
Subjective	Burning pink, follicles	Burning/irritation	Irritation
Objective	Inner canthal involvement Breakup time	Preauricular nodes Pseudomembrane	Hyperacute Hemorrhagic

(Continued)

Conjunctivitis, Viral (continued)	**Mild**	**Moderate**	**Severe**
Assessment	Rule out Staphylococcus/HSV	Rule out Chlamydia/HSV	Rule out gram-negative/HSV
Plan	Advise/Cold	Advise/Cold	Culture
Drug	Lubrications	Lubrications	Steroid (?)
Route	Topical eyedrops	Topical eyedrops	Topical eyedrops
Dosage	q4h	q4h	q2–3h
RTC	7th–8th day	7th–8th day	48 hr
Complications	Contagious	Secondary bacterial Epidemic keratoconjunctivitis	Epidemic keratoconjunctivitis Preseptal
Conjunctival Laceration			
Etiology	Laceration	Laceration to Tenon's	Laceration to sclera
Subjective	Awareness Concern	Concern Mild irritation	Irritation Foreign-body sensation
Objective	Small conjunctival tear	Conjunctival break Subconjunctival hemorrhage	Tenon's capsule tear Bare sclera
Assessment	Rule out foreign matter	Rule out Tenon's tear	Rule out perforation
Plan	Irrigate/Reassure	Irrigate reassure	Irrigate/Dilate/Examine
Drug	Ak-Poly-Bac	Ak-Poly-Bac	Tobramycin
Route	Topical ointment	Topical ointment	Topical ointment
Dosage	1 × or hs	hs	tid to qid
RTC	prn	1 wk	3–5 days
Complications	Subconjunctival hemorrhage	Slow resolution	Lid traction
Episcleritis			
Etiology	Unknown	Collagen vascular (?)	Systemic (?)
Subjective	Awareness	Pain on palpation	Pain (on movement)
Objective	Sector injection	Deep injection/Diffuse infiltration	Nodular formation
Assessment	Rule out inflamed pinguecula	Rule out angular conjunctivitis	Rule out anterior uveitis
Plan	Heat	Heat	Heat
Drug	Ibuprofen (optional)	Steroid/Ibuprofen	Steroid/Ibuprofen
Route	Oral	Topical/Oral	Topical (oral?)/Oral
Dosage	800–1200 mg/day	q4h/400 mg qid	q2–3h/600 mg tid
RTC	1 wk	3–5 days	48 hr
Complications	Chronic	Nodular	Scleritis
Giant Papillary Conjunctivitis			
Etiology	Mechanical trauma (chronic irritation)	Protein on soft lens	Mast cell reaction
Subjective	Mild irritation	Lens/Corneal irritation	Severe irritation
Objective	1–2 + GPC Lens decentration	2–3 + GPC Discharge	3–4 + GPC Heavy mucoid
Assessment	Rule out lens surfaces	Rule out acute inflammation	Rule out vernal, SLK, etc.
Plan	Increase lens replacement	Temporary discontinue soft lens	Temporary discontinue soft lens
Drug	Steroid (optional)	Steroid (e.g., loteprednol)	Loteprednol/Prednisolone
Route	Topical drops	Topical drops	Topical drops
Dosage	bid to qid	qid (without soft lens)	qid 2 wk
RTC	2 wk	2 wk	2 wk
Complications	Lingering	Persistent	Objective signs persist
Cornea			
Abrasion, Epithelial			
Etiology	Squamous epithelium	To basement membrane	50% involvement Diabetes
Subjective	History	Trauma or spontaneous	Trauma or spontaneous Recurrent erosion
Objective	Superficial straining	NaFl pooling	NaFl stromal seepage Loose edges

(*Continued*)

Abrasion, Epithelial (continued)	Mild	Moderate	Severe
Assessment	Rule out foreign body	Rule out foreign-body penetration	Rule out foreign-body, perforation
Plan	Irrigate	Irrigate, patch or bandage soft lens	Irrigate, patch or soft lens
Drug	Tobramycin	Cycloplege-dilate/Tobramycin/ Hypertonics (ibuprofen/aspirin)	Same + soft lens on recurrence
Route	Topical ointment	Topical ointment (oral)	Topical (oral)
Dosage	tid	1 × (prior to patch or BCL)	Lubricant/Soft lens 8–12 wk
RTC	prn or 24–48 hr	24–48 hr	24–48 hr/weekly with prophylaxis
Complications	Secondary infection	Re-erosion	Secondary infection
Burns, Chemical			
Etiology	Acid/Aromatic	Acid/Aromatic/Alkaline	Acid/Aromatic/Alkaline
Subjective	When, What, How much?	Same	Same
	Foreign-body sensation		
Objective	Superficial punctate keratitis, visible iris	Superficial punctate keratitis, hazy iris	Superficial punctate keratitis, obscure iris
	Hyperemia	Chemosis	Ischemic patches
Assessment	Rule out alkaline	Rule out stroma	Rule out collagenolysis
Plan	H_2O irrigation 20–30 min	H_2O irrigation 30–60 min	H_2O irrigation 30–60 min
		Swab cul-de-sac	pH tears
Drug	Cyclo/Dilate/Tobramycin	Cycloplege/Dilate/Tobramycin	Cyclo/Dilate/Tobramycin/ Mucomyst
	Steroid (if secondary uveitis)	Steroid	Steroid
Route	Topical drops	Topical ointment and drops	Topical drops and ointment
Dosage	qid	q4h	q2h
RTC	48–72 hr	24–48 hr	24 hr
Complications	Persistent injection	Symblepharon	Scarring
		Scarring	Corneal melt
Burns, Radiation			
Etiology	Diffuse UV	Concentrated UV	Thermal (Eschar)
Subjective	Dry eye feeling	Corneal pain	Foreign-body sensation
	Sunlight history	History of UV exposure	History of hot particle
Objective	Mild SPK (band) 1–2 + hyperemia	Dense SPK	Focal white charred epithelium
Assessment	Rule out keratitis sicca	Rule out uveitis	Rule out particle(s) embedded
Plan	Lubricate	Bandage soft lens	Remove as foreign body
Drug	Tobramycin (optional)	Tobramycin/Cycloplege/Dilate	Tobramycin, Steroids
		Steroids	Cycloplege/Dilate
Route	Topical ointment	Topical ointment/Drops	Topical ointment/Drops
Dosage	tid	qid	qid
RTC	prn	24 hr	24 hr
Complications	Secondary infection	Secondary infection	Pseudomonas
Dellen			
Etiology	Drying area	Raised conjunctival lesion	Focal dry spot
Subjective	Asymptomatic	Asymptomatic	Asymptomatic
	General examination		
Objective	Hazy epithelium	Depression	Deep peripheral corneal cup with sharp edges
Assessment	Rule out marginal degenerations	Rule out marginal ulcer	Rule out penetrating lesion (very rare)
Plan	Advise	Anti-UV lenses (if pinguecula the cause), thin CL edge	Same
Drug	Lubricate	Patch	Patch/Bandage soft lens
Route	Topical		
Dosage	q2–4h	Constant wear	Extended wear for 1–3 days
RTC	3–5 days	1–2 days	1–2 days
Complications	Tear disruption	Recurrence	Secondary infection

(Continued)

Dry Eye or Keratitis Sicca Syndromes	**Mild**	**Moderate**	**Severe**
Etiology	Aqueous deficiency/Multifactorial	Same	Same
Subjective	Late-day irritation	Advancing symptoms	Aqueous deficiency Pain (> late-day) visual acuity problems
Objective	Hyperemia/Band superficial punctate keratitis/Breakup time	Advancing signs Epithelial breakdown Lissamine green stain	Complications Filaments
Assessment	Rule out epithelial basement membrane disease (EBMD) or Bacterial/Viral/Irritation	Rule out same	Rule out secondary bacterial/Viral
Plan	Advise on chronicity	Check compliance	
Drug	Lubricate, anti-inflammatory?	Lubricants/Anti-inflammatory/Autologous serum/Amniotic membrane extracted drops	Same + Gel tears Bandage soft lens, scleral contacts, moisture chamber goggles
Route	Topical	Topical	Topical
Dosage	PRN	q2h to qid	q3–4h/hs
RTC	2 wk	2 wk	1 wk
Complications	Compliance	Complications (e.g., infection/filaments)	Secondary infection
Epithelial Basement Membrane Disease (EBMD)			
Etiology	Degeneration	Degeneration	Degeneration
Subjective	Asymptomatic	AM syndrome reduced visual acuity	AM syndrome Spontaneous erosion
Objective	Maps/Dots Negative staining	Maps-dots-fingerprint Negative (positive) stain	Anterior stromal haze Brawny edema
Assessment	Rule out dry eye	Rule out infection	Rule out other corneal disorders
Plan	Advise	Advise	Advise
Drug	Hypertonic saline	Hypotonic solution gtts/Oint/Bandage soft lens (7 days max then replace)	Bandage soft lens+ Prophylactic antibiotics/Steroids
Route	Topical drops/Oint	Topical	Topical drops
Dosage	PRN	q3–4h/hs or soft lens	Bandage soft lens + bid drops Bandage soft lens schedule for 8–12 wk (7 days max then replace)
RTC	Routine/PRN	3–4 wk	3–4 wk 1–3 yr duration
Complications	AM syndrome Spontaneous erosion	Visual acuity reduction Spontaneous erosion	Patient despair
Foreign Body			
Etiology	Superficial	Penetration	Perforation
Subjective	History Corneal pain Uveitic pain	History Corneal pain Uveitic pain	History Corneal pain Uveitic pain
Objective	Epithelial	Stroma	Full-thickness corneal signs
Assessment	Rule out penetration	Rule out perforation	Rule out intraocular foreign body
Plan	Irrigate and remove	Refer to corneal specialist	Refer to corneal specialist
Drug	Treat as moderate abrasion	Cyanoacrylate glue and soft lens bandage	Radiography
Route			Ultrasound Dilated fundus examination

(*Continued*)

Foreign Body (continued)	Mild	Moderate	Severe
Dosage			Oral cephalosporin Cyanoacrylate glue and soft lens bandage
RTC	PRN	Per consultant	
Complications	Hemosiderosis	Scarring	Scarring, Panophthalmitis
Fuchs' Dystrophy			
Etiology	Endothelial dystrophy	Edema	Advancing edema
Subjective	Asymptomatic	AM syndrome	Bullous Pain
Objective	Menopausal females, Guttata pigment dusting	Epithelial and stromal edema	Bedewing Bullous keratitis
Assessment	Rule out other dystrophy	Rule out epithelial basement membrane disease (EBMD)	Rule out degeneration Advise/Refer to corneal specialist
Plan	Advise	Advise Antiedema measures	Possible surgical repair Per consultant
Drug	Hypertonic solution	Bandage soft lens/Hypertonic solution/heat	Bandage soft lens (7 days max then replace)/Hypertonic solution
Route	Topical drops /Oint	Topical gtts/oint	Topical gtts
Dosage	prn	3–4 ×/hs	bid
RTC	6 mo/prn	3 mo	Overnight wear schedule q6–12 wk
Complications	AM syndrome	Bullous	Fibrosis
Inclusion Keratoconjunctivitis			
Etiology	Maternal chlamydia	Acquired chlamydia	Prolonged chlamydia
Subjective	Inclusion blennorrhea	Sexually active adult Recurrent	Recurrent Prolonged therapy
Objective	Bacterial/Viral keratoconjunctivitis	Bacterial/Viral keratoconjunctivitis	Bacterial/Viral keratoconjunc tivitis infiltrates
Assessment	Rule out gram-negative (GC or *H. flu*)	Rule out bacterial or viral causes	Rule out other keratites
Plan	Advise mother	Advise patient Inclusion bodies (?)	Advise patient Inclusion bodies (?)
Drug	Azithromycin	Azithromycin or doxycycline	Azithromycin or doxycycline
Route	Oral	Oral	Oral
Dosage	qid (by wt.)	1 g single dose or 100 mg bid ×15 days	1 g single dose/100 mg bid ×15 days
RTC	3–5 days	10 days	3–5 days
Complications	Dacryocystitis/Otitis media	Corneal infiltrates	Scarring
Keratitis, Adenoviral			
Etiology	Non-specific	Pharyngoconjunctival fever/Epidemic keratoconjunctivitis	Epidemic keratoconjunctivitis
Subjective	Mild burning	Burning/irritation	Corneal irritation Reduced visual acuity
Objective	Diffuse superficial punctate keratitis Follicles	Diffuse superficial punctate keratitis (2 +) Follicle	Superficial punctate keratitis/SEI (3–4 +) Pseudomembrane
Assessment	Rule out pharyngoconjunctival fever/Epidemic kerato conjunctivitis, herpes	Rule out Herpes/Thygeson's	Rule out herpes, bacterial
Plan	Advise	Advise	Advise
Drug	Lubricants (optional)	Lubricants/cold	Cyclo/Dilation + steroids
Route	Topical drops	Topical drops	Topical drops
Dosage	q3–4h	q4h	q2–4h (steroids)
RTC	1 wk	3–5 days	48–72 hr
Complications	Secondary bacterial/Toxic Contagious	Secondary toxic Contagious	Infiltrative scarring

(Continued)

Keratitis, HSV, Epithelial	Mild	Moderate	Severe
Etiology	Recurrent HSV	Primary HSV	Postinfection (metaherpetic)
Subjective	Mild or no corneal irritation	Malaise Corneal pain	Resistant HSV
Objective	Dendrite (>75%)	Lymphadenopathy Epithelial	Anterior stromal involvement Indolent epithelial ulcer Basement membrane involvement
Assessment	Rule out infiltrative dendrite	Rule out HSV-2 (genital)	Rule out deep stroma
Plan			Denude ulcer
Drug	Viroptic drops, Zirgan gel or oral antiviral (e.g. Valcyclovir 500 mg)	Viroptic drops, Zirgan gel or oral antiviral, Acyclovir ointment (skin) (e.g. Valcyclovir 500 mg)	Viroptic drops, Zirgan gel, or oral antiviral (e.g. Valcyclovir 500 mg), Prednisolone/ Loteprednol drops
Route	Topical or oral	Topical or oral	Topical or oral
Dosage	Drops q2h/gel q3h Tablets tid	Drops q2h/gel q3h Acyclovir (on skin) qid Tablets tid	Viroptic q2h, Zirgan q3h Prednisolone/Loteprednol drops tid to qid Tablets tid
RTC	48 hr	48–72 hr	48 hr
Complications	Resistant strain (>14 days)	Recurrence Metaherpetica	Scarring Stromal keratitis

Keratitis, HSV, Stromal			
Etiology	Immune response	Unknown etiology	Virulent strain
Subjective	Multiple recurrences Uveitic pain	With or without HSV epithelial keratitis	Multiple recurrences Uveitic pain
Objective	Deep stromal infiltration	Disciform stromal edema	Interstitial keratitis
Assessment	Rule out interstitial keratitis	Rule out bacterial ulcer	Rule out melting
Plan	Refer to corneal specialist	Monitor epithelium	Refer to corneal specialist
Drug	Steroids	Steroids Antiedema	Steroids Penetrating keratoplasty
Route	Topical	Topical	
Dosage	Variable	qid to q4h	
RTC	Per consultant	48–72 hr	
Complications	Scarring, Wessley ring	No response Scarring	Phthisis bulbi

Keratitis, Staphylococcal			
Etiology	Diffuse toxic/Irritative Sterile superficial punctate keratitis	Focal toxic/Hypersensitive infiltrative	Bacterial invasion
Subjective	Lid history Cornea (AM) irritation	AM syndrome Peripheral infiltrate	Hot eye/Pain
Objective	Inferior or diffuse superficial punctate keratitis Staphylococcal lid signs	Edema-island lesion(s) Superficial leash of vessels	Congestion-deep stromal Chemosis-post. Cornea 360° violet anterior chamber Depressed pus
Assessment	Rule out other infection/Stromal keratoconjunctivitis	Rule out ulcer	Rule out endophthalmitis
Plan	Antistaphylococcal (lids)	Antistaphylococcal (lids)	Hospitalize Refer to corneal specialist
Drug	Lubricants	Antibiotic/Steroid combo	Triple aminoglycosides/ 4th generation fluroquinolone
Route	Topical drops	Topical drops	Topical drops/Injectables
Dosage	6–10 × daily	q2–4h	q1h
RTC	7–10 days	48–72 hr	24 hr
Complications	Marginal K	Secondary infection	Scarring/Perforation

(Continued)

Ocular Rosacea	Mild	Moderate	Severe
Etiology	Dermatoblepharitis	Dermatoblepharaconjunctivitis	Dermatoblepharokerto-conjunctivitis
Subjective	Dermatologic history (+/−) (30–60 age range)	Chronic/Nonresponsive Dermatologic history (+/−)	Recurrent Dermatologic (+/−)
Objective	Blepharitis with or without dermatitis	Blepharoconjunctivitis with or without dermatitis	Peripheral corneal involvement (360°)
Assessment	Rule out Staphylococcus seborrhea	Rule out bacterial/Viral	Rule out bacterial/Viral
Plan	Lid anti-staphylococcal Warm compresses	Lid anti-staphylococcal Warm compresses	Refer to dermatology specialist
Drug	Omega-3 fatty acids	Doxycycline 50 mg 6–12 weeks	Doxycycline 50–100 mg 6–12 weeks Prednisolone drops
Route	Oral	Oral	Oral/Topical
Dosage	qd to bid	qd to bid	Qd to bid/q4h
RTC	1–2 wk	1 wk	3–5 days
Complications	Nonresponsive	Corneal involvement	Corneal complications
Superior Limbic Keratoconjunctivitis (SLK)			
Etiology	Hyperthyroid (?)	Unknown/Hyperthyroid	Unknown/Hyperthyroid
Subjective	Mild irritation	Corneal irritation	Superior infection
Objective	Superior injection Superior superficial punctate keratoconjunctivitis Mild tarsal reaction	Pseudodendrites Anterior stromal haze Tarsal involvement	Superior superficial punctate keratoconjunctivitis, SEI Mild tarsal reaction
Assessment	Rule out GPC	Rule out Vernal	Rule out Theodore SLK
Plan	Lubricants		Discontinue soft lens
Drug	Topical NSAID Antihistamine/Mast cell stabilizer	Steroid (first) NSAID (topical and oral)	Silver nitrate Steroid NSAID (topical and oral)
Route	Topical	Topical	Topical/Oral
Dosage	tid to qid	q4h (steroids)/As directed for NSAIDs	q4h (steroids)/As directed for NSAIDs
RTC	1 wk	1 wk	1 wk
Complications	Recurrence	Secondary infection	Deep stromal
Superficial Punctate Keratoconjunctivitis of Thygeson			
Etiology	Unknown	Viral (?)	Viral (?)
Subjective	Asymptomatic (white eye)	Decrease BVA (white eye)	Severe discomfort
Objective	Fine superficial punctate keratoconjunctivitis "No company"	Dense SPK/Epith. opacities "No company"	Bilateral, dense "No company"
Assessment	Rule out bacterial/Viral	Rule out bacterial/Viral	Rule out bacterial/Viral
Plan	Don't discontinue soft lens		
Drug	Lubricants	Lubricants/Steroids/Bandage soft lens	Steroids/Bandage soft lens
Route	Topical drops	Topical drops	Topical drops
Dosage	qid	q3–4h	q2h
RTC	1–2 wk	1 wk	3 days
Complications	Increased superficial punctate keratoconjunctivitis/infiltrates	Exacerbations	Chronicity
Vernal Keratoconjunctivitis			
Etiology	Type I, mild	Seasonal	Eosinophilic
Subjective	Corneal irritation	Itching Discomfort	Severe discomfort Persistent
Objective	Limbal (vernal)	Giant papillae	Psuedodendrites

(*Continued*)

Vernal Keratoconjunctivitis (continued)	**Mild**	**Moderate**	**Severe**
	Mild edema	Superior superficial punctate keratoconjunctivitis	Erosions/Shield ulcer Tranta's dots Mucoid discharge
Assessment	Rule out staphylococcal marginal keratoconjunctivitis	Rule out other immune keratoconjunctivitis	Rule out infection
Plan	Prophylax tid	Antihistamines/Mast cell stabilizer	Oral steroids (?)
Drug	Antihistamine/Mast cell stabilizers	Loteprednol 0.5% gel/Drops	Loteprednol 0.5% gel/drops
Route	Topical	Topical	Topical
Dosage	qd to bid	q2–4h(steroids)	q2–3h
RTC	3–5 days	2–3 days	48 hr
Complications	Recurrence	Maintenance	Recurrence
Anterior Chamber			
Hyphema			
Etiology	Injury/Systemic	Injury/Surgery	Surgery
Subjective	History of injury	Drowsiness	Uveitic pain
Objective	Blood cells in aqueous	Layered blood in anterior chamber	Blood fills anterior chamber
Assessment	Rule out systemic	Rule out increased intraocular pressure	Rule out rebleeds/Increased intraocular pressure
Plan	Reduce activity	Bedrest	Bedrest/Hospital (?)
Drug	None	Atropine 0.5% (?)	Atropine 0.5%, and/or aminocaproic acid
Route	N/A	Topical	Topical/Oral
Dosage	N/A	bid	Aminocaproic 100 mg/kg/day × 5 days
RTC	Daily for 7 days	Daily for 7 days	Daily until reversal
Complications	Risk of systemic condition	Corneal blood staining	Rebleeds/Glaucoma
Intermediate Uveitis			
Etiology	Unknown	Stress/Systemic	Systemic
Subjective	Young adults	Insidious	Reduced visual acuity/Photo phobia/Vitreous floaters
Objective	Cells in the anterior vitreous	Retinal involvement	Peripheral "snowbanking"
Assessment	Rule out systemic	Rule out sarcoidosis	Rule out syphilis
Plan			
Drug	Steroids	Steroids	Steroids Immunosuppressive drugs
Route	Oral	Oral/Injectable	Oral/Injectable
Dosage	PRN	40–60 mg/d and taper after 5 days	Per consultant
RTC	2–4wk	1–2 wk	Per consultant
Complications	Chronicity	Cystoid macula edema (CME) Epiretinal membrane (ERM)	Cataracts/Glaucoma Band keratopathy
Anterior Uveitis			
Etiology	Trauma/Unknown	Trauma/Unknown/Systemic	Unknown/systemic
Subjective	Mild aching	Moderate to severe aching	Mild to no pain
Objective	Circumcorneal flush/Cells in AC/Flare/Keratic precipitates, decreased intraocular pressure	Pseudoptosis/Plasmoid aqueous/Decreased visual acuity	Mutton fats/synechiae
Assessment	Rule out vitreous	Rule out posterior/systemic	Rule out active systemic disease
Plan	Heat/Dark glasses	Heat/Dark glasses/Plus (add)	Medical consultation
Drug	Cycloplege/Steroid (?)/Ibuprofen	Cycloplege/pred/ibuprofen	Cycloplege/Steroid (topical/oral)
Route	Drops/oral	Drops/Oral/Depot (?)	(Drops/Oral)
Dosage	bid to tid (cycloplegia)/800–1600 mg/day (ibuprofen)	q2–3h pred drops/1600 mg/day (ibuprofen)	q1–2h drops (steroid) 40–60 mg/day, taper slowly
RTC	2–3 days	48 hr	48 hr
Complications	Keratic precipitates	Synechiae	Multiple anterior and posterior

APPENDIX 5: POSTOPERATIVE COMPLICATIONS (BY TIME) IN APHAKIC AND PSEUDOPHAKIC INTRAOCULAR LENS (IOL) CARE

(Also see Chapter 7)

Possible Complication	In Operating Room	First 24 Hours	First 2 Weeks	Third Week to Years
Astigmatism				
Continuous sutures			Spherical equivalent	Cut suture(s)
Interrupted sutures			Spherical equivalent	Remove suture(s)
Loose sutures		Tighten or add	Reduce intraocular pressure	Wedge resection
No sutures			Peripheral incisions	Toric lenses
Bullous keratopathy			Bandage soft lens	Bandage soft lens Keratoplasty
Capsular fibrosis				YAG laser
Choroidal effusion		Retinal consultation		
Corneal clouding	Superior 1/3	Follow	Monitor intraocular pressure	Corneal consult
Corneal edema	Superior 1/3	Follow	5% NaCl	Bandage soft lens
Cystoid macular edema				Fluorescein angiography
Diplopia		Follow		Check neurologist
Displaced intraocular lens			Consider visual acuity	Consider visual acuity
Endophthalmitis		Emergent care	Emergent care	Emergent care
Foreign-body sensation			Check sutures	Trim sutures
Hyphema		Follow	Rule out sickle cell	
Hypotony	Check sutures	Resuture	Reconstruct	
Increased intraocular pressure		Timoptic or Diamox	Switch to fluorometholone (FML)/ Lotepredednol	Avoid epinephrine drugs
Infection	Antibiotics	Antibiotics	Rule out Hypopyon	
Iris prolapse		Surgical repair	Surgical repair (and cycloplege/ dilate)	
Iritis	Steroids	Steroids	Steroids and cycloplege/dilate	Standard uveitic therapy (1–3 mo) (see Chapter 6)
Posterior vitreous detachment (PVD)			Visual fields	Rule out retinal detachment
Pseudofibrosis				Scrub or YAG laser
Ptosis		Follow		Check neurologist
Pupillary entrapment			Dilate to reposition	Attempt repositioning
Reduced visual acuity	Follow	Follow	Determine cause	
Retinal detachment		Retinal consultation	Retinal consultation	Binocular indirect ophthalmoscopy examination
Seidel test +		Add suture(s)	Tighten or add	
Vitreal hemorrhage		Retinal consultation	Retinal consultation	Binocular indirect ophthalmoscopy examination

APPENDIX 6: OCULAR CONDITIONS (BY SOAP) REQUIRING ORAL (PO) MEDICATIONS IN PRIMARY CARE OF THE ANTERIOR SEGMENT

(Plans listed include only oral medication considerations. See complete SOAP description in text for additional topical therapies.)

I. Conditions of the Eyelids, Adnexa, and Orbit

A. Irritations and Injuries

1. Blunt Injuries

S: Presenting history
O: Ecchymosis and crepitus
A: Rule out blowout fracture
P: Oral agents to consider:

a. Antihistamine/decongestant (e.g., Diphenhydramine/phenylephrine)
Disp. Benadryl (over the counter [OTC])
Sig. 25–50-mg cap qid for 3 to 5 days
b. Anti-infective (e.g., Keflex)
Disp. 20 500-mg caps
Sig. 1 cap bid 7 to 10 days
Child: 25–50 mg/kg/day
c. Adverse reactions:
Benadryl: drowsiness and ocular dryness
Keflex: gastrointestinal

2. Lacerating Injuries

S: Presenting history and instrument
O: Depth, edges, location, orientation
A: Rule out eyeball involvement
P: Oral agents to consider:

a. Analgesic (e.g., ibuprofen)
Disp. (OTC packaging)
Sig. 2 200-mg tabs qid for 48 hr
b. Adverse reactions: aggravates gastric ulcers

B. Inflammatory Conditions

1. Allergic Blepharitis

S: History and itching
O: Edema and erythema
A: Rule out preseptal cellulitis
P: Oral agents to consider:

c. Antihistamine/decongestant
Disp. (a "million" OTCs)
Sig. per package insert
d. Adverse reactions: drowsiness, ocular dryness

2. Chronic Bacterial Blepharitis/ Meibomian Gland Dysfunction (MGD)

S: Greater than 6- to 12-week history
O: Bacterial signs with inflammation
A: a. Rule out other forms (viral, etc.)
b. Staphylococcal
c. Streptococcal
d. *Haemophilus influenzae*

P: Oral agents to consider:

a. Disp. 20 500-mg tablets (Keflex)
i. If Staph. or Strep: Keflex 500 mg
ii. If *H. flu* in child: Augmentin
iii. If MGD: Doxycycline (adults only) 50 mg caps
Sig. Keflex 1 tab bid for 10 days Doxycycline: 50 or 100 mg cap q12h for 1–2 months
Child: Keflex: 25–50 mg/kg/day
Augmentin: 20–40 mg/kg/ day
b. Adverse reactions: gastrointestinal

3. Dacryocystitis

S: Inferonasal pain
O: Tearing with preseptal cellulitis
A: Rule out Lid or orbital disease
P: Oral agents to consider:

a. Anti-infectives (e.g., Keflex)
Disp. 20 500 mg tablets
Sig. 1 tab bid × 10 days
Child: Keflex: 25–50 mg/kg/day
b. Adverse reactions: gastrointestinal

4. Herpes Simplex Blepharitis

S: Mild to moderate irritation
O: Vesicles to pustules
A: Rule out other forms of blepharitis
P: Oral agents to consider:

a. Valacyclovir (Valtrex)
Disp. 30 500-mg tablets
Sig. 1 tab tid for 7 to 10 days
b. Adverse reactions: very rare

5. Herpes Zoster Blepharitis

S: Variable degree of pain (usually severe)
O: Unilateral vesicles to ulcerations
A: Rule out other blepharitis and systemic causes
P: Oral agents to consider:

a. Valacyclovir (Valtrex)
Disp. 1000-mg tabs
Sig. 1 tab tid for 7–10 days
b. Corticosteroid (e.g., Prednisone)
Disp. 10 mg tabs
Sig. 20–60 mg/day, and slowly taper
c. Narcotic analgesic (e.g., Tylenol w/Codeine #3)
Disp. 12 300/30 mg capsules or tablets
Sig. 1 to 2 caps or tabs q4h or prn
d. Adverse reactions:
Valacyclovir: very rare
Steroids: multiple
Narcotic: dependency

6. Ocular Rosacea

S: Epidemiologic risk factors
O: Dermatologic and ocular signs
A: Rule out other anterior segment disease
P: Oral agents to consider:

a. Doxycycline (50 mg caps)
Disp. 84 50-mg capsules
Sig. 1 50-mg cap qd to bid for 6–12 weeks
b. Adverse reaction: gastrointestinal

7. *Orbital Cellulitis*

S: Diplopia with systemic illness (e.g., sinusitis)
O: Chemosis, proptosis, limitation of ocular movement
A: Rule out sinusitis, cavernous sinus thrombosis, etc.
P: IV drugs required

8. *Preseptal Cellulitis*

S: History of blepharitis, dacryocystitis, hordeolum
O: Painful (on palpation) erythema beyond orbital rim
A: Rule out orbital cellulitis
P: Oral agents to consider:
a. Anti-infectives (e.g., Keflex)
Disp. 20 500-mg tablets
Sig. 1 tab bid for 10 days
Child: Keflex: 25–50 mg/kg/day
b. Adverse reactions: gastrointestinal

II. Conditions of the Conjunctiva, Sclera, and Episclera

A. Irritations and Injuries: Scleral Perforation

S: History of high-velocity projectile
O: Intraocular hemorrhage and/or foreign body
A: Rule out orbit or cranial penetration
P: IV drugs required

B. Inflammatory Conditions

1. *Allergic Conjunctivitis*

S: History and itching
O: Chemosis and hyperemia
A: Rule out sinusitis, orbital cellulitis
P: Oral agents to consider:
Antihistamine/decongestant
Disp. (a "million" OTCs)
Sig. per package insert
a. Adverse reactions: drowsiness, ocular dryness

2. *Hyperacute Bacterial Conjunctivitis*

S: Rapid onset
O: Copious purulent discharge
A: Rule out Streptococcus, Gonococcus, other gram-negatives
P: Oral agents to consider:
a. Anti-infectives (e.g., Keflex)
Disp. 20 500-mg tablets
Sig. 1 tab bid × 10 days
Child: Augmentin: 20–40 mg/kg/day
b. Adverse reactions: gastrointestinal

3. *Episcleritis*

S: Mild to moderate aching type pain
O: Wedge-shaped hyperemic pattern
A: Rule out conjunctivitis, uveitis, scleritis
P: Oral agents to consider:
a. Nonsteroidal anti-inflammatory drugs (naproxen or ibuprofen)
Disp. Meds for 7–10 days
Sig. Naproxen 250–500 mg bid or Ibuprofen 400–600 mg tid (1800 mg/day) or Indomethacin 25–50 mg bid
b. Adverse reactions: gastrointestinal, aggravates gastric ulcers

4. *Scleritis*

S: Severe pain
O: Diffuse, deep inflammation
A: Rule out systemic disease (rheumatoid disease)
P: Oral agents to consider:
a. Anti-inflammatories/immunosuppressive agents
Disp. Meds for 7–10 days
Sig. Mild: Ibuprofen 600 mg tid (1800 mg/day), Naproxen 250–500 mg tid
Moderate: Prednisone 60–80 mg/day for 3 to 5 days, then taper
Severe: Cyclophosphamide (by internist)
b. Adverse reactions: seek medical consultation

III. Conditions of the Cornea

Irritations and Injuries

1. *Abrasions*

S: History of injury
O: Corneal staining
A: Rule out penetration/perforation
P: Oral agents to consider:
a. Analgesic (e.g., ibuprofen)
Disp. (OTC packaging)
Sig. 2 200-mg tabs qid for 48 hr
b. Narcotic analgesic (e.g., Tylenol w/Codeine #3)
Disp. 12 300/30 mg capsules or tablets
Sig. 1 to 2 caps or tabs q4h or prn
c. Adverse reactions:
Ibuprofen: aggravates gastric ulcers
Narcotics: dependency

B. Inflammatory Conditions

1. *Atopic/Vernal Keratoconjunctivitis*

S: History of allergies, dermatites
O: Superior palpebral conjunctival and corneal insult
A: Rule out SLK, viral, chlamydia, rosacea, etc.
P: Oral agents to consider:
a. Oral antihistamine and/or decongestant
Diphenhydramine (Benadryl)
25 mg tabs 1–2 tabs qid
Zyrtec (Cetirizine) 10 mg tab qd
b. Nonsteroidal anti-iflammatory drugs (aspirin or ibuprofen)
Disp. Meds for 7–10 days
Sig. Mild: Aspirin: 2- to 5-grain tabs q4h (12/day) or Ibuprofen 400 mg qid (1600 mg/day)
Mod.: Ibuprofen 600 mg qid (2400 mg/day)
Sev: see Corticosteroid, below
c. Corticosteroid (e.g. Prednisone) (consult pediatrician if a child)
Disp. 10 mg tabs
Sig. 20–40 mg/day, and taper slowly
d. Adverse reactions:
Antihistamines: drowsiness, ocular dryness
Nonsteroidal anti-iflammatory drugs: aggravate gastric ulcers
Steroids: Multiple

2. *Bacterial Keratitis (Corneal Ulcer)*

S: Infectious hx (injury, CL related, etc.)
O: Epithelial break with stromal inflammatory response
A: Determine organism through culturing
P: Oral agents to consider with risk of perforation:

a. Tetracycline (250 mg caps) or
b. Doxycycline 50 or 100 mg caps
   Disp. 60 capsules
   Sig. 1 100 mg cap q12h for 30 days
c. Analgesic (e.g., ibuprofen)
   Disp. (OTC packaging)
   Sig. 2 200 mg tabs qid for 48 hr
d. Narcotic analgesic (e.g., Tylenol w/Codeine #3)
   Disp. 300/30 mg caps or tabs
   Sig. 1 to 2 caps or tabs q4h or PRN
e. Adverse reactions:
   Ibuprofen: gastrointestinal, aggravates gastric ulcers
   Narcotics: dependency

3. *Herpes Simplex Stromal Keratitis*

S: Recurrent disease
O: Stromal immune infiltration
A: Rule out stromal "melting"
P: Oral agents to consider:
a. Valacyclovir (Valtrex)
   Disp. 500 mg tabs
   Sig. 1 cap tid for duration of time on topical steroids
b. Corticosteroid (e.g., prednisone)
   – Disp. 50 to 5 mg tabs
   – Sig. 50 mg/day decreasing by 5 mg daily
c. Adverse reactions:
   Valacyclovir: very rare
   Steroids: multiple

4. *Herpes Zoster Ophthalimicus Keratitis*

S: Severe pain (but may vary in intensity)
O: Anything in the anterior segment!
A: Rule out undiagnosed HIV or cancer
P: Oral agents to consider:
a. Valacyclovir (Valtrex)
b. Disp. 30 1000-mg capsules
   Sig. 1 cap tid for 7 to 10 days
c. Corticosteroid (e.g., prednisone)
   Disp. 10 mg tabs
   Sig. 20–60 mg/day, and taper slowly
d. Narcotic analgesic (e.g., Tylenol w/Codeine #3)
   Disp. 300/30 mg caps or tabs
   Sig. 1 to 2 caps or tabs q4h or PRN
e. Adverse reactions:
   Valacyclovir: very rare
   Steroids: multiple
   Narcotic: dependence

5. *Chlamydial Keratoconjunctivitis*

S: Venereal disease hx
O: Mixed, persisting bacteria/viral presentation
A: Rule out bacterial, viral, chronic keratoconjunctivitis
P: Oral agents to consider:
a. Azithromycin or doxycycline
   Disp. Azithromycin 1 1000-mg cap
   Doxycycline 30 100 mg caps
   Sig. Azithromycin 1000-mg cap 1×
   Doxycycline 100 mg caps bid for 15 days
b. Adverse reactions: gastrointestinal

IV. Conditions of the Anterior Uvea

A. Irritations and Injuries: Hyphema

S: Usually history of blunt trauma or postop
O: Red blood in anterior chamber
A: Systemic causes
P: Oral agents to consider:
a. Aminocaproic acid-fibrinolytic inhibitor (Amicar)
   Disp. 16-oz bottle of 250 mg/ml syrup
   Sig. 50 mg/kg q4h (5×/day) for 2 to 3 days (max.) post bleed or rebleed
b. Analgesic (acetaminophen—**no aspirin**)
   Disp. OTCs (e.g., Tylenol)
   Sig. 325–500 mg q6h or PRN
c. Methazolamide with IOP increase
   Disp. 50 mg tabs
   Sig. 1 50-mg tab bid to tid until IOP normal
d. Adverse reactions:
   Aminocaproic acid: multiple
   Methazolamide: multiple

B. Inflammatory Conditions

1. *Acute and Recurrent Anterior Uveitis*

S: Dull, aching pain
O: Cells and flare
A: Anterior vs intermediate vs posterior
P: Oral agents to consider
a. Nonsteroidal anti-inflammatory drugs (aspirin or ibuprofen)
   Disp. Meds for 7–10 days
   Sig. Mild: Aspirin: 2- to 5 grain tabs q4h (12/day)
   Ibuprofen 400 mg qid (1600 mg/day)
   Mod.: Ibuprofen 600 mg qid (2400 mg/day)
   Mod./Sev: see corticosteroids, below
b. Corticosteroid (e.g., prednisone)
   Disp. 10 mg tabs
   Sig. 40–60 mg/day, and taper slowly
c. Narcotic analgesic (e.g., Tylenol w/Codeine #3)
   Disp. 300/30 mg caps or tabs
   Sig. 1 to 2 caps or tabs q4h or PRN
d. Adverse reactions: NSAIDs: aggravate ulcers
   Aspirin: risk of bleeding and Reye's syndrome (under 12)
   Steroids: multiple
   Narcotics: dependency

2. *Intermediate Uveitis (Pars Planitis)*

S: Insidious onset with dull pain, photophobia
O: Blurred vision with anterior vitreous floaters
A: Rule out systemic diseases
P: Oral agents to consider:
a. Nonsteroidal anti-inflammatory drugs (aspirin or ibuprofen)
   Disp. Aspirin (OTC) 5-grain tabs, Ibuprofen (OTC 200 mg tabs or Rx 400 mg)
   Sig. Mild: Aspirin: 2- to 5-grain tabs q4h (12/day)
   Ibuprofen: 600 mg qid (2400 mg/day)
   Mod./Severe: see b and c, below

b. Corticosteroid (e.g., prednisone)
   Disp. 10-mg tablets
   Sig. 40–60 mg/day, and taper slowly
c. Immunosuppressive agents: e.g., methotrexate
   Referral and co-management with internal medicine
d. Narcotic analgesic (e.g., Tylenol w/Codeine #3)
   Disp. 300/30 mg caps or tabs
   Sig. 1 to 2 caps or tabs q4h or prn
e. Adverse reactions: nonsteroidal anti-inflammatory drugs aggravate ulcers
   Aspirin: risk of bleeding and Reye's syndrome (under 12)
   Steroids: multiple
   Narcotics: dependency

3. Chronic Uveitis

S: Uveitis greater than 6 weeks (with or without drugs)
O: Anterior/intermediate/posterior/disseminated uveitis
A: Systemic disease (often undiagnosed)
P: Oral agents to consider beyond systemic therapies
   a. Corticosteroids co-managed with medical consultant
   b. Immunosuppressive agents co-management with internal medicine consultant
   c. Adverse reactions: multiple drug interactions

INDEX

D

H

I

J

K

L

M

Q

R